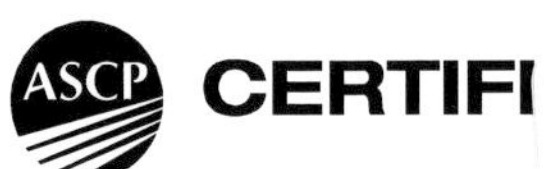

QUICK COMPENDIUM OF MEDICAL LABORATORY SCIENCES

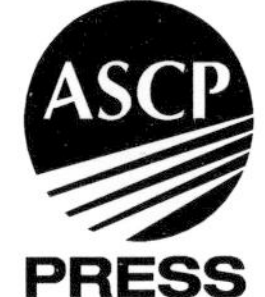

Publishing Team
Erik N Tanck & Annabelle Ulalulae (production)
Joshua Weikersheimer (publishing direction)

Notice
Trade names for equipment & supplies described are included as suggestions only. In no way does their inclusion constitute an endorsement of preference by the Author(s), Editor(s) or the ASCP. The Author(s), Editor(s) & ASCP urge all readers to read & follow all manufacturers' instructions & package insert warnings concerning the proper & safe use of products. The American Society for Clinical Pathology, having exercised appropriate & reasonable effort to research material current as of publication date, does not assume any liability for any loss or damage caused by errors & omissions in this publication. Readers must assume responsibility for complete & thorough research of any hazardous conditions they encounter, as this publication is not intended to be all inclusive & recommendations & regulations change over time.

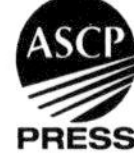

ISBN 978-089189-6616

Printed in Canada

29 25 24 23 22

Table of

Contents

ISBN 978-089189-6616

Chapter 3
Body Fluids

 ISBN 978-089189-6616

Chapter 4

Hematology

Chapter 5
Hemostasis

Chapter 6
Microbiology

ISBN 978-089189-6616

Chapter 7

Laboratory Operations

Chapter 8
Immunology

ISBN 978-089189-6616

Chapter 9

Molecular Biology

Foreword

The Quick Compendium (QC) series began with the publication of Dr Dan Mais' *Quick Compendium of Clinical Pathology* in 2005. QC series titles strive to capture the jewels, the pearls, the essential take away points that are often dispensed by masters during one-on-one teaching and present them in an easily accessed, outline-ordered form.

We considered the situation of the student preparing for the BOC MLS/MLT certification exams: a reading list of many very weighty textbooks....well suited to supplement classroom teaching, but perhaps not particularly easy to use for exam study. A QC textbook for the MLS/MLT student seemed like a good fit, so the editors of the most recent *BOC Study Guide 6e* were asked to take the helm of this ***Quick Compendium of Medical Laboratory Sciences***.

The *QCMLS* is intended to serve as a ready self-instructional textbook companion to the *BOC Study Guide*. The text is organized by subject area, covering all the areas of the most recent MLS/MLT Content Outline and more. The editors decided to retain a separate chapter on Molecular Biology, thinking that it would be useful background information for every aspiring medical laboratory sciences student, but regardless of the particular subject area in any given chapter, cross-references to other pertinent chapters are freely added (eg, in Blood Banking cross-references to specific parts of Immunology, Microbiology, Hematology, Molecular Biology and Laboratory Operations, are found). It is easy to get deeper treatment of topics at many points in every chapter.

Several years ago, Dr George Leonard devised a set of suggestions for residents to use to remember the multitude of facts that one must master to begin well in a medical career....and to be ready for the examination...what comes hereafter, with a nod to his original, are some thoughts for MLS/MLT students to use.

Making Things Memorable

The BOC certification exam can be a daunting prospect. As an adaptive exam, diverse subjects are lumped together in what you may consider the single most difficult exam of your professional training. Even a distilled text like the *QCMLS* is not tiny and each line is concentrated information. The reader must try to absorb each word. There is no filler material to skip over. So how does anyone make it all memorable?

A duo of the most helpful techniques are the preparation of flashcards and question writing/answering. So take a look and see if either might suit you well.

Flashcards

For the purposes of discussion, a flashcard is defined as a 2-sided card with information on one side of the card that the learner is trying to associate with information on the other side of the card. For years, these have been used to learn simple associative facts. How you use the flashcards is crucial:

Spaced (or interval) repetition of flash cards was popularized by an Austrian educator named Sebastian Leitner, who first introduced the method to increase the efficiency of learning. His technique involves the use of categories or boxes into which one sorts "cards" of information. Each box is defined by the degree to which the student rates their own knowledge of the information on the card. If the student knows the information on the card well, the card is placed in a higher box; if the student does not know the information, it is placed in a lower box. An algorithm then presents the well known cards at a longer-spaced interval than the less well known cards. Several popular foreign language courses use this technology to great effect. Flashcards are an extraordinarily effective means of learning, but there are limitations and rules to be followed:

The cards must be made properly

They must be simple and not overloaded with information. For example, on one side of the card one could write, "Preferred growth medium for *Bordetella*," and on the other side "Regan-Lowe medium" (we do realize there are other suitable media, but it's just an example). An example of a poorly written card would be to have "*Bordetella*" on one side and a slew of facts, eg, media, Gram stain, species, diseases, and antibiotic sensitivities. Cards must be simple to be effective.

You have to be honest about your own performance

You aren't doing yourself a favor by upgrading or downgrading your ability to remember a card. For spaced repetition to work, there must be an accurate accounting of whether you know the information or not. If you follow these rules, flashcards are an efficient means to learn a lot of information, at least in the short term.

Question Writing/Answering

A strong method for actively studying is to formulate your own questions and prepare your own brief explanations! This trick is applicable to reading and listening to lectures, with the benefit of increasing retention of the material. When you read, simply write for yourself questions and short answers to review later. So read the material, come up with a question, write down or key in the question and the answer you devise from the text (you can add the *QCMLS* outline number for reference), then later review. This cycle of repetition wears a rut in your mind and aids in rapid "knee-jerk" responses (similar to flash cards).

There is one other advantage to using this method. If you prepare your questions in proper BOC question style, you can submit them to ASCP [joshua.weikersheimer@ascp.org]. The editors will review all crowd-sourced questions. If the editors elect to use your question, you contribute to future generations of MLS/MLT students. Pay it forward to help others who come after you.

Contributors

Our thanks to those who edited/reviewed or otherwise contributed to this book

Blood Bank

Susan L Wilkinson, EdD, MT(ASCP)SBB^{CM}
Associate Professor Emerita
Hoxworth Blood Center
University of Cincinnati
Cincinnati, OH

Contributing Reviewers
Kathleen M Doyle, PhD, MASCP, MLS(ASCP)^{CM}
Medical Laboratory Scientist, Consultant
Professor Emerita
Medical Laboratory Sciences
University of Massachusetts Lowell
Lowell, MA

Janice J Habel BS, MT(ASCP)
Division Director, Quality Assurance
Hoxworth Blood Center\
University of Cincinnati
Cincinnati, OH

Jayanna Slayten, MS, MT(ASCP)SBB^{CM}
Blood Bank Supervisor, Indiana University Health
Indianapolis, IN
Adjunct Instructor
University of Texas Medical Branch SBB Program
Galveston, TX

Chemistry

Vicki S Freeman, PhD, MASCP, MLS(ASCP)^{CM}SC^{CM}, FAACC
Professor, Department of Clinical Laboratory Sciences
Associate Dean for Faculty Development, School of Health Professions
University of Texas
Galveston, TX

Contributing Reviewers
Wendy L Arneson, MS, MASCP, MLS(ASCP)^{CM}
Adjunct Instructor & Former Assistant Professor
University of Texas Medical Branch
Galveston, TX

Muneeza Esani, PhD, MPH, MT(ASCP)
Program Director, CLS Program
Assistant Professor of Instruction
University of Texas Medical Branch
Galveston, TX

Eddie Salazar, PhD, MLS(ASCP)^{CM}
Interim Chair, Clinical Laboratory Sciences
Program Director, DCLS program
Assistant Professor of Instruction
University of Texas Medical Branch
Galveston, TX

Urinalysis/Body Fluids

Takara L Blamires MS, MLS(ASCP)^{CM}
Assistant Professor, Program Director
Department of Pathology
University of Utah
Salt Lake City, UT

Contributing Reviewers
Wendy L Arneson (see Chemistry for credentials)

Karen A Brown (see Hematology for credentials)

Vicki S Freeman (see Chemistry for credentials)

Larry E Schoeff, MS, MT(ASCP)
Formerly Professor, Department of Pathology
University of Utah
Salt Lake City, UT

Hematology

Karen A Brown, MS, MASCP, MLS(ASCP)^{CM}
Adjunct Professor, Department of Pathology
University of Utah
Salt Lake City, UT

Contributing Reviewers
Betty Ciesla MS, MT(ASCP)SH
Formerly Adjunct Professor
Stevenson University
Stevenson, MD

Kathleen Finnegan, MS, MT(ASCP)SH^{CM}
Clinical Associate Professor
Clinical Laboratory Sciences
Stony Brook University
Stony Brook, NY

Hemostasis

Donna D Castellone, MS, MASCP, MT(ASCP)SH
QA Manager, Specialty Testing
Supervisor, Special Coagulation & Hematology
New York Presbyterian-Columbia Medical Center
New York, NY

Contributing Reviewers
Elaine Castelli, BS, MT(ASCP)SH
Section Supervisor, Special Hematology Laboratory
Stony Brook Medicine
Stony Brook, NY

Larry J Smith, PhD, SH(ASCP), HCLD/CC(AAB)
Liaison Manager, Medical & Scientific Affairs
Abbott Diagnostics Division-Hematology

Microbiology

JoAnn P Fenn, MS, MASCP, MT(ASCP)
Professor (Retired) & Division Chief, Medical Laboratory Sciences
Department of Pathology
University of Utah School of Medicine
Salt Lake City, UT

Contributing Reviewers
Karen J Honeycutt, PhD, MASCP, MLS(ASCP)^{CM}SM^{CM}
MLS Program Director
Clarence & Nelle Gilg Professor for Teaching Excellence & Innovation in Allied Health
Varner Educator Laureate
Medical Laboratory Science
University of Nebraska Medical Center
Omaha, NE

Theresa Tellier-Castellone, EdD, MPH, MLS(ASCP)^{CM}
Program Director, School of Medical Technology
University of Rhode Island
Our Lady of Fatima & Rhode Island Hospitals
Kingston, RI

Laboratory Operations

Joanne B Simpson MT(ASCP)DLM
Senior Laboratory Consultant
Laboratory Medicine & Pathology
University of Washington
Seattle, WA

Contributing Reviewers
Diane L Davis, PhD, MLS(ASCP)^{CM}SC^{CM}, SLS^{CM} (re Safety)
Professor of Clinical Laboratory Science
Health Sciences Department, Salisbury University
Salisbury, MD

Lotte Mulder, PhD (re Diversity, Equity & Inclusion)
Director, Leadership & Empowerment
American Society for Clinical Pathology
Chicago, IL

Amy J Spiczka, MS, HTL(ASCP)^{CM}SCT^{CM}, MB^{CM} (re Patient Safety)
Senior Director, Quality & Patient Safety
American Society for Clinical Pathology
Washington, DC

Immunology

Catherine L Gebhart, PhD, MB(ASCP)^{CM}, D(ABHI)
Senior HLA Director
Biomedical Services, American Red Cross
Dedham, MA

Contributing Reviewers
Denise Anamani, MA, I(ASCP)MB^{CM}
Lecturer
Department of Allied Health Sciences
Diagnostic Genetic Sciences Program
Medical Laboratory Sciences Program
University of Connecticut
Storrs, CT

Molecular Biology

Catherine L Gebhart (see Immunology for credentials)

Contributing Reviewers
Varun Kesherwani, MS, PhD, MB(ASCP)
Department of Biomedical Sciences
Creighton University
Omaha, NE

Permissions

The ASCP has accumulated many thousands of illustration and image assets in the ASCPedia warehouse. Many of those assets are repurposed in *QCMLS* and have previously appeared in ASCP publications over time.

ASCP Press books

Ash L, Orihel T. [2007] *Atlas of Human Parasitology 5e*. ISBN 978-089189-1673

Carson FL, Cappellano C [2020] *Histotechnology: A Self-Instructional Text 5e*. ISBN:978-089189-6760

Davis DL [2016] *Laboratory Safety: A Self Assessment Workbook 2e*. ISBN:978-089189-6463

Gulati G, Caro J [2014] *Blood Cells: Morphology & Clinical Relevance 2e*. ISBN:978-089189-6234

Hussong JW, Kjelsberg CR [2015] *Kjeldsberg's Body Fluid Analysis*. ISBN:978-089189-5824

Mais D [2014] *Quick Compendium of Clinical Pathology 3e*. ISBN:978-089189-6159

Schumann GB, Friedman SK [2003] *Wet Urinalysis: Interpretations, Correlations and Implications*. ISBN:978-089189-4438

In spite of the depth of ASCP holdings, we have turned to other sources to make *QCMLS* comprehensive. We are grateful to the following sources for granting permission for figures and images.

Other sources

i6.9a Courtesy of Hans Newman via http://www.bacteriainphotos.com/pyr_test.html

i6.29 Commons.wikimedia.org

i6.30 PHIL 3873

i6.43 PHIL 610

i6.44b PHIL 9927, **c** CDC DPDx Free Living Amebic Infections

i6.69 PHIL 4241

i6.76 PHIL 23016, 23081

i6.77 PHIL 4168

i6.78 PHIL 16296

i6.79 PHIL 23011, 19048

i6.80 PHIL 20861

i6.81 PHIL 23009

i6.82 PHIL 14658a

i6.83 PHIL 14658b

i6.85 PHIL 22123, 21411

i6.86 PHIL 22035

i6.87 PHIL 22030, 22029, 22260

i6.88 PHIL 22025, 21580

i6.89 PHIL 22058, 21485

i6.92 PHIL 4318

i6.93 Momtaz MS, Shamsi S, & Dey T [2019] Association of *Bipolaris* and *Drechslera* Species with Bipolaris Leaf Blight (BPLB) Infected Wheat Leaves. *J Bangladesh Acad Sci*, 43(1), 11-16. https://doi.org/10.3329/jbas.v43i1.42228

i6.94 PHIL 22056

i6.95 PHIL 3784

i6.96 PHIL 15208

i6.97 PHIL 20240

i6.99 Adapted via CC-BY-SA 3.0 license (see creativecommons.org) from commons.wikimedia.org/wiki/File:Ulocladium_conidiophores_40X.png

i6.102 PHIL 21204

i6.103 PHIL 3061

i6.104 PHIL 4238

i6.105 PHIL 2920

i6.108 Courtesy of Lablogatory from Wojewoda C, Bryant, B. Microbiology Case Study: Immunocompromised 65 Year Old Man. Lablogatory. https://labmedicineblog.com/2016/01/15/microbiology-case-study-immunocompromised-65-year-old-man/

i6.109 PHIL 22836

i6.116 Lodha N, Shital Amin Poojary SA [2015] A novel contrast stain for the rapid diagnosis of pityriasis versicolor: A comparison of Chicago Sky Blue 6B stain, potassium hydroxide mount and culture. *Indian J Dermatol*. Jul-Aug 2019;64(4):311-314. doi: 10.4103/ijd.IJD_401_18. Used by permission of Wolters Kluwer Health, Inc

f9.3c,d Adapted via CC-BY-SA 3.0 license (see creativecommons.org) from en.wikipedia.org/wiki/Nucleic acid structure

f9.4a Adapted via CC-BY-SA 4.0 (see creativecommons.org) from en.wikipedia.org/wiki.microRNA

f9.4b Adapted via CC-BY (see creativecommons.org) by Oxford University Press: Agris P. Decoding the genome: a modified view. *Nucleic Acids Research* 2004;32(1):223-238. doi:10.1093/nar/gkh185

f9.4c Adapted with permission from Springer Nature: Gutmann S, Haebel P, Metzinger L, et al [2003] Crystal structure of the transfer-RNA domain of transfer-messenger RNA in complex with SmpB. *Nature* 424**,** 699-703. doi: 10.1038/nature01831

f9.4d Adapted with permission from Springer Nature: Ramaswamy P, Woodson S [2009] S16 throws a conformational switch during assembly of 30S 5' domain. *Nat Struct Mol Biol* 16, 438-445. doi: 10.1038/nsmb.158

f9.6 Modeled after an illustration attributed only to Addison Wesley Longman [1999]

f9.8 Adapted from a public domain figure courtesy of LadyofHats, as found at en.wikipedia.org/wiki/Exon#/media/File:RNA_splicing_diagram_en.svg

f9.30 Courtesy of National Human Genome Research Institute (genome.gov)

f9.33 Reprinted with permission from Springer Nature: Royo,J, Hidalgo M, Ruiz A [2007] Pyrosequencing protocol using a universal biotinylated primer for mutation detection and SNP genotyping. *Nat Protoc* 2**,** 1734-1739. https://doi.org/10.1038/nprot.2007.244

f9.35 Adapted from an original made available by Andy Vierstraete

f9.39 & **f9.40** Adapted via a CC-BY-2.0 license (see creativecommons.org) from Al-achkar, W, Aljapawe, A, Othman, MK [2013] A de novo acute myeloid leukemia (AML-M4) case with a complex karyotype and yet unreported breakpoints. *Mol Cytogenet* 6**,** 18. doi: 10.1186/1755-8166-6-18

f9.41 Adapted via CC-BY-4.0 license (see creativecommons.org) from Colaianni, V, Mazzei, R, Cavallaro, S [2016] Copy number variations and stroke. *Neurological Sciences* (2016). doi: 37. 10.1007/s10072-016-2658-y

f9.42 Reprinted from Neoh HM, Tan XE, Sapri HF, Tan TL [2019] Pulsed-field gel electrophoresis (PFGE): A review of the "gold standard" for bacteria typing and current alternatives. *Infect Genet Evol* Oct;74:103935 doi: 10.1016/j.meegid.2019.103935, with permission from Elsevier

f9.43 Adapted via a CC-BY-4.0 license from Singhal N, Kumar M, Kanaujia PK, Virdi JS [2015] MALDI-TOF mass spectrometry: an emerging technology for microbial identification and diagnosis. *Front Microbiol* 05 August 2015. doi: 10.3389/fmicb.2015.00791

MLS/MLT Examination Content Outline

This content outline was accessed 1 January 2021. In this combined outline, underlined items apply to MLS exams only. Current outlines are found at https://www.ascp.org/content/docs/default-source/boc-pdfs/boc-us-guidelines/mls_imls_content_guideline.pdf?sfvrsn=16

Blood Banking

(17%-22% of MLS exam, 15%-20% of MLT exam)

I. Blood Products
A. Donors
1. Qualification
2. Collection methods
3. Adverse reactions
4. Special donations (eg, autologous)
B. Processing
1. Testing
2. Labeling
C. Storage
1. Anticoagulants/additives
2. Temperature requirements
3. Transportation
4. Properties of stored products
5. Expiration
D. Blood Components
1. Red blood cells
2. Cryoprecipitated AHF
3. Platelets
4. Plasma
5. Leukocyte-reduced components
6. Frozen/deglycerolized red blood cells
7. Apheresis products
8. Fractionation products
9. Whole blood
10. Washed red blood cells
11. Rejuvenated red blood cells
12. Irradiated components
E. Blood Component Quality Control

II. Blood Group Systems
A. Genetics
1. Basic
2. Molecular
3. Inheritance of blood groups
B. Chemistry, Antigens
1. ABO
2. Lewis
3. Rh
4. MNS
5. P1PK/Globoside(P)
6. Ii
7. Kell
8. Kidd
9. Duffy
10. Lutheran
11. Other
12. Antigens of high prevalence
13. Antigens of low prevalence
14. HLA
15. Platelet-specific
16. Granulocyte-specific
C. Role of Blood Groups in Transfusion
1. Immunogenicity
2. Antigen frequency

III. Blood Group Immunology
A. Immune Response
1. Primary & secondary response
2. B & T cells, macrophages
3. Genetics
B. Immunoglobulins
1. Classes & subclasses
2. Structure
3. Biologic & physical properties
C. Antigen-Antibody Interactions
1. Principles
2. Testing
a. Principles
b. Methods
D. Complement
1. Classical & alternative pathway mechanisms
2. Biologic properties

IV. Physiology & Pathophysiology
A. Physiology of Blood
1. Circulation & blood volume
2. Composition & function of blood
a. Normal function
b. Abnormal physiology
3. Cell survival
4. Cell metabolism
B. Hemostasis & Coagulation
1. Coagulation factors & disorders
2. Platelet functions & disorders
C. Hemolytic Disease of the Fetus & Newborn
1. Pathophysiology
2. Detection
3. Treatment
4. Prevention
D. Anemias
1. Congenital & acquired
a. Pathophysiology
b. Detection
c. Treatment
2. Immune hemolytic anemias: warm, cold, drug-induced
a. Pathophysiology
b. Detection
c. Treatment
E. Transplantation
1. Solid organ
2. Hematopoietic progenitor cells (HPC)

V. Serologic & Molecular Testing
A. Routine Tests
1. Blood grouping tests
2. Compatibility tests
a. Antibody detection
b. Crossmatch
3. Antibody identification/clinical significance
4. Direct antiglobulin testing
B. Reagents
1. Antiglobulin sera
2. Blood grouping sera
3. Reagent red cells
C. Application of Special Tests & Reagents
1. Enzymes
2. Enhancement media
3. Lectins
4. Adsorptions
5. Elutions
6. Titrations
7. Cell separations
8. ELISA
9. Molecular techniques
10. Neutralization/inhibition
11. Use of thiol reagents
12. Immunofluorescence
13. Solid phase
14. Column agglutination test
15. Chloroquine diphosphate
16. EDTA glycine acid
D. Leukocyte/Platelet Testing
1. Cytotoxicity
2. Platelet testing
3. Granulocyte testing
E. Quality Assurance
1. Blood samples
2. Reagents
3. Test procedures

VI. Transfusion Practice
A. Indications for Transfusion
B. Component Therapy
C. Adverse Effects of Transfusion
1. Immunologic reactions
2. Nonimmunologic reactions
3. Transfusion-transmitted diseases
D. Apheresis & Extracorporeal Circulation
E. Blood Administration & Patient Blood Management

Urinalysis & Body Fluids

(5%-10% of total exam)

I. Urinalysis
A. Physical
1. Color & clarity
2. Specific gravity/osmolality
B. Chemical
1. Reagent strip
2. Confirmatory tests
C. Microscopic
1. Cells
2. Casts
3. Crystals
4. Microorganisms
5. Contaminants
6. Artifacts
D. Renal Physiology
E. Disease States

II. Body Fluids (eg, CSF, Amniotic, Synovial, Serous, Semen & Feces)
A. Physical
B. Chemical
C. Microscopic
D. Physiology
E. Disease States

Chemistry

(17%-22% of MLS exam, 20%-25% of MLT exam)

I. General Chemistry
A. Carbohydrates
1. Biochemical theory & physiology
a. Metabolic pathways
b. Normal & abnormal states
c. Physical & chemical properties
2. Test procedures
a. Principles
b. Special precautions, specimen collection & processing, troubleshooting & interfering substances
c. Tolerance testing
d. Glycated proteins
3. Test result interpretation
4. Disease state correlation
B. Lipids
1. Biochemical theory & physiology
a. Metabolic pathways
b. Normal & abnormal states
c. Physical & chemical properties
1) Lipoproteins
2) Phospholipids
3) Triglycerides
4) Cholesterol
5) Apolipoproteins
2. Test procedures
a. Principles
b. Special precautions, specimen collection & processing, troubleshooting & interfering substances
3. Test result interpretation
4. Disease state correlation
C. Heme Derivatives
1. Biochemical theory & physiology
a. Metabolic pathways
b. Normal & abnormal states
c. Physical & chemical properties
1) Hemoglobin
2) Bilirubin
3) Urobilinogen
4) Myoglobin
5) Other porphyrins
2. Test procedures
a. Principles
b. Special precautions, specimen collection & processing, troubleshooting & interfering substances
3. Test result interpretation
4. Disease state correlation

II. Proteins & Enzymes
A. Enzymes
1. Biochemical theory & physiology
a. Metabolic pathways
b. Normal & abnormal states
c. Physical & chemical properties
1) LD
2) CK
3) AST/ALT
4) GGT
5) Lipase
6) Amylase
7) Alkaline phosphatase
8) Other enzymes
2. Test procedures
a. Principles
b. Special precautions, specimen collection & processing, troubleshooting & interfering substances
3. Test result interpretation
4. Disease state correlation
B. Proteins & Other Nitrogen-Containing Compounds
1. Biochemical theory & physiology
a. Metabolic pathways
b. Normal & abnormal states
c. Physical & chemical properties
1) Proteins
2) Amino acids
3) Urea
4) Uric acid
5) Creatinine
6) Ammonia
7) Tumor markers
8) Viral proteins
9) Cardiac markers
10) Other compounds
2. Test procedures
a. Principles
b. Special precautions, specimen collection & processing, troubleshooting & interfering substances
c. Clearances
3. Test result interpretation
4. Disease state correlation

III. Acid-Base, Blood Gases & Electrolytes
A. Acid-Base Determinations (Including Blood Gases)
1. Biochemical theory & physiology
a. Henderson-Hasselbach equation
b. pH & H^+ ion concentration
c. CO_2 & O_2 transport
d. Normal & abnormal states
2. Test procedures
a. Analytical principles
b. Special precautions, specimen collection & processing, troubleshooting & interfering substances
3. Test result interpretation
4. Disease state correlation
B. Electrolytes
1. Biochemical theory & physiology
a. Sodium, potassium, chloride, CO_2, bicarbonate
b. Calcium, magnesium, phosphorus, iron, TIBC
c. Trace elements
d. Normal & abnormal states

2. Test procedures
a. Principles
b. Special precautions, specimen collection & processing, troubleshooting & interfering substances
3. Calculations (osmolality, anion gap)
4. Test result interpretation
5. Disease state correlation

IV. Special Chemistry
A. Endocrinology
1. Biochemical theory & physiology
a. Metabolic pathways
b. Normal & abnormal states
c. Mechanism of action
d. Physical & chemical properties
1) Steroid hormones (eg, cortisol, estrogen, hCG)
2) Peptide hormones (eg, insulin, prolactin)
3) Thyroid hormones
4) Other hormones
2. Test procedures
a. Principles
1) Fluorescence
2) Immunoassay
3) Other methods
b. Special precautions, specimen collection & processing, troubleshooting & interfering substances
c. Stimulation/suppression tests
3. Test result interpretation
4. Disease state correlation
B. Vitamins & Nutrition
1. Biochemical theory & physiology
a. Metabolism & action
b. Normal & abnormal states
c. Properties
1) Vitamin D
2) Vitamin B_{12}/folate
3) Other vitamins
2. Test procedures
a. Principles
b. Special precautions, specimen collection & processing, troubleshooting & interfering substances
3. Test result interpretation
4. Disease state correlation
C. Therapeutic Drug Monitoring
1. Pharmacokinetics
a. Therapeutic states
b. Toxic states
c. Metabolism & excretion
2. Chemical & physical properties
a. Aminoglycosides (eg, gentamicin)
b. Cardioactive (eg, digoxin)
c. Anti-convulsants (eg, phenobarbital)
d. Anti-depressants (eg, lithium)
e. Immunosuppressants (eg, tacrolimus)
f. Other drugs
3. Test procedures
a. Principles
1) Immunoassay
2) Other methods
b. Special precautions, specimen collection & processing, troubleshooting & interfering substances
4. Test result interpretation
5. Disease state correlation
D. Toxicology
1. Toxicokinetics
a. Toxic effects, signs & symptoms
b. Metabolism & excretion
2. Chemical & physical properties
a. Alcohols
b. Heavy metals (eg, lead)
c. Analgesics (eg, acetaminophen)
d. Drugs of abuse
e. Other toxins
3. Test procedures
a. Principles
1) Immunoassay
2) Other methods
b. Special precautions, specimen collection & processing, troubleshooting & interfering substances
4. Test result interpretation
5. Disease state correlation

Hematology

(17%-22% of MLS exam, 15%-20% of MLT exam)

I. Physiology (to include blood, body fluids, and bone marrow)
A. Production
B. Destruction
C. Function

II. Disease States
A. Erythrocytes
1. Anemia
a. Microcytic
1) Iron deficiency
2) Thalassemia
3) Sideroblastic
4) Chronic inflammation
b. Normocytic
1) Hereditary hemolytic
2) Acquired hemolytic
3) Hypoproliferative
4) Acute hemorrhage
c. Macrocytic
1) Megaloblastic
2) Non-megaloblastic
d. Hemoglobinopathies
2. Erythrocytosis
a. Relative
b. Absolute
B. Leukocytes (WHO classification)
1. Benign leukocyte disorders
a. Myeloid
b. Lymphoid
2. Myeloid neoplasia
a. Acute leukemia
b. Myelodysplastic syndromes
c. Myeloproliferative neoplasms
3. Lymphoid neoplasia
a. Acute leukemia
b. Chronic leukemia/lymphoma
c. Plasma cell dyscrasias
4. Hereditary anomalies
C. Platelets
1. Quantitative abnormalities
a. Thrombocytopenia
1) Increased destruction (eg, ITP, TTP, HIT)
2) Decreased production
3) Pseudothrombocytopenia
b. Thrombocytosis
2. Qualitative defects
a. von Willebrand disease
b. Bernard-Soulier syndrome
c. Glanzmann thrombasthenia

III. Hematology Laboratory Testing
A. Cell Counts (to include blood & body fluids)
1. Manual
2. Automated
3. Reticulocytes
4. Spurious results
B. Differentials & Morphology Evaluation (to include blood & body fluids)
C. Hemoglobin
1. Quantitative
2. Qualitative
a. Electrophoresis
b. HPLC
c. Sickle solubility
D. Hematocrit
E. Indices
F. Hemolytic Indicators (eg, haptoglobin, LD)
G. Special Stains
1. Esterase
2. Myeloperoxidase
3. Prussian blue
4. Kleihauer Betke
H. Other Studies
1. ESR
2. G6PD
3. Heinz body
I. Flow Cytometry Immunophenotyping
1. Leukemia
2. Lymphoma
3. Lymphocyte subsets
4. PNH
J. Molecular & Cytogenetic Testing
1. Recurring cytogenetic abnormalities (WHO classification)
2. *BCR-ABL*
3. JAK2

IV. Hemostasis
A. Physiology
1. Coagulation pathways
2. Fibrinolytic pathway
3. Vascular system
B. Disease States
1. Coagulation factor deficiencies
a. Acquired
b. Hereditary
2. Inhibitors
3. Fibrinolytic system
4. Hypercoagulable states
5. DIC
C. Laboratory Determinations
1. PT/INR
2. APTT
3. Fibrinogen
4. D-dimer
5. Thrombin time
6. Mixing studies
7. Platelet function (eg, PFA)
8. Inhibitor assays
9. Factor assays
10. von Willebrand assays
11. Platelet aggregation
12. Thromboelastography
13. Hypercoagulability assessment
a. Assays (eg, lupus anticoagulant, protein S, protein C, HIT studies)
b. Molecular (eg, factor V Leiden, prothrombin 20210)
14. Anti-Xa
15. Direct thrombin inhibitors
16. Heparin neutralization

Immunology

(5%-10% of total exam)

I. Principles of Immunology
A. Immune System Physiology
1. Primary & secondary response
2. B & T cells, macrophages
3. Genetics
B. Immunoglobulins
1. Classes & subclasses
2. Structure
3. Biologic & physical properties
C. Antigen-Antibody Interactions
1. Principles
2. Testing
a. Principles
b. Methods
D. Complement
1. Classical & alternative pathway mechanisms
2. Biologic properties

II. Diseases of the Immune System
A. Autoimmunity
1. Systemic (eg, SLE)
2. Organ-specific (eg, Graves disease)
B. Hypersensitivity
1. I, II, III, IV
C. Immunoproliferative Diseases
1. Monoclonal gammopathies (eg, multiple myeloma, Waldenström macroglobulinemia)
D. Immunodeficiency
1. Hereditary (eg, SCID)
2. Acquired (eg, HIV)

III. Transplantation
A. Graft-vs-host Disease
B. HLA Typing
C. Tumor Immunology

IV. Infectious Disease Serology
A. Clinical Significance & Epidemiology of Viral Pathogens (eg, hepatitis [A, B, C], EBV, HIV, CMV, rubella, measles)
B. Stages of Infection of *Treponema pallidum* & *Borrelia burgdorferi*
C. Tuberculosis Infection (eg, interferon gamma release assay, PPD)

V. Serologic & Molecular Procedures
A. ANA
B. Thyroid Antibodies
C. Rheumatoid Factor
D. Direct Detection Methods for Pathogens
E. Labeled Immunoassays (eg, ELISA)
F. Nontreponemal Syphilis Testing (eg, RPR)
G. Treponemal Syphilis Testing (eg, MHATP)
H. Cytokine Testing
I. Target Amplification
J. Nucleic Acid Sequencing
K. Hybridization Techniques
L. Other

VI. Test Results
A. Interpretation
B. Confirmatory Testing
C. Disease State Correlation

Microbiology

(17%-22% of MLS exam, 15%-20% of MLT exam)

I. Preanalytic Procedures
A. Specimen Collection & Transport
1. Patient identification & specimen labeling
2. Specimen collection
3. Specimen transport systems & conditions for all organisms
B. Specimen Processing
1. Specimen prioritization & rejection criteria
2. Biosafety cabinet & personal protective equipment
3. Specimen preparation methods and applications
4. Media
5. Inoculation of media
6. Incubation conditions (eg, temperature, atmosphere, duration)
7. Preparation methods for slides used for stains
C. Stains: Procedure, Principle & Interpretation (KOH & calcofluor-white, trichrome, Giemsa)
1. Gram
2. Acid-fast
3. Modified acid-fast
4. KOH & calcofluor-white
5. Trichrome
6. Giemsa
7. Acridine orange

ISBN 978-089189-6616

II. Analytic Procedures for Bacteriology

A. Blood & Bone Marrow
1. Specimen sources (eg, peripheral, intravenous catheters)
2. Continuous monitoring systems
3. Rapid identification/resistance detection methods
4. Species comprising skin flora & clinical significance
5. Colony morphology & identification of major pathogens (eg, *Staphylococcus aureus*, coagulase-negative staphylococci, beta-hemolytic streptococci, *Enterococcus* spp., *Candida* spp., *Streptococcus pneumoniae*, *Acinetobacter baumannii*, *Enterobacteriaceae*, *Pseudomonas* spp.)
6. Common agents of endocarditis
7. Agents of bone marrow infection (eg, *Brucella* spp., *Salmonella* spp.)
8. Organism pathogenicity (eg, etiology, transmission, virulence mechanisms)

B. Cerebrospinal Fluid
1. Specimen sources (eg, lumbar puncture, shunt, reservoir)
2. Colony morphology & identification of major pathogens associated with acute meningitis (eg, *Streptococcus pneumoniae*, *Haemophilus influenzae*, *Neisseria meningitidis*, *Escherichia coli*, *Listeria monocytogenes*, *Enterobacteriaceae*, *Staphylococcus aureus*, beta-hemolytic streptococci)
3. Common agents of shunt infections (eg, coagulase-negative staphylococci, *Corynebacterium* spp., *Propionibacterium* spp.)
4. Correlation with other lab results (eg, glucose, protein, cell count)
5. Direct detection & molecular methods
6. Organism pathogenicity (eg, etiology, transmission, virulence mechanisms)

C. Body Fluids from Normally Sterile Sites
1. Specimen sources (eg, pleural, peritoneal, pericardial, vitreous & aqueous humor, synovial, amniotic)
2. Indigenous organisms associated with mucosal surfaces & skin
3. Colony morphology & identification of major pathogens (eg, *S. pneumoniae*, *H. influenzae*, *Neisseria* spp., *E. coli*, *Listeria monocytogenes*, *Enterobacteriaceae*, *S. aureus*, beta-hemolytic streptococci, *Enterococcus* spp., *Pseudomonas aeruginosa*, *Acinetobacter*, *Clostridium perfringens*, *Bacteroides fragilis* group)
4. Molecular methods
5. Organism pathogenicity (eg, etiology, transmission, virulence mechanisms)

D. Lower Respiratory
1. Specimen sources (eg, sputum, endotracheal aspirate, bronchoalveolar lavage, bronchial wash, bronchial brush)
2. Significance of quantitative & semiquantitative reporting of results
3. Species comprising oral flora colony & Gram stain morphology
4. Colony morphology & identification of major pathogens
5. Direct detection & molecular methods (eg, *Streptococcus pyogenes*, *Bordetella pertussis*)
6. Organism pathogenicity (eg, etiology, transmission, virulence mechanisms)

E. Upper Respiratory
1. Specimen sources (eg, throat, nasopharynx, middle ear, sinus)
2. Indigenous flora colony & Gram stain morphology
3. Colony morphology & identification of major pathogens
4. Direct detection & molecular methods (eg, *Streptococcus pyogenes*, *Bordetella pertussis*)
5. Organism pathogenicity (eg, etiology, transmission, virulence mechanisms)

F. Gastrointestinal
1. Colony morphology & identification of major pathogens (eg, *Salmonella* spp., *Shigella* spp., toxigenic *E. coli*, *Campylobacter* spp., *Vibrio* spp., *Yersinia enterocolitica*, *Aeromonas* spp., *Plesiomonas shigelloides*)
2. Direct detection & molecular methods (eg, *Clostridium difficile*, Shiga toxin)
3. Serotyping of *E. coli*, *Salmonella*, *Shigella*
4. Organism pathogenicity (eg, etiology, transmission, virulence mechanisms)
5. Detection methods for *Helicobacter pylori*

G. Skin, Soft Tissue & Bone
1. Specimen sources (eg, wound, abscess, biopsy)
2. Indigenous flora colony & Gram stain morphology
3. Colony morphology & identification of major pathogens
4. Organism pathogenicity (eg, etiology, transmission, virulence mechanisms)

H. Genital Tract
1. Specimen sources (eg, vaginal, cervical, urethral, endocervical)
2. Indigenous organisms colony & Gram stain morphology
3. Methods for detection of pathogens associated with vaginitis (eg, *Trichomonas*, *Candida*, bacterial vaginosis)
4. Culture and/or molecular detection (eg, *N. gonorrhoeae*, *C. trachomatis*, *Streptococcus agalactiae* & *Mycoplasma* spp.)
5. Organism pathogenicity (eg, etiology, transmission, virulence mechanisms)

I. Urine
1. Specimen source (eg, mid-stream clean catch, catheterized, suprapubic, nephrostomy)
2. Colony morphology & identification of major urinary pathogens (eg, *Enterobacteriaceae*, *Enterococcus*, *Streptococcus agalactiae*, *Candida* spp., *Staphylococcus saprophyticus*)
3. Correlation of colony counts with clinical significance
4. Correlation of culture with urinalysis results

J. Identification Methods (Theory, Interpretation, and Application)
1. Colony morphology
2. Rapid tests used for presumptive identification (eg, coagulase, catalase, oxidase, indole, PYR)
3. Conventional biochemical identification (eg, TSI, decarboxylases, carbohydrate utilization, motility, urease, XV factors)
4. Commercial kits
5. Automated methods
6. MALDI-TOF MS
7. Multiplex molecular methods
8. Sequencing (eg, 16S)

K. Antimicrobial Susceptibility Testing & Antibiotic Resistance
1. Method, theory, interpretation, and application
2. Phenotypic detection of resistance (eg, beta-lactamase, ESBL, inducible clindamycin resistance, carbapenamases)
3. Mechanisms of action of major antibiotic classes
4. Detection of genetic determinants of resistance (eg, mecA, vanA, blaKPC)
5. Intrinsic resistance patterns for common species

L. MRSA/MSSA, VRE, ESBL/CRE Screening
1. Specimen sources
2. Culture methods
3. Molecular methods

M. BSL-3 Pathogens & Select Agents (Bioterrorism)
1. Specimen source (eg, blood, sputum, tissue, lymph node)
2. Colony morphology & rapid tests used for presumptive identification (eg, *Bacillus anthracis*, *Yersinia pestis*, *Brucella* spp., *Francisella tularensis*)
3. Role of regional laboratory & Laboratory Response Network
4. Organism pathogenicity (eg, etiology, transmission, virulence mechanisms)

III. Analytic Procedures for Mycology, Mycobacteriology, Parasitology & Virology

A. Mycobacteriology & *Nocardia* spp.
1. Specimen source (eg, lower respiratory, blood, soft tissue)
2. Acid-fast reaction, colony morphology and growth characteristics
3. Identification methods (eg, probes, sequencing, MALDI-TOF MS)
4. Direct detection by molecular methods
5. Antimicrobial therapy
6. Organism pathogenicity (eg, etiology, transmission, virulence mechanisms)

B. Virology
1. Specimen sources
2. Major pathogens & disease states (eg, etiology, epidemiology, transmission)
3. Direct detection of pathogens

C. Parasitology
1. Specimen source (eg, stool, respiratory, blood, tissue)
2. Major pathogens & disease states (eg, etiology, epidemiology, transmission)
3. Microscopic & macroscopic identification
4. Direct & molecular detection

D. Mycology
1. Specimen sources
2. Major pathogens & disease states (eg, etiology, epidemiology, transmission)
3. Colony morphology & growth characteristics of major pathogens (eg, temperature, growth rate, length of incubation)
4. Microscopic identification of major pathogens
5. Direct & molecular detection
6. Other identification methods (eg, biochemical, automated methods, MALDI-TOF MS)

IV. Post-Analytic Procedures

A. Documentation Practices
B. Urgent & Critical Value Reporting
C. Result Review & Autoverification
D. Issuing Corrected Reports
E. Reporting to Infection Control/Prevention & Public Health

Laboratory Operations

(5%-10% of total exam)

I. Quality Assessment/Troubleshooting

A. Pre-analytical, Analytical, Post-analytical
B. Quality Control
C. Point-of-care Testing (POCT)
D. Compliance
E. Regulation (eg, proficiency testing, competency assessment, accreditation standards)

II. Safety

A. Safety Programs & Practices
1. Prevention of infection with bloodborne pathogens
2. Use of personal protective equipment (PPE)
3. Safe work practices
4. Safety data sheets (SDS) for chemicals and reagents

B. Emergency Procedures (eg, needlesticks, splashes to mucous membranes, fire)

C. Packaging & Transportation of Specimens & Microorganisms

III. Laboratory Mathematics

A. Concentration, Volume & Dilutions
B. Molarity, Normality
C. Standard Curves
D. Mean, Median, Mode & Confidence Intervals
E. Sensitivity, Specificity & Predictive Value

IV. Manual/Automated Methodology & Instrumentation

A. Microscopy
B. Centrifugation
C. Spectrophotometry & Photometry
D. Mass Spectrometry
E. Osmometry
F. Electrophoresis
G. Chromatography
H. Electrochemistry
I. Molecular Methods
J. Other Methods

V. Basic Management Principles

VI. Education Principles

Examples provided (as indicated by eg) are not limited to those listed.

All Board of Certification examinations use conventional & SI units for results & reference ranges.

You will need to bring a nonprogrammable calculator with logarithmic function to the examination.

Chapter 1

Blood Banking

ISBN 978-089189-6616

Standards and requirements throughout this chapter are based on *AABB Standards for Blood Banks and Transfusion Services*, 32nd ed, 2020, and Food and Drug Administration (FDA) Code of Federal Regulations, Title 21, notably Parts 606, 610, 630 and 640 and applicable FDA guidance documents.

1.1 Blood products

1.1.1 Donors

1.1.1.1 Allogeneic donor requirements & qualification

- Donor must provide form of identification and basic demographic data, including address for any test deferral notification
- Previous donor record (if applicable) assessed for any active donation deferrals
- Age ≥16 years or conform to state law
  - Age 16 and/or 17 years may require parental consent
    - Includes explanation of the donation process and potential adverse events of donation including risk of iron deficiency and mitigation strategies
  - No upper age limit
- If previous red cells donation, confirm donation interval is acceptable
  - ≥8 weeks for single unit Whole Blood donation
  - ≥16 weeks for 2-unit Red Blood Cells donation (apheresis)
- Free of disease (major organs) and cancer
- History and physical
  - Day of donation and before blood collection
- Physical examination requirements are shown in **t1.1**

t1.1 Blood donor physical examination requirements

General appearance	Must appear in good health; donor feels well
Temperature	≤37.5°C (99.5°F)
Blood pressure	90-180 mm Hg systolic; 50-100 mm Hg diastolic
Pulse	50-100 bpm & without pathologic irregularities
Weight	50 kg (110 lb) Variable requirements for 2-unit Red Blood Cells collection (apheresis) For plasmapheresis collections, donor is weighed; other donations accept self-reported weight
Hemoglobin/hematocrit	≥12.5 g/dL (≥125 g/L)/≥38% for women; ≥13.0 g/dL (≥130 g/L)/ ≥39% for men; variable requirements for 2-unit Red Blood Cells collection (apheresis)
Venipuncture site	Free of lesions & evidence of infection; no evidence of drug abuse

- Reasons for donor deferrals and deferral periods are shown in **t1.2**
- Donor educational materials including those related to
  - Donation process
  - Transfusion-transmitted infections
  - Importance of providing accurate information
  - Not to donate to obtain infectious disease testing
  - Risk of postdonation iron deficiency and mitigation strategies
  - Importance of withdrawing from the process if blood may not be safe for transfusion
  - Acknowledgment that the educational materials have been read
- Signed consent for blood donation

1.1.1.2 Autologous donor requirements

- Rigid criteria are not required, and minimum requirements include
  - Physician's order
  - Hemoglobin ≥11 g/dL (≥110 g/L) or hematocrit ≥33%
  - Blood collection completed >72 hours before surgery
  - No risk of bacteremia in donor
  - Unit is only for autologous transfusion
- Infectious disease screening is required if the collecting facility and transfusing facility are different
  - If collecting facility and transfusing facility are the same, infectious disease screening is not required
- The transfusing facility must confirm the ABO and Rh of each autologous unit

1.1.1.3 Directed or designated donors

- For certain limited clinical situations, including those in which rare antigen-negative blood is required, blood donation by a specific donor can be beneficial
- These donors must meet the same eligibility requirements as an allogeneic donor and all laboratory testing of donor blood, including infectious disease screening
  - Exception to donation frequency may be necessary and this must be certified by a physician
  - If the blood component is not needed by intended recipient, it may be used for other patients

Blood products>Donors

t1.2 Donor deferrals & deferral periods

Reason for deferral	Deferral period
Drugs*	
Teratogenic	
Proscar, Propecia	1 month after last dose
Accutane & similar drugs	1 month after last dose
Avodart, Jaylyn	6 months after last dose
Soriatane	3 years after last dose
Tegison	Permanent
Erivedge	24 months after last dose
Odomzo	24 months after last dose
Aubagio	24 months after last dose
Arava	24 months after last dose
Cellcept	6 weeks after last dose
Antiplatelet function	
Aspirin, Feldene	2 days after last dose
Effient	3 days after last dose
Brilinta	7 days after last dose
Plavix, Ticlid	14 days after last dose
Zontivity	1 month after last dose
Warfarin & similar drugs & heparin & its derivatives	For plasma products, 7 days after last dose
Eliquis, Pradaxa, Xarelto & similar drugs	2 days after last dose
HIV prevention drugs (PrEP & PEP)	3 months after last dose
HIV treatment/antiretroviral therapy (ART)	Indefinite
Other medications, including antibiotics & certain vaccinations & immunizations	As defined by facility's medical director
Vaccinations & immunizations	
Hepatitis B immune globulin	12 months
Measles, mumps, polio, typhoid, yellow fever	2 weeks
German measles, chicken pox/shingles (varicella zoster)	4 weeks
Infectious diseases/behavioral questions	
Confirmed positive test for HBsAg	Permanent
Repeatedly reactive test for anti-HBc more than once	Indefinite
Repeatedly reactive test for anti-HTLV more than once	Indefinite
Positive HBV NAT	Indefinite
Present or past clinical or laboratory evidence of infection with HIV, HCV, HTLV, or *Trypanosoma cruzi*	Indefinite
History of a reactive test for *Babesia* spp[†]	At least 2 years from date of reactive test
Use of needle for nonprescription drugs	3 months
Mucous membrane exposure to blood	3 months
Previous blood transfusion or tissue transplant	3 months
Xenotransplantation	Indefinite
Nonsterile skin penetration with instruments contaminated with blood; includes tattoos or permanent make-up unless applied by a state-regulated entity	3 months
Sexual contact or lived with individual who has acute or chronic hepatitis B or has symptomatic hepatitis C	12 months
Sexual contact with an individual with HIV infection or at high risk for HIV	3 months
Incarceration for 72 hours or more consecutively	12 months
Reactive screening test for syphilis	Indefinite
Diagnosis of syphilis or gonorrhea	3 months if completed treatment
Diagnosis of malaria	3 years after becoming asymptomatic
Travel	
Lived longer than 5 years in malaria-endemic country	3 years after departure
Traveled to an area where malaria is endemic	3 months after departure[‡]
Family genetic history of CJD	Permanent
Variant CJD	Indefinite & includes varying amounts of time spent in UK, France & Ireland from 1980-1996 & 1980-2001; history of blood transfusion in UK, France & Ireland from 1980-present[§]
Miscellaneous	
Pregnancy	>6 weeks after
Receipt of allogeneic dura mater transplant	Permanent

CJD, Creutzfeldt-Jakob disease; FDA, Food and Drug Administration; HBsAg, hepatitis B surface antigen; HBV, hepatitis B virus; HCV, hepatitis C virus; HIV, human immunodeficiency virus; HTLV, human T-cell leukemia virus; NAT, nucleic acid testing; PEP, post-exposure prophylaxis; PrEP, pre-exposure prophylaxis

**Refer to http://aabb.org/tm/questionnaires/pages/dhqaabb.aspx for medication deferral updates*

†Question must be asked in states where testing is not required. Licensed NAT testing for Babesia *species is required for each donation in Connecticut, Delaware, Maine, Maryland, Massachusetts, Minnesota, New Hampshire, New Jersey, New York, Pennsylvania, Rhode Island, Vermont, Virginia, Wisconsin, and Washington, DC. Pathogen reduction can be used as an alternative to testing or donor question if all transfusable components are prepared using FDA-approved pathogen reduction technology*

‡There is no deferral period for travel to an area where malaria is endemic for collecting apheresis platelets or plasma if all transfusable components from the donation are prepared using FDA-approved pathogen reduction technology

§See most recent FDA's "Guidance on Recommendations to Reduce the Possible Risk of Transmission of Creutzfeldt-Jakob Disease and Variant Creutzfeldt-Jakob Disease by Blood and Blood Components" for additional details on this complex deferral

ISBN 978-089189-6616

1.1.1.4 Apheresis donor requirements

- Allogeneic donor requirements apply; exceptions/additions as noted below
  - Plasmapheresis
    - Infrequent donations no more than once every 4 weeks
    - Frequent donations ≤2/week at least 2 days apart
    - Weighed at each donation (≥50 kg)
  - Plateletpheresis
    - 2-day donation interval; ≤2 donations/week for single plateletpheresis
    - Once in 7 days donation interval for double and triple plateletpheresis
    - Cannot exceed 24 donations in a rolling 12-month period
    - Platelet count ≥150,000/µL ($\geq 150 \times 10^9$/L); performed before or after procedure to qualify donor
  - 2-unit red cell apheresis
    - Hemoglobin/hematocrit and weight requirements as defined by device manufacturer and cleared by the Food and Drug Administration (FDA)
    - Deferred from all donations for 16 weeks

1.1.1.5 Collection methods

- Blood must be collected into a sterile closed system using aseptic techniques
  - This includes the preparation of the venipuncture site with povidone iodine or isopropyl alcohol and iodine tincture
    - Green soap is not permitted
  - Blood collection containers with diversion pouches will divert the first 30-45 mL of Whole Blood with any potentially contaminated skin plug from entering the final blood components
    - Especially important when producing platelets derived from Whole Blood or apheresis platelets because of room temperature storage conditions
- Manual Whole Blood collections use polyvinyl chloride bags containing anticoagulants including
  - citrate-phosphate-dextrose (CPD)
  - citrate-phosphate-dextrose-dextrose (CP2D)
  - citrate-phosphate-dextrose-adenine (CPDA-1)
- Whole Blood collection volumes can be either 450±45 mL or 500±50 mL
  - Maximum Whole Blood collection is 10.5 mL/kg of donor weight, including samples
- Manual Whole Blood collections can produce the following blood components
  - Whole Blood
  - Red Blood Cells
  - Platelets
  - Fresh Frozen Plasma, Plasma Frozen Within 24 Hours After Phlebotomy, or Plasma Frozen Within 24 Hours After Phlebotomy Held at Room Temperature up to 24 Hours After Phlebotomy
  - Cryoprecipitated AHF
    - During manufacturing, blood components produced from Whole Blood collections may be further modified to include prestorage pooled components, leukocyte-reduced components, or pathogen-reduced plasma components
- Automated or apheresis/cytapheresis collections can produce the following blood components
  - Apheresis Platelets, Apheresis Platelets Leukocytes Reduced, Apheresis Platelets Platelet Additive Solution Added Leukocytes Reduced, Apheresis Platelets Pathogen Reduced
    - Most platelet transfusion in the US are apheresis platelets that are leukocyte-reduced
  - Apheresis Red Blood Cells
  - Apheresis Granulocytes
  - Fresh Frozen Plasma, Plasma Frozen Within 24 Hours After Phlebotomy, or Plasma Frozen Within 24 Hours After Phlebotomy Held at Room Temperature up to 24 Hours After Phlebotomy
  - During or following collections, apheresis products may be further modified to include those that are leukocyte-reduced
  - Platelet and plasma components collected via apheresis methods may also be pathogen-reduced

1.1.1.6 Donor adverse reactions

- Most donor reactions occur at the donation site
  - Donors must be observed during donation and for an appropriate length of time thereafter
- Common reactions include
  - Vasovagal: includes both presyncope and syncope (loss of consciousness)
  - Local injury related to needle: hematoma, nerve irritation, and arterial puncture
  - Apheresis related: citrate toxicity, air embolism, infiltration during blood return, hemolysis of red cells, and hypovolemia
  - Allergic: local and often related to venipuncture site preparation (iodine)

- Postdonation iron deficiency is another adverse effect of blood donation and is of concern in the following populations with increased risk
  - Premenopausal women
  - Young donors
  - Frequent donors
  - Donors with hemoglobin values near the minimum for eligibility

1.1.2 Processing

1.1.2.1 Laboratory testing of donor blood

- Serologic testing
  - ABO typing
    - Forward and reverse
  - Rh(D) typing
    - If D-positive, blood component will be labeled Rh-positive
    - If D-negative, must do weak D testing
    - If D typing and weak D testing are both negative (including control), blood component will be labeled Rh-negative
    - If D typing is negative but weak D testing is positive (and control negative), blood component will be labeled Rh-positive
  - Antibody detection test on donor serum or plasma using methods to detect clinically significant red cell antibodies
- Infectious disease screening
  - Infectious disease screening tests and supplemental assays currently performed are found in **t1.3**
    - Screening tests are performed on samples from every donation, except for antibodies to *Trypanosoma cruzi* which is a 1-time test
    - Screening tests for *Babesia* species in certain geographic locations will be performed on samples from every donation (**t1.2** and **t1.3**)

t1.3 Infectious disease screening & supplemental assays

Agent	Marker detected	Screening test method	Supplemental assay
HBV	Hepatitis B surface antigen	ChLIA or EIA	HBV DNA Neutralization
	Antibody to hepatitis B core antigen	ChLIA or EIA	
	HBV DNA	TMA or PCR	
HCV	Antibody to HCV peptides or recombinant proteins	ChLIA or EIA	HCV RNA
	HCV RNA	TMA or PCR	
HIV-1 & 2	Antibody to HIV-1 & 2	ChLIA or EIA	HIV-RNA HIV-1 IFA or Western blot HIV-2 EIA
	HIV-1 RNA	TMA or PCR	
HTLV-I & II	Antibody to HTLV-I & II	ChLIA or EIA	Western blot
Syphilis	Antibody to *Treponema pallidum* antigens or, nontreponemal test for syphilis	Microhemagglutination or EIA Particle agglutination	Second FDA-cleared test Antigen-specific immunofluorescence or agglutination assay
Trypanosoma cruzi	Antibody to *T cruzi* (1 time)	ChLIA or EIA	Enzyme strip assay
West Nile virus	WNV RNA	TMA or PCR	Repeat or alternate NAT
Zika virus*	ZIKV RNA	TMA or PCR	Repeat or alternate NAT
Babesia spp*†	*Babesia* spp RNA	TMA or PCR	Repeat or alternate NAT

ChLIA, chemiluminescent immunoassay; EIA, enzyme immunoassay; FDA, Food and Drug Administration; HBV, hepatitis B virus; HIV, human immunodeficiency virus; HTLV, human T-cell leukemia virus; IFA, indirect immunofluorescence assay; NAT, nucleic acid testing; PCR, polymerase chain reaction; TMA, transcription-mediated amplification

**Testing for Zika virus and* Babesia *species is not required if all transfusable components from the donation are prepared using FDA-approved pathogen reduction technology*

†Licensed NAT testing for Babesia *species is required for each donation in Connecticut, Delaware, Maine, Maryland, Massachusetts, Minnesota, New Hampshire, New Jersey, New York, Pennsylvania, Rhode Island, Vermont, Virginia, Wisconsin, and Washington, DC*

Adapted from Cohn CS, Delaney M, Johnson ST, Katz LM, eds. Technical Manual. *20th ed; Bethesda, MD: AABB; 2020*

- Bacterial detection in platelet components
  - In addition to minimizing bacterial contamination at the time of collection with adequate disinfection of venipuncture site and diversion of the first 10-40 mL of donor blood which can contain contaminated skin, all platelet components must undergo testing for the detection of bacteria (culture-based or rapid detection device), or be exposed to pathogen reduction technology

 ISBN 978-089189-6616

- Recent FDA Guidance for Industry (Bacterial Risk Control Strategies for Blood Collection Establishments and Transfusion Services to Enhance the Safety and Availability of Platelets for Transfusion, September 2019) establishes new approaches to enhance the safety of all platelet components stored at room temperature
- Based on the type of platelet component and strategy selected for bacterial detection or pathogen reduction, the shelf life of the platelet component can vary between 5 and 7 days
- Various bacterial risk control strategies, platelet components, and shelf lives are summarized in **t1.4**
- Only FDA-cleared or approved bacterial detection devices, pathogen reduction devices, and platelet storage containers can be used in accordance with manufacturers' instructions
- Cultures are incubated and, depending on the procedure used, platelet components may be issued for transfusion after the first 12 hours of incubation
  - Culture continues for the shelf life of the unit
  - Subsequently positive units, if already released, are retrieved
  - All positive cultures are tested to determine the identity of the organism

1.1.2.2 Overview of blood component manufacturing from Whole Blood collections

- Whole Blood to be manufactured into Platelets must be cooled toward 20°C-24°C; otherwise units of Whole Blood are cooled toward 1°C-10°C
- Component preparation from Whole Blood is based on differential centrifugation and the different specific gravities of the cellular and plasma constituents in each unit
- Calibrated, validated, and temperature-controlled large centrifuges deliver the highest product yield in the shortest time and lowest speed, to minimize damage to any component
- Whole Blood is usually leukocyte-reduced in the laboratory and Red Blood Cells are produced following centrifugation of Whole Blood and removal of plasma
  - Red Blood Cells usually have an additive solution, allowing for storage for up to 42 days
  - Levels of 2,3-diphosphoglycerate (2,3-DPG) in Red Blood Cells decline rapidly after 1 to 2 weeks of storage but this does not affect adults and older children because 2,3-DPG is quickly replenished after transfusion
    - The replenishment of 2,3-DPG in children younger than 4 months is less efficient and one of the reasons red cell components for transfusion are usually <5-7 days old
- Fresh Frozen Plasma is produced from the plasma removed from a unit of Whole Blood if placed in a freezer (≤–18°C) within 8 hours of collection
- Plasma Frozen Within 24 Hours After Phlebotomy (PF24) is manufactured if placement in a freezer (≤–18°C) is not possible within 8 hours of collection but is possible within 24 hours; plasma must be placed at 1-6°C within 8 hours of collection
- Plasma Frozen Within 24 Hours After Phlebotomy Held at Room Temperature up to 24 Hours After Phlebotomy (PF24RT24) is manufactured if plasma is held at room temperature for up to 24 hours and then placed in a freezer (≤–18°C)
- Cryoprecipitated AHF is produced from Fresh Frozen Plasma that has been frozen and then thawed at 1°C-6°C
  - The cryoprecipitate is seen as the white material that remains in the bag after thawing
  - Cryoprecipitated AHF is then suspended in 10-15 mL of plasma and frozen (≤–18°C)
- Platelets derived from Whole Blood require a 2-step process
  - The first step uses a low-speed centrifugation (light spin) to separate the Red Blood Cells from the plasma, allowing the platelets to remain in the plasma portion, known as platelet-rich plasma (PRP)
  - The second step uses a higher-speed centrifugation (hard spin) for the PRP, forcing the platelets to the bottom of the bag
  - The plasma is removed and the platelet pellet is resuspended in a small volume of plasma
  - After a resting period, the Platelets are placed on a rotator and maintained at room temperature
    - Platelets derived from Whole Blood may be pooled (prestorage) using a sterile connection device (closed system), allowing for a 5-day expiration based on the oldest unit in the pool
      - Expiration may be extended to 7 days with secondary rapid bacterial detection testing **t1.4** and **t1.7**
    - Platelets derived from Whole Blood may be pooled just before transfusion (poststorage) in an open system, allowing for a 4-hour expiration
    - Pools for adult transfusions typically contain 4-6 units of Platelets

Blood products> Processing

t1.4 Bacterial risk control strategies for platelet components

Bacterial risk control strategy	Product(s)	Expiration	Overview of process & additional comments related to control strategy
Pathogen reduction	Based on current device labeling, only apheresis platelets	5 days	Treat ≤24 hours after collection. May apply to other platelet products in the future if appropriately FDA approved & labeled pathogen reduction devices & storage containers become available
LVDS for culture no sooner than 36 hours after collection	Apheresis platelets & pre-storage pools of WBD platelets	5 days	Sampling volume of at least 16 mL is inoculated evenly into aerobic & anaerobic culture media. Minimum incubation of 12 hours before release of product is recommended
LVDS for culture no sooner than 48 hours after collection	Apheresis platelets	7 days	Sampling volume of at least 16 mL is inoculated evenly into aerobic & anaerobic culture media. Minimum incubation of 12 hours before release of product is recommended
Primary culture performed no sooner than 24 hours after collection AND secondary culture performed no sooner than day 3 of storage	Apheresis platelets & prestorage pools of WBD platelets	5 days	For primary culture, at least 16 mL is inoculated evenly into aerobic & anaerobic culture media. Minimum incubation of 12 hours. For secondary culture, at least 8 mL is inoculated into at least an aerobic medium
LVDS for primary culture no sooner than 36 hours after collection AND secondary culture performed no sooner than day 4 of storage	Apheresis platelets	7 days	Sampling volume of at least 16 mL for primary culture is inoculated evenly into aerobic & anaerobic culture media. Minimum incubation of 12 hours before release of product is recommended. Secondary culture performed with at least 16 mL inoculated evenly between aerobic & anaerobic culture media with a minimum incubation of 12 hours
LVDS for primary culture no sooner than 36 hours after collection AND secondary rapid bacterial detection test (safety measure)	Apheresis platelets & prestorage pools of WBD platelets	7 days	Sampling volume of at least 16 mL for primary culture is inoculated evenly into aerobic & anaerobic culture media. Minimum incubation of 12 hours before release of product is recommended. The secondary rapid bacterial testing is performed in accordance with device labeling at ≤24 hours before transfusion
Rapid bacterial testing	Single units of WBD platelets & poststorage pools of previously untested WBD platelets	Single units of WBD platelets: 5 days Poststorage pools of WBD platelets: 4 hours	Rapid bacterial testing is performed in accordance with device labeling
Single culture with sampling performed no sooner than 36 hours after collection	Single units of WBD platelets	5 days	Inoculation into aerobic culture media. As single unit of WBD platelets is of small volume, the largest practical volume with the range permitted by the bacterial testing device should be used for culture. Minimum incubation period of 12 hours before release for transfusion
Single culture with sampling performed no sooner than 24 hours after collection	Single units of WBD platelets	5 days	Inoculation into aerobic culture media. As single unit of WBD platelets is of small volume, the largest practical volume with the range permitted by the bacterial testing device should be used for culture. Minimum incubation period of 12 hours before release for transfusion. If unit is transfused after day 3 of storage, secondary rapid bacterial testing may be considered

LVDS, large-volume, delayed sampling; WBD, Whole Blood–derived

ISBN 978-089189-6616

1.1.2.3 Pathogen reduction technology

- Treatment with amotosalen (psoralen) plus UVA light phototherapy is currently FDA approved for pathogen reduction in plasma components and apheresis platelets
  - Other pathogen reduction technologies including the use of riboflavin plus UVA light are under development as is technology to treat Whole Blood and Red Blood Cells
- This treatment is effective in preventing nucleic acid replication for bacterial, viral, and parasitic pathogens and mitigates risk for emerging and unknown pathogens
- Apheresis platelets that undergo pathogen reduction treatment are not required to be tested with a culture-based system for bacterial detection
- Pathogen reduction technologies can be used as an alternative to testing or donor questioning for *Babesia* species and Zika virus if all transfusable components from the donation are prepared using FDA-approved pathogen reduction technology, currently only applicable to plasma and apheresis platelets
- Pathogen reduction technologies inactivate white cells and the risk of transfusion-associated graft-versus-host disease (TA-GVHD), negating the need for irradiation

1.1.2.4 Labeling of blood products

- In the US, blood component labeling uses ISBT 128 symbology and follows the United States Industry Consensus Standard for the Uniform Labeling of Blood and Blood Components Using ISBT 128, Version 3.0.0
  - Combination of eye-readable and machine-readable data
  - Labeling process includes second check to ensure accuracy of donation identification number, ABO and Rh, expiration date, and component name and code
  - General ISBT 128 label requirements for blood and blood components are shown in **t1.5**

t1.5 General ISBT 128 blood component labeling requirements

Name of blood component
Collection facility
Unique facility identifier (ie, FDA registration number)
Donation identification number
Anticoagulant or preservative
Approximate volume
Storage temperature
Expiration date, and if needed, expiration time
ABO & Rh
Volunteer or paid donor
Number of units in pool, if needed
Instructions to transfusionist:
Rx only
May transmit infectious agents
Identify intended recipient
See Circular of Information

1.1.2.5 Use of a sterile connection device

- Sterile connection device maintains a functionally closed system when processing blood components
  - Closed system maintains original expiration date of product
  - The weld must be inspected for completeness
    - If weld is incomplete, treated as open system with shortened expiration date of product (see 1.1.4 and **t1.7**)
- Uses in the blood bank include
  - Prestorage pooled Platelets or pooled Cryoprecipitated AHF
  - Split or divided units for pediatric use
  - Attachment of leukocyte reduction filters or processing solutions
  - Sampling blood products for further testing, including those for bacterial culturing

1.1.3 Storage & transport

- Blood component storage and transport requirements are summarized in **t1.6**
  - Storage temperatures are monitored continuously and recorded at least every 4 hours
  - If storage occurs in an open area, ambient temperature is recorded at least every 4 hours

t1.6 Storage & transport requirements for blood components

Component	Storage temperature	Transport temperature
All red blood cell products	1°C-6°C	1°C-10°C
Frozen red blood cells	≤–65°C	Maintain frozen state
Platelet products	20°C-24°C with continuous gentle agitation	As close as possible to 20°C-24°C; maximum time without agitation is 30 hours
Cold stored platelets	1°C-6°C with optional agitation	1°C-10°C
All frozen plasma products & cryoprecipitated AHF	≤–18°C	Maintain frozen state
All thawed plasma products	1°C-6°C	1°C-10°C
Thawed cryoprecipitated AHF	20°C-24°C	As close as possible to 20°C-24°C
Apheresis granulocytes	20°C-24°C	As close as possible to 20°C-24°C

AHF, antihemophilic factor

- Most platelet components are stored and transported at 20°C-24°C
  - Some trauma centers are adopting the use of cold-stored platelets to manage significant bleeding
    - Cold-stored platelets have a storage temperature of 1°C-6°C and a transport temperature of 1°C-10°C

1.1.4 Blood component shelf life (storage time), special attributes & dosage

- Shelf life (storage time), special attributes, and dosages for blood and blood components manufactured from manual Whole Blood collections and apheresis (automated) collections are found in **t1.7**

1.1.4.1 Irradiated cellular blood components

- Red cell-containing components that are irradiated will have the original expiration date or 28 days from date of irradiation, whichever is sooner
- Platelets, Apheresis Platelets, or Apheresis Granulocytes that are irradiated maintain the original expiration date

t1.7 Shelf life (storage times), special attributes & dosages for blood & blood components manufactured from manual Whole Blood collections & apheresis (automated) collections

Component	Shelf life or storage time	Special attributes & dosage
Whole Blood & Whole Blood Leukocytes Reduced	CPD & CP2D: 21 days CPDA-1: 35 days Open system: 24 hours	Not routinely transfused but may be used in certain patients with massive blood loss. ↑Hb 1 g/dL (10 g/L) or ↑Hct 3%, but continued massive blood loss may result in smaller increments
Red Blood Cells	Most will use an additive solution to increase shelf life to 42 days; otherwise as for Whole Blood; open system: 24 hours	↑Hb 1 g/dL (10 g/L) or ↑Hct 3%
Red Blood Cells Leukocytes Reduced	Most will use an additive solution to increase shelf life to 42 days; otherwise as for Whole Blood; open system: 24 hours	CMV-safe component; results in reduced frequency of febrile, nonhemolytic transfusion reaction; ↑Hb 1 g/dL (10 g/L) or ↑Hct 3%
Apheresis Red Blood Cells & Apheresis Red Blood Cells Leukocytes Reduced	Most will use an additive solution to increase shelf life to 42 days. Typically, 2 units of red blood cells are collected during donation. Can also include collection of a single red blood cells with a unit of plasma and/or plateletpheresis component. Some collections are leukocyte-reduced & have additive solution added during the procedure, but others occur offline in the laboratory	Male & female donors meet variable criteria based on both height & weight to undergo these procedures. A double red cell collection results in a minimum deferral of 16 weeks. Each unit ↑ Hb 1 g/dL (10 g/L) or ↑ Hct 3%
Frozen Red Blood Cells	≤–65°C for 10 years; usually frozen with 6 days of collection	High glycerol as cryoprotectant; often used to preserve units with rare red cell phenotypes
Deglycerolized Red Blood Cells	Open system: 24 hours; closed system: 14 days or as FDA approved	↑ Hb 1 g/dL (10 g/L) or ↑ Hct 3%; often provides transfusion support to alloimmunized individuals who require rare red cell phenotype blood
Platelets & Platelets Leukocytes Reduced (Whole Blood derived)	5 days	1 Platelet increases the platelet count in a 70-kg adult by 5000/μL (5×10^9/L). Usually given as a pooled product (see below)
Pooled Platelets & Pooled Platelets Leukocytes Reduced (Whole Blood derived)	Prestorage pooled platelets if pooled using sterile connection device (closed system) & based on oldest unit in pool have 5-day expiration; prestorage pools can be extended to 7-day expiration using a secondary rapid bacterial detection test; 4 hours if pooled in an open system (see **t1.4**)	1 Platelet increases the platelet count in a 70-kg adult by 5000/μL (5×10^9/L). Multiply 5000 × number of units in pool for approximate expected platelet increment
Apheresis Platelets & Apheresis Platelets Leukocytes Reduced	5 days or 7 days, depending on bacterial risk reduction strategy (**t1.4**). Most platelet transfusions in the US are those collected via apheresis methods that are also leukocyte-reduced	Multiple apheresis platelet components may be collected from the donor at a single donation, based on the donor's platelet count. Donors must have a minimum platelet count of 150,000/μL (150×10^9/L). 1 Apheresis Platelet increases the platelet count in a 70-kg adult by 30,000-50,000/μL ($30\text{-}50\times10^9$/L)
Apheresis Platelets Pathogen Reduced	5 days	Dosage equivalent to other apheresis products. FDA-approved pathogen reduction devices used according to manufacturer's instructions need no further measures to control the risk of bacterial contamination, including bacterial detection testing
Apheresis Platelets Platelet Additive Solution Added Leukocytes Reduced	5 days	65% of the plasma volume is replaced with this additive solution. Useful in reducing allergic transfusion reactions while achieving good posttransfusion platelet counts equivalent to other apheresis products
Platelets Cold Stored (could be derived from Whole Blood, but usually from automated apheresis collections)	3 days at 1°C-6°C; FDA variance required to store apheresis platelets for up to 14 days at 1°C-6°C Agitation is optional	Only appropriate for actively bleeding patients because of shorter circulation time after transfusion

ISBN 978-089189-6616

t1.7 Shelf life (storage times), special attributes & dosages for blood & blood components manufactured from manual Whole Blood collections & apheresis (automated) collections

Component	Shelf life or storage time	Special attributes & dosage
Apheresis Granulocytes	24 hours	Red cell compatibility testing must be performed as product usually contains large number of red blood cells (≥2 mL). Product usually given daily
Fresh Frozen Plasma (FFP)	≤–18°C: 12 months from collection; ≤–65°C: 7 years from collection (requires FDA approval); thaw at 30°C-37°C in water bath or FDA-cleared device. Use plastic overwrap in water bath to keep entry port out of water. Once thawed, store for 24 hours at 1°C-6°C	Must be frozen within 8 hours of collection. Manufactured from Whole Blood or apheresis collection. Dose depends on clinical situation. For factor deficiency, 10-20 mL/kg is usual dose
Plasma Frozen Within 24 Hours After Phlebotomy (PF24)	≤–18°C: 12 months from collection; thaw at 30°C-37°C in water bath or FDA-cleared device. Use plastic overwrap in water bath to keep entry port out of water. Once thawed, store for 24 hours at 1°C-6°C	Must be frozen within 24 hours of collection. Manufactured from Whole Blood or apheresis collection. If prepared from apheresis collection, the product is stored at 1°C-6°C within 8 hours of collection. Dose depends on clinical situation. For factor deficiency, 10-20 mL/kg is usual dose
Plasma Frozen Within 24 Hours After Phlebotomy Held at Room Temperature up to 24 Hours After Phlebotomy (PF24RT24)	≤–18°C: 12 months from collection; thaw at 30°C-37°C in water bath or FDA-cleared device. Use plastic overwrap in water bath to keep entry port out of water. Once thawed, store for 24 hours at 1°C-6°C	Held at room temperature for up to 24 hours after collection & then frozen. Manufactured from Whole Blood or apheresis collection. Dose depends on clinical situation. For factor deficiency, 10-20 mL/kg is the usual dose
Thawed Plasma	Thawed FFP, PF24, or PF24RT24 stored beyond 24 hours can be converted to thawed plasma. Expires 4 days after initial 24 hours thaw period	Reduced factor V & factor VIII levels but adequate amounts of other factors. Dose depends on clinical situation
Plasma Pathogen Reduced	≤–18°C: 12 months from collection; thaw at 30°C-37°C in water bath or FDA-cleared device. Use plastic overwrap in water bath to keep entry port out of water	Equivalent to other plasma products
Cryoprecipitated AHF	≤–18°C: 12 months from collection; 6 hours once thawed as single units or pooled in closed system; 4 hours if pooled in open system	Used primarily to replace fibrinogen. Each unit will increase fibrinogen by 5-10 mg/dL in an average-sized adult

1.1.5 Blood component quality control

- Blood component quality control requirements are summarized in **t1.8**

t1.8 Blood component quality control metrics

Component	Quality Control Metrics
Red Blood Cells without additive	Hematocrit ≤80%
Deglycerolized Red Blood Cells	Yield a mean recovery of ≥80% of preglycerolized red cells & minimal free hemoglobin in supernatant
Red Blood Cells Leukocytes Reduced & Whole Blood Leukocytes Reduced	At least 85% of original red cells retained & $<5\times10^6$ leukocytes per unit; ≥95% units sampled must meet criterion
Apheresis Red Blood Cells	Method known to ensure a mean collection of ≥60 g of Hb (180 mL red cell volume) per unit. At least 95% of units sampled shall have >50 g Hb (150 mL red cell volume)
Apheresis Red Blood Cells Leukocytes Reduced	Method known to ensure a mean collection of ≥51 g of Hb (or 153 mL red cell volume) & $<5\times10^6$ residual leukocytes per unit. At least 95% of units sampled shall have >42.5 g Hb (or 128 mL red cell volume) per unit; ≥95% units sampled must meet criterion
Platelets (derived from Whole Blood)	At least 90% of units sampled contain $\geq5.5\times10^{10}$ platelets & have a pH ≥6.2 at the end of allowable storage
Platelets Leukocytes Reduced (derived from Whole Blood)	$\geq5.5\times10^{10}$ platelets in at least 75% of units sampled; $<8.3\times10^5$ leukocytes in 95% of units sampled; at lease 90% of units sampled pH ≥6.2 at end of allowable storage
Pooled Platelets & Pooled Platelets Leukocytes Reduced	For Pooled Platelets Leukocytes Reduced, the residual leukocyte count must be $<5\times10^6$; pH ≥6.2 at the end of allowable storage. Platelet counts as defined for Platelets & Platelet Leukocytes reduced also apply
Apheresis Platelets	At least 90% of units sampled contain $\geq3.0\times10^{11}$ platelets: pH ≥6.2 at the time of issue or at the end of allowable storage
Apheresis Platelets Leukocytes Reduced	At least 90% of units sampled contain $\geq3.0\times10^{11}$ platelets and, at the end of allowable storage or at time of issue, have a pH ≥6.2; 95% of units sampled contain a residual leukocyte count of $<5\times10^6$
Apheresis Granulocytes	Method used yields a minimum of 1.0×10^{10} granulocytes in at least 75% of units tested
Cryoprecipitated AHF	Minimum of 150 mg fibrinogen & a minimum of 80 IU of coagulation factor VIII per container or unit. For prestorage pooled components, minimum of 150 mg of fibrinogen & 80 IU of factor VIII × the number of components in the pool

AHF, antihemophilic factor; Hg, hemoglobin

1.2 Blood group systems

1.2.1 Genetics

- There are 38 blood group systems and 1 provisional blood group system that define 326 antigens
- Each blood group system is controlled by a single gene or by ≥2 very closely linked homologous genes and demonstrates ≥1 antigens within that system **t1.9**

t1.9 Blood group systems

System name	System symbol	Gene(s)	Number of antigens	Chromosome location
ABO	ABO	*ABO*	4	9q34.2
MNS	MNS	*GPA, GPB*	49	4q31.21
P1PK	P1PK	*A4GALT*	3	22q13.2
Rh	RH	*RHD, RHCE*	55	1p36.11
Lutheran	LU	*BCAM*	25	19q13.2
Kell	KEL	*KEL*	36	7q33
Lewis	LE	*FUT3*	6	19p13.3
Duffy	FY	*ACKR1*	5	1q21-q22
Kidd	JK	*SLC14A1*	3	18q11-q12
Diego	DI	*SLC4A1*	22	17q21.31
Yt	YT	*ACHE*	5	7q22
Xg	XG	*XG, MIC2*	2	Xp22.32
Scianna	SC	*ERMAP*	7	1p34.2
Dombrock	DO	*ART4*	10	12p13-p12
Colton	CO	*AQP1*	4	7p14
Landsteiner-Wiener	LW	*ICAM4*	3	19p13.2
Chido/Rodgers	CH/RG	*C4A, C4B*	9	6p21.3
H	H	*FUT1*	1	19q13.33
Kx	XK	*XK*	1	Xp21.1
Gerbich	GE	*GYPC*	11	2q14-q21
Cromer	CROM	*CD55*	20	1q32
Knops	KN	*CR1*	9	1q32.2
Indian	IN	*CD44*	6	11p13
Ok	OK	*BSG*	3	19p13.3
Raph	RAPH	*CD151*	1	11p15.5
John Milton Hagen	JMH	*SEMA7A*	6	15q22.3-q23
I	I	*GCNT2*	1	6p24.2
Globoside	GLOB	*B3GALNT1*	2	3q25
Gill	GIL	*AQP3*	1	9p13
Rh-associated glycoprotein	RHAG	*RHAG*	3	6p12.3
FORS	FORS	*GBGT1*	1	9q34.13-q34.3
JR	JR	*ABCG2*	1	4q22.1
LAN	LAN	*ABCB6*	1	2q36
Vel	VEL	*SMIM1*	1	1p36.32
CD59	CD59	*CD59*	1	11p13
Augustine	AUG	*SLC29A1*	4	6p21.1
KANNO	KANNO	*PRNP*	1	20p13
Sid	SID	*B4GALNT2*	1	17q21.32
CTL2*	CTL2	*SLC44A2*	2	19p13.2

**Provisional status*

- The International Society of Blood Transfusion (ISBT) and one of its Working Parties maintains and updates this information: *http://www.isbtweb.org/working-parties/red-cell-immunogenetics-and-blood-group-terminology/*
  - In this chapter, the ISBT system symbol for each blood group system, eg, KEL instead of Kell, is used **t1.9**
    - The Rh blood group system is the exception
- Most blood group antigens are glycoproteins and specificities are determined by oligosaccharide or carbohydrate epitopes (ABO, H, LE, P1PK, I, GLOB), or amino acid sequences (MNS, KEL, FY, JK)
  - Rh blood group system antigens are protein, but uniquely not glycosylated or phosphorylated; amino acid sequences determine specificity
- Carbohydrate and protein antigens and their respective antibodies have some unique and different attributes **t1.10**

t1.10 Comparison of carbohydrate & protein blood group antigens & their antibodies

Carbohydrate antigens	Protein antigens
ABO, H, LE, I, P1PK & GLOB	FY, JK, KEL, Rh, MNS
Often naturally occurring antibodies	Usually produced as a result of exposure to foreign antigens through pregnancy, transfusion, or transplantation
Usually IgM antibodies to respective antigens; can be IgG, or both	Usually IgG antibodies to respective antigens
IgM antibodies usually react best at room temperature	IgG antibodies usually react best at 37°C
IgM antibodies usually cause direct agglutination with respective antigens	IgG antibodies attach to respective antigens, failing to demonstrate direct agglutination
Some IgM antibodies may initiate the activation of complement, noting this on the surface of red cells if AHG reagent contains anti-C3	AHG reagent used to demonstrate agglutination (indirect method) when antibody attaches to respective antigen

AHG, antihuman globulin

- Antigens within a blood group system are polymorphic, usually the result of a single nucleotide polymorphism (SNP) in either a glycosyltransferase or extracellular domain of a red cell membrane protein
  - The *KEL* gene that produces the K antigen encodes Met193 (methionine at amino acid 193) but the *KEL* gene that produces the k antigen encodes Thr193 (threonine at amino acid 193)

1.2.1.1 Modes of inheritance

- The inheritance of blood group genes and the resulting antigens follow the principles of independent segregation and independent assortment
  - Only 1 member of an allelic pair from each parent is passed to the next generation
- Most blood group antigens are expressed as autosomal dominant or autosomal codominant traits

ISBN 978-089189-6616

- A group AB individual who inherits an *A* and *B* gene will demonstrate A and B antigens on their red cells as an autosomal codominant trait
- Individual who inherits a *B* and *O* gene will demonstrate B antigens on their red cells as an autosomal dominant trait
- When identical alleles for a given locus are inherited, the individual is homozygous for the trait, eg, MM
- When alternate alleles for a given locus are inherited, the individual is heterozygous for the trait, eg, MN

- Some blood group system genes express their antigens as autosomal recessive traits
  - Group O individuals inherit 2 *O* genes as an autosomal recessive trait
- One blood group, XG, expresses its genetic product as an X-linked dominant trait
  - Heterozygous females pass the trait to 50% of offspring whether male or female and homozygous females pass the trait to all offspring regardless of sex
  - Hemizygous males (inherit X-linked trait) pass the trait to all daughters

1.2.1.2 Hardy-Weinberg equation

- Gene frequencies tend to remain constant and maintain equilibrium over generations and can be expressed as follows

$$p^2 + 2pq + q^2 = 1$$

- If 2 alleles, typically referred to as A and a, have gene frequencies of p and q, the homozygotes and heterozygotes are represented as follows

$$AA = p^2;\ Aa = 2pq\ ;\ aa = q^2$$

- In this 2-allele system, if the gene frequency for 1 allele (p) is known, the gene frequency for the other allele (q) can be calculated as follows

$$p + q = 1$$

The Hardy-Weinberg equation also allows the calculation of genotype frequency from gene frequency

An example of calculating gene frequency and genotype frequency using the Hardy-Weinberg equation is shown in **f1.1**

1.2.2 ABO & H blood group systems

1.2.2.1 Clinical importance

- The ABO system is the most important blood group system because individuals routinely demonstrate clinically significant ABO antibodies in their serum to the ABO antigens they lack on their red cells **t1.11**

determine the gene frequencies of the alleles *K* & *k* in a population where the K+ phenotype is observed in 9% of individuals tested

determine the genotype frequencies for those that are *KK*, *Kk*, and *kk*

2 equations necessary to solve the gene frequencies & genotype frequencies are:

$$p^2 + 2pq + q^2 = 1$$
$$p + q = 1$$

where:
p = frequency of *K* gene
q = frequency of *k* gene
p^2 = frequency of *KK* genotype
2pq = frequency of *Kk* genotype
q^2 = frequency of *kk* genotype

$p^2 + 2pq$ = the frequency of K+, which is 9% or 0.09

$$p^2 + 2pq + q^2 = 1$$
$$q^2 = 1 - (p^2 + 2pq)$$
$$q^2 = 1 - 0.09$$
$$q^2 = 0.91$$
$$q = \sqrt{0.91}$$
$$q = 0.95$$
$$p + q = 1$$
$$p = 1 - q$$
$$p = 1 - 0.95$$
$$p = 0.05$$

therefore, the gene frequency for *K* (p) is 0.05 & the gene frequency for *k* (q) is 0.95

based on this information, the genotype frequencies for *KK*, *Kk* and *kk* can now be calculated

$p^2 = (0.05)^2 = 0.0025$ = frequency for *KK*
$2pq = 2 \times 0.05 \times 0.95 = 0.0950$ = frequency for *Kk*
$q^2 = (0.95)^2 = 0.9025$ = frequency for *kk*

f1.1 Hardy-Weinberg equation

- ABO antibodies occur without exposure to RBCs and likely result from exposure to bacteria with structures similar to A and B antigens
  - Detectable in infants at 3-6 months of age but may not reach adult levels until 5 years of age
- Transfusion with ABO-incompatible blood can cause acute and immediate hemolysis of red cells, leading to renal failure and death

1.2.2.2 Genes & interactions

- The ABO locus is found on chromosome 9
  - Inheritance follows simple Mendelian genetics as 1 ABO gene is inherited from each parent: *A*, *B*, *O*
  - ABO phenotype prevalence varies by ethnicity **t1.12**
- *A* and *B* genes are dominant or codominant and *O* is recessive
  - The *O* gene is amorphic and produces no detectable antigen

- The inheritance of a single *O* gene with an *A* or *B* gene is serologically indistinguishable from those who inherit 2 *A* or 2 *B* genes
- The *H* gene (*FUT1*) and *h* (absence of *H*) alleles are located on chromosome 19 and interact with the *ABO* genes
- The *H* gene produces H antigen and H antigens must be present to produce A and/or B antigens when *A* and/or *B* genes are inherited
- The *H, A,* and *B* genes produce glycosyltransferase enzymes that add specific sugars to preformed structures (oligosaccharide chains) that give rise to A, B, and H antigens **t1.13**
- On RBCs, these antigens are type 2 oligosaccharide chains that demonstrate β 1→4 linkages between galactose and N-acetylglucosamine, whereas in the secretions, these soluble antigens will be type 1 oligosaccharide chains with β 1→3 linkages between galactose and N-acetylglucosamine **f1.2**

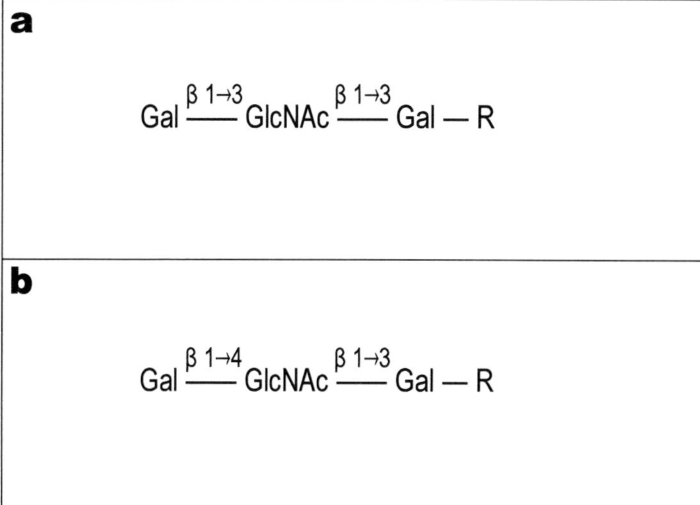

f1.2 **a** Type 1 oligosaccharide chains as found in secretions
b Type 2 oligosaccharide chains as found on red blood cells
Gal, galactose; GlcNAc, N-acetylglucosamine

t1.11 ABO forward & reverse typing

ABO forward typing		**ABO reverse typing**		**Result**
Test patient red cells with reagent antisera		Test patient serum with reagent red cells		ABO type
Anti-A	Anti-B	A_1 cells	B cells	
0	0	+	+	O
+	0	0	+	A
0	+	+	0	B
+	+	0	0	AB

t1.12 ABO phenotype prevalence (%) by ethnicity

ABO	**White**	**Black**	**Hispanic**	**Asian**
O	45	49	56	40
A	40	27	31	28
B	11	20	10	25
AB	4	4	3	7

t1.13 ABO & H system genes, enzyme produced, immunodominant sugar & terminal antigenic structure

Gene	**Glycosyltransferase or gene product**	**Immunodominant sugar responsible for ABH antigens**	**Terminal antigenic structure**
H (*FUT1*)	α-2-L-fucosyltransferase	Fucose	Gal —(β 1-3 or β 1-4)— GlcNAc — Gal — R; Gal |α 1-2 Fuc
A	α-3-N-acetylgalactosaminyltransferase	N-acetylgalactosamine	GalNAc —(α 1-3)— Gal —(β 1-3 or β 1-4)— GlcNAc — Gal — R; Gal |α 1-2 Fuc
B	α-3-D-galactosyltransferase	Galactose	Gal —(α 1-3)— Gal —(β 1-3 or β 1-4)— GlcNAc — Gal — R; Gal |α 1-2 Fuc
O	None	Expresses only H antigen	

ISBN 978-089189-6616

1.2.2.3 Amount of H antigen on red cells

- The *O* gene (amorph) does not produce a transferase enzyme and group O red cells demonstrate the most amount of H antigen
- The *A2* gene has a less efficient transferase when compared to *A1* so less A antigen is produced in A_2 individuals, giving rise to increased amounts of H antigen
- *B* genes and *A* and *B* genes inherited together convert H antigen to A and B antigen with varying degrees of efficiency
  - ↑H 0, > A_2, > B, > A_2B, > A_1, > A_1B ↓H

1.2.2.4 ABO subgroups

- Two most widely recognized ABO subgroups are A_1 and A_2
  - 80% of group A individuals will be A_1 and 20% will be A_2
  - Differentiate with anti-A1 lectin (*Dolichos biflorus*)
  - Some A_2 individuals (5%) will demonstrate anti-A1 in their serum that is usually clinically insignificant
  - Similarly, A_1B and A_2B individuals can be differentiated with anti-A1 lectin
    - Some A_2B individuals (35%) will demonstrate anti-A1 in their serum that is usually clinically insignificant
- Other subgroups of A exist and demonstrate variable serologic results **t1.14**
  - Anti-A,B and anti-H (*Ulex europaeus*) can be useful in differentiating various subgroups of A
- Subgroups of B also exist and demonstrate variable serologic results including reactivity with anti-A,B and anti-H (**t1.14**)
- The presence of weak A and/or weak B antigens is sometimes confirmed by adsorbing anti-A or anti-B onto red cells and subsequently eluting the antibody from those red cells
- Studies of soluble A, B, or H antigens in saliva may also be useful in confirming ABO type

1.2.2.5 ABO discrepancies

- Red cell related: ABO forward typing has missing, reduced, or unexpected antigen reactions
  - ABO subgroup
  - Unusual ABO phenotypes like cis AB, B(A), A(B)
  - Out-of-group transfusion or hematopoietic progenitor cell (HPC) transplantation
  - Genetic chimera
  - Autoagglutination, abnormal serum proteins, reagent-dependent antibody, neutralization by excess blood group substance
    - Washing red cells and repeat testing may resolve
  - Polyagglutination including T activation and acquired B phenotype
  - Technical errors
    - Too heavy or too light red cell suspensions
    - Over- or undercentrifugation
    - Failure to add reagent
    - Incorrect interpretation
- Serum related: ABO reverse typing has missing, reduced, or unexpected antibody reactions
  - ABO subgroup
  - Age of patient including the very young or very old
  - Hypogammaglobulinemia
  - Out-of-group transfusion or HPC transplantation
  - Cold allo- or cold autoantibody
  - Rouleaux from abnormal serum proteins or infusion of high-molecular-weight volume expanders
  - Infusion of intravenous immunoglobulin
  - Technical errors as listed before

t1.14 Subgroups of A & B

	Red cell reactions					Serum reactions	
Phenotype	Anti-A	Anti-B	Anti-A,B	Anti-A1	Anti-H	A_1 cells	B cells
A_1	4+	0	4+	4+	0	0	4+
A_2	4+	0	4+	0	2+	0/2+	4+
A_3	$3+^{mf}$	0	$3+^{mf}$	$+^{mf}$	3+	0/2+	4+
A_x	0/±	0	1-2+	0	4+	0/2+	4+
A_{el}	0	0	0	0	4+	0/2+	4+
B	0	4+	4+	NT	0/1+	4+	0
B_3	0	$3+^{mf}$	$3+^{mf}$	NT	4+	4+	0
B_{weak}	0	±/2+	±/2+	NT	4+	4+	0

mf, mixed-field agglutination

- ABO discrepancies need to be resolved and strategies might include
  - Antibody identification studies
  - Testing with lectin reagents including anti-A1 and anti-H
  - Collection of new blood sample
  - Repeat testing with washed red cells
  - Adsorption and elution studies to prove the presence of ABO antigens
  - Autoadsorption of serum to remove suspected autoantibody followed with repeat testing
  - Evaluation of clinical history
  - Adherence to standard operating procedures

1.2.2.6 Bombay (O_h) phenotype

- Arises from the inheritance of a nonfunctional *FUT1* (*H*) gene and a nonfunctional *FUT2* (*Se* or *Secretor*) gene
  - May also be described as inheriting 2 "*h*" genes
- Although normal *A* and/or *B* genes may be inherited, they are unable to produce A and/or B antigens because of a lack of H antigen
  - A and/or B transferase can be detected
- Red cells lack all ABH antigens and demonstrate potent and clinically significant anti-A, anti-B, anti-A,B, and anti-H in their serum
  - On initial routine ABO forward and reverse typing, these individuals appear to be group O, but their serum will be strongly reactive with antibody detection cells and the red cells of every group O donor because of the potent anti-H alloantibody
- Studies with anti-H lectin (*Ulex europaeus*) will demonstrate that cells lack H antigen
- Only blood from other O_h individuals will be suitable for transfusion therapy
- Other rare H-deficient individuals with a functional *FUT2* gene are identified as para-Bombay phenotype

1.2.2.7 ABH antigens in secretions & plasma

- Soluble ABH antigens can be found in secretions, including saliva, tears, and plasma
  - Presence or absence of soluble antigens defined by genes at the *Secretor* locus on chromosome 19
  - Alleles of the *Secretor* locus are *Se (FUT2)* and *se*
  - Inheritance of at least 1 *Se* gene (autosomal dominant) gives rise to individuals defined as secretors and found in 80% of the population
  - Inheritance of 2 *se* genes (autosomal recessive) gives rise to individuals defined as nonsecretors and found in 20% of the population
  - The *Secretor* locus is not a blood group system, but genes at this locus interact with ABO, H & LE blood group systems
  - The *Se* gene does not affect the formation of A, B & H antigens on the red cells
- *Se* (*FUT2*) gene codes for α-fucosyltransferase enzyme that adds fucose to type 1 oligosaccharide chains with β 1→3 linkage between galactose and N-acetylglucosamine to form soluble H antigen in the secretions
  - Soluble A and B antigen can then be made if the corresponding gene is inherited

1.2.3 LE (Lewis) blood group system

- Alleles of the *LE* locus include *Le* (*FUT3*) and *le*
- *Le* is autosomal dominant whereas *le* is autosomal recessive
- The product of the *Le* (*FUT3*) gene is an α-fucosyltransferase that adds fucose to soluble type 1 oligosaccharide chains
- There are 2 LE antigens, Le^a and Le^b and 3 LE phenotypes, Le(a+b–), Le(a–b+), and Le(a–b–), and phenotype prevalence varies by ethnicity **t1.15**
  - LE antigens are not synthesized by the red cell but are passively adsorbed onto the red cell from soluble antigens present in plasma
  - The addition of a single fucose molecule from the *Le* (*FUT3*) gene gives rise to the Le^a antigen
  - The addition of 2 fucose molecules gives rise to the Le^b antigen
    - The *Se (FUT2)* gene must first add fucose to type 1 oligosaccharide chains to produce soluble H antigen
    - The *Le* (*FUT3*) gene adds a second fucose to type 1 H antigen to produce the Le^b antigen

t1.15 LE phenotype prevalence (%) by ethnicity

Phenotype	White	Black
Le(a+b–)	22	23
Le(a–b+)	72	55
Le(a–b–)	6	22

- The *Le* gene gives rise to 2 different LE red cell phenotypes that are also dependent upon the inheritance of 1 or 2 *Se* genes or 2 *se* genes
  - If *Le* and 2 *se* genes inherited, red cells will be Le(a+b–)
    - Le^a antigen will be found in the secretions, but not soluble A, B, or H antigen
    - Termed nonsecretors

 ISBN 978-089189-6616

- If *Le* and 1 or 2 *Se* genes inherited, red cells will be Le(a–b+)
    - Le^a and Le^b antigens will be found in the secretions as well as soluble A, B, or H antigen
    - Termed secretors
- Two *le* genes give rise to the Le(a–b–) phenotype and these individuals can be secretors or nonsecretors based on the *Secretor* genes inherited

1.2.3.1 LE system antibodies

- LE antibodies are naturally occurring and can be produced by Le(a–b–) individuals
- Anti-Le^a may occur as the only antibody
    - More commonly detected if testing is performed at room temperature
    - Usually IgM and clinically insignificant but examples of clinically significant anti-Le^a have been well documented
- Anti-Le^b is seen as a less avid antibody and may be found with anti-Le^a
    - More commonly detected if testing is performed at room temperature
    - Usually IgM and clinically insignificant
    - Some examples of anti-Le^b react preferentially with Le(b+) red cells that express the greatest levels of H antigen (group O)
        - Identified as anti-Le^{bH}
    - Other examples of anti-Le^b react equally well with all Le(b+) red cells, regardless of the amount of H antigen
        - Identified as anti-Le^{bL}
- Pregnant women may transiently appear as Le(a–b–) and can produce LE antibodies
    - No harm to fetus because fetal red cells are Le(a–b–) and most LE antibodies are IgM and unable to cross the placenta

1.2.3.2 Interaction of *ABO, H, Secretor* & *LE* genes

- **t1.16** summarizes the interactions between these genetic loci and the antigens present on the red cell and in the secretions

t1.16 Interaction of *ABO*, *H*, *Secretor* & *LE* genes

Genes	RBC phenotype	Antigens in secretions
Le, Se, A/B/H	A, B, H, Le(a–b+)	A, B, H, Le^a, Le^b
lele, Se, A/B/H	A, B, H, Le(a–b–)	A, B, H
Le, sese, A/B/H	A, B, H, Le(a+b–)	Le^a
lele, sese, A/B/H	A, B, H, Le(a–b–)	None
Le, sese, hh, A/B	O_h, Le(a+b–)	Le^a
Le, Se, hh, A/B	Para-Bombay (A/B), Le(a–b+)	Le^a, Le^b, A, B, H

1.2.4 I blood group system & Ii blood group collection

- I blood group system has a single antigen, I
- Ii blood group collection has a single antigen, i
    - A blood group collection is related to a blood group system, but the genetic basis is not fully resolved
- Adult red cells are generally I-positive
    - Some rare adult red cells are i-positive (i_{adult})
- Cord blood red cells are i-positive
    - Gradually become I-positive over the first 18 months of age
    - Linear carbohydrate structures become more branched and complex as I antigen develops

1.2.4.1 I system & Ii collection antibodies

- Anti-I
    - Harmless and common IgM autoantibody, often detected if tests are done at 4°C and may be detected at room temperature
    - May be pathologic and the causative autoantibody in cold agglutinin disease (CAD) and may be seen in association with *Mycoplasma pneumoniae* infections
- Anti-IH
    - Harmless and common IgM autoantibody, often detected if tests are done at 4°C and may be detected at room temperature
    - Reacts preferentially with adult I-positive cells that express the greatest amounts of H antigen (group O)
    - Usually detected in the serum of A_1 individuals
    - May be pathologic and the causative autoantibody in CAD
- Anti-i
    - Less common IgM autoantibody that preferentially reacts with i_{adult} red cells and cord blood red cells
    - May be pathologic and the causative autoantibody in CAD secondary to infectious mononucleosis

1.2.5 P1PK & GLOB (globoside) blood group systems

- P1PK (previously P blood group) blood group system has 3 antigens: P1, P^k, and NOR
- GLOB blood group system has 2 antigens: P and PX2
- Three of these antigens, P1, P, and P^k are most relevant to the blood bank and give rise to 5 phenotypes: P_1, P_2, p, P_1^k, and P_2^k **t1.17**
    - The p, P_1^k, and P_2^k phenotypes are rare

t1.17 Phenotypes, antigens & antibodies in the P1PK & GLOB blood group systems

Phenotype	Antigens on RBCs	Antibodies in serum
P_1	P1, P, P^k (trace amount)	None
P_2	P, P^k (trace amount)	Anti-P1 (25% will have)
p	None	Anti-PP1P^k
P_1^k	P1, P^k	Anti-P & anti-PX2
P_2^k	P^k	Anti-P, -P1 & anti-PX2

- Four of these 5 phenotypes produce antibodies with the following specificities
  - Anti-P1 is usually naturally occurring, IgM, and clinically insignificant
    - Reactivity with P1+ red cells may be variable because P1 antigen expression differs from person to person
    - Reactivity can be inhibited in the presence of hydatid cyst fluid or P1 substance derived from pigeon eggs
  - Anti-PP1P^k is IgM or IgM and IgG and clinically significant
    - Separable mixture of anti-P, anti-P1, and anti-P^k
    - Antibody is naturally occurring in p phenotype
    - Associated with recurrent spontaneous abortions
  - Anti-P is IgM or IgM and IgG and clinically significant
    - Antibody is naturally occurring in P_1^k and P_2^k phenotypes
    - Associated with recurrent spontaneous abortions
    - Anti-P is frequently the autoantibody specificity in paroxysmal cold hemoglobinuria (PCH)

1.2.6 Rh blood group system

- Most important system after ABO because of the highly immunogenic properties of the D antigen
  - When large amounts of D-positive (≥200 mL) red cells are transfused to D-negative recipients, approximately 85% respond and produce anti-D
- Every blood donor routinely typed for the presence or absence of D antigen
  - Initial D-negative donors will also be tested for weak D
    - Must be weak D-negative for donor unit to be labeled as Rh-negative
    - If weak D-positive, donor unit will be labeled as Rh-positive
    - Must avoid potential alloimmunization to D antigen in D-negative recipients
- Every blood recipient routinely typed for the presence or absence of D antigen
  - Initial D-negative recipients do not require weak D testing
- In general, give D-positive recipients D-positive blood and D-negative recipients D-negative blood
  - Some laboratories may do weak D testing on D-negative recipients, followed with *RHD* genotyping on those who are weak D-positive
    - Depending on the type of weak D, some recipients may receive D-positive transfusions
  - May need to transfuse D-positive blood to D-negative recipients under certain circumstances and need policies to address this transfusion decision
  - Best to avoid transfusing D-positive blood to D-negative women of child-bearing age because of more severe hemolytic disease of the fetus and newborn (HDFN) seen with anti-D
- Rh blood group system currently has 55 different antigens

1.2.6.1 Molecular basis of the Rh blood group system

- Two closely linked genes on chromosome 1 control the expression of the 5 most commonly tested for Rh antigens D, C, E, c, and e **t1.18**
- These codominant genes are termed *RHD* and *RHCE* **t1.19**
- *RHD* gene codes for the presence of RhD protein and the D antigen
  - D-positive individuals inherit 1 or 2 *RHD* genes and 2 *RHCE* genes
- *RHCE* gene codes for the presence of C, E, c, and e antigens
  - Most D-negative individuals are the result of a complete deletion of the *RHD* gene and inherit only 2 *RHCE* genes

t1.18 5 most commonly identified Rh antigens & relative prevalence (%) by ethnicity

Antigen	White	Black
D	85	92
C	68	27
E	30	21
c	80	97
e	98	99

t1.19 Rh genes & 8 common haplotypes

1st locus	2nd locus	Haplotype Fisher-Race	Haplotype Wiener	Antigens
RHD	*RHCE*Ce*	CDe	R_1	D, C, e
RHD	*RHCE*cE*	cDE	R_2	D, E, c
RHD	*RHCE*CE*	CDE	R_z	D, E, C
RHD	*RHCE*ce*	cDe	R_0	D, c, e
-	*RHCE*Ce*	Ce	r'	C, e
-	*RHCE*cE*	cE	r''	c, E
-	*RHCE*CE*	CE	r^Y	C, E
-	*RHCE*ce*	Ce	r	c, e

 ISBN 978-089189-6616

- *RHCE* has several alternate alleles to explain the 4 combinations of the C/c and E/e antigens
  - *RHCE*Ce* produces C and e antigens
  - *RHCE*ce* produces c and e antigens
  - *RHCE*cE* produces c and E antigens
  - *RHCE*CE* produces C and E antigens

1.2.6.2 Rh haplotypes & most probable genotypes

- Although the genetic basis for the Rh blood group system is well defined, both Fisher-Race and Wiener terminologies continue to be used in the laboratory to express Rh haplotypes
  - Haplotype is a single term used to denote the inherited allele from each parent that expresses the 5 Rh antigens D, C, E, c, and e **t1.20**
- Typing results for these 5 Rh antigens can be used with the prevalence of the haplotypes to predict most probable genotype (**t1.20**)
  - An example of predicting this is shown using the following red cell typing results:

Anti-D	Anti-C	Anti-E	Anti-c	Anti-e
+	+	0	0	+

  - Based on these results, there are 2 possible genotypes written in Wiener or Fisher-Race terminology 1) R^1R^1 or *CDe/CDe* and 2) R^1r' or *CDe/Ce*
    - The actual genes would be *RHDRHCE*Ce/RHDRHCE*Ce* or *RHDRHCE*Ce/RHCE*Ce*
    - As shown in **t1.20**, the prevalence of the R^1 gene is far greater than the *r'* gene, making the most probable genotype R^1R^1

t1.20 Fisher-Race & Wiener terminologies used to express haplotypes & racial/ethnic prevalence for those haplotypes

			Prevalence		
	Fisher-Race	**Wiener**	**White**	**Black**	**Asian**
D-Positive	DCe	R_1	42	17	70
	DcE	R_2	14	11	21
	Dce	R_0	4	44	3
	DCE	R_z	<0.01	<0.01	1
D-Negative	ce	r	37	26	3
	Ce	r'	2	2	2
	cE	r"	1	<0.01	<0.01
	CE	r^y	<0.01	<0.01	<0.01

1.2.6.3 Rh antibodies

- Immune in origin and the result of exposure to red cells through transfusion, pregnancy, or transplantation to antigens genetically absent in the antibody producer
  - Most often IgG and usually IgG1 or IgG3, but do not readily activate complement
  - Usually react at the antiglobulin phase of testing (indirect antiglobulin testing)
  - Reactivity can be enhanced with the use of enzymes
  - Reactivity may be stronger with red cells that express a double dose of the respective antigen
- Rh antibodies are clinically significant
  - Capable of causing HDFN
    - Anti-D had been the most frequent cause of severe HDFN before the introduction of RhIG prophylaxis
    - Many other Rh antibody specificities have caused HDFN
  - Capable of causing acute and delayed transfusion reactions
  - If transfusion therapy is needed, antigen-negative blood must be provided

1.2.6.4 Rh Typing Reagents

- Low protein reagents
  - Routine monoclonal reagents used most commonly today
  - Anti-D may be from several clones to enhance reactivity with multiple D epitopes
  - Usually IgM and IgG are blended to enable weak D testing at the anti-human globulin (AHG) phase
  - Used in tube, slide, solid phase and gel technology testing
  - ABO forward typing serves as the negative control for this reagent
    - An AB, D-positive sample must have a separate negative control tested (always consult the manufacturer's directions)
    - This could include the patient's red cells and autologous serum or an inert control such as 6%-10% albumin or manufacturer's monoclonal control reagent
- High protein reagents
  - Not used frequently in routine Rh typing
  - Contains IgG anti-D obtained from immunized individuals
  - Contains approximately 20%-24% protein and other high-molecular-weight additives

- Enables reactions at immediate spin (IS) and can be used at AHG phase of testing
- Used in tube, slide, and microplate testing
- Requires the use of an Rh control from the same manufacturer
  - Rh control is of the same composition as the anti-D but uses serum from nonimmunized persons (no anti-D)
  - Must be negative for valid interpretation of D typing
- Testing using anti-D
  - 85%-92% of red cells will react at IS with anti-D and are identified as D-positive
  - 8%-15% of red cells will fail to react at IS and are identified as D-negative
    - Weak D testing may be performed on red cells that are identified as D-negative
    - Requires incubation of red cells with anti-D at 37°C and the addition of AHG
    - Appropriate weak D control using the patient's red cells and their serum, 6%-10% albumin, or manufacturer's Rh control, must be negative at the AHG phase of testing to correctly interpret weak D test
    - Weak D testing is required on blood donor samples to determine how to label collected blood components and prenatal/postnatal samples to assess RhIG candidacy, but optional on other patient/recipient samples
- Weak D classifications
  - Weak D-quantitative difference
    - All pieces of the D epitope are present, but in reduced quantities
    - Individuals of this type do not make alloanti-D
    - Increased testing of individuals in the prenatal/postnatal population with *RHD* genotyping to assess RhIG candidacy as weak D types 1, 2, 3 & 4.1 will not produce anti-D and do not require RhIG
      - Weak D type 4.0 should receive RhIG out of an abundance of caution
  - Partial D-qualitative difference
    - Inheritance of unique *RHD* genes that produce some, but not all, epitopes of the D protein
    - Can make alloantibody to the portion(s) of the D antigen missing from D protein
    - Can type as D-positive and demonstrate alloanti-D in their serum
    - Need to receive D-negative blood for transfusion and should receive RhIG prophylaxis during and after pregnancy if other criteria are met
- False-positive Rh typing
  - Positive direct antiglobulin test (DAT) result because of IgG-sensitized red cells
    - Less common with the use of low-protein Rh reagents
  - Rouleaux or fibrin
  - Wrong reagent or contaminated reagent
  - Overcentrifugation
  - Polyagglutination
  - Failure to follow manufacturer's directions
- False-negative Rh typing
  - Positive DAT and "blocked" or "saturated" D antigen sites
  - Specific reagent nonreactive with a variant or weak form of the antigen
  - Cell suspension too heavy
  - Failure to add reagent or wrong reagent added
  - Failure to follow the manufacturer's directions
  - Centrifugation too short or revolutions per minute (rpm) too low
  - Deterioration of reagents or contamination
  - Vigorous shaking of tubes

1.2.6.5 Other Rh antigens & unusual Rh phenotypes

- Compound antigens ce (f), Ce (rh_i), CE (Rh22), and cE (Rh27) (**t1.21**)
  - Define epitopes that depend on conformational changes resulting from amino acids associated with C, E, c, and e antigens
  - Can be useful in determining the most probable genotype from an observed phenotype

t1.21 Compound Rh antigens

Antigen	Gene producing antigen
ce or f	*RHCE*ce*
Ce or rh_i	*RHCE*Ce*
cE or Rh27	*RHCE*cE*
CE or Rh22	*RHCE*CE*

- G antigen
  - Found on red cells that express the D antigen and/or C antigen
  - Antibodies to G appear as anti-D plus anti-C but cannot be separated
  - D-negative individuals exposed to C+ (but D-negative) red cells via transfusion, pregnancy, or transplantation may demonstrate an apparent anti-D plus anti-C that is anti-G (or anti-G plus anti-C)

ISBN 978-089189-6616

        - D-negative women with only anti-G may still be candidates for RhIG prophylaxis during and after pregnancy if other criteria are met
    - D-deletion phenotypes
        - Rh phenotypes that suggest pieces of genetic material that make C, E, c, and e antigens have been deleted
        - Have enhanced expression of D antigen
        - Inherited *RHCE* genetic material replaced by *RHD* genetic material resulting in a hybrid gene with increased amounts of D antigen, decreased amounts of C, E, c, and e antigens and negative for several high-prevalence Rh antigens
        - Phenotypes include
            - D– –
            - D. .
            - Dc-
            - DC^w–
    - Rh_{null} phenotypes
        - Red cells lack all Rh antigens
        - Two different genetic backgrounds
            - Regulator type (more common)
                - *RHAG* (Rh-associated glycoprotein) gene is absent or mutated
                - The *RHD* and *RHCE* genes that are inherited are unable to make their respective antigens because of the absent or mutated Rh-associated glycoprotein
            - Amorph type
                - Arises from inheritance of mutated *RHCE* gene and deleted *RHD* gene
        - Rh_{null} red cells express decreased levels of glycophorin B (structure responsible for the S, s, and U antigens), and lack Fy5, LW^a, and LW^b antigens
        - Rh_{null} individuals who become immunized through transfusion, pregnancy, or transplantation produce complex Rh antibodies and must be transfused with Rh_{null} red cells
        - Persons who are Rh_{null} experience a type of anemia with hereditary stomatocytosis

1.2.7 MNS blood group system

1.2.7.1 MNS antigens

- Two linked genes on chromosome 4 are responsible for this blood group system
    - The first gene is *GYPA* and it produces glycophorin A (GPA) on the red cell membrane
        - GPA is the structure that carries the M and N antigens
        - M and N antigens are destroyed when red cells are treated with trypsin, ficin, or papain
        - M antigen demonstrates serine and glycine at the 1st and 5th positions respectively; N antigen demonstrates leucine and glutamic acid
    - The second gene is *GYPB* and it produces glycophorin B (GPB) on the red cell membrane
        - GPB carries the S and s antigens
        - S and s antigens may be destroyed when red cells are treated with ficin and papain
        - S antigen demonstrates methionine at the 29th position; s antigen demonstrates threonine at this position
    - This highly complex blood group system consists of 49 different antigens, all produced on either GPA or GPB
    - Very rare individuals lack all or part of GPA and the high-prevalence antigen(s) called En or En^a
    - About 2% of Blacks lack GPB and the S and s antigens and the high-prevalence antigen U
    - A rare gene in the MNS system called *Mk* produces neither GPA or GPB and lacks all MNS system antigens
    - MNS system phenotypes vary by ethnicity, and their prevalence is shown in **t1.22**

t1.22 MNS system phenotype prevalence (%) by ethnicity

Phenotype	White	Black
M+N–	30	25
M+N+	49	49
M–N+	21	26
S+s-	10	6
S+s+	42	24
S–s+	48	68
S–s–	0	2

1.2.7.2 MNS antibodies

- Most examples of anti-M are IgM, naturally occurring, react at room temperature and clinically insignificant
    - Some examples of anti-M react more strongly with cells expressing a double dose of the antigen when compared to those that express a single dose
    - Reactivity of some examples of anti-M may be enhanced at a pH of approximately 6.5
- Unusual examples of anti-M react at 37°C and the antiglobulin phase of testing and are considered clinically significant
- Most examples of anti-N are IgM, occur naturally, react at room temperature, and are clinically insignificant
- The vast majority of anti-S and anti-s antibodies are IgG, immune in origin, and considered clinically significant
- Antibodies to the high-prevalence antigens En^a and U are usually immune in origin, IgG, and considered clinically significant

1.2.8 KEL (Kell) blood group system

1.2.8.1 KEL system antigens

- The *KEL* gene is located on chromosome 7
- The KEL system consists of 36 unique antigens and 6 of these antigens are of interest
  - the low-prevalence antigen Js^a and its antithetical high-prevalence antigen Js^b
  - the low-prevalence antigen Kp^a and its antithetical high-prevalence antigen Kp^b
  - the low-prevalence antigen K and its antithetical high-prevalence antigen k
- Within certain races, these low-prevalence antigens occur more frequently (**t1.23**)

t1.23 KEL system phenotype prevalence (%) by ethnicity

Phenotype	White	Black
K–k+	91	98
K+k+	8.8	2.0
K+k–	0.2	Rare
Kp(a-b+)	97.7	100
Kp(a+b+)	2.3	Rare
Kp(a+b–)	Rare	0.0
Js(a–b+)	100	80
Js(a+b+)	Rare	19
Js(a+b–)	0.0	1.0

  - Js^a antigen is found in 20% of Blacks, but rare in Whites
  - Kp^a antigen is found in over 2% of Whites, but rare in Blacks
  - 9% of Whites are K+, but only 2% of Blacks are K+
  - When an individual inherits 2 *KEL* genes that both produce the same low-prevalence antigen, the antithetical high-prevalence antigen is absent from their red cells
    - Such individuals are at risk to produce alloantibody to the high-prevalence antigen absent from their red cells (see below)
- K_0 red cells lack all KEL system antigens and are considered a null phenotype
  - Immunized individuals produce anti-K_u, requiring transfusion with K_0 red cells
- McLeod red cells express diminished amounts of KEL antigens and lack the high-prevalence antigens K_x and K_m
  - McLeod syndrome is a rare X-linked condition associated with acanthocytosis, chronic granulomatous disease, and various neurologic and muscular symptoms
  - Depending on the genetic basis for McLeod syndrome, complex antibodies including anti-K_x and/or anti-K_m can be produced in immunized individuals and require transfusion with either K_0 or McLeod red cells
- KEL system antigens can be destroyed if red cells are treated with disulfide bond-reducing agents like dithiothreitol and 2-amonoethylisothiouronium bromide (AET)

1.2.8.2 KEL system antibodies

- A K+k– individual can make anti-k
- A Kp(a+b–) individual can make anti-Kp^b
- A Js(a+b–) individual can make anti-Js^b
  - Finding compatible blood for such alloimmunized individuals can be difficult and the services of a rare donor registry may be necessary
- Anti-K is a common alloantibody because the K antigen is highly immunogenic
- KEL system antibodies are usually IgG and clinically significant
  - Must provide antigen-negative blood for transfusion therapy
- KEL system antibodies have been associated with acute and delayed hemolytic transfusion reactions and HDFN

1.2.9 FY (Duffy) blood group system

1.2.9.1 FY system antigens

- The gene responsible for the FY antigens is *ACKR1* (atypical chemokine receptor 1), located on chromosome 1
- There are 5 FY system antigens: Fy^a, Fy^b, Fy3, Fy5, and Fy6
- The 4 common FY system phenotypes vary by ethnicity, and their prevalence is shown in **t1.24**

t1.24 FY system phenotype prevalence (%) by ethnicity

Phenotype	White	Black
Fy(a+b–)	20	10
Fy(a+b+)	48	3
Fy(a–b+)	32	20
Fy(a–b–)	0	67

- The Fy(a–b–) phenotype is common in Blacks and these cells demonstrate resistance to invasion by *Plasmodium vivax* merozoites (**t1.24**)
- The Fy^a, Fy^b, and Fy6 antigens are destroyed by proteolytic enzymes including ficin, papain, and bromelin
- Fy3 and Fy5 antigens are resistant to proteolytic enzymes

ISBN 978-089189-6616

1.2.9.2 FY system antibodies

- Anti-Fy^a is seen more frequently than anti-Fy^b
- Anti-Fy^a or anti-Fy^b often occur in the presence of other alloantibodies
- Anti-Fy3 fails to react with Fy(a–b–) red cells
- FY antibodies are immune in origin and IgG
- FY antibodies have been responsible for acute or delayed transfusion reactions and HDFN

1.2.10 JK (Kidd) blood group system

1.2.10.1 JK system antigens

- The gene responsible for the JK antigens is *SLC14A1*, located on chromosome 18
- There are 3 JK system antigens: Jk^a, Jk^b, and Jk3
- The 3 common JK system phenotypes vary by ethnicity, and their prevalence is shown in **t1.25**

t1.25 JK system phenotype prevalence (%) by ethnicity

Phenotype	White	Black	Asian
Jk(a+b–)	26	52	23
Jk(a+b+)	50	40	50
Jk(a–b+)	24	8	27

- Jk^a and Jk^b are resistant to proteolytic enzymes
- Jk^a and Jk^b are poor immunogens
- Rare Jk(a–b–) phenotype is found more frequently in Polynesian and Chinese populations
  - Lack the Jk3 antigen and are at risk to produce anti-Jk3

1.2.10.2 JK system antibodies

- Anti-Jk^a and anti-Jk^b are clinically significant IgG antibodies, capable of activating complement
- Anti-Jk^a or anti-Jk^b often occur in the presence of other alloantibodies
- Reactivity of JK system antibodies with respective antigens may be enhanced if red cells are treated with proteolytic enzymes
- Because of the difficulty in identifying some examples of anti-Jk^a and anti-Jk^b in pretransfusion antibody detection testing, these antibodies are often associated with delayed transfusion reactions
  - Antibody levels decline over time and may go undetected
  - Antibody may preferentially react with cells expressing a double dose of the antigen and react weakly or not at all with cells expressing a single dose
  - Antibody may activate more C3 than IgG molecules, but may go undetected based on type of antiglobulin reagent in routine use
- These characteristics of JK antibodies highlight the importance of checking past patient records and honoring historical findings

1.2.11 LU (Lutheran) blood group system

1.2.11.1 LU system antigens & antibodies

- The gene responsible for the LU antigens is *BCAM*, located on chromosome 19
- There are 25 LU system antigens, but those most familiar include the low-prevalence antigen Lu^a and the high-prevalence antigen Lu^b
- Antibodies in the LU system are most often IgG, immune in origin and have been associated with delayed transfusion reactions and mild HDFN
- Anti-Lu^a may be naturally occurring and can be IgM, IgG, or IgA; anti-Lu^a may demonstrate direct agglutination and show mixed-field reactivity and may also react at the antiglobulin phase of testing
- Anti-Lu^b is formed in individuals who are Lu(a+b–) and transfusion therapy requires units that are also Lu(a+b–)
- Very rare individuals may be Lu(a–b–) and produce anti-Lu3, reactive with all red cells except other Lu(a–b–) red cells

1.2.12 LW (Landsteiner-Wiener) blood group system

- The gene responsible for the LW antigens is *ICAM4*, located on chromosome 19
- There are 3 LW system antigens including the low-prevalence antigen LW^b, the high-prevalence antigen LW^a, and the high-prevalence antigen LW^{ab}
- There is an extremely rare LW-null phenotype, LW(a–b–), that lacks the LW^{ab} antigen
- Rh_{null} cells are also LW(a–b–) and lack the LW^{ab} antigen
- D-positive red cells express more LW antigen than do D-negative red cells

1.2.13 Antigens of low prevalence & antigens of high prevalence

- Antigens of low prevalence occur in <10% of the population and antigens of high prevalence occur in >98% of the population
- Some antigens of low prevalence assigned to a blood group system and not mentioned previously include C^W, C^X, Go^a, Rh32, Mi^a, Mur, Wr^a, Di^a, Sw^a, Yt^b, and Co^b
- Some antigens of high prevalence assigned to a blood group system and not mentioned previously include Hr, Hr_o, Rh29, Wr^b, Di^b, Yt^a, Co^a, Ch, Rg, Vel, and Lan
  - Antibodies to these antigens are typically clinically significant, but noted exceptions include anti-Ch and anti-Rg

- Seventeen antigens of low prevalence (700 series) not assigned to a blood group system are noted in **t1.26**
- Six antigens of high prevalence (901 series) not assigned to a blood group system are noted in **t1.27**

t1.26 Antigens of low prevalence not assigned to a blood group system

Name	Symbol
Batty	By
Christiansen	Chr^a
Biles	Bi
Box	Bx^a
Torkildsen	To^a
Peters	Pt^a
Reid	Re^a
Jensen	Je^a
Livesay	Li^a
Milne	
Rasmussen	RASM
	JFV
Katagiri	Kg
Jones	JONES
	HJK
	HOFM
	REIT

t1.27 Antigens of high prevalence not assigned to a blood group system

Name	Symbol
	Emm
Anton	AnWj
	PEL
	ABT1
	MAM
	LKE

1.2.14 Role of blood groups in transfusion

1.2.14.1 Immunogenicity

- Foreign red cell antigens can evoke an antibody response in transfusion recipients
- Transfusion of some foreign red cell antigens to antigen-negative recipients are more likely to evoke an immune response and include
  - D+ to D– and production of anti-D
  - K+ to K– and production of anti-K
  - c+ to c– and production of anti-c
  - E+ to E– and production of anti-E
  - k+ to k– and production of anti-k

1.2.14.2 Calculations for finding compatible blood

- Finding compatible blood is based on the incidence of being antigen-negative
  - If a patient has anti-c, the incidence of being c– is 20% so 20% of random units will lack the c antigen and be compatible with this antibody
  - If a patient has anti-c (20% are c–) and anti-S (45% are S–), the incidence of units lacking both antigens will be 0.20 × 0.45 or 0.09 or 9.0%
  - Should this patient be group O (45%), multiply 0.09 × 0.45. This reduces the incidence of antigen-negative units to 0.04 or 4.0%

1.2.15 Other genetic systems in blood banking

1.2.15.1 The HLA System

- (See also Immunology 8.1.1.3, 8.1.1.4, 8.3.2 & 8.3.3)
- Major histocompatibility complex (MHC) genes on chromosome 6 are responsible for human leukocyte antigens or HLA
- HLA is divided into 2 classes, I and II; MHC class III also is identified
  - Class I products are HLA-A, HLA-B, and HLA-C
    - Expressed on all nucleated cells
  - Class II products are HLA-DP, HLA-DQ, and HLA-DR
    - Expressed on antigen-presenting cells including B lymphocytes, dendritic cells, and macrophages
  - Class III products are non-HLA genes on the MHC that encode other molecules involved in immune responses including complement proteins and tumor necrosis factor
- The HLA system is important in transplantation (see 1.4.3 and Immunology 8.3.4 & 8.3.5) and in TA-GVHD (see 1.6.3.2)
- The HLA system is also important in platelet refractoriness
  - Patients fail to achieve a therapeutic increment in platelet count after platelet transfusion
  - Most common alloantibodies are directed against HLA class I antigens which are expressed on platelets
    - HLA-matched donors or family members as a source of platelets can be beneficial
    - Platelet crossmatching of patient serum with donor platelets may also be useful

1.2.15.2 Human platelet antigens (HPA)

- Thirty-five different HPAs have been described
  - HPA-1a is the most familiar platelet antigen

ISBN 978-089189-6616

- >80% of HPA-specific antibodies detected are anti-HPA-1a
- Clinical conditions related to HPA antibodies
  - Fetal and neonatal alloimmune thrombocytopenia (FNAIT)
    - Maternal IgG HPA antibodies cross the placenta and destroy fetal platelets
    - Anti-HPA-1a is most frequently implicated
    - Treatment includes the administration of intravenous immunoglobulin (IVIG), with or without antigen-negative platelets that can include maternal washed platelets
  - Posttransfusion purpura
    - Occurs 5-10 days after a red cell transfusion in patients with HPA antibodies
    - Produces profound thrombocytopenia and destruction of the patient's own platelets
    - Anti-HPA-1a is most frequently implicated
    - Treatment includes the administration of IVIG
  - Platelet transfusion refractoriness
    - Most frequently associated with HLA antibodies
    - HPA antibodies can cause platelet refractoriness

1.2.15.3 Human neutrophil antigens (HNA)

- Nine HNAs have been described
- Clinical conditions related to HNA antibodies
  - Neonatal alloimmune neutropenia (NAN)
    - Maternal IgG HNA antibodies cross the placenta causing neonatal neutropenia
    - Most frequent specificities include anti-HNA-1a, anti-HNA-1b, and anti-HNA-2
  - Transfusion-related acute lung injury (TRALI)
    - Respiratory distress, hypo- and hypertension, and noncardiogenic pulmonary edema that can be life-threatening
    - Usually within 6 hours of receiving a blood component
    - The presence of HNA and HLA antibodies from the donor can initiate TRALI

1.3 Blood group immunology

- See chapter 8 Immunology for foundational information on this topic

1.3.1 Immune response in blood banking

- (See also Immunology 8.1.2.5)
- Blood group antibodies may occur naturally or from exposure to substances in the environment with structures similar to RBC antigens
  - Include ABO, LE, I, P1PK, GLOB, and some MNS system antibodies
- Blood group antibodies may be immune in origin and the result of RBC antigen exposure from transfusion, pregnancy, or transplantation
  - Includes Rh, KEL, JK, FY, and some MNS system antibodies
  - B lymphocytes, when stimulated by antigen, evolve into plasma cells that secrete antibody
- Primary immune response after exposure to foreign RBC antigens by transfusion
  - Occurs days to months after a transfusion event
  - Initial antibody produced is IgM, followed by IgG
  - IgM eventually disappears, but IgG persists indefinitely
- Secondary (anamnestic) response in previously immunized recipients
  - Occurs in hours to days after a transfusion event
  - Large quantities of IgG antibody produced
  - Often associated with delayed hemolytic and serologic transfusion reactions

1.3.2 Immunoglobulins in blood banking

- (See also Immunology 8.1.2)
- Blood group antibodies are IgG, IgM, and IgA (rare) immunoglobulins
  - These immunoglobulins and their characteristics are shown in **t1.28**

t1.28 Characteristics of blood group immunoglobulins (Ig)

Immunoglobulin characteristic	IgM	IgG	IgA
Heavy chain isotype	μ	γ	α
Light chain type	κ & λ	κ & λ	κ & λ
Molecular weight (kD)	900-1000	150	180-500
Serum concentration (mg/dL)	85-205	1000-1500	200-350
Antigen-binding sites	10	2	2 or 4
Fixes complement	Often	Some	No
Hemolytic in vitro	Often	Rare	No
Placental transfer	No	Yes	No
Direct agglutinin	Yes	Rare	Rare
Biologic half-life (days)	5	21	6

- IgG immunoglobulins can be subdivided into 4 subclasses: IgG1, IgG2, IgG3, and IgG4
  - IgG1 and IgG3 are the most efficient at activating complement
  - IgG4 does not activate complement

- IgG1 and IgG3 bind strongly to Fc receptors (FcγRs)
- All IgG subclasses can cross the placenta

1.3.3 Antigen-antibody interactions in blood banking

- (See also Immunology 8.1.3)
- First phase is binding of antibodies to antigens on the red cell membrane
  - Utilizes hydrogen bonds, van der Waals interactions, and electrostatic charges
- Second phase is formation of an agglutination (hemagglutination) lattice by antibody-sensitized red cells
  - Antibody molecules must be able to span the distance between adjacent red cells to form this lattice
  - Red cells naturally repel each other because of negative charges (ζ potential)
- IgM antibodies reacting with their respective antigens are of sufficient size to span the distance between red cells and cause direct agglutination after centrifugation
  - Each IgM molecule has 10 antigen-binding sites
- IgG antibodies generally do not support direct agglutination and must rely on an indirect method (AHG, see below) to demonstrate their presence and support agglutination
  - Each IgG molecule has 2 antigen-binding sites
- Many IgM antibodies and some IgG antibodies, after incubation at 37°C, may demonstrate in vitro hemolysis during blood bank testing, including antibody detection, antibody identification, and crossmatching
  - Agglutination may be noted, but sometimes hemolysis is the only indication of reactivity of an antibody with its antigen
  - Associated with ABO antibodies
  - Associated with alloantibodies including anti-Le^a, anti-H, anti-PP1P^k, and anti-Vel
  - Activation of the classic complement pathway through the membrane attack complex leads to red cell hemolysis
  - Two Fc sites are necessary for complement pathway initiation
  - The pentameric IgM molecules facilitates complement activation
  - Two IgG molecules must be in close proximity on the RBC membrane to initiate complement activation
  - Activation of the classic pathway may not always result in hemolysis, but may stop with the activation of C3
    - In vitro, anti-Jk^a, and anti-Jk^b may demonstrate complement on antigen-positive cells at the AHG phase of testing if the AHG reagent contains anti-C3d/C3b

1.3.4 Factors affecting agglutination

- Centrifugation brings reactants closer together and helps overcome ζ potential between red cells, facilitating agglutination
- Antigen-antibody concentrations and ratios can affect agglutination
  - Excess unbound immunoglobulin can lead to a prozone effect and a false-negative result
  - Excess antigen can lead to a postzone effect and a false-negative result
  - Increasing the serum-to-cell ratio may enhance antibody reactivity
- pH can affect agglutination because some antibodies react more strongly with their antigens at a pH of <6.5 and can include some examples of anti-M
- Temperature and immunoglobulin class of antibody also affect agglutination
  - IgM blood group antibodies preferentially bind to their respective antigens at IS or following an incubation at room temperature (22°C)
  - IgG blood group antibodies preferentially bind to their respective antigens following an incubation at 37°C
- Increased incubation times can enhance antibody reactivity
- Enhancement media also affect agglutination
  - Albumin (usually 22%) increases the dielectric constant and subsequently reduces the ζ potential
  - Low-ionic-strength saline (LISS) reduces the ζ potential
  - Polyethylene glycol (PEG) increases the dielectric constant, excludes water, and subsequently reduces the ζ potential
  - Proteolytic enzymes (ficin and papain) used to modify red cells may enhance agglutination or negate the ability of an antibody to agglutinate red cells because of antigen degradation
    - Antibody reactions that are enhanced after enzyme treatment include those directed to antigens in the following blood group systems: Rh, P1PK, I, JK, and LE
    - Antibody reactions that are negated after enzyme treatment include those directed to the following antigens: M, N, Fy^a, Fy^b, Ch, Rg, and Xg^a

1.3.5 Antiglobulin or AHG reagents & tests

- Antibody to immunoglobulin or complement components that facilitate hemagglutination as the visual indicator that sensitization of red cells has occurred
    - AHG is produced via a hybridoma process with clonal selection for increased specificity for IgG or components of complement
    - May be derived from monoclonal or polyclonal source material
- Polyspecific reagent (pooled or blended)
    - Anti-IgG and anti-C3d/C3b
- Monospecific reagent
    - Anti-IgG
    - Anti-C3d
    - Anti-C3d/C3b
- DAT is used to detect immunoglobulin and/or complement components bound to RBCs in vivo
    - Cells washed with normal saline to remove unbound immunoglobulin/complement and then tested with AHG
    - No saline washing required if using gel column technology
    - Used to detect the following clinical conditions
        - HDFN
        - Autoimmune hemolytic anemias
        - Drug-induced immune hemolytic anemias
        - Hemolytic transfusion reactions
- The indirect antiglobulin test (IAT) or method is used to detect immunoglobulin and/or complement bound to red cells in vitro following an incubation at 37°C
    - Cells washed with normal saline to remove unbound immunoglobulin/complement and then tested with AHG
    - No saline washing required if using gel column technology
    - Used in the following tests
        - Antibody detection or antibody screening studies
        - Antibody identification studies
        - Crossmatching/compatibility testing
        - Weak D testing
        - Red cell antigen typing
        - Titration studies
- In manual tube testing, IgG-sensitized red cells (check cells) are added to each negative AHG test (DAT and IAT) to ensure that
    - AHG (anti-IgG) reagent was not neutralized because of insufficient saline washing to remove unbound immunoglobulin
    - AHG (anti-IgG) was added to the test system
    - The use of IgG-sensitized red cells does not ensure that the test was read correctly
    - IgG-sensitized red cells are not needed with gel column technology
- False-positive AHG test
    - Potent agglutinins; saline control may also be positive
    - Fibrin or other contaminating particles such as dirt or dust
    - Overcentrifugation
    - Samples collected in silica gel tubes
    - Sample from infusion lines used to administer dextrose-containing solutions
- False-negative AHG test
    - Inadequate washing to remove patient serum and unbound immunoglobulin
    - Neutralized AHG reagent
    - Failure to add AHG reagent
    - Interruption of saline washing, leading to dissociation of bound immunoglobulin
    - Overcentrifugation
    - Undercentrifugation
    - Failure to add patient serum to tests that include IAT phase
    - Red cell suspension too heavy
    - Tube shaking/resuspension too vigorous

1.3.6 Testing modalities used in the blood bank

- Tube testing
    - Low technology and minimal equipment
    - Tube shaking/resuspension technique must be acquired
    - More subjective endpoint
- Solid-phase red cell adherence
    - Requires specialized equipment
    - Adaptable to automated platform
    - Less subjective endpoint
        - A strong (4+) positive reaction shows a diffuse monolayer of red cells across the well
        - A negative reaction shows a button of red cells at the center of the well
        - Intermediate positive reactions show varying degrees of a diffuse monolayer and button of red cells

- Gel column technology
  - Common technology used in blood banks
  - Does require specialized equipment
  - Adaptable to automated platform
  - Saline washing and check cells not needed
  - Less subjective endpoint
    - A strong (4+) positive reaction shows a layer of agglutinated cells at the top of the gel media
    - A negative reaction shows a button of cells at the bottom of the gel media
    - Intermediate positive reactions show agglutinated cells dispersed throughout the gel media and depending on the strength of the reaction, unagglutinated red cells at the bottom of the gel media
  - Results are stable and allow for later review of work output

1.3.7 Inhibition or neutralization technique

- This immunologic technique can be useful in antibody identification
- Soluble forms of some blood group antigens exist in body fluids, including saliva, urine, and plasma
- Incubation of soluble antigen (body fluid) with its respective antibody (patient serum) will result in inhibition or neutralization of the antibody
  - After incubation, use antigen-positive RBCs to determine if neutralization has occurred
  - If neutralization has occurred, the red cells will no longer be reactive, or fail to demonstrate agglutination
  - If neutralization has not occurred, the red cells will continue to be reactive, or demonstrate agglutination
  - Must include a saline control with identical dilution factor used in the neutralization test to account for possible dilution of the antibody
    - For valid interpretation of test results, saline control must continue to react with antigen-positive red cells
- Soluble substances and their sources include
  - LE substance found in the saliva of individuals who are Le(a+b-) (Le^a substance) and individuals who are Le(a-b+) (Le^a and Le^b substance)
    - Commercially prepared LE substance is available
  - P1 substance present in hydatid cyst fluid and the ovalbumin of pigeon eggs
    - Commercially prepared P1 substance is available
  - Sd^a substance found in the urine of Sd(a+) individuals
  - Chido (Ch) and Rodgers (Rg) substance found in the plasma of Ch+ and Rg+ individuals

1.4 Physiology & pathophysiology

- Refer to chapter 4 Hematology for information on normal and abnormal physiology of blood (see 4.1, 4.2, 4.3, 4.4, 4.5, 4.7, 4.8 & 4.9).
- Refer to chapter 5 Hemostasis for an overview of hemostasis and coagulation.
- Refer to chapter 4 Hematology for additional congenital and acquired anemias (4.7.1).

1.4.1 Hemolytic disease of the fetus & newborn

- (See also Hematology 4.7.1.3.2)
- HDFN is the destruction of fetal and newborn red cells by maternal antibodies
  - Maternal antibody crosses the placenta and must be IgG
    - IgG1 and IgG3 maternal antibodies more efficient at crossing the placenta than IgG2 and IgG4
  - Fetal and newborn red cells must express the antigen to which the antibody is directed
    - Antigen will be paternally inherited
  - HDFN can be clinically benign and only demonstrate a positive DAT
  - Anemia is the greatest concern to the fetus in utero
    - Maternal antibody and fetal antigen interaction lead to red cell destruction
    - Results in the release of immature nucleated red cells from fetal liver and spleen
    - Severe cases of anemia can result in hydrops fetalis, characterized by generalized edema, heart failure, and death
  - Bilirubinemia is of great concern to the newborn after birth
    - In utero, indirect bilirubin from fetal red cells destruction is conjugated in the maternal liver and excreted
    - The newborn's immature liver is unable to conjugate bilirubin effectively
    - Indirect bilirubin in the newborn can reach toxic levels, resulting in permanent damage to the brain and central nervous system, known as kernicterus

ISBN 978-089189-6616

1.4.1.1 Maternal alloimmunization & causative antibodies

- Maternal alloimmunization occurs after a red cell transfusion, pregnancy, or transplantation
  - Fetomaternal hemorrhage (FMH) can occur during pregnancy but most likely at delivery
  - Generally, first pregnancy rarely affected by HDFN
- Anti-D
  - Before the advent of Rh-immune globulin (RhIG), anti-D was the causative antibody in 95% of HDFN cases and those that were most severe
    - D antigen is the most potent red cell immunogen
    - Although today responsible for <0.2% of all cases, HDFN caused by anti-D continues to be the most severe
    - ABO incompatibility between the mother and fetus protects against sensitization to the D antigen because ABO incompatible fetal red cells are destroyed by maternal ABO antibodies
- ABO antibodies
  - Primarily seen in group O mothers and their group A or group B infants
    - Most common cause of HDFN
    - Maternal antibodies are naturally occurring so HDFN can occur during the first pregnancy
    - Usually a clinically mild disease that may require no treatment or only phototherapy
    - Fetal ABO antigens are poorly developed at birth and maternal antibody may be neutralized by soluble ABO antigens
- Other antibodies
  - Any maternal IgG antibody has the potential to cause HDFN if the antigen is expressed on fetal red cells
  - Specificities associated with HDFN have included anti-K, -E, -C, -c, -e, -Fy^{a}, -Fy^{b}, -Jk^{a}, -Jk^{b}, -S, -s, and -U
  - Disease may be mild, moderate, or severe

1.4.1.2 Diagnosis & management

1.4.1.2.1 Maternal history & testing

- Transfusion and pregnancy histories, including the presence of alloantibodies, previous births, stillbirths, miscarriages, abortions, and newborns with HDFN
- ABO and Rh
  - Includes weak D test if the woman is D-negative
  - Weak D-positive individuals are more frequently undergoing *RHD* genotyping to identify those weak D phenotypes (including weak D types 1, 2, 3 & 4.1) that will not produce alloanti-D and do not require RhIG
- Antibody detection studies and antibody identification studies (if indicated)
  - May need to differentiate IgG from IgM alloantibody with sulfhydryl reagents such as dithiothreitol for certain alloantibodies such as anti-M
- Titration studies with maternal alloantibody
  - Rely less on titration studies
  - Semiquantitative and does not necessarily predict severity of disease or the need for fetal intervention
  - In those cases where it can be useful, usually looking at a critical titer of 16-32 or a rise in titer (2-tube or 4-fold rise) to indicate significance

1.4.1.2.2 Fetal monitoring, testing & treatment

- Antepartum
  - Doppler fetal ultrasonography of the middle cerebral artery (MCA) is used to assess fetal anemia based on reduced blood viscosity
    - Noninvasive procedure that replaces amniocentesis
  - Cordocentesis may be used to secure a fetal blood sample that can be tested for hemoglobin, hematocrit, bilirubin, DAT, ABO, and Rh or other blood group system phenotype/genotype
    - Increased risk of FMH or premature birth
    - For phenotyping/genotyping, easier and safer to evaluate paternal sample or secure fetal DNA from maternal blood sample
  - Ultrasonography
    - Aids in cordocentesis sampling
    - Used to detect hydrops fetalis
  - Intrauterine transfusion may be indicated at 24-26 weeks' gestation
    - MCA indicates anemia, or
    - Cordocentesis indicates hemoglobin <10 g/dL (<100 g/L), or
    - Fetal hydrops noted on ultrasonography
    - RBCs usually injected directly into fetal umbilical vein
    - Attributes of RBCs selected for intrauterine transfusion are shown in **t1.29**

t1.29 Attributes of red blood cells for neonatal intrauterine, postpartum & exchange transfusions

Group O, Rh-negative
Antigen negative for implicated antibodies
Crossmatch compatible with maternal serum
CMV seronegative or leukocyte-reduced (CMV safe)
Fresh, usually <5-7 days old
Irradiated to prevent transfusion-associated graft-vs-host disease
Hgb S-negative

CMV, cytomegalovirus; Hgb, hemoglobin

- Premature delivery may also be performed at 32-34 weeks' gestation
  - Not recommended if lungs are not fully developed
- Postpartum
  - ABO/Rh testing and DAT on cord blood
    - Interpretation of results must take into consideration antepartum interventions, including intrauterine transfusion, the ABO and Rh of units used, and administration of antepartum RhIG
      - D-positive infants could have a weakly positive DAT because of antepartum RhIG crossing the placenta and sensitizing fetal red cells
    - If HDFN is unexpected or the maternal antibody detection results are negative in the presence of a positive DAT result on the cord blood, there may be a need to prepare an eluate from the cord RBCs and further evaluate materal serum to identify the antibody responsible for the positive DAT
      - Evaluate potential for ABO HDN
      - Consider the presence of maternal antibody to a low-prevalence antigen (eg, anti-Kp^a, anti-C^w) and fetal inheritance of the low-prevalence antigen
  - Phototherapy
    - Used for mild HDFN or as additional treatment in moderate/severe HDFN
    - Ultraviolet florescent light metabolizes unconjugated bilirubin at the skin's surface into a nontoxic water-soluble form, excreted by the kidneys
  - Exchange transfusion
    - Exchange the infant's blood with Whole Blood or reconstituted Whole Blood (usually group O Red Blood Cells and group AB plasma)
    - Indicated for anemia (hemoglobin <11 g/dL [<110 g/L]) and bilirubinemia (>20 mg/dL [>342 μmol/L])
    - A 2-volume exchange removes 80%-90% of infant's sensitized RBCs, maternal antibody, and 50% of the bilirubin
    - Attributes of Whole Blood or reconstituted Whole Blood are shown in **t1.29**
  - Simple or small-volume transfusion
    - Used if infant well-managed from previous intrauterine transfusions, or if anemia is the primary concern
    - Use Red Blood Cells with attributes as described in **t1.29**
- Infant blood needs in the presence of maternal antibody to a high-prevalence antigen
  - Antibodies could include anti-U, -Kp^b, -Js^b, -k, -Vel
  - If blood is not available, could use maternal washed or frozen and deglycerolized red cells
    - Must be irradiated
  - May also consider testing maternal siblings and searching rare donor registries for appropriate antigen-negative units

1.4.1.3 Prevention of D alloimmunization with RhIG

- RhIG is prepared from pooled human plasma from individuals who have made anti-D
  - Comes as a 50-μg dose and a 300-μg dose
  - 300-μg dose of RhIG protects against alloimmunization to the D antigen after exposure to 15 mL of fetal red cells or 30 mL of fetal whole blood

1.4.1.3.1 Antepartum RhIG

- Administered as a 300-μg dose at 28 weeks' gestation to D-negative, weak D-negative mothers who have not formed alloanti-D
  - Should also be given to D-negative, weak D-positive mothers who are partial D and can produce anti-D to the portions of the D epitope genetically absent from their red cells
  - *RHD* genotyping can be used to differentiate certain D-negative, weak D-positive phenotypes including weak D types 1, 2, 3 & 4.1 who will not produce anti-D
    - Weak D types 1, 2, 3 & 4.1 for purposes of RhIG administration can be managed as if D-positive
    - Weak D type 4.0 should receive RhIG out of an abundance of caution
  - Important to have policies and procedures to address RhIG administration to weak D-positive mothers if the genetic background is unknown or cannot be determined

1.4.1.3.1.1 Other antepartum clinical situations where RhIG administration is appropriate

- During the first 12 weeks of gestation, a 50-μg microdose of RhIG can be used for
  - Abortion
  - Miscarriage
  - Termination of ectopic pregnancy
- For the aforementioned clinical situations occurring after 12 weeks' gestation, a 300-μg dose of RhIG should be administered
- A 300-μg dose of RhIG should also be administered for
  - Abdominal trauma
  - Following amniocentesis/cordocentesis
  - Antepartum hemorrhage

ISBN 978-089189-6616

anti-D + maternal RBC incubate @ 37°C ↓ **wash 4× with saline** ↓ **add D+ indicator cells** ↓ **examine microscopically for rosettes**	**sensitivity** can detect FMH of ≥10 mL **negative rosette test** administer 1 vial RhIG **positive rosette test** requires quantitation of FMH using Kleihauer-Betke (or flow cytometry) to determine how many vials of RhIG are needed

f1.3 Rosette test to detect fetomaternal hemorrhage (FMH)

prepare thin maternal blood smear
fix in alcohol ↓
expose to acid buffer
fetal Hgb is resistant to acid treatment where adult Hgb is not
↓
stain with eosin
stains fetal cells pink
↓
counterstain with hematoxylin
(stains "ghost" adult cells purple)

f1.4 Principle & general procedure for Kleihauer-Betke test

1.4.1.3.2 Postpartum RhIG

- Administered as a 300-µg dose within 72 hours of delivery to D-negative, weak D-negative mothers
  - Should also be administered to D-negative, weak D-positive mothers who are partial D and to D-negative, weak D-positive mothers where the genetic background of their weak D is unknown or cannot be determined
- Infant must be D-positive
- Maternal serum does not demonstrate alloanti-D
  - Maternal serum may demonstrate weak anti-D from antepartum dose of RhIG
  - Titer of this anti-D will generally be <4
- Maternal serum may demonstrate other alloantibody specificities (eg, anti-K), but this does not exclude RhIG candidacy if other criteria are met

1.4.1.4 Evaluation for postpartum FMH & dosage of RhIG

- Each maternal sample is screened for FMH with a rosette test
  - Qualitative test
  - Can detect ≥10 mL of fetal red cells
  - The rosette test procedure is summarized in **f1.3**
- If the rosette test result is negative, a single vial of RhIG is given
- If the rosette test result is positive, a quantitative assay, such as the Kleihauer-Betke test or flow cytometry assessment, must be performed and the FMH calculated
- Flow cytometry
  - Can include the measurement of fetal hemoglobin and/or D-positive cells
  - Turnaround times and equipment requirements limit common usage
- Kleihauer-Betke test
  - More common quantitative assay
  - Based on acid elution and the resistance of fetal hemoglobin **f1.4**
  - Once staining is completed, the blood smear is viewed microscopically, fetal and adult cells are counted, and the number of vials of RhIG to administer is calculated **f1.5**
  - Because the Kleihauer-Betke assay is subjective, additional safeguards in calculating the number of vials of RhIG are needed and are shown in **f1.6**

count a total of 2000 cells
keep track of how many fetal cells seen

 # fetal cells/2000 × 5000 mL = FMH (mL)

5000 mL is approximate maternal blood volume

FMH (mL)/30 mL = # vials of RhIG to administer

each vial of RhIG protects against 30 mL of fetal whole blood

f1.5 Calculating the number of vials of RhIG to administer

when calculating # vials of RhIG, go out to 1 decimal place **if the digit to the right of the decimal is <5, round down & add 1 vial of RhIG** **if the digit to the right of the decimal ≥5, round up & add 1 vial of RhIG**	**example calculation** 26 fetal cells seen in 2000 cells counted 26/2000 × 5000 mL = 65 mL FMH 65 mL/30 mL = 2.2 vials RhIG round down to 2, add 1 2 + 1 = give 3 vials of RhIG

f1.6 Additional safeguards in calculating the number of vials of RhIG to administer

1.4.2 Immune hemolytic anemias

- (See also Hematology 4.7.1.3.3)
- Almost always demonstrates a positive DAT result
  - Polyspecific AHG (anti-IgG + anti-C3d/C3b) must be used when performing a DAT on the red cells of patients suspected of having immune hemolytic anemia
  - The positive DAT result may present other serologic challenges including determinations for ABO & Rh typing
    - Ensure appropriate control is included when performing ABO typing
    - Use of low-protein, monoclonal Rh reagents are less likely to cause false-positive results than high-protein polyclonal Rh reagents
    - Removal of some bound immunoglobulin (chloroquine diphosphate or gentle heat elution) may further facilitate red cell typing
  - Because of the positive DAT result, any test with patient red cells that requires the use of AHG reagent will show positive results
    - Use of monoclonal typing reagents (including anti-Fy^a, -Fy^b, -Jk^a, -Jk^b, -K, -S, and -s) that react at IS or following an incubation at 37°C and do not require an AHG phase of testing can be useful in red cell phenotyping
- Immune hemolytic anemias can be categorized as
  - Warm autoimmune hemolytic anemia (WAIHA)
  - Cold agglutinin disease (CAD)
  - Paroxysmal cold hemoglobinuria (PCH)
  - Mixed-type autoimmune hemolytic anemia (warm and cold autoantibodies)
  - Drug-induced immune hemolytic anemia (DIIHA)
- WAIHA, CAD, PCH, and mixed-type autoimmune hemolytic anemia all demonstrate autoantibodies; DIIHA (including one that produces autoantibodies) demonstrates 4 serologically distinct drug-related categories. Serologic findings are summarized in **t1.30**

t1.30 Serologic findings in autoimmune hemolytic anemia & drug-induced immune hemolytic anemia

	DAT			
	IgG	**C3**	**Serum**	**Eluate**
WAIHA			57% present with IgG warm autoantibody; may demonstrate alloantibody or alloantibody & autoantibody	IgG & reactive with normal red cells
67%	+	+		
20%	+	0		
13%	0	+		
CAD	0	+	IgM autoantibody always present; may demonstrate alloantibody or alloantibody & autoantibody	Nonreactive
PCH	0	+	IgG biphasic hemolysin	Nonreactive
Mixed-type autoimmune hemolytic anemia	+	+	IgG warm reacting autoantibody & IgM cold reacting autoantibody; alloantibody may also be present	IgG & reactive with normal red cells
DIIHA				
Drug-dependent or drug adsorption	+	(+)	IgG antibody only reactive with drug-bound red cells	IgG antibody only reactive with drug-bound red cells
Drug-dependent & formerly known as immune complex type	(+)	+	Drug antibody reacts with untreated red cells only if drug incorporated into test	Nonreactive
Drug-independent with production of autoantibodies indistinguishable from WAIHA	+	(+)	IgG warm autoantibody may be present; may demonstrate alloantibody or alloantibody & autoantibody	IgG & reactive with normal red cells
Nonimmunologic protein adsorption	+	+	Nonreactive unless alloantibody present	Nonreactive

CAD, cold agglutinin disease; DIIHA, drug-induced immune hemolytic anemia; PCH, paroxysmal cold hemoglobinuria; WAIHA, warm autoimmune hemolytic anemia; (+), occasionally positive

- Decisions regarding the need for blood transfusion therapy in the presence of autoantibodies must be made by the patient's physician and the blood bank medical director
  - If transfusion therapy becomes necessary, the blood specimen selected must be negative for any antigen(s) to which patient alloantibodies is directed

ISBN 978-089189-6616

1.4.2.1 Mechanisms of immune red cell destruction

1.4.2.1.1 Intravascular destruction

- (See also Hematology 4.6.2 & 4.6.3)
- Complement-mediated red cell destruction in the bloodstream
  - Classic pathway of complement activation
  - Formation of membrane attack complex (MAC), or C5b through C9, and red cell lysis
- Although uncommon in immune hemolytic anemias, can be seen in
  - PCH
  - CAD
  - Mixed-type autoimmune hemolytic anemia
  - DIIHA with certain drug-dependent antibodies
  - WAIHA, but more frequently in children than adults

1.4.2.1.2 Extravascular destruction

- (See also Hematology 4.6.1 & 4.6.3)
- More common mechanism for red cell destruction in immune hemolytic anemias
- Red blood cells sensitized with IgG or complement only, or IgG and complement are destroyed or damaged by macrophages within the reticuloendothelial system (RES)
  - Red cells sensitized with complement do not necessarily proceed through the complement cascade to lysis
  - Macrophage interaction with sensitized red cells occurs primarily in the spleen and liver due to Fc-γ receptors (FcγRs) & complement receptor 3 (CR3) on the macrophage
    - IgG1 and IgG3 antibodies have the strongest affinity for FcγRs
    - CR3 is the receptor for C3b
    - Macrophage may phagocytize the sensitized red cell
    - Macrophage may only internalize a portion of the red cell, releasing spherocytes that are susceptible to early destruction
    - Complement-sensitized cells that are not phagocytized by macrophages are released into the circulation with C3d on their surface and may continue to survive nearly normally
    - Red cells sensitized with IgG and complement tend to demonstrate the greatest degree of extravascular destruction

1.4.2.2 Warm autoimmune hemolytic anemia (WAIHA)

- General characteristics
  - 60%-70% of immune hemolytic anemias will be of this type
  - Autoantibodies are optimally reactive with red cell antigens at 37°C
  - Autoantibodies are usually IgG, but rare cases of IgM and IgA autoantibodies have been described
  - May manifest as a primary disease or secondary to other disease states, including leukemia, lymphoma, and lupus

1.4.2.2.1 WAIHA serology

- DAT result is most always positive when tested with polyspecific AHG
  - DAT-negative cases of WAIHA have been described
- DAT done with monospecific AHG reagents demonstrate the following frequencies in cases of WAIHA
  - IgG: 20%
  - IgG & C3: 67%
  - C3: 13%
- Eluates prepared from red cells generally react with all cells tested
  - Autoantibody specificities are complex and often directed against high-prevalence antigens in the Rh, LW, MNS, and DI blood group systems
  - On occasion, autoantibody specificities may be simple and include autoanti-e, autoanti-c, autoanti-K, autoanti-Jk^a, and autoanti-Jk^b
- Antibody detection studies may be negative or positive
  - 57% of cases of WAIHA demonstrate free, or unbound, IgG autoantibody in patient serum
  - Autoantibody may be present with IgG alloantibody
    - Antibody detection studies may be positive because only IgG alloantibody is present
  - If transfusion therapy is required and antibody detection is positive, antibody identification studies must be performed to determine the presence and specificity of
    - Autoantibody
    - Alloantibody
    - Autoantibody and alloantibody
  - These differences may require adsorption using autologous red cells (autoadsorption) or allogeneic red cells (alloadsorption)
- Adsorption with autologous red cells
  - Patient's own red cells are modified to remove bound immunoglobulin using methods that can include
    - 56°C heat elution followed with enzyme treatment

- ZZAP (dithiothreitol and cysteine-activated papain)
- Chloroquine diphosphate
- Citric acid
- Acid glycine/EDTA
- PEG

- Modified patient cells are incubated with patient serum at 37°C
- Serum autoantibody will bind to the modified red cells, but alloantibody will remain in the serum
- Following autoadsorption, the serum is retested for reactivity and studies are performed to determine the presence and identity of any alloantibodies

- Adsorption with allogeneic red cells
  - May be necessary if the patient has received a transfusion recently or if the patient is severely anemic
  - Use allogeneic red cells that will be negative for antigens to clinically significant alloantibodies and therefore fail to adsorb them from patient serum, but adsorb warm autoantibody
  - Select group O red cells that are R_1R_1, R_2R_2, and rr to ensure that anti-D, anti-C, anti-E, anti-c, or anti-e (if any are present as alloantibodies) will remain after adsorption
  - With the 3 previously stated cells selected, ensure that at least one is K–, Jk(a–), Jk(b–), S–, s–, Fy(a–), and Fy(b–)
    - To facilitate adsorption of the autoantibody, these cells will usually be premodified with enzymes or ZZAP and these methods render cells Fy(a–) and Fy(b–)
  - After the 3 adsorption procedures, the serum is retested for reactivity and studies are performed to determine the presence and identity of any alloantibodies

1.4.2.3 Cold agglutinin disease

- General characteristics
  - 16%-32% of immune hemolytic anemias will be of this type
  - Autoantibodies are usually IgM, but rare cases of IgA and IgG autoantibodies have been described
  - Cold autoantibodies responsible for CAD facilitate red cell destruction because of their thermal range
    - These pathologic antibodies bind to red cell antigens at temperatures between 30°C and 32°C (and occasionally at higher temperatures) in the peripheral circulation
    - As temperatures in the body increase to 37°C, these IgM autoantibodies dissociate from the red cell and activate complement
    - Red cells may be hemolyzed or continue to circulate with cell-bound C3
  - May be a primary disease, but more frequently seen as a secondary disease associated with
    - *Mycoplasma pneumoniae* (anti-I and anti-IH)
    - Infectious mononucleosis (anti-i)

1.4.2.3.1 CAD serology

- The DAT is positive, and cells demonstrate only C3d
  - Eluate prepared from these cells is nonreactive
- Antibody detection studies are always positive
  - Because these autoantibodies can cause significant autoagglutination, it may be necessary to collect and maintain samples at 37°C to perform serologic testing, including ABO and Rh typing
- Autoantibody specificities include
  - Anti-I (most common)
  - Anti-IH
  - Anti-i
  - Anti-Pr
    - These autoantibody specificities may also be found as harmless cold autoantibodies
    - Harmless cold autoantibodies are more common than those responsible for CAD
    - Harmless cold autoantibody characteristics are quite different from those of the pathologic autoantibodies associated with CAD and these are summarized in **t1.31**

t1.31 Characteristics of pathologic cold autoantibodies in cold agglutinin disease & harmless cold autoantibodies

Characteristic	Pathologic cold autoantibodies	Harmless cold autoantibodies
Immunoglobulin class	IgM & rarely IgA or IgG	IgM
Thermal range	30°C-32°C (and occasionally at higher temperatures)	4°C-22°C
Specificity	Usually anti-I & rarely anti-i, anti-IH, or anti-Pr	Usually anti-I
Titer	Usually >1000 at 4°C	Usually <64 at 4°C
Clonal origin	Monoclonal in primary disease; usually polyclonal in secondary disease	Polyclonal
Reactivity enhanced with albumin	Usually	Not usually

ISBN 978-089189-6616

- Adsorption with autologous red cells
  - Because antibody detection studies are always positive, it may be necessary to determine the presence of underlying alloantibodies especially if transfusion therapy is needed
  - Patient red cells are premodified with proteolytic enzymes
  - Perform adsorption at 4°C using patient premodified red cells and patient serum
  - Repeat antibody detection studies with autoadsorbed serum and perform antibody identification studies if indicated
- Adsorption with allogeneic red cells
  - If the patient has received a transfusion recently or if the patient is severely anemic, allogeneic red cells as described earlier for WAIHA can be used to remove autoantibody and determine the presence of alloantibody

1.4.2.4 Paroxysmal cold hemoglobinuria

- General characteristics
  - Also known as Donath-Landsteiner hemolytic anemia
  - Rarest form of immune hemolytic anemia
  - If it occurs, generally seen in children and as a secondary disease to transient viral infection
  - Can be seen in adults as an idiopathic disease

1.4.2.4.1 PCH serology

- The DAT result is positive and cells only demonstrate C3d
  - Eluate prepared from these cells is nonreactive
- The autoantibody is always IgG and is described as biphasic
  - IgG autoantibody binds to the red cells at low temperatures in the peripheral blood and activates complement as the blood is warmed to 37°C
  - The IgG autoantibody dissociates from the red cells as the blood is warmed to 37°C
  - Antibody detection tests may be nonreactive as the autoantibody is cold-reactive
  - The characteristics of this autoantibody provide the basis for the diagnostic test for this disease, the Donath-Landsteiner test
- The most frequent autoantibody specificity is anti-P
  - Less frequent autoantibody specificities have included anti-I, anti-i, and anti-Pr

1.4.2.5 Mixed-type autoimmune hemolytic anemia

- General characteristics
  - Seen in approximately 8% of immune hemolytic anemias
  - Has serology of both WAIHA and CAD
  - Usually associated with severe hemolysis
  - DAT result is positive and most frequently, IgG and C3d are detected
  - An eluate prepared from patient red cells will be reactive with all cells as seen in WAIHA
  - Antibody detection studies will be positive and antibody identification studies typically demonstrate IgG warm autoantibody and IgM cold autoantibody
    - The cold autoantibody has a thermal range between 30°C and 32°C in the peripheral circulation and efficiently activates complement as the blood is warmed to 37°C
      - Specificities include those seen in CAD
    - The IgG warm autoantibody in the serum can be complex and identical to those seen in WAIHA
      - If transfusion therapy is necessary, studies needed to detect clinically significant alloantibodies, including autologous or allogeneic adsorption, may be required

1.4.2.6 Drug-induced immune hemolytic anemia

- General characteristics
  - Seen in approximately 10% of immune hemolytic anemias
  - Some patients have profound hemolysis, but others show no hemolysis and present with only serologic findings including a positive DAT result
  - DAT results can be variable
  - Accurate drug history is important
  - Once the drug is discontinued, hemolysis and/or serology resolve
  - Multiple theories as to how drugs induce red cell-related antibodies have been proposed and the following is a useful serologic classification
- Serologic classification
  - Drug-dependent antibodies that react with drug-treated cells (also known as drug adsorption mechanism)
  - Drug-dependent antibodies that react with untreated cells in the presence of a solution of drug (formerly known as immune complex mechanism)
  - Drug independent because the drug does not need to be added to the test system and these antibodies behave like, and are indistinguishable from, the autoantibodies responsible for WAIHA
  - Nonimmunologic protein adsorption independent of antibody production

1.4.2.6.1 Drug-dependent antibodies that react with drug-treated cells (drug adsorption mechanism)

- Serology and associated drugs
  - Associated with penicillin, ampicillin, and many cephalosporins
  - Drug-induced antibody is directed against drug or one of its metabolites
  - DAT most frequently demonstrates IgG immunoglobulin, but some demonstrate IgG and C3d
  - Can result in severe hemolysis, but may only be a serologic finding
  - Tests to confirm this form of DIIHA in the laboratory include the preparation of red cells where suspect drugs, such as penicillin or cephalosporin, are bound to red cells
    - The patient serum and an eluate prepared from patient red cells will be reactive with these drug-bound or drug-treated red cells
    - The patient serum and eluate will be nonreactive with the same red cells that are not bound or treated with drug
      - Make sure the patient does not have an alloantibody directed against an antigen on the red cells used to prepare drug-bound or drug-treated red cells

1.4.2.6.2 Drug-dependent antibodies that react with untreated cells in the presence of a solution of drug

- Serology and associated drugs
  - Associated with quinine, piperacillin, and second- and third-generation cephalosporins
  - Drug-induced antibody is directed against drug or one of its metabolites
  - DAT most frequently demonstrates only C3d on the red cell, but some also demonstrate IgG
  - Serum drug antibody can be IgG or IgM or a combination of both
  - These patients often have profound hemolysis that can be life-threatening
  - Tests to confirm this form of DIIHA in the laboratory require the incubation of patient serum, untreated red cells, and a solution of the drug
    - If present, drug antibodies may cause agglutination, hemolysis, or sensitization
    - Untreated red cells and patient serum without the solution of drug should be negative
      - Make sure the patient does not have an alloantibody directed against an antigen on the untreated red cells

1.4.2.6.3 Drug-independent antibodies with autoantibody production

- Serology and associated drugs
  - Historically, methyldopa was associated with this type of DIIHA and today, seen with fludarabine
  - Drug-induced autoantibody is directed against intrinsic red cells antigens
  - DAT usually demonstrates only IgG, but weak C3d in addition to IgG has also been observed
  - An eluate prepared from patient red cells will react with all red cells tested and the drug is not required to be present
    - Eluate results will be indistinguishable from those seen in patients with WAIHA
  - Studies with patient serum may be nonreactive, but can demonstrate autoantibody, alloantibody, or autoantibody plus alloantibody
    - The drug is not required to be present
    - May require adsorption studies as described for WAIHA to differentiate autoantibody from alloantibody

1.4.2.6.4 Nonimmunologic protein adsorption

- Serology and associated drugs
  - Associated with cephalothin, cisplatin, and diglycoaldehyde
  - Hemolysis associated with this phenomenon is rare
  - Drug modifies the patient red cell membrane allowing nonimmunologic adsorption of serum proteins that can include IgG, IgA, IgM, C3, and albumin, resulting in a positive DAT result if corresponding antiglobulin/antiprotein serum is used to test patient red cells
  - An eluate prepared from patient red cells will be nonreactive

1.4.3 Transplantation

- (See also Immunology 8.3.1, 8.3.4 & 8.3.5)

1.4.3.1 Solid organ

1.4.3.1.1 Kidney

- ABO compatibility is the most important factor in determining immediate outcomes in kidney transplantation
  - ABH antigens are ubiquitous and of particular importance for vascular endothelial cells and rejection
  - Use of A_2 organs for group B and group O recipients with low-titer anti-A can be acceptable
- Renal transplant recipients are typed for ABO and HLA and assessed for HLA antibodies

ISBN 978-089189-6616

- Recipient serum and donor lymphocytes are crossmatched, typically using flow cytometry
- Long-term graft survival is longer with living donors versus cadaveric donors

1.4.3.1.2 Other solid organs

- For liver, heart, lung, and heart/lung transplants, ABO compatibility is the biggest concern related to donor selection
- HLA typing and HLA antibody screening of potential recipients and HLA crossmatching with intended donor are usually done in heart, lung, and heart/lung transplantation
  - These studies are performed less frequently in liver transplantation

1.4.3.2 Hematopoietic progenitor cells (HPC)

- HPC transplantation is undertaken for
  - Bone marrow rescue following ablation of the marrow with irradiation and/or chemotherapy
  - Replacement of diseased or destroyed marrow
- Used to treat a variety of hematologic malignancies and nonneoplastic immune disorders
  - Myeloid leukemias
  - Lymphoid leukemias
  - Hodgkin and non-Hodgkin lymphoma
  - Multiple myeloma
  - Aplastic anemia
  - Immune deficiencies like severe combined immunodeficiency
  - Sickle cell disease

1.4.3.2.1 Types of HPC transplants

- Autologous
  - Patient is the source of HPC
  - Collected while patient in remission and stored
  - If relapse occurs and patient undergoes ablation therapy, can be used for hematopoietic rescue
- Allogeneic
  - May be a related or unrelated donor
  - High-resolution allele-level HLA typing and matching is important in unrelated transplant to achieve good outcomes
    - Donor registries exist to facilitate identification of HLA-matched unrelated potential donors
    - In general, an HLA-matched related donor is selected over an HLA-matched unrelated donor
    - If an HLA-matched unrelated donor is not available, a haploidentical related donor may be considered
  - Typically considered when patient experiences a relapse

1.4.3.2.2 Sources of HPC

- Bone marrow
  - May be used for autologous or allogeneic donors
  - Invasive procedure performed under anesthesia
- Peripheral blood
  - Most common source of HPC
  - Requires mobilization of HPC from the marrow into the peripheral circulation after the administration of hematopoietic growth factors such as granulocyte-colony stimulating factor
  - HPC collected using apheresis devices and procedures
  - May be used for autologous or allogeneic donors
- Umbilical cord blood
  - Rich source of HPC
  - HLA-typed cord blood stored for public use
  - HPCs are immunologically naïve, and HLA mismatches are often better tolerated in the recipient with less GVHD
  - This source for HPC is increasing in frequency, but because of the stem cell dose, more frequently used in pediatric transplantations unless performing double cord blood transplantation

1.4.3.2.3 Laboratory testing of HPC products

- CD34 antigen testing is used as a surrogate marker to assess the quality of HPC products
  - Goal is $2\text{-}5\times10^6$ CD34+ cells/kg of recipient body weight
- Cell count and differential and test for viability (trypan blue or acridine orange) performed
- Clonogenic assay including a count of colony-forming units correlates the speed and likelihood of engraftment
- Cultures for bacteria and fungus

1.4.3.2.4 Engraftment

- Neutrophils and platelets are the first cell lines to show engraftment
  - Neutrophil count >500/μL (>0.50×10^9/L) at 9-30 days
  - Platelet count >20,000/μL (>20×10^9/L) at ≥15 days
- Red blood cell engraftment and immune reconstitution usually require ≥90 days

- Standard measurement of success is engraftment of all 3 cell lines at 100 days
  - Variability of engraftment depends on quality of HPC product transplanted
- Between HPC product infusion and engraftment, recipient is supported by blood and platelet transfusions that will be
  - Leukocyte reduced to prevent HLA alloimmunization
  - Irradiated to prevent TA-GVHD
  - Cytomegalovirus (CMV) safe to prevent CMV infection

1.4.3.2.5 ABO group & transfusion support following HPC transplantation

- ABO incompatibility of HPC donor and recipient are no longer barriers to successful transplantation, especially if HLA compatibility is very good
- Pretransplant strategies to avoid marked incompatibility may include
  - Red cell reduction in donor HPC product
  - Reduction of ABO antibodies in recipient through apheresis
  - Immunosuppressive drug therapies for the recipient
- Transfusion therapy and selection of the appropriate ABO type for red cell-containing and plasma-containing products is very important
- If transplantation is successful, the recipient will slowly become the donor's ABO type
- ABO incompatibilities between donor and recipient may be classified as
  - Major (recipient ABO antibodies directed against donor ABO antigens) and would include
    - Group A donor to a group O recipient
    - Group B donor to a group O recipient
    - Group AB donor to a group O recipient
    - Group AB donor to a group A recipient
    - Group AB donor to a group B recipient
  - Minor (donor ABO antibodies directed against recipient ABO antigens) and would include
    - Group O donor to a group A recipient
    - Group O donor to a group B recipient
    - Group O donor to a group AB recipient
    - Group A donor to a group AB recipient
    - Group B donor to a group AB recipient
  - Major and minor and would include
    - Group A donor to a group B recipient
    - Group B donor to a group A recipient
- t1.32 summarizes ABO blood component selections for transfusion support in ABO-mismatched HPC transplants

t1.32 ABO & blood component support in ABO-mismatched hematopoietic progenitor cell transplantations

Type of ABO incompatibility	ABO of red blood cell components	ABO of plasma components	ABO of platelet components*
Major Recipient ABO antibodies directed to donor ABO antigens	Recipient	Donor	Donor
Once recipient ABO antibodies are no longer detected	Donor	Donor	Donor
Minor Donor ABO antibodies directed to recipient ABO antigens	Donor	Recipient	Recipient
Once recipient red cells are no longer detected	Donor	Donor	Donor
Major & minor Recipient ABO directed to donor ABO antigens & donor ABO antibodies directed to recipient ABO antigens	Group O	Group AB	Group AB
Once recipient ABO antibodies & recipient red cells are no longer detected	Donor	Donor	Donor

**Because of limited availability of group AB platelets, group A, B, or O platelets may be necessary*

1.5 Serologic & molecular testing

- See chapter 9 Molecular Biology: 9.3 for information on molecular testing

1.5.1 Routine tests

1.5.1.1 Serologic confirmation of donor blood component ABO & Rh

- Testing from an integrally attached segment
- ABO group of each unit of Whole Blood, Red Blood Cells and Apheresis Granulocytes will be confirmed before it is made available for transfusion
- Rh(D) type of units labeled Rh-negative will also be confirmed
  - Weak D testing is not required for Rh(D) confirmation
- Any discrepancies in ABO and Rh testing will be reported to the collecting facility and must be resolved before components are available for transfusion

1.5.1.2 Transfusion requests

- Must be complete, accurate, and legible
  - Also contains 2 independent patient identifiers (eg, patient name, unique facility identification number, date of birth) for accurate recipient identification
- Specific type and amount of blood component requested with any special processing requirements (eg, irradiation, fresh, volume reduction, CMV-negative)
- Name of ordering physician or authorized health professional

1.5.1.3 Collection of pretransfusion blood sample

- Identification of patient before phlebotomy with precautions in place to prevent misidentification
- Written/printed label affixed to sample before it leaves the patient's side that includes the 2 independent patient identifiers
- Mechanism to identify date and time of collections and who collected the sample
- Acceptance of samples that are accurate, legible, complete, and in agreement with transfusion request

1.5.1.4 Pretransfusion testing of recipient blood sample

- ABO forward RBC typing with anti-A and anti-B
- ABO reverse serum typing with A_1 and B RBCs
- *AABB Standards for Blood Banks and Transfusion Services* requires 2 determinations of the intended recipient's ABO group
  - First determination shall be performed on a current sample
  - Second determination may include 1 of the following
    - Comparison with previous records
    - Testing a second sample collected at a time different from the first sample, including a new verification of patient identification
    - Retesting the same sample if patient identification was verified using a validated electronic identification system
- Rh typing
  - Rh type is determined with anti-D reagent
  - Weak D testing is optional in D-negative recipients
- Tests for unexpected antibodies to RBCs antigens (antibody detection test or antibody screening test) with patient's serum
  - Group O reagent red cells (2-4 vials) that express antigen combinations to maximally detect antibodies
  - Reagent red cells for antibody detection testing must not be pooled
  - Method used must detect clinically significant antibodies
  - Method must include 37°C incubation before performing an antiglobulin test (IAT)
  - If clinically significant antibodies are detected, additional tests must be performed, including antibody identification and the selection of red cell-containing components for transfusion that lack the antigens to which the antibodies are directed
- Once pretransfusion testing is complete, results must be compared with historical records for
  - ABO and Rh
  - Difficulty in blood typing
  - Clinically significant antibodies
  - Significant adverse events to transfusion
  - Special transfusion requirements or attributes
- Any discrepancies discovered between historical records and the current results need to be evaluated and resolved before blood is issued for transfusion
- Sample age
  - If pregnant or if red cell-containing products were transfused within the previous 3 months, or if unknown, sample for pretransfusion testing must be no more than 3 days old
    - Day of collection is day 0
  - If no pregnancy or red cell-containing transfusions in the previous 3 months and the history is known with certainty, pretransfusion testing may be completed in advance and in accordance with facility policies and procedures

1.5.1.5 Selection of blood & blood components for transfusion

- An overview of ABO-compatible components for transfusion is shown in **t1.33**

t1.33 Overview of ABO compatibility & blood components for transfusion

Component	ABO requirement
Whole Blood	ABO identical to recipient or use low-titer group O
Red Blood Cells	ABO compatible with recipient plasma
Granulocytes	ABO compatible with recipient plasma
Plasma	ABO compatible with recipient RBCs
Platelets	All ABO groups are acceptable, but ABO identical platelets are preferred. Platelets express ABO antigens so ABO compatibility with recipient plasma is optimal. Additionally, donor plasma that is compatible with recipient RBCs is preferred, especially if large volumes of plasma are given; can consider volume reduction to avoid excess donor ABO antibody if directed to recipient RBCs
Cryoprecipitated AHF	All ABO groups are acceptable

AHF, antihemophilic factor

- Recipients receive ABO group-compatible Red Blood Cells, ABO group-specific Whole Blood, or low-titer group O Whole Blood for non-group O recipients or for recipients whose ABO type is unknown
    - If an ABO discrepancy is noted and transfusion is necessary before resolution, only group O Red Blood Cells should be transfused
- D-negative recipients receive D-negative Whole Blood or Red Blood Cells
    - Policies should exist to describe the use of D-positive red cell-containing components to D-negative recipients
    - If an Rh typing discrepancy is noted and transfusion is necessary before resolution, only D-negative red cell-containing products should be transfused to recipients of child-bearing age

1.5.1.6 Serologic crossmatch/compatibility testing

- Uses recipient serum and donor red blood cells (major crossmatch) from integrally attached segment from red cell-containing components
- If recipient demonstrates no clinically significant antibodies, the IS crossmatch method used to detect ABO incompatibilities is all that is required
- If recipient demonstrates clinically significant antibodies, or has a history of clinically significant antibodies, the serologic crossmatch must include incubation at 37°C and an antiglobulin (IAT) phase of testing
    - Red cell-containing components selected for transfusion must not express the corresponding antigen to which the clinically significant antibody is directed
- Recipient sample and segment from red cell-containing components are stored at refrigerated temperatures for at least 7 days after each transfusion

1.5.1.7 Use of computer to detect ABO incompatibility (computer crossmatch)

- Can only be used if
    - Recipient fails to demonstrate clinically significant antibodies
    - There is no record of previous detection of such antibodies
- If the computer system is used as the method to detect ABO incompatibility, the following requirements also apply
    - Computer system validated on-site to ensure only ABO-compatible Whole Blood or Red Blood Cells have been selected for transfusion
    - The computer system must contain the donation identification number, component name, ABO and Rh of component; the confirmed blood component ABO group; the 2 unique recipient identifiers; recipient ABO and Rh type and antibody screen results; and interpretation of compatibility
    - A method exists to verify correct entry of data before blood components are released
    - The system contains logic to alert the user to discrepancies between
        - Donor ABO group and Rh type on the unit label and those determined on blood group confirmatory testing
        - ABO incompatibility between the recipient and the donor unit

1.5.1.8 Inspection & issue of blood & blood components for transfusion

- Every blood container has an attached label or tie tag indicating
    - Intended recipient's 2 independent identifiers
    - Donation identification number or pool number
    - Interpretation of crossmatch testing, if performed
- At the time of issue, a check of records and each blood component is performed and includes the following
    - Intended recipient's 2 independent identifiers, ABO group, and Rh type
    - Donor identification number, donor ABO, and if required, Rh type
    - Interpretation of crossmatch tests, if performed
    - Special transfusion requirements
    - The expiration date and, if applicable, time
    - Date and time of issue
    - Final visual inspection of the product
        - Abnormal color, foam, bubbles, particulate matter or other unusual findings negate the issue of that component; follow-up is necessary to investigate cause

1.5.1.8.1 Reissue of blood & blood components

- Blood components returned to the transfusion service can be reissued if the following conditions have been met
    - The container closure has not been disturbed
    - Appropriate temperature has been maintained
    - At least one sealed segment of integral donor tubing has remained attached to the container
        - Removed segments may be attached if the tubing identification numbers on both the removed segment (s) and the container are identical

ISBN 978-089189-6616

- Records indicate the components have been inspected and they are acceptable for reissue

1.5.1.9 Basic antibody identification

- After a positive result with antibody detection tests (antibody screening tests), antibody identification studies are undertaken using the patient's serum
- Group O reagent red cells (10-14 vials) that express antigen combinations to maximally identify antibody specificities
- Usually include an autocontrol with these identification studies
  - Patient red blood cells plus patient serum
  - May facilitate identification of alloantibody, autoantibody, or alloantibody plus autoantibody
  - May also need to perform a DAT if autocontrol is positive at the antiglobulin phase of testing
- Although procedures for antibody identification studies may vary from facility to facility, they typically include an IS phase of testing, 37°C phase of testing, and an IAT phase of testing with the intent to detect clinically significant antibodies
  - May also include a room temperature phase of testing, though this phase of testing is more likely to detect clinically insignificant antibodies
  - Testing usually includes the addition of enhancement media such as LISS or PEG
- At each phase of testing, it is important to grade the reactivity
  - This can suggest the presence of >1 antibody
  - It may also be helpful in identifying antibodies that preferentially react with cells expressing a double dose of an antigen versus those expressing a single dose of an antigen
- The use of proteolytic enzymes (usually ficin or papain) may destroy certain red cell antigens including the blood group antigens M, N, Fy^a, and Fy^b
  - Antibodies directed to any of these antigens will no longer react with these enzyme premodified red cells
- Enzymes may also enhance the reactivity of certain antigens (Rh and JK blood group systems) with their respective antibodies
- Phenotyping the patient's own red cells will help define those antibodies the patient can produce, while eliminating those the patient cannot produce
  - If patient received a transfusion recently, DNA-based phenotyping or genotyping may be useful
  - Cell separation techniques also may be used for recovering younger autologous red cells for red cell phenotyping in the presence of transfused red cells
- If the patient has a known antibody, consider testing an abbreviated or selected cell panel to identify other antibodies the patient could produce
  - For example, in the presence of known anti-e, select e-negative red cells that express various other red cell antigens and test these with the patient's serum
- Cross-out or rule-out strategies are an additional aid for antibody identification
  - If an antigen is present on a specific red cell used in antibody identification studies and that cell is nonreactive with the patient's serum, the corresponding antibody to that antigen may be excluded
    - Exercise caution because some antibodies only react with cells expressing a double dose of their respective antigen and fail to react with those expressing a single dose of the antigen
    - If working with such an antibody, cross-out results will most likely be inaccurate
    - Some laboratories follow more complex cross-out or rule-out procedures that concurrently evaluate the expression of a single vs a double dose of an antigen for each nonreactive antibody identification panel cell
  - Following a cross-out or rule-out exercise, additional selected cells may need to be tested to further rule out antibody specificities that could not be eliminated from the original panel
- Once antibody specificity is determined (or very likely determined), it is accepted practice to confirm that 3 antigen-positive red cells are reactive with the patient's serum and 3 antigen-negative red cells are nonreactive with the patient's serum (3+3 rule)
  - Based on the Fisher exact method, the 3+3 rule provides 95% confidence in antibody identification
  - Some facilities may only require the testing of 2 antigen-positive red cells that are reactive and 2 antigen-negative red cells that are nonreactive to confirm specificity

1.5.1.9.1.1 Antibody identification studies

- **f1.7-f1.13** review antibody identification studies that incorporate some of the concepts described earlier

1.5.1.10 Direct antiglobulin testing

- The basic principle and clinical uses for the DAT are found in other sections of this chapter
  - 1.3.5
  - 1.4.1 & 1.4.2
  - 1.6.3.1

Serologic & molecular testing>Routine tests

a

Cell	D	C	E	c	e	K	k	Fy^a	Fy^b	Jk^a	Jk^b	Le^a	Le^b	P1	M	N	S	s	IS	LISS 37°C	IAT
1	+	+	0	0	+	0	+	+	+	+	+	0	+	+	+	+	+	0	0	0	3+
2	+	+	0	0	+	0	+	0	+	+	0	0	+	+	+	0	+	+	0	0	3+
3	+	0	+	+	0	+	+	+	0	0	+	+	0	+	+	0	0	+	0	0	0
4	+	+	0	+	+	0	+	+	+	+	0	0	+	0	+	+	+	+	0	0	3+
5	+	0	+	+	+	0	+	0	+	0	+	0	+	0	0	+	+	0	0	0	0
6	0	+	0	+	+	0	+	+	+	+	+	0	+	+	+	+	+	+	0	0	3+
7	0	0	+	+	0	+	+	0	+	+	0	+	0	+	0	+	0	+	0	0	0
8	0	0	0	+	+	0	+	+	+	0	+	+	0	+	+	0	+	+	0	0	0
9	0	0	0	+	+	+	+	+	0	+	0	0	+	0	0	+	0	+	0	0	0
10	+	0	0	+	+	0	+	0	0	0	+	0	+	0	+	0	+	0	0	0	0
AC																			0	0	0

b

Cell	D	C	E	c	e	K	k	Fy^a	Fy^b	Jk^a	Jk^b	Le^a	Le^b	P1	M	N	S	s	IS	LISS 37°C	IAT
1	+	+	0	0	+	0	+	+	+	+	+	0	+	+	+	+	+	0	0	0	3+
2	+	+	0	0	+	0	+	0	+	+	0	0	+	+	+	0	+	+	0	0	3+
3	+	0	+	+	0	+	+	+	0	0	+	+	0	+	+	0	0	+	0	0	0
4	+	+	0	+	+	0	+	+	+	+	0	0	+	0	+	+	+	+	0	0	3+
5	+	0	+	+	+	0	+	0	+	0	+	0	+	0	0	+	+	0	0	0	0
6	0	+	0	+	+	0	+	+	+	+	+	0	+	+	+	+	+	+	0	0	3+
7	0	0	+	+	0	+	+	0	+	+	0	+	0	+	0	+	0	+	0	0	0
8	0	0	0	+	+	0	+	+	+	0	+	+	0	+	+	0	+	+	0	0	0
9	0	0	0	+	+	+	+	+	0	+	0	0	+	0	0	+	0	+	0	0	0
10	+	0	0	+	+	0	+	0	0	0	+	0	+	0	+	0	+	0	0	0	0
AC																			0	0	0

f1.7 Antibody identification with single specificity; **a** Initial results of antibody identification studies
b Applying a cross-out or rule-out strategy to the panel; by utilizing a cross-out or rule-out strategy based on the antigens expressed on the nonreactive panel cells, anti-C is identified. There are at least 3 reactive C+ panel cells & at least 3 nonreactive C– panel cells. The patient is confirmed to be C–.
AC, auto control; IAT, indirect antiglobulin test

a

Cell	D	C	E	c	e	K	k	Fy^a	Fy^b	Jk^a	Jk^b	Le^a	Le^b	P1	M	N	S	s	IS	LISS 37°C	IAT
1	+	+	0	0	+	0	+	+	0	0	+	0	+	+	+	+	+	0	0	0	0
2	+	+	0	0	+	0	+	0	+	+	0	0	+	+	+	0	0	+	0	0	0
3	+	0	+	+	0	+	+	+	0	0	+	+	0	+	+	0	0	+	0	0	3+
4	+	+	0	+	+	0	+	+	+	+	0	0	+	0	+	+	+	+	0	0	3+
5	+	0	+	+	+	0	+	0	+	0	+	0	+	0	0	+	+	0	0	0	3+
6	0	+	0	+	+	0	+	+	+	+	+	0	+	+	+	+	+	+	0	0	3+
7	0	0	+	+	0	+	+	0	+	+	0	+	0	+	0	+	0	+	0	0	3+
8	0	0	0	+	+	0	+	+	+	0	+	+	0	+	+	0	+	+	0	0	3+
9	0	0	0	+	+	+	+	+	0	+	0	0	+	0	0	+	0	+	0	0	3+
10	+	0	0	+	+	0	+	0	0	0	+	0	+	0	+	0	+	0	0	0	3+
AC																			0	0	0

b

Cell	D	C	E	c	e	K	k	Fy^a	Fy^b	Jk^a	Jk^b	Le^a	Le^b	P1	M	N	S	s	IS	LISS 37°C	IAT
1	+	+	0	0	+	+	+	+	0	0	+	0	+	+	+	+	+	0	0	0	0
2	+	+	0	0	+	0	+	0	+	+	0	+	0	+	+	0	0	+	0	0	0
3	+	+	+	0	0	0	+	+	0	0	+	0	+	+	+	+	+	0	0	0	2+
4	+	+	+	0	0	0	+	0	+	+	0	0	+	+	+	0	+	+	0	0	2+
5	+	+	0	0	+	+	+	+	0	0	+	+	0	+	+	+	+	0	0	0	0
6	+	+	+	0	+	0	+	0	+	+	0	0	+	+	+	0	+	+	0	0	2+

f1.8 Antibody identification requiring a selected cell panel; **a** There are only 2 nonreactive panel cells (cells 1 & 2). Based on a cross-out or rule-out strategy, we can eliminate anti-D, -C, -e, -k, -Fy^a, -Fy^b, -Jk^a, -Jk^b, -Le^b, -P1, -M, -N, -S & -s. There is evidence that anti-c is present, but additional antibodies including anti-E, -K & -Le^a cannot be ruled out. A selected cell panel will be of value to confirm antibody identification.
b Selected c– cell panel: Anti-K & anti-Le^a can now be eliminated & this selected c– cell panel demonstrates the presence of anti-E in addition to the anti-c. The patient is shown to be c– & E–.
AC, auto control; IAT, indirect antiglobulin test

Cell	D	C	E	c	e	K	k	Fy^a	Fy^b	Jk^a	Jk^b	Le^a	Le^b	P1	M	N	S	s	IS	LISS 37°C	IAT
1	+	+	0	0	+	0	+	+	0	0	+	0	+	+	+	+	+	0	0	0	0
2	+	+	0	0	+	0	+	0	+	+	0	0	+	+	+	0	+	+	0	0	0
3	+	0	+	+	0	+	+	+	0	0	+	+	0	+	+	0	0	+	2+	2+	4+
4	+	+	0	+	+	0	+	+	+	+	0	0	+	0	+	+	+	+	0	0	0
5	+	0	+	+	+	0	+	0	+	0	+	0	+	0	0	+	+	0	0	0	3+
6	0	+	0	+	+	0	+	+	+	+	+	0	+	+	+	+	+	+	0	0	0
7	0	0	0	+	+	+	+	0	+	+	0	+	0	+	0	+	0	+	2+	2+	4+
8	0	0	0	+	+	0	+	0	+	0	+	+	0	+	+	0	0	+	0	0	0
9	0	0	0	+	+	+	+	+	0	+	0	0	+	0	0	+	0	+	2+	2+	4+
10	0	0	+	+	+	0	+	0	0	0	+	0	+	0	+	0	+	0	0	0	3+
AC																			0	0	0

f1.9 Antibody identification studies showing reactivity in different phases of testing in addition to variability in reaction strength. Variability in reaction strength & reactivity at different phases of testing can indicate that multiple antibodies are present. Cells 3, 7 & 9 react at all phases of testing & these 3 cells all express the K antigen. Cells 5 & 10 are reactive only at the antiglobulin phase of testing & both cells react less strongly than cells 3, 4 & 9. Cells 5 & 10 express the E antigen. Cell 3 expresses both the E antigen & the K antigen. Cross-out or rule-out strategies further suggest the presence of anti-K & anti-E. Testing of an additional E+ & K– cell (in order to test 3 E+ cells) will confirm the presence of anti-K & anti-E. The patient is also K– & E–.
AC, auto control; IAT, indirect antiglobulin test

a

Cell	D	C	E	c	e	K	k	Fy^a	Fy^b	Jk^a	Jk^b	Le^a	Le^b	P1	M	N	S	s	IS	LISS 37°C	IAT
1	+	+	0	0	+	0	+	+	0	0	+	0	+	+	+	+	+	0	0	0	0
2	+	+	0	0	+	0	+	0	+	+	0	0	+	+	+	0	+	+	2+	1+	0
3	+	0	+	+	0	+	+	+	0	0	+	+	0	+	+	0	0	+	2+	1+	0
4	+	+	0	+	+	0	+	+	+	+	0	0	+	0	+	+	+	+	0	0	0
5	+	0	+	+	+	0	+	0	+	0	+	0	+	0	0	+	+	0	0	0	0
6	0	+	0	+	+	0	+	+	+	+	+	0	+	+	+	+	+	+	0	0	0
7	0	0	0	+	+	+	+	0	+	+	0	+	0	+	0	+	0	+	0	0	0
8	0	0	0	+	+	0	+	0	+	0	+	+	0	+	+	0	+	+	2+	1+	0
9	0	0	0	+	+	+	+	+	0	+	0	0	+	0	0	+	0	+	0	0	0
10	0	0	+	+	+	0	+	0	0	0	+	0	+	0	+	0	+	0	2+	1+	0
AC																			0	0	0

b

Cell	D	C	E	c	e	K	k	Fy^a	Fy^b	Jk^a	Jk^b	Le^a	Le^b	P1	M	N	S	s	IS	RT	LISS 37°C	IAT
1	+	+	0	0	+	0	+	+	0	0	+	0	+	+	+	+	+	0	0	1+	0	0
2	+	+	0	0	+	0	+	0	+	+	0	0	+	+	+	0	+	+	2+	3+	1+	0
3	+	0	+	+	0	+	+	+	0	0	+	+	0	+	+	0	0	+	2+	3+	1+	0
4	+	+	0	+	+	0	+	+	+	+	0	0	+	0	+	+	+	+	0	1+	0	0
5	+	0	+	+	+	0	+	0	+	0	+	0	+	0	0	+	+	0	0	0	0	0
6	0	+	0	+	+	0	+	+	+	+	+	0	+	+	+	+	+	+	0	1+	0	0
7	0	0	0	+	+	+	+	0	+	+	0	+	0	+	0	+	0	+	0	0	0	0
8	0	0	0	+	+	0	+	0	+	0	+	+	0	+	+	0	+	+	2+	3+	1+	0
9	0	+	0	+	+	+	+	+	0	+	0	0	+	0	0	+	0	+	0	0	0	0
10	0	0	+	+	+	0	+	0	0	0	+	0	+	0	+	0	+	0	2+	3+	1+	0
AC																			0	0	0	0

f1.10 Antibody identification with antibody reacting preferentially with red cells expressing a double-dose of the antigen. **a** If a cross-out or rule-out strategy is used with this antibody, every potential specificity is eliminated. But, cells 2, 3, 8 & 10 all express a double-dose of the M antigen. Some antibodies react preferentially with red cells expressing a double-dose of the antigen & this is likely what is happening here
b Repeat testing that included a 15 minute room temperature incubation: the antibody now reacted with the M+ red cells expressing only a single-dose of antigen (MN or M+N+), although much weaker than those red cells expressing a double-dose of antigen (MM or M+N–).
AC, auto control; IAT, indirect antiglobulin test

ISBN 978-089189-6616

a

Cell	D	C	E	c	e	K	k	Fy^a	Fy^b	Jk^a	Jk^b	Le^a	Le^b	P1	M	N	S	s	IS	LISS 37°C	IAT
1	+	+	0	0	+	0	+	+	0	0	+	0	+	+	+	+	+	0	0	0	3+
2	+	+	0	0	+	0	+	0	+	+	0	0	+	+	+	0	+	+	0	0	0
3	+	0	+	+	0	+	+	+	0	0	+	+	0	+	+	0	0	+	0	0	3+
4	+	+	0	+	+	0	+	+	+	+	0	0	+	0	+	+	+	+	0	0	3+
5	+	0	+	+	+	0	+	0	+	0	+	0	+	0	0	+	+	0	0	0	0
6	0	+	0	+	+	0	+	+	+	+	+	0	+	+	+	+	+	+	0	0	3+
7	0	0	0	+	+	0	+	0	+	+	0	+	0	+	0	+	0	+	0	0	0
8	0	0	0	+	+	0	+	0	+	0	+	+	0	+	+	0	+	+	0	0	0
9	0	0	0	+	+	+	+	+	0	+	0	0	+	0	0	+	0	+	0	0	3+
10	0	0	+	+	+	0	+	0	0	0	+	0	+	0	+	0	+	0	0	0	0
AC																			0	0	0

b

Cell	D	C	E	c	e	K	k	Fy^a	Fy^b	Jk^a	Jk^b	Le^a	Le^b	P1	M	N	S	s	IS	LISS 37°C	IAT
1	+	+	0	0	+	0	+	+	0	0	+	0	+	+	+	+	+	0	0	0	0
2	+	+	0	0	+	0	+	0	+	+	0	0	+	+	+	0	+	+	0	0	0
3	+	0	+	+	0	+	+	+	0	0	+	+	0	+	+	0	0	+	0	0	0
4	+	+	0	+	+	0	+	+	+	+	0	0	+	0	+	+	+	+	0	0	0
5	+	0	+	+	+	0	+	0	+	0	+	0	+	0	0	+	+	0	0	0	0
6	0	+	0	+	+	0	+	+	+	+	+	0	+	+	+	+	+	+	0	0	0
7	0	0	0	+	+	0	+	0	+	+	0	+	0	+	0	+	0	+	0	0	0
8	0	0	0	+	+	0	+	0	+	0	+	+	0	+	+	0	+	+	0	0	0
9	0	0	0	+	+	+	+	+	0	+	0	0	+	0	0	+	0	+	0	0	0
10	0	0	+	+	+	0	+	0	0	0	+	0	+	0	+	0	+	0	0	0	0
AC																			0	0	0

f1.11 Antibody identification where enzyme-treated panel cells may be useful:
a Initial antibody identification studies indicate the presence of anti-Fy^a but anti-K cannot be ruled out & may also be present. While a selected cell panel could be created to rule out the presence of anti-K, an enzyme premodified panel could also be used. The Fy^a antigen would be destroyed, but the K antigen would not be destroyed.
b Repeat panel studies with enzyme-treated red cells: The enzyme-treated panel cells are no longer reactive with anti-Fy^a. The K+ cells are nonreactive, eliminating the presence of anti-K
AC, auto control; IAT, indirect antiglobulin test

1.5.2 Reagents described in other sections of this chapter

- Antiglobulin sera
  - 1.3.5
- Blood grouping sera
  - 1.2.2.1
  - 1.2.6.4
  - 1.5.1.4
- Reagent red cells
  - 1.2.2.1
  - 1.5.1.4
  - 1.5.1.9

1.5.3 Applications of special tests & reagents

- Special tests and reagents, their principle and/or mechanism, and applications in the blood bank are summarized in **t1.34**

Cell	D	C	E	c	e	K	k	Fy^a	Fy^b	Jk^a	Jk^b	Le^a	Le^b	P1	M	N	S	s	IS	LISS 37°C	IAT
1	+	+	0	0	+	0	+	+	0	0	+	0	+	+	+	+	+	0	0	0	3+
2	+	+	0	0	+	0	+	0	+	+	0	0	+	+	+	0	+	+	0	0	3+
3	+	0	+	+	0	+	+	+	0	0	+	+	0	+	+	0	0	+	0	0	3+
4	+	+	0	+	+	0	+	+	+	+	0	0	+	0	+	+	+	+	0	0	3+
5	+	0	+	+	+	0	+	0	+	0	+	0	+	0	0	+	+	0	0	0	3+
6	0	+	0	+	+	0	+	+	+	+	+	0	+	+	+	+	+	+	0	0	3+
7	0	0	0	+	+	0	+	0	+	+	0	+	0	+	0	+	0	+	0	0	3+
8	0	0	0	+	+	0	+	0	+	0	+	+	0	+	+	0	+	+	0	0	3+
9	0	0	0	+	+	+	+	+	0	+	0	0	+	0	0	+	0	+	0	0	3+
10	0	0	+	+	+	0	+	0	0	0	+	0	+	0	+	0	+	0	0	0	3+
AC																			0	0	3+

DAT on patient red cells = 3+

f1.12 Antibody identification studies in a patient with warm autoimmune hemolytic anemia & warm autoantibody in their serum. This type of serology is discussed in more detail in the Physiology & Pathophysiology section of this chapter where warm autoimmune hemolytic anemia & its serology are described. Of importance in situations such as shown in this panel is to differentiate autoantibody from alloantibody & adsorption studies may be necessary in order to make that determination. Such samples may need referral to an immunohematology reference laboratory for antibody identification & resolution.
AC, auto control; IAT, indirect antiglobulin test

Cell	D	C	E	c	e	K	k	Fy^a	Fy^b	Jk^a	Jk^b	Le^a	Le^b	P1	M	N	S	s	IS	LISS 37°C	IAT
1	+	+	0	0	+	0	+	+	0	0	+	0	+	+	+	+	+	0	0	0	3+
2	+	+	0	0	+	0	+	0	+	+	0	0	+	+	+	0	+	+	0	0	3+
3	+	0	+	+	0	+	+	+	0	0	+	+	0	+	+	0	0	+	0	0	0
4	+	+	0	+	+	0	+	+	+	+	0	0	+	0	+	+	+	+	0	0	2+
5	+	0	+	+	+	0	+	0	+	0	+	0	+	0	0	+	+	+	0	0	0
6	0	+	0	+	+	0	+	+	+	+	+	0	+	+	+	+	+	+	0	0	3+
7	0	0	0	+	+	0	+	0	+	+	0	+	0	+	0	+	0	+	0	0	0
8	0	0	0	+	+	0	+	0	+	0	+	+	0	+	+	0	+	+	0	0	0
9	+	0	0	+	+	+	+	+	0	+	0	0	+	0	0	+	0	+	0	0	0
10	0	0	+	+	+	0	+	0	0	0	+	0	+	0	+	0	+	+	0	0	0
AC																			0	0	0

f1.13 Additional approach to cross-out or rule-out strategies focused on a single vs a double dose of an antigen. Some laboratories require that antibody identification studies focus on whether a nonreactive cell expresses a single or a double dose of each antigen. Cross-out or rule-out strategies begin with each nonreactive cell within the body of the antibody identification panel. As shown in the panel above, if a single dose of antigen is present on a nonreactive cell, a single line is drawn through the antigen. If a double dose of antigen is present, 2 lines are drawn. For example, cell #5 expresses a single dose for D, E, e, S & s, and a double dose of c, k, Fy^b, Jk^b & N. Continued evaluation of the other nonreactive cells (#3, #7, #8, #9 & #10) collectively express a double dose of D, E, c, e, K, Fy^a, Jk^a, M & s. There is no nonreactive cell that expresses a double dose of S

This is also summarized in the top row of the antibody identification panel where a single line rules out specificity using only heterozygous cells but a double line rules out specificity with homozygous cells; the cell with S is the only cell with a single line

P1, Le^a & Le^b do not express zygosity but multiple antigen-positive cells were nonreactive, allowing their elimination

The patient appears to have anti-C, but this laboratory would test a C-cell that expressed a double dose of the S antigen with the patient's serum to ensure a weak anti-S only reacting with cells expressing a double dose of the antigen is not present

AC, auto control; IAT, indirect antiglobulin test

Serologic & molecular testing>Applications of special tests & reagents

t1.34 Applications of special tests & reagents in the blood bank

Special test or reagent	Principle and/or mechanism	Application in the blood bank
Enzymes	Proteolytic enzymes, including ficin, papain, bromelin & trypsin, target certain glycoproteins on the red cell membrane. The removal of some glycoproteins may destroy an antigen or modify the red cell membrane in such a way as to enhance antigen-antibody reactions	Certain antigens including Fy^a, Fy^b, M, N, Ch, Rg & Xg^a are destroyed with enzyme treatment. Enhanced antigen-antibody activity may be seen with Rh, JK, LE & I system antibodies. These techniques can be useful in antibody identification studies & premodifying red cells for adsorption studies
Enhancement media	Includes LISS, albumin & PEG. In general, these reagents bring sensitized red cells closer to each other to enhance antigen-antibody reactions	Used in procedures including antibody detection & identification studies and crossmatching to maximize antigen-antibody interactions
Lectins	Protein extracts primarily from plants (seeds) that bind to red cell membrane carbohydrate antigens & support agglutination	Lectin prepared from the seeds of *Dolichos bifloris* is commonly used as anti-A1 reagent
Adsorption	Under optimal conditions, providing a serum antibody with its corresponding antigen & removing the antibody from serum	May be used to remove autoantibody after modification of autologous red cells to optimize antigen-antibody interaction. May also be used to remove alloantibody or autoantibody after modification of allogeneic red cells to optimize antigen-antibody interaction. The adsorbed serum with antibody of interest now removed is then tested to evaluate the presence of antibodies not removed through the adsorption process. May also be used to verify the presence of a red cell antigen, including the weak expression of A & B antigens
Elution	Red cells sensitized with antibody are treated to disrupt the bonds between antigen & antibody, recovering the antibody in a diluent that can be further tested. Methods to free antibody include those that are physical (heat & freeze-thaw) or chemical such as organic solvents or acid. The resulting antibody-containing fluid is called an eluate	Removal & identification of red-cell-bound antibody can be useful in evaluating HDFN, delayed or serologic transfusion reactions, and autoimmune & drug-induced immune hemolytic anemias
Titration	The serial dilution (usually 2-fold) of an antibody to determine its relative amount. Semiquantitative. Endpoint is the titer, reported as the reciprocal of the last 1+ or $+^w$ reactive dilution	Used occasionally to monitor the antibody in pregnant women to follow potential HDFN situations. May also be used to determine if the weak anti-D seen in a maternal postpartum blood sample is from antepartum RhIG. May be used as part of complex serologic investigations to characterize reactivity, such as a high-titer, low-avidity antibody
Cell separations	Separating different red cell populations as occurs in individuals who received transfusions recently. Recovery of younger autologous red cells in the presence of transfused cells is based on cell density differences	If red cell phenotyping is needed in a recipient of a recent transfusion, separation studies & recovery of younger autologous red cells may be useful
ELISA	May be used to detect antibody or antigen & always incorporates a secondary antibody with bound enzyme. After incubation & washing, enzyme substrate is added & enzymatically converted to a color & analyzed spectrophotometrically	Methodology may be used in the HLA laboratory or specialized laboratories that work with granulocyte & platelet antigens & antibodies
Neutralization/ inhibition	Inactivation or neutralization of an antibody by binding with its soluble antigen, negating the ability of the antibody to bind with red cell antigens & support agglutination. Sources of soluble antigen could include saliva or serum	Neutralization may be helpful in confirming antibody specificity. Anti-Le^a specificity might be confirmed by incubating the antibody with saliva from an Le(a+) individual & then testing with Le(a+) red cells. If neutralization occurred, the saliva/serum mixture will no longer react with these Le(a+) red cells. Must include a saline control to account for dilution factor. This control should continue to react with the Le(a+) red cells for valid test results. Neutralization studies can also be used for anti-P1 & anti-Sd^a using P1 substance & pooled urine, respectively
Use of thiol reagents	Includes DTT & 2-ME, capable of cleaving disulfide bonds of IgM molecules, but not IgG molecules. DTT may also be used to cleave disulfide bonds of certain red cell antigens, such as those in the KEL blood group system & CD38 molecule	Differentiation of IgM & IgG serum antibodies may be useful in studies of pregnant women to determine potential fetal risk for HDFN. Modification of certain red cell antigens may be useful in determining or confirming antibody specificity such as antibodies in KEL blood group system or verification of use of monoclonal antibodies such as anti-CD38
Solid phase	Solid-phase immunoassays (SPRCA) use microtiter wells bound with antibody or antigen, based on the test being performed. Includes centrifugation to enhance reactivity	Full automation based on solid-phase technology is now common in the blood bank. Tests that can be performed include ABO, Rh, antibody detection, antibody identification, DAT (IgG only) & an IgG crossmatch
Column agglutination test or gel technology	More commonly referred to as gel technology, uses microtubes containing dextran-acrylamide gel & antibody or antigen, based on the test being performed. Includes centrifugation to enhance reactivity	Full automation based on gel technology is now common in the blood bank. Tests that can be performed include ABO, Rh, antibody detection, antibody identification, titration studies, DAT & an IgG crossmatch. Saline washing for antiglobulin testing is not required. Antiglobulin control cells (check cells) are also not required

DAT, direct antiglobulin test; DTT, dithiothreitol; EDTA, ethylenediaminetetraacetic acid; ELISA, enzyme-linked immunosorbent assay; HDFN, hemolytic disease of the fetus & newborn; HLA, human leukocyte antigen; LISS, low ionic strength saline; PEG, polyethylene glycol; RhIG, Rh immune globulin; SPRCA, solid-phase red cell adherence; 2-ME, 2-mercaptoethanol

ISBN 978-089189-6616

t1.34 Applications of special tests & reagents in the blood bank (continued)

Special test or reagent	Principle and/or mechanism	Application in the blood bank
Chloroquine diphosphate	Dissociates IgG antibodies from their RBC antigens	May be used to dissociate some bound immunoglobulin from the RBCs in cases of autoimmune hemolytic anemia, leaving intact red cells that may be used for phenotyping. Rh & Bg antigens may be denatured
Glycine-HCl/EDTA	Dissociates IgG antibodies from their RBC antigens	May be used as an elution procedure in the blood bank. May also be used to dissociate some bound immunoglobulin from the RBCs in cases of autoimmune hemolytic anemia, leaving intact red cells that may be used for red cell phenotyping. Some red cells antigens are destroyed, including those of the KEL blood group system, and Bg & Er antigens
Saline replacement test	Differentiates rouleaux from red cell agglutination Rouleaux is often noted with the serum of patients who have abnormal or high serum protein concentrations	If rouleaux is suspected, centrifuge the serum & cell mixture & remove the serum, leaving the red cell button. Replace the serum with an equal volume of saline & resuspend the red cell button. Saline will disperse rouleaux, but not true agglutination

DAT, direct antiglobulin test; DTT, dithiothreitol; EDTA, ethylenediaminetetraacetic acid; ELISA, enzyme-linked immunosorbent assay; HDFN, hemolytic disease of the fetus & newborn; HLA, human leukocyte antigen; LISS, low ionic strength saline; PEG, polyethylene glycol; RhIG, Rh immune globulin; SPRCA, solid-phase red cell adherence; 2-ME, 2-mercaptoethanol

1.5.3.1 Applications of DNA-based testing in the blood bank

- See also Molecular Biology 9.5.5
- Determination of red cell phenotypes in patients who received transfusions recently to
  - Identify potential alloantibodies the blood recipient might produce
  - Match extended phenotype of recipient to those of phenotyped donors to avoid alloimmunization or additional alloimmunization
- Determination of red cell phenotypes in patients with a positive DAT result
  - Red cell phenotype to distinguish alloantibody from autoantibody if transfusion therapy is required
  - Replaces physical and chemical modifications of red cells that can be ineffective and labor-intensive
- Antigen typing to evaluate risk for HDFN
  - Testing of fetal DNA to determine the presence or absence of the antigen to which maternal IgG antibody is directed
  - Testing of paternal DNA to determine zygosity and therefore the likelihood that the infant will inherit the antigen of interest
- Differentiation of weak D and partial D in the prenatal population and administration of RhIG
  - Weak D types 1, 2, 3, and 4.1 can be managed as if D-positive and do not require RhIG
  - Partial D individuals should be managed as D-negative and receive RhIG
- Screening blood donors for extended antigen profiles and those that lack certain high-incidence antigens to ensure an adequate registry of rare donors
- Identify the genetic basis for unusual serologic typing results including ABO discrepancies related to a subgroup, aberrant Rh typing results, or situations such as a e+ individual with apparent alloanti-e

1.5.4 Leukocyte/platelet testing

- For current DNA-based and serologic tests used for HLA, see Immunology 8.3.3 and Molecular Biology 9.5.6
- Historically, cytotoxicity (cell-based) testing was common in HLA testing, but is rarely used today
  - Cells, serum, and a source of complement are incubated, followed by the addition of a vital dye and examined microscopically
  - Undamaged cells exclude the vital dye, where damaged cells (antigen and antibody reaction) allow the dye to enter the cell
- Platelet testing
  - Assays include solid-phase red cell adherence using microtiter wells coated with immobilized platelets, flow cytometry, and platelet glycoprotein antigen capture assays for platelet antibody detection
  - DNA-based genotyping is the most reliable method for determining platelet-specific (HPA) antigens
- Granulocyte testing
  - Granulocyte antibodies can be detected using an agglutination test, immunofluorescence test, and microbeads coated with granulocyte (HNA) antigens
  - DNA-based genotyping is used to determine HNA antigens
  - Testing is often included in the evaluation of suspected TRALI transfusion reactions

1.5.5 Quality assurance & quality control in the blood bank

- See Laboratory Operations for information on legislation, regulation, agencies and oversight 7.1; for quality management 7.5; for laboratory safety 7.8

1.5.5.1 Blood samples

- Quality assurance strategies for prevention of wrong blood in tube (WBIT) because of recipient misidentification or pretransfusion sample labeling errors include
  - Identification of intended recipient before sample collection including
    - Two independent identifiers
  - Affixing label to sample before leaving the side of the patient
  - Mechanism to identify date and time of collection and who collected the sample
  - Acceptance of legible, accurate, and completely labeled samples in the blood bank
  - Two determinations of the patient's ABO group
  - Comparison of current results with previous records

1.5.5.2 Reagents

- Quality control strategies for blood bank antiserum
  - Testing with a known antigen-positive control cell each day of use
  - Testing with a known antigen-negative control cell each day of use
- Quality control strategies for blood bank reagent red cells such as ABO reverse grouping cells
  - Testing with known antisera directed to an antigen present on the red cells each day of use
  - Testing with known antisera directed to an antigen absent from the red cells each day of use
- Quality control of antiglobulin serum
  - Testing the antiglobulin reagent with red cells sensitized with IgG immunoglobulin each day of use
  - Testing the antiglobulin reagent with red cells sensitized with complement each day of use

1.5.5.3 Selected test procedures

- Antiglobulin sera and use of check cells in tube testing
  - IgG sensitized red cells (check cells) added to each negative antiglobulin test and then shown to give a positive result to ensure that
    - Antiglobulin reagent was added
    - Neutralization of the antiglobulin reagent did not occur
    - It does not ensure the test was read correctly
- Last wash analysis when performing an elution
  - Evaluation of the last saline wash for nonreactivity helps ensure that antibody detected in an eluate was bound to the RBCs and not residual antibody in the saline wash solution
- ABO forward and ABO reverse typing
  - Agreement between an ABO forward and ABO reverse typing provides its own form of quality control
  - The blood group systems section in this chapter reviews many of the causes of ABO discrepancies and strategies for resolution (1.2.2.5)
- Control of D typing
  - With the use of monoclonal (low-protein) anti-D, the ABO forward typing will usually serve as the control for this reagent
    - In an AB, D-positive individual, the manufacturer will usually recommend an additional control such as an autocontrol (patient red cells and serum) or the patient's red cells with 6% albumin or monoclonal control from the manufacturer, and this must be negative to interpret typing results
  - With high protein, polyclonal anti-D reagents, an additional Rh control reagent is provided, and it must be negative to correctly interpret the Rh typing results
  - The blood group systems section in this chapter reviews many of the causes for inaccurate Rh typing results

ISBN 978-089189-6616

1.5.5.4 Quality control performance intervals for blood bank equipment t1.35

t1.35 Suggested quality control performance intervals for selected blood bank equipment

Equipment	Frequency of Quality Control Checks
Blood component storage devices (refrigerators, freezers & platelet incubators)	
Temperature recording device	Daily
Manual temperature recording	Daily
Temperature charts	Daily & with a weekly review
Alarm activation	Quarterly
Centrifuges	
Speed	Quarterly
Timer	Quarterly
Temperature (refrigerated centrifuge)	Day of use
Temperature verification (refrigerated centrifuge)	Monthly
Automated cell washers	
Speed	Quarterly
Timer	Quarterly
Tube fill level	Day of use
Saline fill volume	Weekly
Serologic calibration for centrifuge & shortest time for:	New equipment, after repair & periodically as defined by facility
Clear supernatant	
Cell button clearly delineated	
Cell button easily resuspended	
Agglutination in positive tube is as strong as expected	
Negative reactions are as expected	
Water baths	
Temperature	Day of use
Blood component thawing device	Day of use
Timers	Twice yearly
Sterile connection device	
Weld	Each use
Functionality	Yearly
Blood irradiator (γ rays)	
Dose delivery verification (indicator)	Each use
Turntable visual check	Each use
Timer	Monthly to quarterly
Leak test	Twice yearly
Calibration & turntable check	Yearly
Dose delivery verification	
Cesium-137	Yearly
Cobalt-60	Twice yearly
Blood irradiator (x-rays)	
Dose delivery verification (indicator)	Each use
Leak test	Yearly
Dose delivery verification	Yearly
Pipette recalibration	Quarterly
Blood warmers	
Effluent temperature	Quarterly
Heater temperature	Quarterly
Alarm activation	Quarterly
Thermometers	Yearly or based on manufacturer's directions
Scales/balances	Day of use

These are suggested quality control frequencies. The manufacturer's suggested or required intervals should always take precedence

Adapted from Cohn CS, Delaney M, Johnson ST, Katz LM, eds. Technical Manual. *20th ed; Bethesda, MD: AABB; 2020*

1.6 Transfusion practice

1.6.1 Indications for transfusion

- Indications for transfusing red cell, platelet, granulocyte, plasma, and cryoprecipitated AHF blood components are summarized in **t1.36**
- See **t1.7** for a more detailed summary of various blood components, including dosage and expected increments after a transfusion

t1.36 Blood components & indications for use

Blood component	Indications for use
Red cell components	Used to treat symptomatic anemia; increase oxygen-carrying capacity & red cell mass
Platelet components	Treatment of bleeding associated with thrombocytopenia; prophylactic transfusions in certain patient populations with low platelet counts; some congenital & acquired disorders with abnormal platelet function; massive transfusion protocols
Granulocytes	Treatment of profound neutropenia (<500/μL [0.5×10^9/L]) in the presence of bacterial or fungal infection unresponsive to antimicrobials
Plasma components	Used in bleeding patients or those undergoing invasive procedures where there are coagulation factor deficiencies secondary to DIC, liver disease, and massive blood component transfusion or volume replacement; can be used for reversal of warfarin effect; congenital factor deficiencies where there is no coagulation concentrate (factor V or XII); primary replacement fluid for therapeutic plasma exchange procedures
Cryoprecipitated AHF	Used to treat congenital or acquired fibrinogen deficiency

AHF, antihemophilic factor; DIC, disseminated intravascular coagulation

1.6.2 Transfusion in special clinical situations

1.6.2.1 Sickle cell disease & other chronic recipients of transfusions

- These recipients of chronic transfusions have high rates of alloimmunization
- It is common to perform extended phenotype or genotype analysis on these patient groups and provide antigen-matched red cells for transfusion
    - If transfusion recipient is negative for the C, E, and K antigens, provide blood for transfusion that also lacks the C, E, and K antigens
    - If transfusion recipient becomes alloimmunized, antigen-matched red cells for transfusion will also include those in the FY, JK, and MNS systems to avoid further alloimmunization

1.6.2.2 Urgent request for transfusion or emergency release of blood components

- If transfusion is deemed medically necessary and blood is released before testing is complete, the record must contain a signed statement from the requesting physician indicating the clinical situation was sufficiently urgent to release blood components
  - Such documentation can be obtained after the transfusion begins
  - Blood bank personnel need to issue properly labeled blood that is ABO compatible
    - Issue group O Red Blood Cells or low-titer group O Whole Blood if recipient's ABO is unknown
    - Usually issue Rh-positive units; Rh-negative units for female recipients of child-bearing age
      - May consider use of RhIG to prevent alloimmunization to D antigen in D-negative recipients who receive D-positive Red Blood Cells
    - Label on unit states that compatibility testing has not been completed
- Finish all testing and notify patient's physician immediately if incompatibility detected

1.6.2.3 Massive transfusion

- Defined as the administration of 8-10 units of Red Blood Cells or approximately the total blood volume in an adult in <24 hours, or the acute administration of 4-5 Red Blood Cells within 1 hour
  - Institutions with a massive transfusion protocol standardize the response to hemorrhage, balancing the ratio of Fresh Frozen Plasma, Platelets, and Red Blood Cells at 1:1:1 or 1:1:2
  - For red cell components, typically transfusing group O Red Blood Cells and AB Fresh Frozen Plasma (or group A Fresh Frozen Plasma) or low-titer group O Whole Blood
    - Usually issue Rh-positive units
    - If recipient is D-negative and depending on patient's age and sex, may consider initially using Rh-negative units, switching to Rh-positive units, and then completing the protocol with Rh-negative units
      - May consider administration of RhIG to prevent formation of anti-D
  - Important to determine patient's true ABO and Rh type with an early blood sample
- Complications of massive transfusion may include
  - Citrate toxicity and hypocalcemia
  - Hemostatic abnormalities related to dilution of platelets and coagulation factors
  - Hypothermia
  - Hyperkalemia or hypokalemia
  - Air embolism

1.6.2.4 Transfusion in neonates

- Preliminary testing in the blood bank for newborns
  - Only ABO forward typing using anti-A and anti-B is required
  - Rh testing using anti-D is required
  - Antibody detection studies can be done with neonatal or maternal serum or plasma
    - If negative, it is unnecessary to crossmatch donor red cells for the initial or subsequent transfusions
    - If positive, units for transfusion will be shown to be negative for the antigen to which the antibody is directed, or are compatible on antiglobulin crossmatching
  - Repeat ABO, Rh typing, and crossmatching may be omitted for the remainder of the neonate's hospital admission or until the neonate reaches the age of 4 months, whichever is sooner
    - Pediatric patients older than 4 months require ABO, Rh testing, and antibody detection studies at the same frequency as adult patients
  - If a non-group O neonate is to receive non-group O Red Blood Cells that are not compatible with the maternal ABO group, the neonate's serum or plasma shall be tested for anti-A or anti-B
    - Test methods will include the antiglobulin phase of testing
    - If test results are positive, Red Blood Cells lacking the corresponding ABO antigen must be transfused
- The attributes for red cell transfusions in neonates are described in **t1.29**
  - Transfusions are typically given in small-volume aliquots from the same unit to limit donor exposures and donor-related risks, and minimize circulatory overload
    - Many configurations for preparing these small-volume transfusions exist and the use of a sterile connection device allows for maximum storage of units
    - Use of citrate phosphate dextrose adenine 1 (CPDA-1) units only versus those containing additive solutions are facility dependent and practices vary
    - All cellular transfusions must be irradiated to prevent transfusion-associated GVHD in this population

ISBN 978-089189-6616

t1.37 Transfusion-related adverse events

Type	Incidence	Signs & symptoms	Selected additional comments
Intravascular, hemolytic	ABO/Rh mismatch: 1:40,000 AHTR: 1:76,000 Fatal HTR: 1:1.8 million	Hemoglobinemia & hemoglobinuria, fever, chills, anxiety, shock, DIC, dyspnea, chest pain, flank pain, oliguria	Stop transfusion; clerical check; DAT & repeat ABO on pre- & post-transfusion sample; check patient sample for free hemoglobin; further tests to define possible incompatibility & hemolysis
Extravascular, hemolytic (acute or delayed)	1:2500-11,000 transfusions	Fever, malaise, decreased hematocrit, indirect hyperbilirubinemia	DAT, review historical records, verify sample & recipient, look for newly formed alloantibody
Febrile, nonhemolytic	0.1%-1% with universal leukocyte reduction	Fever, chills/rigor, headache, vomiting	Rule out hemolysis & bacterial contamination; reaction caused by antibodies to leukocytes or plasma proteins
Allergic/urticarial	1%-3%	Urticaria, pruritis, flushing, angioedema	Antihistamines to resolve symptoms
Anaphylactic or severe allergic	<1%	Hypotension, urticaria, angioedema, bronchospasm, abdominal pain	Evaluate for IgA deficiency, antibodies to plasma proteins. Pretransfusion use of antihistamines, epinephrine, or steroids & use of washed blood products or those from IgA-deficient donors
TACO	1%	Orthopnea, dyspnea, hypertension, pulmonary edema, cardiac arrhythmias	Avoid rapid & excessive transfusion volume; symptoms variable
TRALI	1:1200 to 1:190,000 transfusions	Dyspnea, fever, hypoxia, bilateral pulmonary edema, hypotension	Donor HLA or HNA antibody; male sources for plasma & plateletpheresis products; female donors screened for HLA & HNA antibodies
Bacterial contamination	Varies by type of transfusion; still more frequent with platelet products	Rigor, fever, chills, shock. Usually after infusion of minimal amount of blood product infusion	Gram stain & culture of product & patient Rule out other reasons for reaction including ABO mismatch
Nonimmune hemolysis	Rare	Physical/chemical destruction of RBCs. Hemoglobinuria/hemoglobinemia	Rule out other causes of overt hemolysis
Air embolus	Rare. Air infusion via line	Sudden shortness of breath, acute cyanosis, pain, cough, hypotension	X-ray for intravascular air
Hypocalcemia	Uncommon. Rapid infusion of citrate as seen in massive transfusion	Paresthesia, tetany, arrhythmia	Ionized calcium levels Supplement with calcium
Hypothermia	Uncommon. Rapid infusion of cold blood	Cardiac arrhythmia	Use blood warmer
Alloimmunization to red cell antigens	1:100 transfusions	Weeks to months after transfusion, alloantibodies present in blood recipient	Antibody detection & antibody identification studies are performed. Document in patient record
Graft-vs-host disease	Rare. Donor lymphocytes engraft in recipient & attack host tissues	Erythroderma, vomiting, diarrhea, pancytopenia; nearly always fatal	Skin biopsy, HLA typing. Irradiation of blood components for patients at risk
Posttransfusion purpura	Rare. Recipient platelet antibodies destroy autologous platelets	Thrombocytopenic purpura, bleeding 8-10 days after transfusion	Platelet antibody detection & identification Usually anti-HPA-1a
Iron overload	Can occur after >20 Red Blood Cell transfusions	Diabetes, cirrhosis, cardiomyopathy	Liver & cardiac iron concentration noted with MRI; provide iron chelators

AHTR, acute hemolytic transfusion reaction; DAT, direct antiglobulin test; HLA, human leukocyte antigen; HNA, human neutrophil antigens; MRI, magnetic resonance imaging; RBC, red blood cell; TACO, transfusion-associated circulatory overload; TRALI, transfusion-related acute lung injury

Adapted from Cohen CS, Delaney M, Johnson ST, Katz LM, eds. Technical Manual. *20th ed; Bethesda, MD: AABB; 2020*

1.6.3 Transfusion-related adverse events

- There are many types of transfusion-related adverse events and their incidence, signs and symptoms, and selected additional comments are summarized in t1.37
- Several transfusion-related adverse events are discussed here in further detail

1.6.3.1 Serologic & immunologic adverse events primarily related to red cell transfusions

- Suspected transfusion reaction
  - Defined and written processes for transfusing staff to recognize and respond
  - Discontinue transfusion immediately
  - Verify label on product and identity of patient
  - Notify ordering physician of possible reaction
  - Send blood container/bag to the laboratory/transfusion service
  - Collect posttransfusion sample and send to the laboratory/transfusion service
- Laboratory evaluation of suspected transfusion reaction
  - Inspect pretransfusion and posttransfusion sample labels, test results, and blood component patient identification tags and paperwork for discrepancies and errors
  - Inspect posttransfusion sample for evidence of hemolysis and compare with pretransfusion sample
  - Repeat ABO on posttransfusion sample
  - Perform a DAT on posttransfusion sample
    - If positive, perform DAT on pretransfusion sample
  - Perform additional testing as needed that could include
    - Antibody identification studies
    - Preparation and testing of eluate
    - Compatibility testing
  - Additional laboratory studies as defined in facility policies and procedures that could include plasma hemoglobin, haptoglobin, lactate dehydrogenase, and urine hemoglobin
  - Results reviewed by blood bank medical director and reported to patient's physician
  - Fatalities must be reported to the FDA

1.6.3.1.1 Acute hemolytic transfusion reaction within 24 hours of transfusion

- Intravascular destruction typically associated with complement-activating ABO antibodies, usually the result of human error including wrong sample in tube or transfusion given to the wrong patient
  - Abrupt onset of fever, chills, back pain, pain at infusion site, hypotension, and disseminated intravascular coagulation (DIC)
    - Can be a fatal transfusion reaction
    - Important to treat hypotension and DIC, and minimize renal damage
  - DAT result is positive or negative because the incompatible red cells may have been completely hemolyzed
  - Hemolysis usually seen in posttransfusion sample
  - Hemoglobinuria is also usually noted
- Extravascular destruction occurs when the causative antibody does not activate complement, or only activates complement to C3
  - Usually non-ABO antibodies including those of the Rh, MNS, KEL, FY, and JK blood group systems
  - Patient may demonstrate fever, positive DAT result, and a decreased hematocrit without any overt signs of bleeding
    - May note mixed-field agglutination because of circulating transfused red cells sensitized with patient antibody
    - Can be a fatal transfusion reaction
  - Preparation of an eluate from the patient sample may be helpful in antibody identification
  - Antibody detection test may be negative if recipient antibody is completely attached to donor red cells

1.6.3.1.2 Delayed hemolytic transfusion reaction & delayed serologic transfusion reaction within days to weeks following transfusion

- Patients experiencing a delayed hemolytic transfusion reaction may present with unexplained fever and anemia
  - DAT result is usually positive and demonstrates a mixed-field reaction
  - Preparation of an eluate may be helpful in antibody identification
  - Antibody detection test result may be negative if recipient antibody is completely attached to donor red cells
    - Antibody detection test result may also be positive
  - Usually extravascular removal of sensitized donor red cells
  - May be a primary immune response, but more commonly a secondary or anamnestic response to previously formed alloantibody that was at undetectable levels in pretransfusion testing, or not detected in pretransfusion testing because of human error

- JK blood group system antibodies are particularly notorious for this type of transfusion reaction
- Rh, KEL, FY, and MNS blood group system antibodies are also noted

- Patients experiencing a delayed serologic transfusion reaction have no clinical evidence of hemolysis and are usually asymptomatic
  - The serology is an accidental laboratory finding and is generally the same as is found in a delayed hemolytic transfusion reaction

1.6.3.2 Transfusion-associated graft-vs-host disease (TA-GVHD)

- The transfusion recipient shows rash, fever, enterocolitis with watery diarrhea, and pancytopenia with profound marrow aplasia, usually 8-10 days posttransfusion
- Mortality rate >90%
- The following conditions contribute to the development of TA-GVHD in a transfusion recipient
  - Immunocompetent T lymphocytes are present in the blood component
  - The recipient is immunoincompetent and could include patients who are immunosuppressed as part of their disease management process, immunodeficient or of neonatal age
  - HLA-homozygous donors to HLA-heterozygous recipient where transfused donor lymphocytes attack recipient cells
    - Population's genetic diversity and if donor and recipient are related play a role
- TA-GVHD is preventable with irradiation of all cellular blood components with γ rays (cesium-137 or cobolt-60 source) or X-rays
  - Radiation dose targeted to the midplane of the irradiation container must be 25 gray (Gy) and 15 Gy elsewhere
  - Red cell products: Original expiration or 28 days from the date of irradiation, whichever is sooner
  - Platelet and granulocyte products: No change from original expiration date
- Pathogen reduction technologies inactivate white cells and mitigate TA-GVHD

1.6.3.3 Transfusion-related acute lung injury (TRALI)

- Fever, chills, dyspnea, cyanosis, hypotension, and bilateral pulmonary edema
  - Commonly within 2-6 hours of transfusion
  - Most common cause of transfusion mortality
- Associated with the infusion of donor antibodies to leukocyte antigens (HLA Class I or HLA class II) or HNA
  - Often blood components from multiparous women
- TRALI mitigation strategies now include the transfusion of plasma products, Whole Blood, and apheresis platelets from
  - Men
  - Never-pregnant women
  - Women tested since their last pregnancy and found to be negative for HLA and HNA antibodies

1.6.3.4 Transfusion-associated circulatory overload (TACO)

- Headache, cough, shortness of breath, congestion of pulmonary vasculature, increased central venous pressure, congestive heart failure, and systolic hypertension
  - Commonly within 1-2 hours of transfusion
  - Patients >70 years, those with congestive heart failure, end-stage renal disease, and infants at greatest risk
    - Policy needed to respond to requests for blood products for patients at increased risk for TACO
  - Reduction in infusion rates for blood products can help reduce TACO
- Frequency of TACO is likely underreported because the presentation can be variable
  - Can be associated with transfusion fatalities

1.6.3.5 Febrile nonhemolytic transfusion reactions (FNHTR)

- Fever >38°C and a change of ≥1°C from the pretransfusion temperature; may also include chills and/or rigors
  - Change in temperature not attributable to other reasons
  - Occurs during transfusion or within 4 hours of transfusion
- Febrile reactions may be attributed to patient antibodies to leukocyte antigens or accumulated cytokines in stored blood products
  - Prestorage leukocyte-reduced blood components mitigate FNHTR

1.6.3.6 Allergic reactions

- Generally occur within minutes of starting the transfusion and are common
- Presentation can be highly variable and includes itching and hives, angioedema and anaphylactic reactions

- Pathophysiology of most allergic reactions is poorly understood but some are attributed to the presence of allergens in the blood component and IgE antibodies in the recipient
  - Mild allergic reactions, antihistamine may prevent or resolve symptoms
- IgA-deficient recipients with anti-IgA are typically associated with anaphylactic reactions presenting with severe respiratory problems and/or hypotension
  - Reaction occurs after infusion of only a few milliliters of blood
  - Treat with epinephrine
  - Require transfusion with components from other IgA-deficient donors or saline-washed blood components such as washed Red Blood Cells

1.6.3.7 Bacterial contamination

- Fever (≥38.5°C), chills, rigors, and hypotension during or shortly after transfusion
- Gram-negative organisms often cause more severe symptoms that can include shock, renal failure, and DIC, and may be fatal
- Evaluation includes visual assessment of suspect blood component for color changes (brown or purple) or particulate matter in red cell components and foam/bubbles, particulate matter, or cloudiness in platelet components
  - Gram staining performed on suspect blood component
  - Culture suspect blood component and patient
- Mitigation strategies to prevent bacterial contamination include (**t1.4**)
  - Disinfecting donor venipuncture site with approved agents
  - Diverting the first few milliliters of blood from phlebotomy into a pouch to capture the skin plug that may possess residual bacteria, keeping these bacteria from the blood components
  - Performing bacterial cultures on all platelet components
  - Implementing secondary rapid bacterial detection tests before transfusion
  - Providing plasma and apheresis platelet components that have undergone pathogen reduction processes

1.6.3.8 Transfusion-transmitted diseases

- Infectious disease screening assays and supplemental tests currently performed on US blood donors are summarized in **t1.3**
- Despite this extensive donor testing, blood transfusions may transmit infectious agents and disease
  - The primary cause of residual disease transmission is donations from individuals in the window period of early infection and before current testing can demonstrate a positive result
  - The residual risk and window periods for hepatitis B virus, hepatitis C virus, and human immunodeficiency virus infection are shown in **t1.38**
  - Pathogen reduction processes for blood components are effective in preventing disease transmission and it is anticipated that in the future, additional technologies that include treatment for red cell-containing components will be approved by the FDA for use in the US

t1.38 HBV, HCV & HIV: residual risk & infectious window period

Infectious agent	Infectious window period (days)	Residual risk per donated unit
HBV	18.5-26.5	1:843,000 to 1:1,208,000
HCV	7.4	1:1,149,000
HIV	9.1	1:1,467,000

HBV, hepatitis B virus; HCV, hepatitis C virus; HIV, human immunodeficiency virus

Adapted from Cohen CS, Delaney M, Johnson ST, Katz LM, eds. Technical Manual. *20th ed; Bethesda, MD: AABB; 2020*

1.6.3.9 Platelet refractoriness

- The incidence of HLA alloimmunization as a cause of platelet refractoriness has been substantially reduced because of universal leukocyte-reduction strategies for cellular transfusion products
- Can still be noted in patients and is related to antibodies against HLA class I antigens
  - May require transfusion with platelets from donors known to lack HLA class I antigens to which the patient antibody is directed to see acceptable corrected count increments for platelets after transfusion

1.6.4 Therapeutic apheresis

- Uses automated cell and plasma-separating devices to process large quantities of blood, often replacing what is removed, to achieve clinical benefit

1.6.4.1 Therapeutic plasma exchange

- Removes patient alloantibodies, autoantibodies, immune complexes, abnormal proteins, or other toxic substances by removing patient plasma and replacing patient plasma with albumin, plasma components, or a mixture of fluids

ISBN 978-089189-6616

- Diseases treated with therapeutic plasma exchange include
  - Thrombotic thrombocytopenic purpura
  - Myasthenia gravis
  - Macroglobulinemia
  - Removal of HLA and ABO antibodies in preparation for solid organ and stem cell transplantation

1.6.4.2 Cytapheresis

- Reduces and removes excessive or abnormal cellular elements in the blood
  - Normal cellular elements may be infused as in a red cell exchange
- Diseases treated with cytapheresis include
  - Erythrocytapheresis or red cell exchange in acute complications of sickle cell disease
  - Leukocytapheresis in certain leukemias with leukostasis
  - Thrombocytapheresis in myeloproliferative disorders with thrombocytosis

1.6.4.3 Extracorporeal photopheresis

- Patient leukocytes are collected, exposed to 8-methoxypsoralen and ultraviolet light to prevent DNA replication and RNA transcription, and reinfused
- Diseases treated with extracorporeal photopheresis include
  - Cutaneous T-cell lymphoma
  - Sézary syndrome
  - Steroid-resistant chronic GVHD following stem cell transplantation
  - Solid organ transplant rejection

1.6.4.4 Selective adsorption

- Selective adsorption column removes substances such as low-density lipoprotein cholesterol in patients with familial hypercholesterolemia

1.6.5 Blood administration

- All transfusion components must be ordered (prescribed) and administered under medical direction
- Each intended recipient must sign a consent to transfusion that includes
  - A description of the risks, benefits, potential side effects, and treatment alternatives (including nontreatment)
  - The opportunity to ask questions
  - The right to accept or refuse transfusion
  - If recipient is unable to give consent, a legally authorized representative may do so
- After issue of blood products from the blood bank and immediately before a transfusion begins, the following information needs to be verified
  - Recipient's 2 independent identifiers (such as name, date of birth, and unique facility identification number) and recipient's ABO and Rh
  - Donation identification number on the blood product and donor's ABO and Rh
  - Interpretation of crossmatch tests, if performed
  - Special transfusion attributes (CMV-negative, irradiated, etc)
  - Blood product has not expired
  - The transfusionist and another individual (or an electronic identification system), in the presence of the recipient, positively identify the recipient and match the blood component to the recipient through the use of the 2 independent identifiers
    - This verification matches the recipient's 2 independent identifiers on the patient's armband to the same 2 independent identifiers present on the blood component label or tietag
    - Some facilities have implemented additional systems to prevent misidentification of blood recipients that can include bracelets with bar codes or radiofrequency devices, biometric scanning, and mechanical or electronic locks
- The blood or component must be transfused through a sterile, pyrogen-free transfusion set with the appropriate filter designed to retain particles harmful to the recipient
  - For red cell-containing products, 0.9% sodium chloride is usually the only acceptable accompanying fluid
  - In a stable adult, platelet and plasma components are usually administered over 1-2 hours and Red Blood Cells usually over 1-2 hours and not to exceed 4 hours

- Blood warming devices may be used in the rapid transfusion of multiple blood units, exchange transfusion, cardiopulmonary bypass surgery, severe CAD, and in some pediatric transfusions
- Infusion devices or blood pumps designed to deliver blood components at a predetermined flow rate also may be used

- The recipient needs to be closely observed for possible adverse events during the start of transfusion (usually the first 15 minutes) with periodic monitoring throughout the transfusion
- All identification attached to the blood product container needs to remain attached until the transfusion has been terminated
- The recipient's medical record needs to include the following documentation
  - Transfusion order
  - Patient consent for transfusion
  - Component name and donation identification number
  - Donor ABO/Rh
  - Date and time of transfusion
  - Vital signs taken at facility-defined intervals including before, during, and after transfusion
  - Amount of blood product transfused
  - Identification of transfusionist
  - If applicable, any transfusion-related adverse events

1.6.6 Patient blood management (PBM)

- Approach to improved patient care and safety by eliminating or reducing unnecessary allogeneic blood transfusion
  - Identifying alternative strategies to manage anemia and hemostasis
  - Identifying, developing, and following best practices or guidelines that are evidence based
  - Providing feedback and education to physicians through blood utilization review
  - Promoting a team-based approach to transfusion therapy that encompasses multiple medical disciplines and stakeholders within a health-care organization

1.6.6.1 Basic elements of a PBM program

1.6.6.1.1 Preoperative strategies

- Identification of preoperative anemia and if appropriate, pharmacologic strategies for its correction
- Identification of bleeding risk and as appropriate, discontinuation or dose adjustment of implicated drug
- Preoperative autologous blood donation
  - Used much less frequently than in the past
  - May still be appropriate for patients with complex red cell alloantibodies or for others who refuse allogeneic blood
- Maximum surgical blood order schedule (MSBOS)
  - Best if based on actual blood utilization data for specific surgical procedures to reduce unnecessary preoperative blood orders

1.6.6.1.2 Intraoperative strategies

- Acute normovolemic hemodilution
  - Whole Blood is removed at the beginning of the surgical procedure and reinfused, typically at the end of the procedure
  - Most beneficial in high-blood-loss procedures and in patients with a high hematocrit
- Intraoperative blood recovery
  - Shed blood is recovered during certain high-blood-loss surgical procedures, centrifuged, washed with normal saline, and red blood cells returned to the patient
- Point-of-care testing and the use of transfusion algorithms or protocols as might be seen in cardiac surgery or massive transfusion protocols
- Pharmacologic agents that includes the use of antifibrinolytics to reduce blood loss, desmopressin to stimulate release of von Willebrand factor and factor VIII or topical hemostatic sealants

1.6.6.1.3 Postoperative strategies

- Postoperative blood recovery
  - Blood is collected from surgical drains or wound sites, usually washed with normal saline, concentrated, and reinfused
- Limiting the quantity and frequency of laboratory testing to reduce iatrogenic blood loss
- Less reliance on a transfusion trigger and more reliance on patient clinical signs and symptoms
- More consideration of single-unit Red Blood Cell transfusion vs 2-unit Red Blood Cell transfusion

ISBN 978-089189-6616

1.6.6.1.4 Blood utilization audit programs

- Required by accrediting agencies including the Joint Commission and the AABB
- Often managed by the institutional transfusion committee or other type of peer-review process
  - Develop audit criteria designed to identify inappropriate transfusion decisions
  - Develop evidence-based transfusion guidelines and monitor deviations
  - Monitor other transfusion metrics that could include
    - Usage and discard rates
    - Ordering practices
    - Patient identification
    - Sample collection and labeling
    - Infectious and noninfectious adverse events of transfusion
    - Near-miss events
    - Appropriateness of use including group O and group O D-negative Red Blood Cells and AB plasma
    - Informed consent for blood transfusion
    - Intraoperative blood recovery use and quality control
    - Effectiveness of transfusion protocols
    - Results of external assessments and preventive and corrective actions
    - Compliance with peer-review recommendations
  - Implement and monitor blood ordering practices for utilization review that can include 1 of the following 3 methods
    - Prospective review of all blood orders in real-time and before it is issued
      - Very effective way to prevent unnecessary transfusions or inappropriate blood orders and change physician practice
      - Labor intensive
    - Concurrent review of transfusions within the previous 12-24 hours
      - Provides opportunity for consultative review if transfusion appears to be outside of accepted guidelines or good clinical practice in order to change physician practice
      - May also be labor intensive based on blood bank staffing levels
    - Retrospective review within days to weeks of transfusions
      - Performed by internal staff or external third party
      - Review transfusions that do not meet objective criteria
      - Easiest approach
  - Use of computerized provider order entry with or without clinical decision support facilitates blood utilization review and additional opportunity to change physician practice relative to blood transfusions
    - Often incorporates transfusion guidelines with some systems having "hard stops" where the physician must select a transfusion rationale before the order is accepted, if order is outside the guidelines

1.6.6.1.5 Medical education

- Education for physicians, executives, blood bank staff, nursing staff, and pharmacy staff is vital for a successful PBM program
- Educational efforts must be evidence-based
- The development of transfusion guidelines and subsequent educational efforts need a multidisciplinary approach
- A variety of educational interventions, including one-on-one interactions and lectures or online courses developed by respected colleagues and peers can be successful
- Feedback from blood utilization review or other types of audits and assessments are also educational

1.7 Selected readings

1.7.1 Books

Bandarenko N, King K (eds). *Blood Transfusion Therapy: A Physician's Handbook.* 12th ed. AABB Press. 2017. ISBN 978-1563959431

Cohn CS, Delaney M, Johnson ST, Katz LM (eds). *Technical Manual.* 20th ed. AABB Press. 2020. ISBN 978-1563953705

Harmening DM. *Modern Blood Banking and Transfusion Practices.* 7th ed. FA Davis. 2018. ISBN 978-0803668881

Howard PR. *Basic and Applied Concepts of Blood Banking and Transfusion Practices.* 5th ed. Mosby. 2020. ISBN 978-0323697392

Johns G, Zundel W, Gockel-Blessing E, Denesiuk L. *Clinical Laboratory Blood Banking and Transfusion Medicine: Principles and Practices.* Pearson. 2014. ISBN 978-0130833310

Reid ME, Lomas-Francis C, Olsson ML. *The Blood Group Antigen Factsbook.* 3rd ed. Academic Press. 2012. ISBN 978-0124258498

Standards for Blood Banks and Transfusion Services. 32nd ed. AABB Press. 2020. ISBN 978-1563953675

1.7.2 Online

Blood Banking Tutorial. https://webpath.med.utah.edu/TUTORIAL/BLDBANK/BLDBANK.html#INDEX

Chapter 2

Chemistry

2.1 Carbohydrates

2.1.1 Classification of carbohydrates

- Hydrates of carbon, aldehyde, or ketone derivatives
- Major food source & energy supply
- Chiefly stored as liver & muscle glycogen
- Forms
  - Monosaccharides

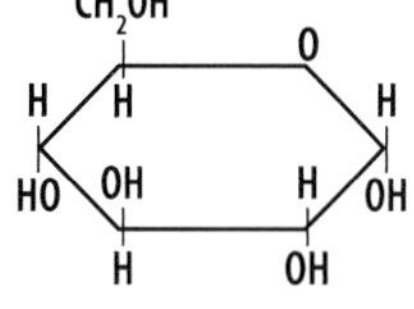

    - Simplest form of sugars
    - Cannot be hydrolyzed further
    - Contain 3, 4, 5 & 6 or more carbon atoms (known as trioses, tetroses, pentoses, hexoses, etc)
    - Most common include glucose, fructose, galactose
  - Disaccharides

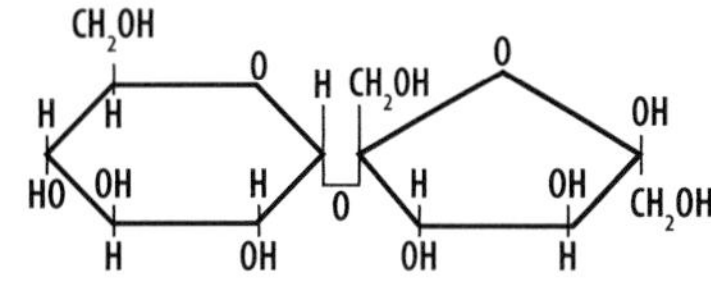

    - Contain 2 monosaccharides linked together—still considered simple sugars
    - Upon hydrolysis, will yield 2 monosaccharides
    - Formed upon the interaction of groups between 2 monosaccharides with the loss of a molecule of water
    - Most common
      - Maltose (glucose + glucose)
      - Lactose (glucose + galactose)
      - Sucrose (glucose + fructose)
  - Polysaccharides

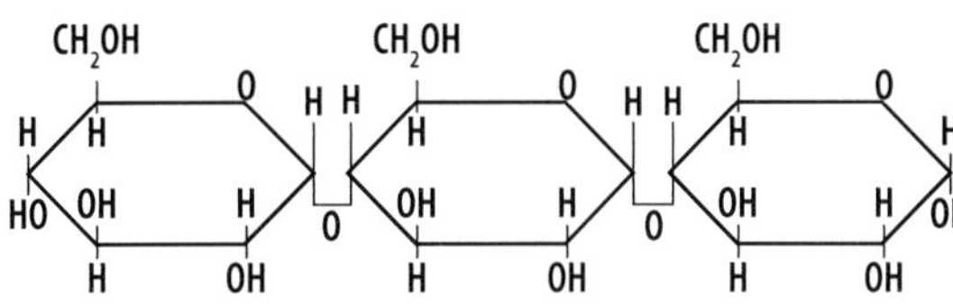

    - Upon hydrolysis, will yield more than 10 monosaccharides
    - Formed by the linkage of many monosaccharide units together
    - Most common
      - Starch (glucose molecules)
      - Glycogen
      - High fiber
  - Stereoisomers
- Digestion & absorption
  - Polysaccharides
    - Amylase hydrolyzes starch to disaccharides in the duodenum
  - Disaccharides
    - Split into monosaccharides by disaccharide enzymes (such as lactase) located on the microvilli of the intestine
    - These monosaccharides are then actively absorbed
  - Monosaccharides
    - Absorbed by specific active transport mechanisms

2.1.2 Chemical properties of carbohydrates

2.1.2.1 Nonreducing substances

- Do not have an active ketone or aldehyde group
- Will not oxidize or reduce other compounds
- Most common: Sucrose (table sugar)

2.1.2.2 Reducing substances

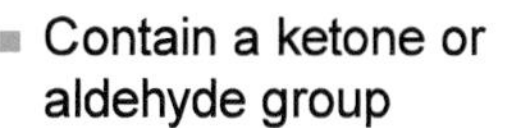

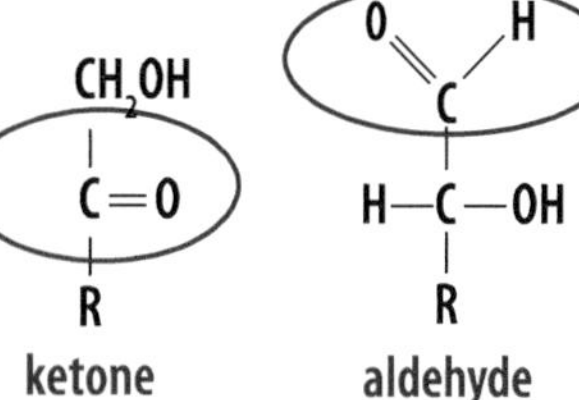

- Contain a ketone or aldehyde group
- Can oxidize or reduce other compounds
- This property is used in many methods in the determination of carbohydrates
- Most common
  - Glucose
  - Fructose
  - Galactose
  - Maltose
  - Lactose
- Can form glycosidic bonds with other carbohydrates and with noncarbohydrates
  - The aldose or ketone group on the carbohydrate forms an oxygen bond
  - If the bond is formed with the anomeric carbon on the other carbohydrate, the resulting compound is NO longer a reducing substance
  - If the bond forms with 1 of the other carbons on the carbohydrate, the anomeric carbon (functional group) is unaltered and the resulting compound remains a reducing substance

2.1.3 Glucose metabolism

2.1.3.1 Glycolysis

- Metabolism of glucose molecule to pyruvate or lactate for production of energy
  glucose→ G6P→ triose P→ pyruvate → lactate or acetyl CoA
- Embden-Meyerhof pathway
  glucose → pyruvate
- Aerobic pathway (requires oxygen)
  pyruvate→ acetyl CoA→ H_2O + CO_2 + ATP (TCA cycle)

- Anaerobic pathway (when pyruvate cannot enter the aerobic pathway)

pyruvate⟶ lactate

2.1.3.2 Glycogenesis

- Conversion of glucose to glycogen for storage
- Major tissues involved in storage: Liver & muscle

glucose ⟶ G6P⟶ glycogen

2.1.3.3 Glycogenolysis

- Breakdown of glycogen to glucose for use as energy

glycogen⟶ G6P⟶ triose P⟶ pyruvate

2.1.3.4 Lipogenesis

- Conversion of carbohydrates to fatty acids
- Occurs in adipose tissue and the liver
- Lipolysis: Decomposition of fat

G6P ⟶ triose P⟶ pyruvate

2.1.3.5 Gluconeogenesis

- Formation of glucose-6-phosphate from non-carbohydrate sources

fatty acids⟶ acetyl CoA *OR* amino acids⟶ Krebs cycle⟶ acetyl CoA

2.1.4 Regulation of carbohydrate metabolism

2.1.4.1 Major hormones from pancreas are involved in carbohydrate metabolism

2.1.4.1.1 Insulin

- Source: β islets cells of Langerhans in pancreas
- Normally released when glucose levels are high, not released when glucose levels are decreased
- Only hormone that decreases glucose levels
- A hypoglycemic agent
- Mode of action
  - ↓ plasma glucose levels by:
    - Glycogenesis
    - Lipogenesis
    - Glycolysis
  - ↑ transport entry of glucose in muscle and adipose tissue via nonspecific receptors
    - Inhibits glycogenolysis

2.1.4.1.2 Glucagon

- Source: α islet cells of Langerhans in pancreas
- Regulation: Released in stress & fasting states
- Referred to as a hyperglycemic agent
- Mode of action: Increases plasma glucose levels by
  - Glycogenolysis in liver
  - Increased gluconeogenesis

2.1.4.1.3 Somatostatin

- Source: D cells of the islets of Langerhans in pancreas
- Regulation: SST1-5 receptors
- Mode of action: Increases plasma glucose levels by:
  - Inhibition of insulin, glucagon, growth hormone, and other endocrine hormones
- If one had to summarize the effects of somatostatin in 1 phrase, it would be: "Somatostatin inhibits the secretion of many other hormones"

2.1.4.2 Hormones produced by the adrenal gland affect carbohydrate metabolism

2.1.4.2.1 Epinephrine

- Produced by the adrenal medulla
- Regulation: Release stimulated by physical or emotional stress (fight or flight)
- Mode of action
  - Inhibits insulin secretion
  - Promotes lipolysis
  - Increases plasma glucose by glycogenolysis

2.1.4.2.2 Cortisol

- Produced by the adrenal cortex
- Regulation: Release stimulated by adrenocorticotropin hormone (ACTH)
- Increases plasma glucose levels by
  - ↑ gluconeogenesis
  - ↑ lipolysis
  - ↓ intestinal absorption
  - ↓ entry into cell
  - ↑ liver glycogen

2.1.4.3 Hormones from anterior pituitary gland

2.1.4.3.1 Growth hormone

- Regulation
  - Release stimulated by ↓ glucose levels and ↓ cortisol levels (ACTH)
  - Inhibited by increased glucose
  - Mode of action: ↑ plasma glucose by:
    - ↓ glycolysis
    - ↓ entry into cells

ISBN 978-089189-6616

2.1.4.3.2 ACTH

- Mode of action
  - Stimulates the adrenal cortex to release cortisol
  - ↑ liver enzymes
  - Promotes gluconeogenesis

2.1.4.4 Other hormones

2.1.4.4.1 Thyroxine

- Source: Thyroid gland
- Regulation: Release stimulated by production of thyroid-stimulating hormone (TSH)
- Mode of action: Increases plasma glucose levels by:
  - ↑ glycogenolysis
  - ↑ gluconeogenesis
  - ↑ intestinal absorption

2.1.4.4.2 Leptin

- A protein hormone with important effects in regulating body weight, metabolism, and reproductive function
- Expressed predominantly by adipocytes, which fits with the idea that body weight is sensed as the total mass of fat in the body
- Affects the hypothalamic centers that control feeding behavior, hunger, body temperature, and energy expenditure
- Blood concentrations of leptin are usually increased in obese humans, suggesting an insensitive to, rather than deficiency

2.1.5 Hyperglycemia

- This is caused by an increase in fasting plasma glucose levels
- Normal values <100 mg/dL ([<5.5 mmol/L]) fasting
- It is also caused by an imbalance of hormones

2.1.5.1 Diabetes mellitus

- This is a group of metabolic diseases characterized by hyperglycemia resulting from defects in insulin secretion, insulin action, or both

2.1.5.1.1 Symptoms

- Polyuria
- Polydipsia
- Polyphagia
- Blurred vision
- Pruritis
- Increased susceptibility to infection
- Hyperventilation
- Mental confusion
- Loss of consciousness (due to ↑ glucose to brain)

2.1.5.1.2 Laboratory findings

- ↑ glucose in plasma & urine
- ↑ urine specific gravity and serum & urine osmolality
- Ketones in serum & urine (ketonemia & ketonuria)
- ↓ blood & urine pH (acidosis)
- Electrolyte imbalance

2.1.5.1.3 Type 1 diabetes

- Autoimmune islet β cell destruction, causing a deficiency of insulin in 5%-10% of diabetics; most commonly presents in childhood
- Usually insulin dependent
- Autoantibodies include
  - Islet cell antibodies (ICA)
  - Insulin autoantibodies (IAA)
  - Antibodies to glutamic acid decarboxylase (GAD)
  - Insulinoma-associated protein (IA2, ICA512)
- Strong association with the HLA DR and DQ loci, with particular alleles having either predisposing or protective effects

2.1.5.1.4 Type 2 diabetes

- Progressive insulin resistance
- Most common form of diabetes; typically presents in adulthood
- Usually noninsulin dependent

2.1.5.1.5 Gestational diabetes mellitus (GDM)

- Onset of diabetes during pregnancy, even if persists beyond pregnancy

2.1.5.1.6 Acute complications of diabetes mellitus

2.1.5.1.6.1 Diabetic ketoacidosis (DKA)

- Occurs in insulin-dependent diabetics because of lack of insulin/stress
- Can result in death (association with type 1 diabetes), hyperglycemia, ketosis, and metabolic acidosis
- ↓HCO3-, ↓ pH, ↑ glucose
- Glucose usually ≥200 mg/dL (≥11.1 mmol/L), and the venous pH <7.30 (or bicarbonate 15 mEq/L [15 mmol/L])

- Often left-shifted neutrophilia, hyperamylasemia, and hyperlipasemia
- Increased anion gap
- Serum potassium initially elevated but severe hypokalemia may follow treatment
- Ketone bodies
  - Produced in cases of carbohydrate deprivation or decreased carbohydrate utilization
  - Products of incomplete fat metabolism (β oxidation)
  - The 3 ketone bodies are
    - Acetone (2%)
    - Acetoacetic acid (20%)
    - β-hydroxybutyric acid (78%)

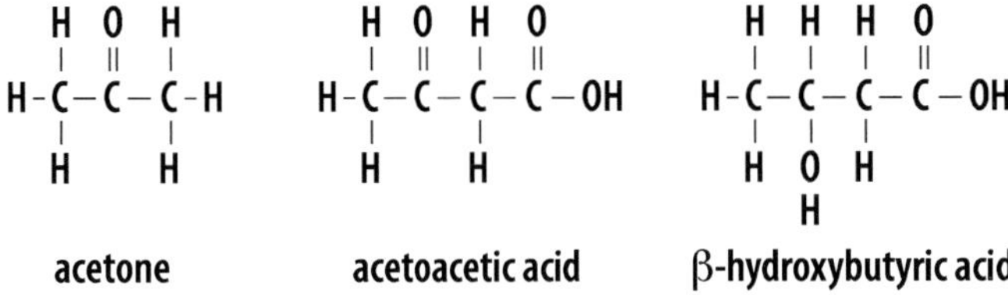

  - Ketonemia: Accumulation of ketones in blood
  - Ketonuria: Accumulation of ketones in urine

2.1.5.1.6.2 Hyperglycemic hyperosmolar nonketotic coma (HHNC)

- Occurs in patients with non-insulin-dependent diabetes
- Altered mental status, profound hyperglycemia, hyperosmolarity, dehydration & essentially normal pH
- ↑ blood osmolarity—osmolarity >330 mOsm/L
- ↑ glucose (>1,000 mg/dL [55.5 mmol/L])
- Normal bicarbonate & ketones
- Lactic acid
- O_2 deprivation of tissues results in blockage of aerobic oxidation of pyruvic acid in TCA cycle
- Anaerobic reduction of pyruvate to lactate results
- Severe O_2 deprivation will result in very high levels of lactate (lactic acidosis) and increased pyruvate
- Severe O_2 deprivation is caused by:
  - Shock
  - Hemorrhage
  - Gram-negative septicemia
- Mild O_2 deprivation may be caused by exercise
- High mortality

2.1.5.1.6.3 Insulin overdose hypoglycemia

- Excessive insulin administration may result in hypoglycemic coma

2.1.5.1.7 Long-term complications

- Retinopathy: Blindness 50% after 10 years
- Nephropathy: Renal disease—proteinuria, increased blood urea nitrogen (BUN) & creatinine
- Neuropathy: Poor sensation, ulceration of skin, may lead to amputation of limbs
- Accelerated macrovascular disease: Coronary artery disease (CAD), cerebral vascular accident (CVA)

2.1.5.1.8 Criteria for testing for prediabetes & diabetes

- Screening tests should be performed for:
  - All adults beginning at age 45 years every 3 years
  - Every year for individuals with ≥1 risk factor
    - Habitually physically inactive
    - Family history of diabetes in a first-degree relative
    - In a high-risk minority population (eg, African American, Latino, Native American, Asian American & Pacific Islander)
    - History of GDM or delivering an infant weighing more than 9 lb (4.1 kg)
    - Hypertension (blood pressure ≥140/90 mm Hg)
    - Reduced high-density lipoprotein (HDL) cholesterol concentrations (<35 mg/dL [<0.90 mmol/L])
    - Elevated triglyceride (TG) concentrations >250 mg/dL (>2.82 mmol/L)
    - A1c concentration ≥5.7% (33 mol/mol), impaired glucose tolerance (IGT) or impaired fasting glycemia (IFG) on previous testing or history of IGT/IFG
    - Women with polycystic ovarian syndrome
    - Other clinical conditions associated with insulin resistance (eg, severe obesity & acanthosis nigricans)
    - History of cardiovascular disease

ISBN 978-089189-6616

2.1.5.1.9 Criteria for the diagnosis of diabetes mellitus

- Four routes to the diagnosis of (nongestational) diabetes mellitus (see t2.1):
  - Fasting plasma glucose (FPG)
  - 75 g oral glucose tolerance test (OGTT)
  - Hemoglobin A1c (HbA1c)
  - Random plasma glucose in patients with classic symptoms

t2.1 Diagnostic criteria for diabetes

One of the following	Notes
HbA1c ≥6.5%	Test should be performed in a laboratory using a method certified by the NGSP & traceable to the DCCT reference assay; point-of-care HbA1c assays are not adequate
FPG ≥126 mg/dL (7 mmol/L)	Fasting = no caloric intake for ≥8 hours
OGTT 2-hour plasma glucose ≥200 mg/dL (≥11.1 mmol/L)	75 g oral glucose load
Random plasma glucose ≥200 mg/dL (≥11.1 mmol/L)	In a patient with classic symptoms of diabetes or in hyperglycemic crisis

DCCT, Diabetes Control & Complications Trial; FPG, fasting plasma glucose; HbA1c, hemoglobin A1c; NGSP, National Glycohemoglobin Standardization Program; OGTT, oral glucose tolerance test

- FPG is the recommended test
- Diagnostic tests with abnormal results should be repeated before a diagnosis is established; alternatively, another test result that is concurrently beyond the threshold renders repeat testing unnecessary
- Three prediabetes/intermediate categories
  - IGT result of 140-200 mg/dL at 2 hours
  - IFG result 110 mg/dL - 126 mg/dL
  - HbA1c of 5.7%-6.4%

2.1.5.1.10 Criteria for the testing & diagnosis of GDM

- In pregnancy, the American Diabetes Association (ADA) recommendations are as follows
  - Women with risk factors are to be tested for type 2 diabetes at the 1st prenatal visit (standard criteria for type 2 diabetes applied)
  - Pregnant women not previously known to have diabetes should be screened for GDM at 24-28 weeks' gestation using a 75 g 2-hour OGTT, after an overnight fast of at least 8 hours, applying the criteria listed t2.2

t2.2 Gestational diabetes diagnostic criteria using 75 g oral glucose tolerance test

Time of collection	Plasma glucose
Fasting	≥92 mg/dL (5.1 mmol/L)
1 hour	≥180 mg/dL (10.0 mmol/L)
2 hours	≥153 mg/dL (8.5 mmol/L)

- After the diagnosis of diabetes is made
  - Day-to-day control
  - Self-monitoring blood glucose
- Long term
  - HbA1c
    - Used to monitor glycemic control
    - ADA recommends at least twice a year in stable patients; goal of therapy is a HbA1c <7%
    - Shows a direct relationship with the glucose level over the preceding 2-3 months
      - <6% is optimal
      - 10%—fair
      - 13%-20%—poor control
  - Glycosylated albumin
  - Microalbumin
    - Monitors kidney function
    - Also a marker of increased risk of cardiovascular morbidity & mortality
    - Annual testing should be performed
    - Serum creatinine should be measured for calculation of the estimated glomerular filtration rate (eGFR)
    - Microalbuminuria defined as excretion of
      - 30-300 mg of albumin/24 hrs or 20-200 µg/min or
      - 30-300 µg/mg creatinine on 2 of 3 urine collections
  - Adult patients should be screened annually for lipid disorders

2.1.6 Hypoglycemia t2.3

2.1.6.1 Symptoms of hypoglycemia

- Neuroglycopenic: Related to the reliance of the brain on glucose for metabolism, such that hypoglycemia directly leads to altered mental status. These symptoms predominate in so-called "fasting" hypoglycemia, in which the drop in serum glucose is moderate and gradual
- Adrenergic: Sweating, palpitations, tachycardia & nervousness. These symptoms predominate in "reactive" hypoglycemia, which tends to be more profound and rapid in onset
- Drug-induced hypoglycemia may be caused by insulin, sulfonylureas (oral hypoglycemic agents), alcohol & quinine

2.1.6.2 Spontaneous (fasting) hypoglycemia

- Gradual onset of hypoglycemia occurs after a prolonged fast

2.1.6.2.1 Characteristics of hypoglycemia

- Nonsuppressible insulinlike activity
- Glucose level drops below normal fasting levels
- Glucose level does *not* spontaneously recover—must give glucose to relieve symptoms

2.1.6.2.2 Causes of hypoglycemia

- These include proliferations of islet β cells (nesidioblastosis or insulinoma), several inherited metabolic defects, certain large sarcomas & end-stage liver disease

2.1.6.2.2.1 Insulinomas: β islet cell tumors

- Neoplasms of β islet cells, resulting in high insulin levels
- Typically presents with Whipple triad of hypoglycemic symptoms, plasma glucose <45 mg/dL (<2.5 mmol/L) & relief of symptoms with glucose administration

t2.3 Hypoglycemia, differential diagnosis

Insulinoma
Nesidioblastosis
Advanced malignancy
Anti-insulin receptor antibodies
Autoimmune insulin syndrome
Post-gastric surgery
Alcohol consumption
Drug induced (exogenous insulin, sulfonylureas, salicylates, quinine, haloperidol, β blockers)
Hepatic failure
Inborn errors of metabolism (glycogen storage disease, hereditary fructose intolerance, galactosemia, carnitine deficiency)
Starvation

2.1.6.3 Reactive (postprandial) hypoglycemia

- Rapid onset hypoglycemia following a meal
- Excessive release of insulin
- Glucose level drops below normal fasting levels
- Spontaneous recovery of glucose level because of insulin levels returning to normal

2.1.6.3.1 Types

- Alimentary: Accelerated absorption of glucose
- Functional: Occurs in fasting states
- Causes: Hereditary fructose intolerance, galactosemia, postvagotomy states (dumping syndrome), and (sometimes) early type 2 diabetes mellitus

2.1.6.4 Signs & symptoms

- Increased hunger
- Sweating
- Nausea & vomiting
- Dizziness
- Nervousness & shaking
- Blurring of speech & sight
- Mental confusion

2.1.6.5 Laboratory findings

- Decreased plasma glucose levels during hypoglycemic episode
- Extremely elevated insulin levels in β cell tumors (insulinoma)

2.1.6.6 Diagnosis

- Diagnosis is made:
  - If the patient complains of symptoms of hypoglycemia
  - If blood glucose levels are measured while the person is experiencing those symptoms and found to be ≤45 mg/dL (≤2.5 mmol/L) in a woman or ≤55 mg/dL (≤3.0 mmol/L) in a man
  - If the symptoms are promptly relieved on ingestion of sugar

2.1.6.7 Other laboratory tests

- Insulin production
- C-peptide levels

2.1.7 Genetic defects in carbohydrate metabolism

2.1.7.1 Glycogen storage disease

- This occurs with a deficiency of 1 of the 8 enzymes that break down glycogen

2.1.7.2 Glucose-6-phosphatase deficiency type 1 (von Gierke disease)

- This is an autosomal recessive disease characterized by severe hypoglycemia, metabolic acidosis, ketonemia, and elevated lactate & alanine
- Hypoglycemia occurs because glycogen cannot be converted back to glucose by way of hepatic glycogenolysis and glycogen buildup is found in the liver, causing hepatomegaly
- The patients usually have severe hypoglycemia, hyperlipidemia, uricemia & growth restriction

ISBN 978-089189-6616

2.1.7.3 Galactosemia

- Definition: Deficiency of 1 of 3 enzymes involved in galactose metabolism, resulting in increased levels of galactose in plasma
- Most common enzyme deficiency is galactose-1-phosphate uridyl transferase (type 1)
- Other enzymes include:
  - Galactokinase deficiency (type II)
  - Uridine diphosphate 4 epimerase (UDPG-epimerase) deficiency (type III)
- Signs & symptoms: Failure to thrive, intestinal problems, jaundice
- Laboratory findings: Hypoglycemia, hyperbilirubinemia, galactose accumulation in blood, tissues & urine following milk ingestion
- Prognosis & treatment
  - Controlled by a galactose-free diet
  - If left untreated, the patient will develop intellectual disability and cataracts

2.1.8 Principles of measurement

2.1.8.1 Specimen collection & handling

- The preferred specimen is drawn early in the morning after an 8-hour fast
- Plasma glucose levels are 10% lower in the afternoon
- Current diagnostic criteria for diabetes are based on plasma glucose levels in blood samples obtained in the morning after an overnight fast, with a value of ≥126 mg/dL (≥7.0 mmol/L) indicating diabetes
- Plasma or serum can be used
- Preferred: Sodium fluoride (NaF), anticoagulated (oxalate)
- If not drawn in gray top tubes, the specimen must be separated from cells within 1 hour of draw time
- When the blood specimen is left in an unseparated test tube, glycolysis will reduce the glucose by ~5-10 mg/dL per hour depending on the temperature and white cell count
- NaF arrests this process for 24 hours; however, the initial arrest of glycolysis takes 1-2 hours to take effect, so an initial decrement of 5-10 mg/dL can be expected even in the presence of NaF
- Uncalibrated whole blood glucose usually runs 10%-15% lower than plasma glucose (depending on the hematocrit)
- After a glucose load, capillary values ↑ ~20 mg/dL

2.1.8.2 Methods

2.1.8.2.1 Glucose oxidase reaction

- Step 1: Enzymatic

$$\text{glucose} + O_2 + H_2O \xrightarrow{\text{glucose oxidase}} \text{gluconic acid} + H_2O_2$$

- Step 2: Spectrophotometric measurement

$$H_2O_2 + \text{reduced chromogen} \xrightarrow{\text{peroxidase}} \text{oxidized chromogen} + H_2O$$

- Spectrophotometric measurement of oxidized chromogen is proportional to the amount of glucose
- Most automated analyzers use this reaction (note: home glucose analyzers use this principle with capillary whole blood)
- Increased levels of ascorbic acid and uric acid depress the glucose oxidase reaction (falsely decreased)

2.1.8.2.2 Oxygen consumption electrode

$$\text{glucose} + O_2 + H_2O \xrightarrow{\text{glucose oxidase}} \text{gluconic acid} + H_2O_2$$

- Oxygen *depletion* is measured, which is proportional to the amount of glucose present

2.1.8.2.3 I-Stat

- Glucose is measured amperometrically
- Oxidation of glucose, catalyzed by the enzyme glucose oxidase, produces hydrogen peroxide (H_2O_2)
- H_2O_2 is oxidized at an electrode to produce an electric current that is proportional to the glucose concentration
- Increased levels of ascorbic acid and uric acid depress the glucose oxidase reaction (falsely decreased)

2.1.8.2.4 Hexokinase reaction

- This is generally accepted as the reference method

$$\text{glucose} + \text{ATP} \xrightarrow{\text{hexokinase}} \text{glucose-6-}PO_4 + \text{ADP}$$

$$\text{glucose-6-}PO_4 + \text{NADP} \xrightarrow{\text{G6PD}} \text{NADPH} \rightarrow + H^+ + \text{6-phosphogluconate}$$

- The amount of *NADPH* is measured and is proportional to amount of glucose present and is not affected by ascorbic acid or uric acid
- Gross hemolysis and extremely elevated bilirubin may cause a false decrease in results

2.1.8.2.5 Chemical analysis (nonspecific reactions)

- In this method, concentrations of glucose and other substances are measured
- Copper reduction methods

$$\text{glucose (and other reducing substances)} + Cu^{+2} \rightarrow \text{(brick red ppt)}$$

- Benedict modification = Clinitest reaction
  - Used in urine glucose measurements to detect the presence of reducing sugars other than glucose (inborn errors)

2.1.8.2.6 Glucose tolerance & 2-hour postprandial tests

- 2-hour test
  - This is performed using a standardized load of glucose (75 mg/dL [4.1 mmol/L]) or performed 2 hours after eating
  - Measure plasma fasting glucose at 2 hours
- Oral glucose tolerance test
  - This is not recommended for routine use
  - Only the fasting and the 2-hour sample measurements are recommended, except in pregnant women
  - The adult dose of glucose solution is 75 g
  - Children receive 1.75 g/kg of glucose to a maximum dose of 75 g

2.1.8.2.7 Glycosylated hemoglobin/HbA1c

- Glycosylated hemoglobin is formed when hemoglobin undergoes nonenzymatic reaction with glucose
- One type of glycosylated hemoglobin is HgbA1c; normal HgbA1c is <6%
- HgbA1c depends on the concentration of serum glucose and the lifespan of the red cells (shortened red cell survival leads to relatively decreased HgbA1c)
- Conditions that result in decreased lifespan of RBCs will cause falsely decreased HbA1c values: Hemolytic anemia, polycythemia, homozygous hemoglobin S (HbS) & hemoglobin C (HbC)
- HbA1c is an indicator of glucose concentrations over the preceding 3 months
- HbA1c can be translated into average blood glucose (AG) through the use of a formula:

$$\text{AG (in mg/dL)} = (28.7 \times \text{HbA1c}) - 46.7$$

2.1.8.2.7.1 Specimen requirement

- EDTA whole blood sample
- A hemolysate must be prepared before analysis

2.1.8.2.7.2 Methods of measurement

- Methods based on structural differences:
  - Affinity chromatography (preferred method)
    - Separation is based on chemical structure
    - Glycosylated hemoglobin attaches to the boronate group of resin
    - Glycosylated hemoglobin is selectively eluted from the resin bed by using a buffer
    - This method is not temperature dependent
    - Not affected by hemoglobin F (HbF), hemoglobin S (HbS), or hemoglobin C (HbC)
  - Immunoassays
    - Poly or monoclonal antibodies toward glycated N-terminal group of β chain on hemoglobin
    - Latex immunoagglutination inhibition methodology
    - Mouse monoclonal antibody specific for HbA1c is used
    - HbA1c and total hemoglobin concentrations are measured, and the ratio between the 2 is reported as "percent HbA1c"
    - Immunoassays do not measure glycated HbF
    - <10% HbF indicates that the patient's glycemic control is accurate
    - >10% HbF HbA1c amount will be lower than expected
- Methods based on charge differences:
  - Cation exchange chromatography
    - Negatively charged hemoglobins attach to positively charged resin bed
    - Uses specific pH buffer to selectively elute from resin bed
    - This method is highly temperature dependent
    - Effected by hemoglobinopathies
    - HbF yields falsely increased levels
    - HbS & HbC yield falsely decreased levels
  - High-pressure liquid chromatography (HPLC)
    - Separation of all forms of glycosylated hemoglobin: A1a, A1b, A1c
  - Electrophoresis
    - Separation based on charge of each hemoglobin type
    - HbF values >7% causes interference

2.1.8.2.8 Ketones

- Specimen requirement
  - **Fresh** serum or urine samples may be analyzed
  - The sample should be tightly stoppered and analyzed immediately
  - Limitation: No method used for determination of ketones reacts with all 3 ketone bodies
- Methods of measurement
  - Sodium nitroprusside [$NaFe(CN)_5NO$] reaction

$$\text{acetoacetic acid + nitroprusside} \xrightarrow{\text{Alk OH}} \text{purple color}$$

ISBN 978-089189-6616

- This method is used with reagent strip test and Acetest tablets
- The addition of glycine to the reagent allows measurement of both acetoacetic acid and acetone
- This method is sensitive to acetone and acetoacetic acid but not β hydroxybutyrate, which, in DKA, is often 80% of serum ketones

- Enzymatic method

$$NADH + H^+ + \text{acetoacetic acid} \xrightarrow{B\text{-}HBD} NAD + \beta\ \text{hydroxybutyric acid}$$

- Detects β hydroxybutyric acid or acetoacetic acid
- Enzyme = β hydroxybutyrate dehydrogenase (B-HBD)
- pH-dependent reaction
  - pH 7.0: Reaction proceeds to the right (decreasing absorbance)
  - pH 8.5-9.5: Reaction proceeds to left (increasing absorbance)

2.1.8.2.9 Microalbuminuria

- This is measured as a ratio of albumin to creatinine
- Albumin
  - Dye binding is performed using a high-affinity sulfonephthalein dye
- Creatinine
  - This is based on the peroxidaselike activity of a copper creatinine complex that catalyzes the reaction of di-isopropylbenzene dihydroperoxide and 3,3',5,5'-tetramethylbenzidine
  - This method has fewer false reactions caused by extremes in urine concentration
- Immunoassays
  - In the reaction, urine albumin combines with specific antibody to form insoluble antigen-antibody complexes
  - The system monitors the change in absorbance at 380 nm
  - This change in absorbance is proportional to the amount of albumin

2.1.8.2.10 C peptide

- This is a substance that the pancreas releases into the bloodstream in equal amounts to insulin
- Although C peptide and insulin are produced in equimolar quantities, the ratio of C peptide to insulin is ~5-15:1 (when both insulin and C peptide are expressed in SI units [picomoles per liter])
- The major clinical use of C-peptide measurement is for the detection of exogenous insulin administration

2.1.8.2.11 Islet autoantibody & insulin testing

- Insulin testing
  - Primarily performed to determine cause of hypoglycemia and to monitor treatment
  - Man be used to identify an individual with insulin resistance
  - May also be performed in conjunction with C-peptide to differentiate between exogenous and endogenous insulin levels
- Islet autoantibodies (3 types)
  - Presence of autoantibodies to the β-islet cells of the pancreas is characteristic of type 1 diabetes
  - Testing is not currently recommended for routine screening for diabetes diagnosis
- Insulin autoantibodies
  - Detected in about 50% of type 1 diabetic children; not commonly detected in adults
  - Test does not differentiate between exogenous and endogenous insulin

2.2 Lipids

2.2.1 Typical classification

- Lipids comprise a heterozygous group of compounds that are related to fatty acids

2.2.1.1 Simple

- This group includes esters of the fatty acids with various alcohols
  - This category includes esters of fatty acids with glycerol
- Simple lipids contain 3 carbon atoms
  - Saturated: These simple lipids contain no double bonds
  - Unsaturated: These contain ≥1 double bonds
- These can be hydrolyzed by strong alkalis or acids or by enzymes known as lipases
- If acid is used for hydrolysis, free fatty acid + glycerol are liberated
- If an alkali is used, a soap is formed along with glycerol (called saponification)
- Triglycerides
  - Neutral glycerides
  - Can be hydrolyzed by strong alkalis or acids or by enzymes known as lipases
  - Are liquid
  - Prevalent tissue storage fat
  - Form in adipose tissue

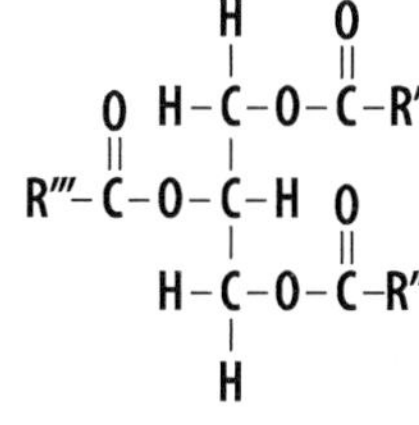

- Waxes-esters of the fatty acids with alcohols other than glycerol cholesterol

2.2.1.2 Conjugated

- Esters of the fatty acid-containing groups in addition to an alcohol & fatty acid
- Phospholipids
  - Substituted fats containing phosphoric acid and nitrogen
  - Lecithin, cephalin, sphingomyelin
- Glycolipids
  - These are compounds of the fatty acids with a carbohydrate and contain nitrogen but no phosphoric acid
  - Cerebrosides, sphingolipids, sphingosine
    - Sphingolipids: Sphingomyelin is of primary importance in the structure of cell membranes and the central nervous system (CNS)
- Lipoproteins
  - These are responsible for lipid transport
  - These include chylomicrons, low-density lipoproteins (LDL), HDL & very-low-density lipoproteins (VLDL)
- Aminolipids, sulfolipids
  - These comprise groups that are at present not sufficiently well characterized for classification

2.2.1.3 Derived

- Derived lipids include substances derived from the aforementioned groups by hydrolysis
- Fatty acids
  - These include straight chain carboxylic acids, free fatty acids & essential fatty acids such as oleic acid, linoleic acid, arachidonic
  - They are a source of energy when carbohydrate metabolism is unavailable by means of β oxidation to ketones
  - Fatty acids are precursors of prostaglandins
- Alcohols
  - Sterols: Derived from the primary sterol (cholesterol) our bodies produce, such as bile acids, steroid hormones & vitamin D
    - Alcoholic lipids include in their molecular structures a skeleton of tetracyclic perhydrocyclopentanophenanthrene
    - Cholesterol (sterol ester)
  - Bile acids
    - They emulsify fats
  - They activate gastrointestinal (GI) lipases

cholesterol

2.2.1.4 Lipoproteins

2.2.1.4.1 Transport form of lipids

- Ingested lipids are internalized by small bowel enterocytes and packaged into chylomicrons; they transport lipid from enterocytes to hepatocytes, into which they are endocytosed via apolipoprotein E
- In the liver, cholesterol and triglycerides (TG) undergo additional metabolism before being packaged into VLDL, which is the vehicle for transport into the bloodstream
- In blood, the TG in VLDL undergoes progressive hydrolysis by the endothelium-bound lipoprotein lipase (LPL), producing intermediate-density lipoprotein (IDL) and, eventually, LDL
- LDL is the main vehicle for transporting cholesterol from the bloodstream to somatic cells, where LDL particles undergo endocytosis mediated by the LDL receptor and apolipoprotein B100
- The liver also produces HDL, a scavenger of cholesterol

2.2.1.4.2 Lipid-protein complex

- Every lipoprotein contains cholesterol, TG, phospholipids & apolipoproteins
- 5 different lipoprotein classes are identified based on the various proportions of these 4 constituents and the particular apolipoproteins they possess **t2.4**

t2.4 Lipoprotein classes

Lipoprotein	Electrophoretic mobility	Average density (g/mL)	Major lipid	Protein (%)	Apolipoproteins
Chylomicrons	Origin	0.95	TG	1	B-48, A-1, CII, E
VLDL	pre-β	1	TG	8	B-100, C, E
IDL	pre-β/β	1.02	Cholesterol	15	B-100, E
LDL	β	1.04	Cholesterol	20	B-100
HDL	α	1.1	Cholesterol	50	A-1, C, E

HDL, high-density lipoprotein; IDL, intermediate-density lipoprotein; TG, triglyceride; VLDL, very-high-density lipoprotein

ISBN 978-089189-6616

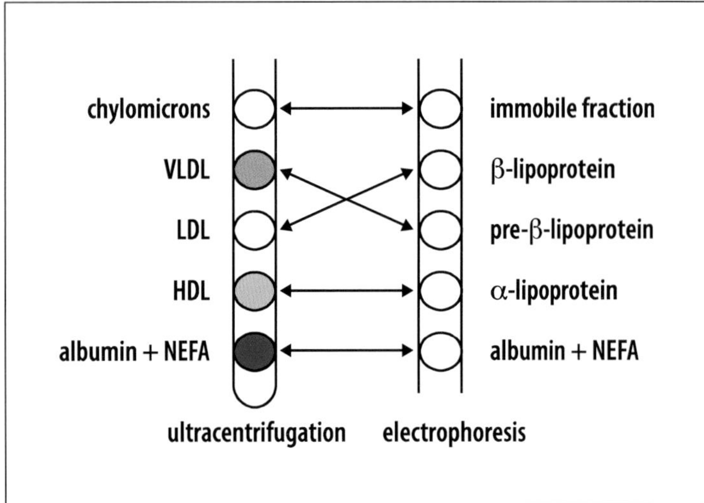

f2.1 Comparison of ultracentrifugation & lipoprotein electrophoresis
NEFA, nonesterified fatty acids

2.2.1.4.3 Classification of lipoproteins

- Lipoproteins are classified using the following methods

2.2.1.4.3.1 Ultracentrifugation

2.2.1.4.3.2 Lipoprotein electrophoresis

- Difference because of relative lipid-protein ratio f2.1
- Increasing density correlates with increasing protein content
- Chylomicrons are major carrier of exogenous trigycerides (TG); do not move from the point of application
- Very-low-density lipoproteins (VLDL) are seen in the pre-β region
- Intermediate-density lipoproteins (IDL)
- Low-density lipoproteins (LDL) migrate in the β region
- High-density lipoproteins (HDL) are in the α region

2.2.1.4.3.3 Electrophoresis (order of migration)

- This is based on electrophoretic mobility
- This is based on both charge and molecular size decreasing
- Lipoproteins separated by alkaline electrophoresis migrate anodically
- (+) alpha, pre-β, β, chylomicrons (at origin) (–)

2.2.1.4.3.4 Overnight refrigeration produces characteristic patterns in plasma

- A creamy layer atop the plasma indicates excess chylomicrons
- Turbidity or opacity of the plasma indicates abundant VLDL
- LDL and HDL, even when present in excess, do not visibly alter the plasma

2.2.1.5 Apolipoproteins

- They act as receptor sites
- Protein moieties are associated with plasma lipoproteins
- Protein units found in lipoproteins but not yet incorporated into a lipoprotein molecule include
  - Apoprotein A1 (major constituent of HDL), apoprotein B (B-100 predominantly in LDL)
  - Apoprotein C (associated with VLDL and HDL, activates LPL, leading to breakdown of TG)
  - Apoprotein D (a glycoprotein, transfers protein molecules)
  - Apoprotein E (primarily a marker for hepatic receptors, synthesized in the liver and incorporated into HDL and then transferred to VLDL and chylomicrons to initiate binding and catabolism)

2.2.2 General function of lipids

- Lipids are the structural and functional element of cell membranes
- They serve as precursors for other essential compounds
- They act as a source of energy
- Lipids act a storage form of energy and as insulators against heat loss and organ damage
- They allow for nerve conduction in the CNS

2.2.3 Metabolism of lipids

2.2.3.1 Dietary source & liver synthesis

- The liver synthesizes 1.5 g of lipids per day (90%)
- Dietary sources contribute 150-300 mg/day
- Lipids constitute 40% of the typical American diet including
  - 35% saturated animal lipids, 98%-99% TG, with the rest being cholesterol and other lipids, and 5% polyunsaturated vegetable lipids
- The body produces most of its cholesterol by endogenous synthesis in the liver from acetyl CoA

2.2.3.2 Exogenous pathway

2.2.3.2.1 Digestive phase

- Most digestion of dietary fats occurs in the intestine
- Bile salts "emulsify" or break up the large dietary TG molecules into very small particles (1 μm) that can be acted upon by digestive enzymes
- Only a small percentage of the lipids are hydrolyzed to free fatty acids and glycerol

- Pancreatic and intestinal enzymes "digest" cholesterol and the emulsified TG so that they can enter the mucosal cell as small aggregates called micelles (5 nm)

2.2.3.2.2 Absorptive phase

- Once in the mucosal cell of the intestine, a reassembly process regenerates TG and cholesterol
- Lipids are released into circulation in 2 forms:
  - chylomicrons, a lipoprotein
  - free fatty acids bound to albumin

2.2.3.2.3 Transport phase

- Chylomicrons are transported to all tissues in the body
- Chylomicrons, heavily laden with TG, are rapidly cleared (within minutes)
- Primary site of uptake is adipose tissue

2.2.3.2.4 Lymphatic transport

2.2.3.2.5 Intracellular metabolism

- Chylomicron catabolism occurs in 2 phases
  - Phase 1
    - Occurs at extrahepatic tissue sites
    - Chylomicrons are hydrolyzed by an enzyme yielding a remnant particle which is relatively TG-poor and cholesterol-rich
  - Phase 2
    - Occurs in the liver
    - Chylomicron remnant is degraded to VLDL
- VLDL catabolism
  - VLDL is released into the bloodstream, where it "gives up" some of its lipid content, resulting in an IDL particle
  - IDL is recognized by the liver and degraded to LDL
  - Hepatocytes and peripheral tissue cells recognize and bind to regions on the LDL membrane
  - The cholesterol-rich LDL is engulfed by cells (including smooth muscle cells), leading to deposits of cholesterol in the cytoplasm of tissue cells
  - Smooth muscle accumulation of LDL cholesterol results in atherosclerotic plaques in arterial walls
- HDL production
  - HDL is produced in both the liver and intestinal wall (and enter peripheral circulation via the thoracic duct)
  - HDL serves to transport cholesterol away from tissues and thus provides some protection against CAD

2.2.3.3 Endogenous pathway

- This includes the following processes:
  - Hepatic lipoprotein synthesis

    chylomicrons → VLDL
  - Cellular metabolism

    VLDL → IDL

    IDL → LDL
  - Hepatic metabolism

    LDL → bile acids
  - HDL metabolism
    - HDL "reverse cholesterol transport": excess cholesterol is transported back to the liver
    - Sythesizes HDL

2.2.4 Clinical significance

2.2.4.1 Cholesterol

- This is dependent on many factors, including genetics, age, sex, diet, physical activity, hormones & primary disease states
- American Heart Association recommendation is for levels to be <200 mg/dL (5.1 mmol/L)
- It is suggested that at least 3 cholesterol measurements be obtained to establish a baseline value (diurnal variation)
- Increased cholesterol is usually a result of:
  - Hypothyroidism (endocrine disease)
  - Liver disease
  - Renal disease (nephrotic syndrome)
  - Diabetes
- Decreased cholesterol is usually a result of
  - Hyperthyroidism
  - An inherited deficiency
  - Malabsorption problems
  - Impaired liver function

2.2.4.1.1 HDL cholesterol

- This is considered the hero; it is inversely correlated with coronary artery disease (CAD)
- HDL cholesterol transfers cholesterol from the cells back to the liver
- Reference range: >45 mg/dL (1.1 mmol/L) in men and >55 mg/dL (1.4 mmol/L) in women
- Factors that increase HDL include:
  - Estrogen (women)
  - Exercise
  - Alcohol
  - Blood pressure medicine

ISBN 978-089189-6616

- Factors that decrease HDL include:
  - Progesterone
  - Obesity
  - Smoking
  - Triglycerides
  - Diabetes

2.2.4.1.2 LDL cholesterol

- This is considered the villain; it is directly correlated with coronary artery disease (CAD)
- It carries cholesterol from its site of origin into the blood vessels
- Reference ranges
  - Optimal: <100 mg/dL (2.6 mmol/L)
  - Near or above optimal: 100-129 mg/dL (2.6-3.3 mmol/L)
  - Borderline high: 130-159 mg/dL (3.3-4.1 mmol/L)
  - High: 160-189 mg/dL (4.1-4.9 mmol/L)
  - Very high: >190 mg/dL (>4.9 mmol/L)

2.2.4.1.3 Triglycerides (TG)

- The role of TG as a risk factor remains unsettled
- They are considered an independent risk factor
- Definite positive association between TG & CAD: <150 mg/dL desired
- Although high TG levels may not cause atherosclerosis, they may indirectly accelerate atherogenesis by influencing the concentration and composition of other lipoproteins
- Conditions that may cause increased glycerol levels include:
  - Collection of sample in test tube containing glycerol (glycerol-stoppered tube)
  - Stress (epinephrine effect)
  - Mannitol infusion
  - Treatment with nitroglycerine
  - Diabetes mellitus
  - Hemodialysis for kidney disease
- Increased TG are usually a result of:
  - A nonfasting sample
  - Pancreatitis
  - Diabetes mellitus
  - Acute alcohol consumption
  - Certain liver disease

2.2.4.1.4 Non-HDL cholesterol

- The sum of VLDL+LDL cholesterol is called non-HDL cholesterol
- It is calculated routinely as total cholesterol – HDL cholesterol
- Non-HDL cholesterol includes all lipoproteins that contain apo B. Persons with high non-HDL cholesterol have a higher risk for atherosclerosis
- It includes other lipid compounds
  - Non-HDL cholesterol
  - If TG >200 mg/dL (2.2 mmol/L) and LDL cholesterol <100 mg/dL (2.6 mmol/L), then look for non-HDL cholesterol
  - Lipoprotein A (a)
    - It is similar in structure to LDL
    - It is a unique protein apo(a) linked to apolipoprotein B-100, with a structure similar to that of plasminogen
    - It is directly correlated with CAD; it is not affected by lifestyle factors such as diet, exercise, or smoking
    - Risk increases at levels >30 mg/dL (0.78 mmol/L)

2.2.4.1.5 Apolipoprotein A

- This is associated with HDL

2.2.4.1.6 Apolipoprotein B-100

- This is associated with LDL

2.2.5 Lipid disorders t2.5

- Premature atherosclerosis is the most notorious consequence of hyperlipidemia, particularly when cholesterol (LDL and/or IDL) is high
- Eruptive xanthomas, presenting as crops of yellow, pruritic papulonodules, are seen with elevated TG (chylomicrons or VLDL)
- Xanthelasma are yellow periorbital papules that are associated with high cholesterol (LDL)
- Acute pancreatitis is associated with elevated TG (chylomicrons or VLDL), particularly when TG exceeds 500 mg/dL (5.6 mmol/L)

2.2.5.1 Predominant hypercholesterolemia

- This occurs when plasma total cholesterol exceeds 200 mg/dL (5.1 mmol/L)
- This condition is usually related to elevated LDL
- Most common primary cause of hypercholesterolemia is familial hypercholesterolemia, an autosomal dominant deficiency of LDL receptors or LDL receptor activity

t2.5 Classification of lipid disorders by predominant lipids

Disorder	Phenotype	Cholesterol	TG	Clinical features
Familial lipoprotein lipase deficiency	I	↑	↑↑↑	Eruptive xanthomas, pancreatitis
Familial apo C-II deficiency	I or V	↑	↑↑↑	Pancreatitis
Familial hypercholesterolemia	IIa	↑↑↑	→↑	Tendinous xanthomas, premature atherosclerosis
Familial dysbetalipo-proteinemia	III	↑↑↑	↑↑↑	
Familial combined hyperlipidemia	IIb or IV	↑↑	↑↑	Premature atherosclerosis
Familial hypertriglyceridemia	IV or V	↑	↑↑↑	Eruptive xanthomas, pancreatitis

- Secondary causes of hypercholesterolemia are hypothyroidism, diabetes mellitus, nephrotic syndrome, cholestasis, cyclosporine, thiazide diuretics, or loop diuretics

2.2.5.2 Predominant hypertriglyceridemia

- This is related to elevated chylomicrons or VLDL
- Secondary causes include heavy alcohol consumption, obesity, diabetes mellitus, hepatitis, pregnancy, renal failure, β-blockers, isotretinoin, corticosteroids, nephrotic syndrome & gout
- Primary causes include familial combined hyperlipidemia, familial LPL deficiency, familial apo C II deficiency & familial hypertriglyceridemia
- Mixed cases of hypertriglyceridemia and hypercholesterolemia are seen
- It is most common in severe diabetes mellitus, hypothyroidism, or nephrotic syndrome; it also may be seen with thiazides, loop diuretics & β-blockers
- Primary causes include familial combined hyperlipidemia and type III hyperlipidemia (dysbetalipoproteinemia)

2.2.5.3 Low levels of HDL cholesterol

- HDL levels <35 mg/dL (0.9 mmol/L) are an independent risk factor for premature atherosclerosis
- Tangier disease: Autosomal recessive disorder characterized by low cholesterol, normal to increased TG, absent HDL, and absence of Apo A1; cholesterol esters deposit in the tonsils, lymph nodes, vasculature & spleen, and corneal opacities develop
- Secondary causes: Smoking, obesity, sedentary lifestyle & anabolic steroids

2.2.5.4 Lipids in the assessment of CAD risk

- The Third Adult Treatment Panel report (ATP III) lists the major risk factors for CAD: smoking, hypertension, low HDL, family history of premature CAD & age (<45 years for men and <55 years for women)
- ATP III recommends a fasting lipoprotein profile (including total cholesterol, LDL cholesterol, HDL cholesterol & TG) for all patients
- ATP III recommends specific cholesterol and LDL targets **t2.6** & **t2.7**

t2.6 ATP III cholesterol classification

Total cholesterol, mg/dL (mmol/L)	Desirable <200 (<5.1) Borderline 200-239 (5.1-6.1) High >240 (>6.2)
LDL (mg/dL)	Optimal <100 (<2.6) Near optimal 100 129 (2.6-3.3) Borderline 130 159 (3.3-4.1) High 160 189 (4.1-4.9) Very high >190 (>4.9)
HDL (mg/dL)	Low <40 (<1) High >60 (1.5)

ATP III, Third Adult Treatment Panel; HDL, high-density lipoprotein; LDL, low-density lipoprotein

t2.7 ATP III recommended LDL targets

Risk group	Notes	Target LDL
Presence of coronary artery disease (CAD) or CAD equivalents	CAD equivalents: Diabetes, noncoronary atherosclerotic vascular disease, Framingham risk of MI within 10 years of >20% (a complex formula determines this risk)	<100 mg/dL (<2.6 mmol/L)
2 or more major risk factors	Major risk factors: Smoking, hypertension (>140/90 mm Hg), HDL <40 mg/dL (1 mmol/L), family history of premature CAD (male 1st degree relative <55 y or female 1st degree relative <65 y), age (men >45 y, women >55 y)	<130 mg/dL (<3.3 mmol/L)
0-1 major risk factors		<160 mg/dL (<4.1 mmol/L)

ATP III, Third Adult Treatment Panel; HDL, high-density lipoprotein; LDL, low-density lipoprotein

2.2.6 Measurement of lipids & lipoproteins

2.2.6.1 Cholesterol

2.2.6.2 Enzyme method

- Free cholesterol in the presence of O_2 reacts with cholesterol oxidase to yield H_2O_2
- At this point measure the rate of O_2 consumption or obtain a reaction of H_2O_2 with a chromogen and read spectrophotometrically

ISBN 978-089189-6616

- Interferences: Reducing substances (ascorbic acid, bilirubin), turbidity

2.2.6.3 HDL cholesterol

- Analytical ultracentrifugation
  - HDL density = 1.063-1.21 g/mL (densest) is considered accurate; it is the classic method and can separate/fractionate all lipoproteins
- Selective precipitation
  - The less dense lipoprotein fractions are precipitated, leaving HDL in the supernatant. The supernatant is measured for cholesterol level
  - Common precipitating reagents include:
    - Heparin-manganese-chloride (method of choice)
    - Dextran sulfate-magnesium chloride
    - Sodium phosphotungstate Mg^{2+}
- Homogeneous enzyme assays (block non-HDL)
  - α cyclodextrin (nonprecipitation method)
    - Makes LDL and VLDL less reactive with cholesterol reagent
    - Makes HDL more reactive with cholesterol reagent

2.2.6.4 LDL cholesterol

- Total cholesterol, HDL, and TG are typically measured, and LDL is calculated using the Friedewald equation:

  calculated LDL = total cholesterol – (HDL + TG/5)
- This calculation is not valid for TG level >400 mg/dL (4.5 mmol/L), if chylomicrons are present, in cholestasis, or in type III dyslipidemia
- Direct measurement
  - This method uses an apolipoprotein antibody that separates LDL from other lipid fractions, then the measurement is taken using total cholesterol methods
    - HDL cholesterol + apo A Ab-bead
    - HDL-Ab bead complex
    - VLDL cholesterol + apo E Ab-bead > VLDL-Ab bead complex

2.2.6.5 VLDL cholesterol

- VLDL cholesterol is often estimated as TG ÷ 5 (when expressed in milligrams per deciliter) or TG ÷ 2.2 (when expressed in millimoles per liter); the estimation is invalid when TG is >400 mg/dL (4.5 mmol/L), when chylomicrons are present, or when there is β VLDL characteristic of the very rare type III dyslipidemia

2.2.6.6 Triglycerides

- Specimen collection
  - Serum, plasma levels generally 2%-5% lower because of efflux of water from red cells (dilutional effect) resulting from the effect of anticoagulant (EDTA)
  - 12- to 16-hour fast, peak lipemia in the plasma is reached 2-4 hours after a meal. It takes approximately 10-12 hours to clear the plasma of exogenous TG (chylomicrons)
  - Blood sample must be collected in a glycerol-free tube
- Visual assessment of appearance
  - Serum appearance after standing overnight in refrigerator: Creamy layer on top of serum indicates the presence of chylomicrons
  - Lactescence indicates the creamy appearance of serum because of TG excess
  - Refrigerator test: Use a serum sample, let set for 18 hours at 4°C. A creamy layer floating on the surface with a clear infranate indicates chylomicrons
- Enzymatic determination of glyceride glycerol
  - This is a common first step in all assays

    triglyceride lipase ⟶ glycerol + FFA & protease
- Glycerol can then be measured based on:
  - NADH consumption or formation (decreasing abs. at 340 nm)
  - Formation of FORMAZON compound (colorimetric)
  - Formation of fluorescent compound
- Fasting >12 hours

2.3 Hemoglobin & porphyrins

2.3.1 Basic structure & solubility of porphyrins

- Porphyrins are cyclic compounds formed by the linkage of 4 pyrrole rings through methylene bridges
  - Only 3 porphyrins are of clinical significance: Uroporphyrin, coproporphyrin & protoporphyrin

2.3.1.1 Structures

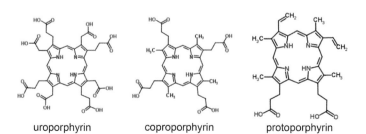

uroporphyrin | coproporphyrin | protoporphyrin

2.3.1.2 Solubility

- Uroporphyrin is highly soluble in H_2O
- Coproporphyrin is soluble in H_2O
- Protoporphyrin is insoluble in H_2O

2.3.2 Heme synthesis

- This occurs in a series of enzymatic reactions beginning with coenzyme A and glycine pyridoxal phosphate, leading to the formation of heme
- Succinyl coenzyme A and glycine pyridoxal phosphate condense to form δ-aminolevulinic acid (DALA)
- Two molecules of DALA condense to form porphobilinogen (PBG)
- Four molecules of PBG condense and cyclize to form uroporphyrinogen (UPG) III
- UPG III is then converted to coproporphyrinogen (CPG) III
- The major portion of UPG III is converted to CPG III, but a small fraction is oxidized to uroporphyrin(URO) III, the form usually found in urine
- Similarly, a small fraction of CPG III is oxidized to coproporphyrin III and is excreted in the urine
- The major portion of coprophyrinogen III is converted to protoporphyrinogen IX which is oxidized to protoporphyrin IX
- The addition of a ferrous ion forms heme. Further addition of protein and globin produces hemoglobin

2.3.2.1 Metabolic pathway

glycine + succinyl Co A
↓ σ-ALA synthase
aminolevulinic acid
↓ σ-ALA dehydratase
porphobilinogen
↓ UPG synthase
uroporphyrin ← UPG
↓ UPG decarboxylase
coproporphyrin ← CPG
↓ CPG oxidase
protoporphyrinogen
↓ protoporphyrinogen oxidase
protoporphyrin
↓ Fe + heme synthetase or ferrochelatase
heme
↓ + protein
hemoglobin

2.3.2.2 Effect of lead on heme synthesis

- Lead poisoning inhibits σ-ALA dehydrase, ferrochelatase, and coproporphrinogen oxidase enzymes

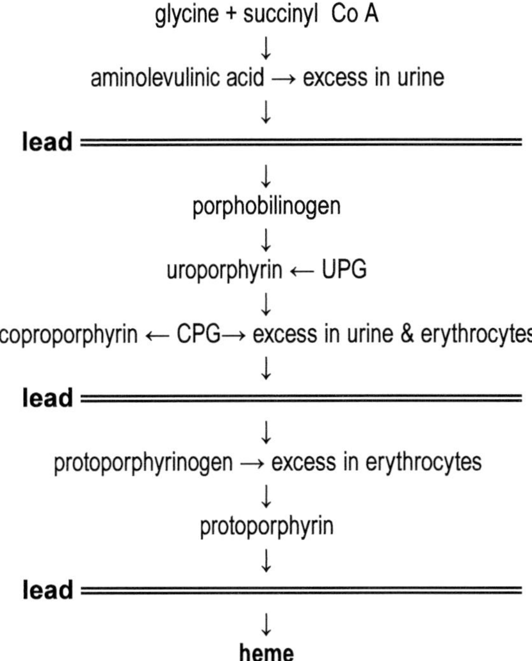

2.3.2.2.1 Laboratory findings

- Increased δ-ALA in urine
- Increased urinary porphyrins
- Free erythrocyte protoporphyrin assay lends itself to mass screenings for lead poisoning

2.3.3 Common causes of porphyrin disorders

2.3.3.1 Porphyrinuria

- This includes secondary conditions with moderate increase in urine coproporphyrin production
- Causes include liver damage, accelerated erythropoiesis, infection & lead intoxication

ISBN 978-089189-6616

2.3.3.2 Porphyria

- This includes a group of inherited disorders that involve a defect in the heme biosynthetic pathways (conversion of glycine to heme)
- It results in overproduction or accumulation of heme precursors
- Each is a result of a deficiency of 1 of the enzymes in the pathway
- Classification is based on the organ involved (ie, the liver or bone marrow). For example,
  - Acute intermittent porphyrin
  - Porphyria variegata
  - Porphyria cutanea tarda
  - Erythropoietic protoporphyria
  - Erythropoietic porphyria

2.3.3.3 Porphyrinemia

- This is a secondary condition with moderate increase in RBC protoporphyrin concentration
- Causes include iron deficiency, chronic infection, impaired iron absorption & lead intoxication

2.3.4 Laboratory measurement

2.3.4.1 Properties of porphyrins

- Dark red or purple
- Irreversibly oxidized on exposure to light
- Fluoresce in organic solutions under UV light

2.3.4.2 Specimen collection & handling

- Random urine sample is collected and must be protected from the light

2.3.4.3 Watson-Swartz test (porphobilinogen [PBG])

- Major reagent: Ehrlich (p-dimethylaminobenzaldehyde)
- PBG + Ehrlich → red color
- Addition of sodium acetate buffers and enhances color
- There are many interferences, therefore extraction must be used
- Initial reaction
  - Urine + Ehrlich + Na acetate
  - If pink color develops, continue
- Primary extraction
  - Add chloroform and shake
  - PBG stays in upper aqueous urine layer
- Confirmatory extraction
  - Add n-butanol and shake
  - This extracts urobilinogen (UBG) into upper (n-butanol) layer
  - PBG stays in lower (urine) layer
- For verification, HCl is added to a fresh urine aliquot. If color develops, it indicates the presence of interfering substances

2.3.4.4 Porphyrin tests

- Based on the principle that porphyrins fluoresce in an organic solution under UV light
- A mixture of amyl alcohol, ethel ether & glacial acetic acid is shaken with an urine aliquot. The upper organic phase is irradiated with a long UV wavelength light and observed for fluorescence (pink) relative to a standard
- Drugs and metabolites may cause interfering fluorescence in the organic layer

2.3.4.5 Free erythrocyte protoporphyrin assay

- Specimen of choice: Whole blood
- Fluorometric measurement

2.4 Liver functions

2.4.1 Anatomy

- The liver anatomy comprises 2 lobes, dual blood supply, portal vein, hepatic artery, lymph vessels & bile ducts
- Liver components include parenchymal cells, sinusoid capillaries, Kupffer cells, portal triad, biliary tree (bile ducts)

2.4.2 Basic functions

- The basic functions of the liver include carbohydrate, protein & lipid metabolism; conjugation, detoxification & excretion; vitamin storage; digestion & formation of bile; hepatocellular & biliary enzyme distribution; and bilirubin metabolism

2.4.2.1 Bilirubin metabolism

- Hemoglobin breakdown **f2.2a**
  - The reticuloendothelial cells break down hemoglobin into bilirubin as follows:

hemoglobin → verdohemoglobin → biliverdin + Fe + globin → bilirubin

  - Hemobglobin forms a complex with albumin to be transported to the liver
- Bilirubin conjugation **f2.2b**
  - The bilirubin-albumin complex is transported by the bloodstream to the liver where it is conjugated

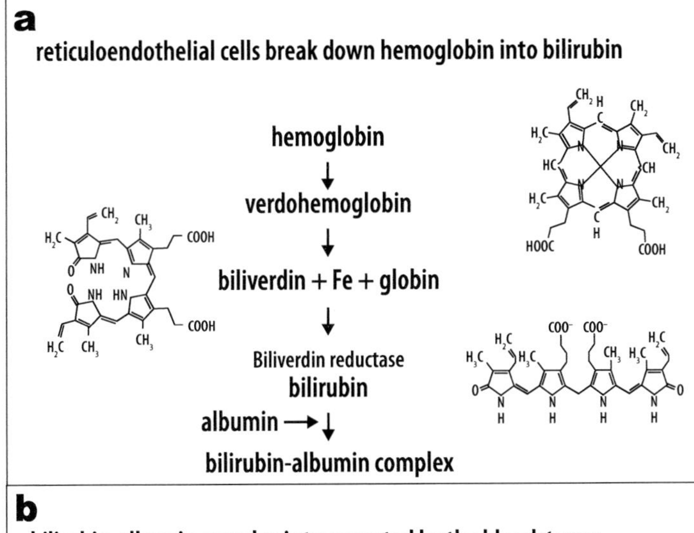

b
bilirubin-albumin complex is transported by the bloodstream to the liver where it is conjugated

bilirubin-albumin complex
to the liver-albumin removed
bilirubin
to parenchymal cells
bilirubin + UDP-glucuronic acid
glucuronyltransferase
bilirubin diglucuronide

c bilirubin diglucuronide excreted to the intestines through the bile ducts where it is converted further for excretion

bilirubin diglucuronide
to intestine
converted to urobilinogen by bacterial enzymes

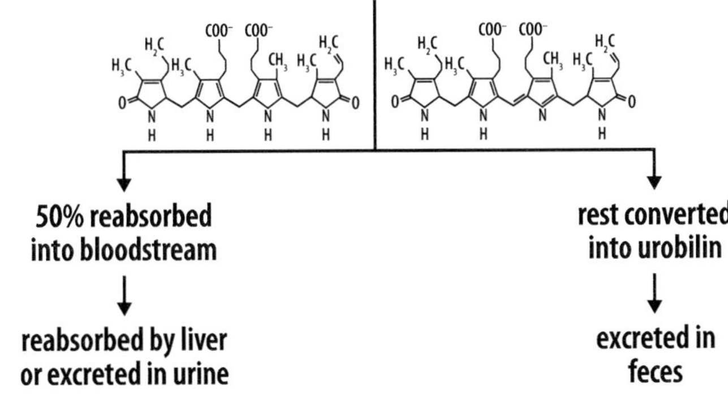

f2.2 Bilirubin metabolism:
a hemoglobin breakdown
b bilirubin conjugation
c urobilinogen formation

UDP, uridine diphosphate

- In the liver
  bilirubin-albumin complex > albumin removed > bilirubin
- In parenchymal cells of liver
  bilirubin + UDP glucuronic acid ⟶ bilirubin diglucuronide

- Urobilinogen formation f2.2c
  - Bilirubin diglucuronide is excreted to the intestines through the bile ducts where it is converted to urobilinogen by bacterial enzymes for excretion
  - Bilirubin diglucuronide > excreted in bile into intestine where bacteria convert some of it to urobilinogen
  - 50% reabsorbed into bloodstream to be reabsorbed by liver or excreted in urine
  - The rest is converted to urobilin and excreted in feces

2.4.3 Definitions

2.4.3.1 Jaundice

- Condition in which the skin, sclerae and mucous membranes are stained yellow because of a prolonged high level of bilirubin in the blood

2.4.3.2 Kernicterus

- Brain damage resulting from high bilirubin levels in infant's blood that can cause athetoid cerebral palsy and hearing loss

2.4.3.3 Icteric

- Yellowing of skin, sclerae and mucous membranes from high bood bilirubin levels; results in jaudice when prolonged

2.4.3.4 Conjugated (direct) bilirubin

- Water soluble
- Without an accelerator (alcohol), mainly conjugated bilirubin is measured (direct reaction)
- Bilirubinuria indicates conjugated hyperbilirubinemia

2.4.3.5 Unconjugated (indirect) bilirubin

- Water insoluble
- Bound to albumin in blood
- Accelerators permit unconjugated bilirubin to react as well, providing total bilirubin
- Difference between total and direct is unconjugated (indirect) bilirubin
- Unconjugated bilirubin does not appear in urine

2.4.3.6 Total bilirubin = conjugated + unconjugated

2.4.3.7 δ bilirubin

- Bilirubin covalently bound to albumin, forming after prolonged hyperbilirubinemia
- Very slowly excreted

ISBN 978-089189-6616

2.4.4 Hyperbilirubinemia

- Conjugated hyperbilirubinemia (>30% of serum bilirubin conjugated) is caused primarily by an excretory defect
- Unconjugated hyperbilirubinemia is caused by increased production (hemolysis) or a hepatic defect that prevents uptake or conjugation

2.4.4.1 Prehepatic

- This is caused by increased hemoglobin breakdown
- It is also caused by hemolytic anemia

2.4.4.1.1.1 Bilirubin levels

- Serum
  - Levels are increased in indirect hyperbilirubinemia
  - Levels are normal to increased in direct hyperbilirubinemia
- Urine: Levels should be negative
- Urobilinogen: Levels are increased in both stool and urine

2.4.4.2 Hepatic

- Causes include conjugation failure, transport failure & cell damage

2.4.4.2.1.1 Bilirubin levels

- Serum
  - Levels are increased in both indirect and direct hyperbilirubinemia
- Urine: Levels are positive
- Urobilinogen: Levels are variable in stool and increased in urine

2.4.4.3 Posthepatic

- This is caused by obstruction of bile duct

2.4.4.3.1.1 Bilirubin levels

- Serum
  - Levels are increased in both direct indirect hyperbilirubinemia
- Urine levels are positive

2.4.4.4 Neonatal jaundice t2.8

- Benign (physiologic) jaundice
  - This is usually noted between days 2 and 3 of neonatal life
  - Bilirubin concentration rarely rises at a rate >5 mg/dL (>88.5 µmol/L) per day
  - Benign jaundice usually peaks by day 4-5
  - Bilirubin concentration rarely exceeds 20 mg/dL (342 µmol/L)
- Pathologic jaundice
  - This may appear within the first 24 hours of life
  - Bilirubin concentration may continue rising beyond 1 week of age
  - Jaundice may persist past 10 days
  - Total bilirubin exceeds 12 mg/dL (205.2 µmol/L)
  - Bilirubin rises quickly, with single day increase of >5 mg/dL (>88/5 µmol/L)
  - Conjugated (direct reacting) bilirubin exceeds 2 mg/dL (34.2 µmol/L)
  - Most common causes of neonatal jaundice include hemolytic disease of the fetus & newborn (HDFN) and sepsis
- Urobilinogen
  - Level is decreased to negative in both stool and urine

t2.8 Causes of neonatal hyperbilirubinemia

Unconjugated	Conjugated
Physiologic jaundice	Biliary obstruction (extrahepatic biliary atresia)
Breast milk jaundice	Sepsis or TORCH infection
Polycythemia	Neonatal hepatitis (idiopathic, Wilson disease, α_1-antitrypsin deficiency)
Hemolysis (HDFN, hemoglobinopathies, inherited membrane or enzyme defects)	Metabolic disorders (galactosemia, hereditary fructose intolerance, glycogen storage disease)
Increased enterohepatic circulation (Hirschsprung disease, cystic fibrosis, ileal atresia)	Inherited disorders of bilirubin transport (Dubin-Johnson syndrome, Rotor syndrome)
Inherited disorders of bilirubin metabolism (Gilbert syndrome, Crigler-Najjar syndrome)	Parenteral alimentation

HDFN, hemolysis disease of the fetus & newborn; TORCH, toxoplasmosis, rubella, cytomegalovirus & herpes simplex

2.4.4.5 Clinical correlation (see t2.9 & t2.10)

t2.9 Pathophysiologic differential diagnosis of hyperbilirubinemia

Step of bilirubin metabolism	Pathologic processes	Type of hyperbilirubinemia
Excess conversion of heme to unconjugated bilirubin	Hemolysis (extravascular) Ineffective hematopoiesis (intramedullary hemolysis) Large hematoma (resorbed heme)	Unconjugated hyperbilirubinemia
Excess delivery of unconjugated bilirubin to liver	Blood shunting (cirrhosis) Right heart failure	Unconjugated hyperbilirubinemia
Poor uptake of unconjugated bilirubin into hepatocyte	Gilbert syndrome Drugs, especially rifampin & probenecid	Unconjugated hyperbilirubinemia
Impaired conjugation of bilirubin in hepatocyte	Crigler-Najjar syndrome Hypothyroidism	Unconjugated hyperbilirubinemia
Impaired transmembrane secretion of conjugated bilirubin into canaliculus (hepatocellular jaundice) **t2.10**	Hepatitis/hepatic injury Endotoxin (sepsis) Pregnancy (estrogen) Drugs: Estrogen, cyclosporine Dubin-Johnson syndrome Rotor syndrome	Conjugated hyperbilirubinemia
Impaired flow of conjugated bilirubin through canaliculi & bile ducts (cholestatic jaundice) **t2.10**	Intrahepatic: Primary biliary cirrhosis, medication, alcohol, pregnancy, sepsis Extrahepatic: Primary sclerosing cholangitis, tumor, stricture, stone, AIDS choledochopathy	Conjugated hyperbilirubinemia

t2.10 Differential diagnosis of conjugated hyperbilirubinemia

	Hepatocellular jaundice	Cholestatic jaundice
Alkaline phosphatase	<3× upper limit of normal	>3× upper limit of normal
Transaminases	>3× upper limit of normal	<3× upper limit of normal
Serum cholesterol	Normal	Increased
Pruritus	Absent	Present

2.4.5 Liver enzymes

- See also 2.6 Enzymes
- Alkaline phosphatase (ALP): This is greatly increased in obstructive jaundice
- γ-glutamyltransferease: It is greatly increased in cirrhosis
- Aspartate aminotransferase (AST; also known as serum glutamic oxaloacetic transaminase [SGOT]): Greatly increased in hepatitis
- Alanine aminotransferase (ALT; also known as serum glutamic pyruvic transaminase [SGPT]): Greatly increased in hepatitis
- Lactate dehydrogenase (LD) (especially LD 4 & 5)

2.4.6 Hereditary defects in bilirubin metabolism

2.4.6.1 Unconjugated forms

- Gilbert syndrome
    - This is the most common hereditary cause of increased bilirubin
    - The activity of the enzyme glucuronyltransferase is reduced
    - The main symptom is jaundice caused by mild elevated levels of unconjugated bilirubin in the bloodstream
    - It does not require treatment
    - It does not result in kernicterus
- Crigler-Najjar syndrome
    - It is an inherited form of nonhemolytic jaundice
    - Intense jaundice appears in the first days of life and persists thereafter
    - Type 1 is characterized by a serum bilirubin usually >20.7 mg/dL (>345 μmol/L), mainly in unconjugated levels
    - It leads to brain damage—kernicterus—in infants

2.4.6.2 Conjugated forms

- Dubin-Johnson syndrome
    - This is a benign autosomal recessive disorder
    - It is a defect in the ability of hepatocytes to transport conjugated bilirubin into the bile
    - No increase is seen in liver enzymes
    - It is associated with a factor VIII deficiency
- Rotor syndrome
    - This is a benign autosomal recessive bilirubin disorder
    - It is similar to Dubin-Johnson syndrome
    - Liver cells are not pigmented
    - The main symptom is a nonitching jaundice

ISBN 978-089189-6616

- An increase in bilirubin is seen in the patient's serum, mainly of the conjugated type
- Biliary atresia
  - Rare condition in newborn infants in which the common bile duct between the liver and the small intestine is blocked or absent
  - It is characterized by obliteration or discontinuity of the extrahepatic biliary system
  - It results in obstruction to the bile flow

2.4.7 Bilirubin measurement

- Specimen requirements
  - Serum/heparinized plasma
  - Hemolysis interferes with diazo reaction
  - Protect from light
- Bilirubin properties
  - Unconjugated (bilirubin bound to albumin)
    - Water insoluble
    - Alcohol soluble
    - Van den Bergh reaction—indirect
    - Affinity for brain tissue—high
  - Conjugated (bilirubin diglucoronide)
    - Water soluble
    - Alcohol soluble
    - Van den Bergh reaction—direct
    - Affinity for brain tissue—low
- Diazo reagent
  - Sulfanilic acid + HCl + sodium nitrite ($NaNO_3$)
  - Conjugated (direct) bilirubin gives an immediate reaction
  - Unconjugated bilirubin must have albumin bond broken with methanol
- Evelyn Malloy
  - Principle: Bilirubin + diazo reagent → azobilirubin
- Jendrassik-Grof
  - Principle: Na acetate (buffer) + caffeine-Na benzoate (accelerator) + diazo
  - Ascorbic acid (stop reaction)
  - Alkaline tartrate (changes pH)
  - Omit caffeine-Na benzoate in direct
- Dimethyl sulfoxide (DMSO)
  - Principle: Total bilirubin reagent consists of sulfanilic acid, sodium nitrite, DMSO
  - DMSO solubilizes the indirect (unconjugated) form of bilirubin
- Bilirubinometer
  - Principle: Serum color is read at 2 wavelengths: 575 nm for hemoglobin and 455 nm for bilirubin
  - Subtract hemoglobin ABS from bilirubin ABS
  - Can only be used for newborns because dietary pigments can interfere
- Urine bilirubin
  - Reminder: Only conjugated bilirubin can be excreted
  - Methods
    - Foam test
    - Fouchet reagent—ferric chloride
    - Ictotest—uses diazo reagent

2.4.8 Urobilinogen measurement

- Specimen requirements—2 hours (alkaline tide)
- Erhlich test
  - Erhlich reagent (P-dimethylaminobenzaldehyde) & Na acetate
  - Forms a red color
  - Interference—porphobilinogen

2.5 Proteins

- 20 amino acids required as the building blocks of proteins

2.5.1 General characteristics of proteins

- Proteins are macromolecules that consist of covalently linked polymers of amino acids
- Amino acids are linked to each other through peptide bonds, with carboxyl group of 1 amino acid combining with amino group of another

2.5.2 Aminoacidopathies

- These are inherited enzyme defects that inhibit metabolism of certain amino acids
- They exist either in the activity of specific enzymes in metabolic pathway or in the membrane transport system for amino acids
- Some states require screening for up to 26 amino acids
- Over 100 diseases result from aminoacidopathies
- They can cause severe medical complications because of the buildup of toxic amino acids & byproducts of amino acid metabolism in blood, such as
  - Phenylketonuria
  - Tyrosinemia
  - Alkaptonuria
  - Maple syrup urine disease

- Isovaleric acidemia
- Homocystinuria
- Citrullinemia
- Argininosuccinic aciduria
- Cystinuria

2.5.3 Amino acid analysis

- Blood samples should be drawn after at least a 6-hour to 8-hour fast
- Sample is collected in a heparin tube and plasma removed promptly from cells
- Take care not to aspirate platelet and white cell layer, no hemolysis
- Analysis is performed immediately or sample frozen at –20°C to –40°C
- Urinary amino acid analysis is performed on random specimen for screening
- Method of choice for screening is thin-layer chromatography

2.5.4 Protein structure

- This is determined by the number and types of amino acids and their sequence in the polypeptide chain
- Secondary structure
    - This is determined by winding of polypeptide chain—α helix, β pleated sheet, or random coil
- Tertiary structure
    - This is determined by the way the twisted chain folds back on itself to form a 3-dimensional structure
    - Tertiary structure is the result of hydrophobic Interactions
- Quaternary structure
    - 2 or more polypeptide chains attract to form functional protein molecules (aggregates), eg, hemoglobin has 4 subunits: 2 α chains and 2 β chains

2.5.5 Protein components

- Carbon
- Hydrogen
- Oxygen
- Sulfur
- Nitrogen (16%—differentiates from carbohydrates and lipids)

2.5.6 Important terms

- Ampholyte or zwitterion
    - Amino acids contain 2 ionizable sites and at a particular pH, also known as isoelectric point, (such as pH 6.0 for glycine), both carboxyl and amino sites are ionized
    - An amino acid with both sites ionized (have positive and negative charges on the same molecule) is called an ampholyte or zwitterion
- Isoelectric point (pI)
    - pH at which amino acid is neutral, having no net surface charge
    - Key factor for consideration in protein electrophoresis

2.5.7 Functions of proteins

- Carrier molecules
- Maintenance of osmotic pressure
- Immune response agents
- Enzymes
- Acts as a marker for nutrition
    - Albumin, transferrin, transthyretin or thyroxine-binding prealbumin
- Acts as a marker for liver function
- Important in assessment of renal function
- Acute-phase reactant (APR) **t2.11**

t2.11 Acute-phase reactants

	Protein	Acute inflammation	Chronic inflammation
	Prealbumin	↓	↓
	Albumin	↓	↓
α_1	α_1-antitrypsin	↑	↑
	α_1-antichymotrypsin	↑	↑
	α_1-acid glycoprotein	↑	↑
α_2	Haptoglobin	↑	↑
	Ceruloplasmin	↑	↑
β	Complement (C_3)	↑	↑
	Transferrin	↓	↑
	Fibrinogen	↑	↑
	Ig (IgA, IgM)	→↓	↑
γ	Ig (IgG, IgA, IgM)	→↓	↑
	CRP	↑	↑

CRP, C-reactive protein; Ig, immunoglobulin

- Proteins that increase in response to inflammation
- Frequently occurs as a result of infection, myocardial infarction (MI), tumor growth, surgery, or trauma
- APRs play a role in host defense

ISBN 978-089189-6616

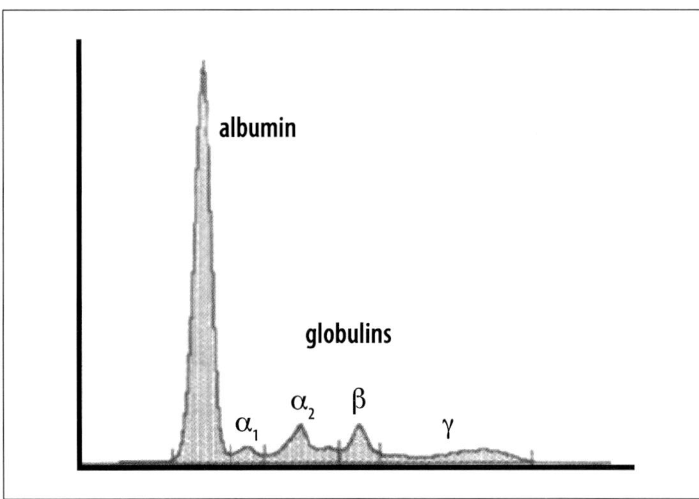

f2.3 Serum protein electrophoresis

- Examples include C-reactive protein (CRP), α_1-antitrypsin (AAT), C3, α_1-acid glycoprotein, haptoglobin & ceruloplasmin
- As APR proteins increase, levels of negative APR proteins (albumin, prealbumin & transferrin) decrease. Total protein concentration changes very little, as a result

2.5.8 Total protein measurement

- Biuret reaction uses alkaline copper sulfate solution to react with peptide bonds in the proteins

2.5.9 Specific protein fractions by serum protein electrophoresis (SPEP) t2.12

- 2 main groups: Albumin & globulins f2.3
- Prealbumin
- Albumin
- α_1 proteins
- α_2 proteins
- β proteins (β_1 and β_2)
- γ proteins

2.5.9.1 Prealbumin

- Thyroxine-binding protein, also called transthyretin, or TBPA (transports T3 and T4)
- Molecular weight is ~54,000 g/mol
- Synthesized by liver
- Clinical utility
  - Negative APR
  - Sensitive marker of poor nutritional status, because it has a half-life of only 2 days
  - Decreased in hepatic damage, burns, salicylate ingestion & tissue necrosis
  - Functions in serum to bind thyroxine (also called transthyretin [TTR]) and the retinol-binding protein vitamin A complex)
- Migrates anodal (ahead of) albumin in routine electrophoresis
- Rarely seen on cellulose acetate (unless cerebrospinal fluid [CSF]), prealbumin band is a hallmark of CSF protein electrophoresis

t2.12 Serum proteins

Electrophoretic band	Major constituent(s)	Notes
Prealbumin	Prealbumin	Indicator of nutritional status Binds thyroid hormones, binds retinol-binding protein Negative APR
Albumin	Albumin	Maintains serum oncotic pressure Binds numerous substances Negative APR
Alb-α_1 interface	α_1-lipoprotein	High-density lipoprotein
α_1	α_1-antitrypsin	Positive APR α1 antitrypsin deficiency detectable with serum protein electrophoresis
α_1-α_2 interface	Gc globulin	Binds vitamin D
	α_1-antichymotrypsin	Positive APR
	α_1-acid glycoprotein	Positive APR
α_2	α_2-macroglobulin	Elevated in nephrotic syndrome
	Haptoglobin	Positive APR
	Ceruloplasmin	Binds copper Low ceruloplasmin not detectable with SPEP Positive APR
α_2-β interface	Usually empty	Hemoglobin, usually absent from serum, may be present here when there is hemolysis—a possible pseudo-M-spike
β_1	Transferrin	Transferrin may be high in iron deficiency—a possible pseudo-M-spike
β_1-β_2 interface	β-lipoprotein	LDL
β_2	IgA	Fibrinogen, usually absent from serum, may be present in the β-γ interface when there is incomplete clotting—a possible pseudo-M-spike
	C3	Positive APR, C3 breakdown products—a possible pseudo-M-spike
γ_1	γ globulins	Positive APR
γ_2	CRP	Positive APR

2.5.9.2 Albumin

- This is the most abundant serum protein
- Molecular weight is ~66,000 g/mol
- It is synthesized in the liver

- Its half-life is 15-19 days
- It is present in the highest concentration in serum (~ half of total protein is 3.5-5.0 g/dL)
- Analbuminemia results in mild edema and hyperlipidemia
- Several albumin alleles exist, most common of which is albumin A; variant albumin alleles may result in bisalbuminemia, a benign condition

2.5.9.2.1 Clinical utility

- Assessment of nutritional status: Half-life of albumin is 17 days
- Assessment hepatic synthetic function
- Assessment of renal glomerular function
- Negative APR
- Diabetic control: Glycated albumin is an indicator of short-term glycemic control

2.5.9.2.2 Functions

- Maintains fluid balance (80% of osmotic pressure)
- Transports molecule for less soluble substances such as fatty acids, bilirubin, hormones, calcium, metals, drugs & vitamins
- Has antioxidant activity
- Buffers pH

2.5.9.2.3 Clinical significance of albumin

- Hyperalbuminemia—increased albumin
  - Dehydration
  - Rare and of no clinical significance
- Hypoalbuminemia—decreased albumin
  - Caused by impaired synthesis (liver function), inflammatory responses, or protein loss (renal or in burns)
- Analbuminemia—absence of albumin
  - Rare genetic abnormality
  - Asymptomatic except for slight edema
- Bisalbuminemia
  - Congenital conditions characterized by the presence of albumin that has unusual molecular characteristics—2 identical albumin bands on electrophoresis

2.5.9.2.4 Measurement principles

- Bromcresol green (BCG) dye binding
- Bromcresol purple (BCP) dye binding
- Immunochemical

2.5.9.3 α_1 proteins

2.5.9.3.1 α_1-antitrypsin

- This is a group of serine protease inhibitors synthesized in the liver
- It is a protease inhibitor that binds to, and inactivates, trypsinlike enzymes that cause hydrolytic damage to structural proteins
- It migrates directly following albumin and comprises 90% of the α_1 band in electrophoresis
- SPEP can detect AAT deficiency (homozygous for PiZZ), in which the serum will display a markedly diminished α_1 band
- AAT gene (*SERPINA1*) highly polymorphic, with >100 alleles; most common allele is PiM, and the most common genotype is PiMM
- Clinical utility
  - Deficiency is inherited in homozygous or heterozygous state and is linked to pulmonary emphysema and cirrhosis
  - Increased levels in inflammatory reactions, pregnancy & oral contraceptive use
- Measurement principles
  - Immunochemical

2.5.9.3.2 α_1-fetoprotein (AFP)

- This is synthesized by the fetal liver
- It is the major fetal protein during 2nd trimester of pregnancy
- Increased AFP in maternal serum indicates twins or high risk for open neural tube defects (ONTD)
- Decreased levels indicate increased risk for down syndrome
- It also is used as a tumor marker and is elevated in cancers of liver
- Measurement principles
  - Immunochemical

2.5.9.3.3 α_1-acid glycoprotein (AAG)

- It is synthesized by the liver
- Its biological function is unknown
- It is a minor component of the α_1 band normally but a major component of the increased α_1 band in acute inflammatory states
- Measurement principles
  - Immunochemical
- It inactivates progesterone and binds basic drugs

ISBN 978-089189-6616

2.5.9.4 α_2 proteins

2.5.9.4.1 α_2-macroglobulin

- It is the largest nonimmunoglobulin in serum (723 kD)
- It inhibits proteases such as trypsin, pepsin & plasmin and binds to some hormones such as insulin and is removed by the reticuloendothelial system
- Clinical utility
  - Relative concentration is elevated in liver and renal disease
  - Its large size prevents its loss in nephrotic syndrome, leading to a relative 10-fold rise in concentration
- Measurement principles
  - Immunochemical

2.5.9.4.2 Haptoglobin (α_2)

- 3rd major component of the α_2 band
- Binds free hemoglobin and transports it to the reticulo-endothelial system where hemoglobin is degraded
- Does not bind myoglobin
- Acute-phase reactant
- Prevents loss of hemoglobin and its iron into the urine
- Clinical utility
  - Decreased in hemolytic diseases, such as hemolytic disease of the newborn and transfusion reactions, because it is rapidly depleted in intravascular hemolysis
  - Increased in inflammatory conditions, burns & nephrotic syndrome
- Measurement principles
  - Immunochemical

2.5.9.4.3 Ceruloplasmin (α_2)

- Copper-containing α_2-glycoprotein, synthesized in the liver
- Acute-phase reactant
- Decreased levels found in:
  - Wilson disease because of inhibition of synthesis
  - Menkes disease because of decreased absorption
- Measurement principles
  - Immunochemical

2.5.9.5 β proteins

2.5.9.5.1 Transferrin (β)

- This is a major β globulin
- Negative APR
- Synthesized in the liver
- Transports ferric (Fe^{3+}) iron; normally ~30% saturated; markedly increased in iron deficiency
- Asialated (unique form and physical structure) transferrin (so-called *tau* protein) and a double transferrin peak are hallmarks of CSF electrophoresis
- Carbohydrate-deficient transferrin a marker for alcohol use
- Binds and transports iron and prevents its loss through the kidneys
- Clinical utility
  - Increased in iron-deficiency anemia, pregnancy & estrogen therapy
  - Decreased in infection, inflammation, liver disease, kidney disease, malignancy & hereditary atransferrinemia
- Measurement principles
  - Immunochemical

2.5.9.5.2 β_2-microglobulin (B2M)

- Small protein (molecular weight 11,800 g/mol)
- Found on the surface of most nucleated cells, particularly lymphocytes
- Filtered by the renal glomerulus but most (>99%) is reabsorbed
- Clinical utility
  - Urinary B2M is used to measure renal tubular function
  - Elevated in renal failure, inflammation & malignancies
- Measurement principles
  - Immunochemical

2.5.9.5.3 Fibrinogen

- This is a β globulin that is usually absent from serum
  - Forms fibrin clot when activated by thrombin
  - Seen only if plasma is used instead of serum because fibrinogen is used up in the clotting process
  - If specimen clots incompletely, fibrinogen may be seen; may produce pseudo M spike
- It is synthesized in the liver
- It is an APR
- Peak seen between β and γ fractions (may straddle the β-γ interface)
- Increased in pregnancy and with use of birth control pills
- Clinical utility
  - Decreased in extensive coagulation
- Measurement principles

- Fibrinogen activity using Clauss method for clot formation
- Immunochemical method detects amount but not function

2.5.9.5.4 Complement

- This is a protein that participates in the immune reaction and serves as a link to the inflammatory response
- Its peak is seen in the β fraction
- Increased in inflammatory conditions
- Decreased in malnutrition, lupus & intravascular coagulopathies
- Measurement principles
  - Immunochemical

2.5.9.5.5 C-reactive protein (CRP)

- It is synthesized in the liver
- It is the first APR to rise in response to inflammatory disease
- It is recognized as an independent risk factor in cardiovascular disease
- hsCRP assay is used to assess risk groups
- Found in the β region; can produce a small apparent band
- High sensitivity assays can detect CRP concentrations as low as 0.05 mg/dL (<0.5 mg/L), resulting in 3 tiers of CRP
- Clinical utility
  - Marker of inflammation
  - Significantly increased in acute rheumatic fever, bacterial infections, MI & viral infections
  - Normal CRP: <0.2-0.3 mg/dL (<2-3 mg/L)
  - High level CRP elevation: >1 mg/dL (>10 mg/L); usually indicates active inflammation, eg, collagen vascular disease, infection
  - Low level CRP elevation: 0.3-1 mg/dL (3-10 mg/L); indicative of cellular stress and correlated with higher mortality regardless of cause, poor outcome following cardiovascular events
- Measurement principles
  - Immunochemical

2.5.9.5.6 Troponin (Tn)

- Highly cardiospecific; has largely replaced creatine kinase (CK) measurement for a myocardial infarction (MI) diagnosis
- Reference interval includes all values up to the 99th percentile of healthy adults
- Elevated in nonischemic states
- Nonischemic pathology: Pulmonary embolus, myocarditis, pericarditis, heart failure, intracranial insults, rhabdomyolysis, sepsis, shock & renal insufficiency
- 1% of healthy adults have troponin I (TnI) above the 99th percentile
- Analytical false positives: Interferences, eg, fibrin, heterophile antibodies
- Current universal definition of MI
  - Alteration in troponin with ≥1 value above the 99th percentile
  - Clinical evidence of ischemia, including any 1 of the following
    - Symptoms of ischemia
    - New significant ST-T changes or new left bundle branch block
    - Development of pathologic Q waves
    - Imaging showing new loss of viable myocardium or new regional wall motion abnormality
    - Identification of an intracoronary thrombus on angiography or autopsy
- In patients whose initial cardiac troponin I (cTnI) value is abnormal
  - >20% change in cTnI values at 3 or 6 hours indicates myocardial necrosis. This combination plus clinical evidence of ischemia indicate MI
  - In patients with normal initial cTnI value, >50% change in cTnI values at 3 or 6 hours indicates myocardial necrosis. This plus clinical evidence of ischemia indicates MI
  - Note that the demonstration of a rising and/or falling pattern is needed to distinguish acute from chronic elevations in cTn concentrations. Troponin elevations related to conditions such as chronic renal failure or congestive heart failure do not change acutely
- Measurement principles
  - Immunochemical

2.5.9.5.7 B-type natriuretic peptide (BNP)

- The main source of BNP is ventricular myocytes
- Synthesis of BNP correlates directly with ventricular wall tension
- Rapidly degraded following production with $t_{1/2}$ of 20 minutes; N-terminal peptide fragment (NT-proBNP) is more stable ($t_{1/2}$ of 1-2 hours)
- BNP and NT-proBNP are elevated in patients with heart failure
- Measurement principles
  - Immunochemical

ISBN 978-089189-6616

2.5.9.6 γ proteins

2.5.9.6.1 γ globulins

- Includes immunoglobulins (IgG, IgM, IgA, IgD & IgE)
- Synthesized by plasma cells from the B-lymphocyte lineage in bone marrow
- Immunoglobulins are composed of 2 identical heavy and 2 identical light (κ and λ) chains
- Single sharp peak in γ (or sometimes β) region indicates monoclonal (coming from 1 cell line) gammopathy; also known as M-protein
- Increased in plasma cell malignancy (multiple myeloma), infection etc
- Broad peak, homogenous γ fraction or multiple bands indicate polyclonal (from multiple cell lines) gammopathy
- Indicates inflammation
- IgG is increased in liver disease, autoimmune diseases & infections
- Autoimmune hepatitis associated with marked polyclonal increase in IgG
- IgM is the first to appear in response to antigen stimulation
  - Monoclonal increase in IgM is seen in Waldenström macroglobulinemia
  - Primary biliary cirrhosis is associated with polyclonal increase in IgM
- IgA is a secretory antibody found in saliva, tears, sweat & nasal secretions
- Polyclonal increase is seen in liver disease, infections & autoimmune disease
- β-γ bridging is seen in cirrhosis
- IgD is increased in infections, liver disease & connective tissue disorders
- IgE is associated with allergic and anaphylactic reactions
- Decreased albumin-globulin (A/G) ratio (<1.0) usually is the result of liver disease
- Measurement principles
  - Serum protein electrophoresis (SPEP)
  - Immunofixation electrophoresis to confirm SPEP results
  - Immunochemical such as immunonephelometry

2.5.10 Protein abnormalities

2.5.10.1 Hypoproteinemia

- It is caused by excessive loss related to renal disease, leakage into the GI tract & bleeding. Decreased intake because of malnutrition and malabsorption is also a cause

2.5.10.2 Hyperproteinemia

- It is caused by dehydration from vomiting and diarrhea and excessive protein production such as Bence Jones protein in multiple myeloma

2.5.10.3 Urine protein & urine albumin

- Normal proteinuria does not exceed 150 mg/day (mainly Tamm-Horsfall glycoprotein)
- Significant proteinuria usually defined as exceeding 300 mg/day
- Assessment of proteinuria traditionally is based on a 24-hour urine collection
- Random urine samples ("spot urine") can be misleading, because protein handling by the kidney varies throughout the day. But when compared to a simultaneous urine creatinine determination, the spot urine protein measurement is as good as the 24-hour urine measurement
- Urine dipstick result (1+ to 3+) is semiquantitative and most sensitive to albumin; it is not sensitive enough to detect microalbuminuria
- Microalbumin assay
  - It is capable of detecting as little as 0.3 mg/dL of albumin (dipstick sensitive to ~30 mg/dL)
  - Significant microalbuminuria is currently defined in terms of the albumin-creatinine ratio of a spot urine rather than a 24-hour timed urine collection
  - Albumin-creatinine ratio is reported in units of milligrams per gram (protein-creatinine ratio is reported as milligrams per milligram, a possible source of confusion)

2.5.11 Protein analysis

- Reference range: 0.6-0.8 mg/dL (6.5-8.3 g/dL)
- Serum, plasma, CSF & urine samples can be used
- Separating serum proteins
  - Chromatography
  - Gel
  - High-performance liquid chromatography
  - Ion exchange
  - Immunoaffinity

Proteins>Protein analysis

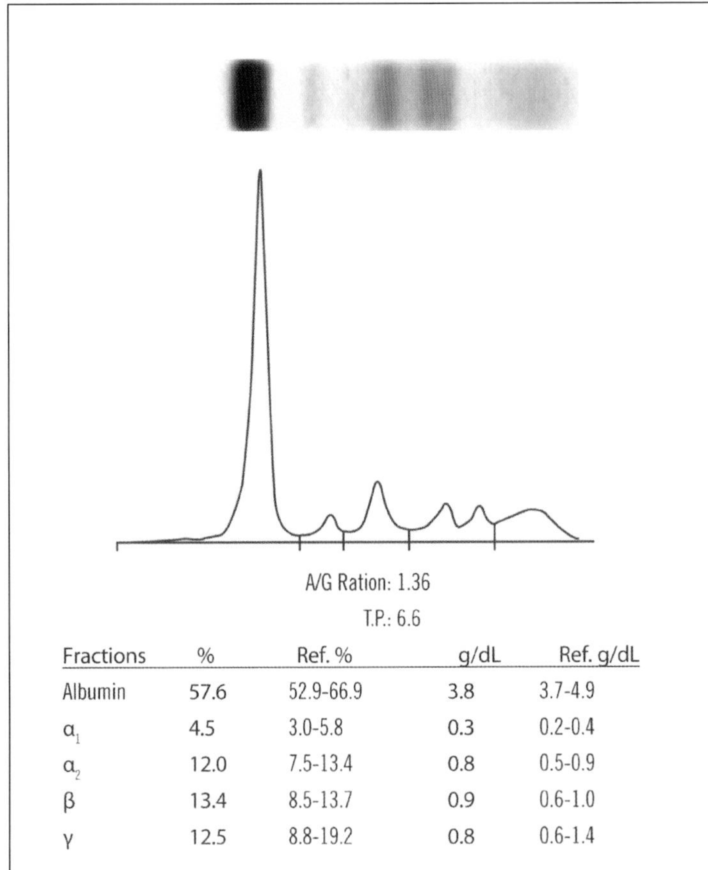

Fractions	%	Ref. %	g/dL	Ref. g/dL
Albumin	57.6	52.9-66.9	3.8	3.7-4.9
α_1	4.5	3.0-5.8	0.3	0.2-0.4
α_2	12.0	7.5-13.4	0.8	0.5-0.9
β	13.4	8.5-13.7	0.9	0.6-1.0
γ	12.5	8.8-19.2	0.8	0.6-1.4

f2.4 Normal high resolution serum protein electrophoresis; the most anodal band is albumin, followed by α_1, α_2, β_1, β_2, and the broad, faint γ region

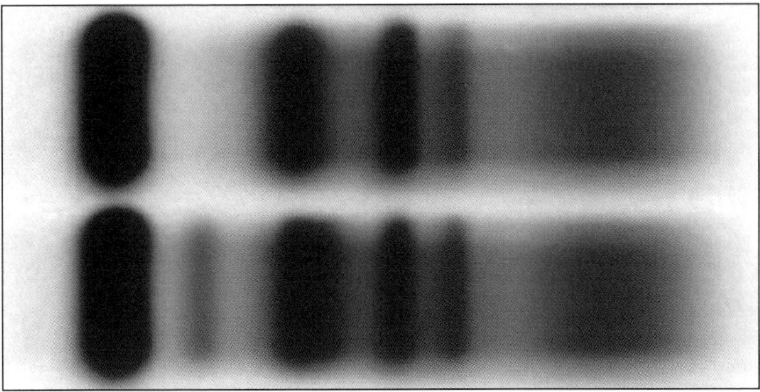

f2.5 Serum protein electrophoresis (SPEP) showing patient with α_1-antitrypsin deficiency (top) & normal SPEP for comparison (bottom)

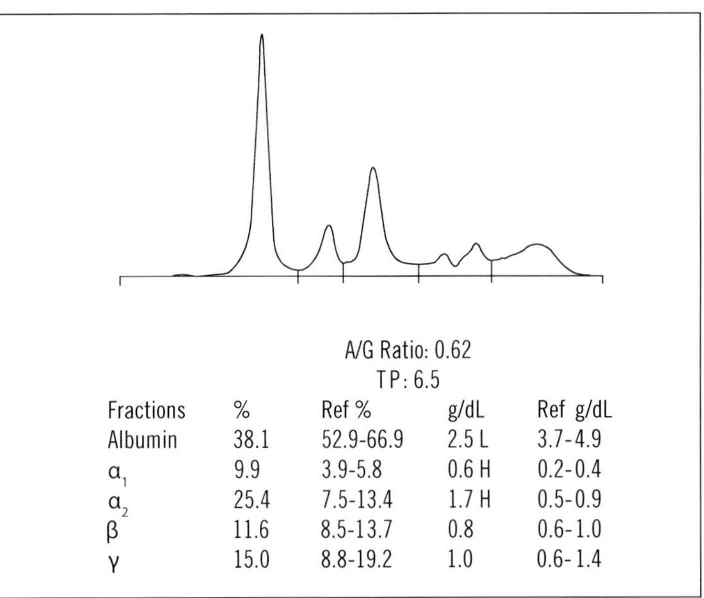

Fractions	%	Ref %	g/dL	Ref g/dL
Albumin	38.1	52.9-66.9	2.5 L	3.7-4.9
α_1	9.9	3.9-5.8	0.6 H	0.2-0.4
α_2	25.4	7.5-13.4	1.7 H	0.5-0.9
β	11.6	8.5-13.7	0.8	0.6-1.0
γ	15.0	8.8-19.2	1.0	0.6-1.4

f2.6 Acute inflammation pattern

- Electrophoresis
  - Starch gel
  - Agarose gel
  - Cellulose acetate
  - Polyacrylamide gel
- Serum protein electrophoresis
  - Electrophoresis of serum at pH 8.6 become negatively charged and migrates to an anode, while the buffer particles migrate to a cathode
  - Results in 5 bands: Albumin, α_1, α_2, β, γ
  - Bands are measured using densitometry
  - Normal serum **f2.4**
    - Nearly invisible prealbumin band, very large albumin band, small peaked α_1 band, broad α_2 band, bimodal β, and broad γ
  - Bisalbuminemia
    - Seen in heterozygotes for albumin alleles; SPEP shows double albumin spike
    - No clinical consequence
  - α_1-antitrypsin deficiency **f2.5**
    - Can be detected with SPEP (not the most sensitive or specific assay)
  - Nephrotic syndrome
    - Loss of small serum proteins, particularly albumin
    - Large protein molecules are retained
    - The result is a decrease of all bands, with the exception of the α_2 band, which contains the α_2 macroglobulin
  - Acute inflammation **f2.6**
    - Decreased albumin, increased α_1 and α_2 bands, and normal to increased γ globulins
  - β-γ bridging
    - Indicative of cirrhosis and caused by increased serum IgA
    - Additional features include hypoalbuminemia and blunted α_1 and α_2 bands

ISBN 978-089189-6616

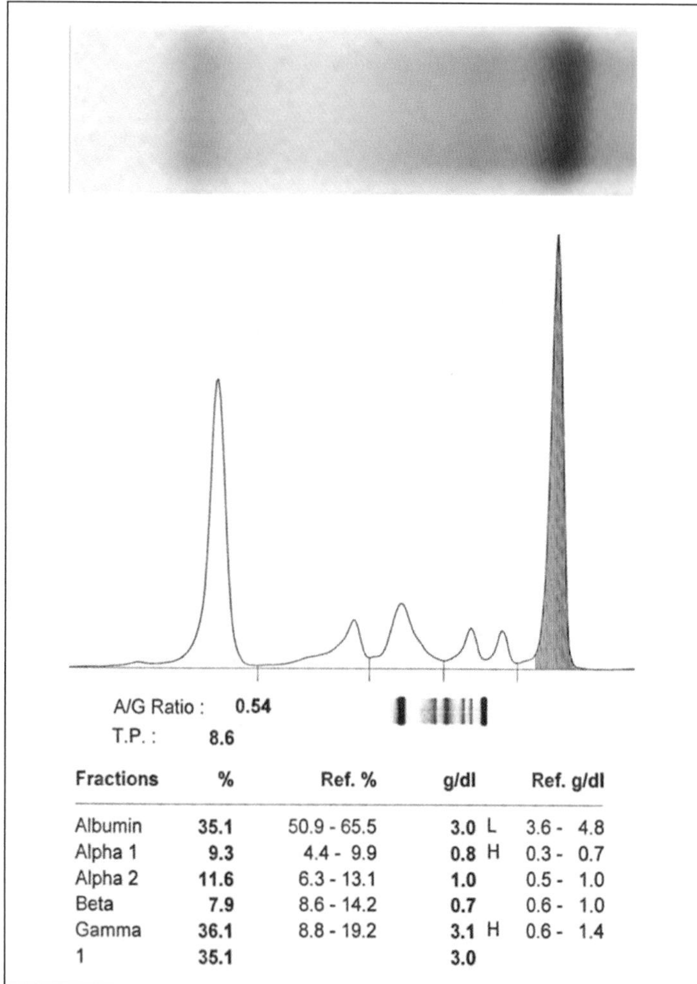

Fractions	%	Ref. %	g/dl		Ref. g/dl
Albumin	35.1	50.9 - 65.5	3.0	L	3.6 - 4.8
Alpha 1	9.3	4.4 - 9.9	0.8	H	0.3 - 0.7
Alpha 2	11.6	6.3 - 13.1	1.0		0.5 - 1.0
Beta	7.9	8.6 - 14.2	0.7		0.6 - 1.0
Gamma	36.1	8.8 - 19.2	3.1	H	0.6 - 1.4
1	35.1		3.0		

f2.7 SPEP showing typical M spike; most IgG paraproteins are found in the γ region on the gel (above) & densitometry tracing (below)

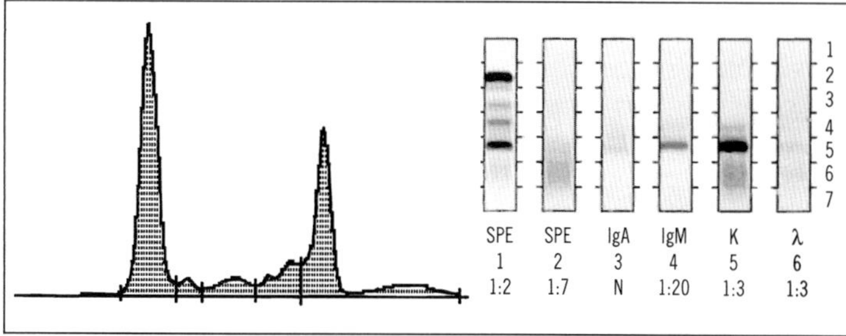

f2.8 SPEP & IFE showing IgM κ M protein; note that IgM paraproteins tend to migrate near the β-γ interface

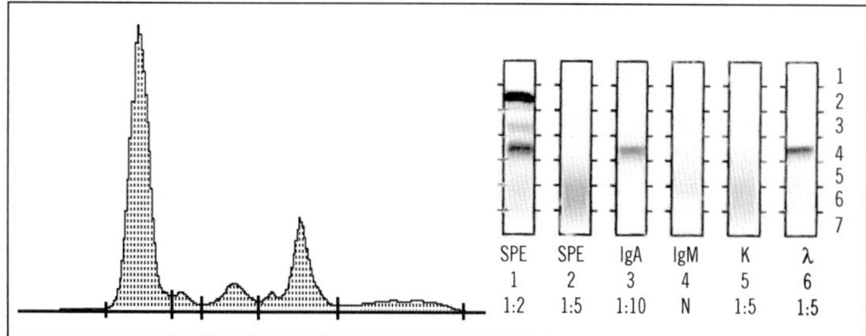

f2.9 SPEP & IFE showing IgA λ M protein; note that IgA paraproteins tend to migrate into the β region

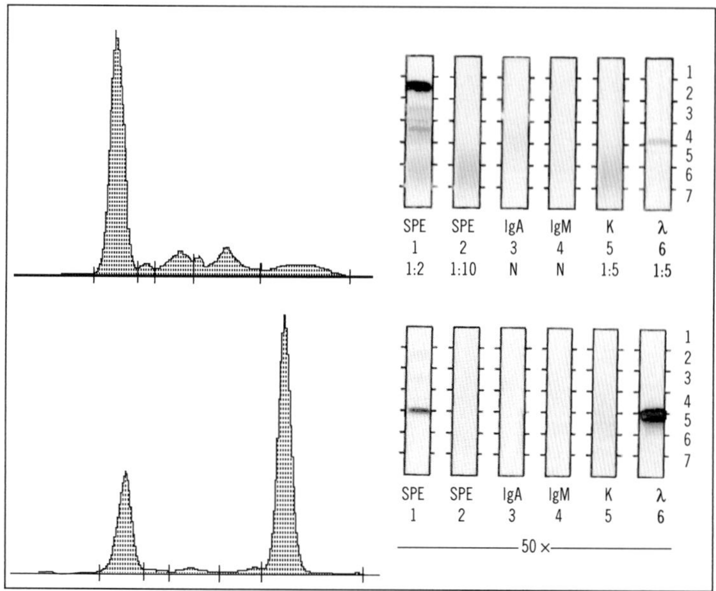

f2.10 SPEP (upper left), serum immunofixation electrophoresis (IFE) (upper right), Urine protein electrophoresis (UPEP) (lower left), urine IFE (lower right) showing λ light chain only M protein

- Monoclonal gammopathy **f2.7-f2.10**
  - An immunochemically homogeneous immunoglobulin (M protein) in the serum
  - The serum protein electrophoresis (SPEP) shows a prominent, discrete, dark band within γ, β, or rarely α_2
  - M protein usually is an intact immunoglobulin, composed of 2 heavy and 2 light chains
  - Sometimes light chain only
  - Rarely a heavy chain only
  - Biclonal gammopathy in 3%-4% of cases (if IgA, especially if single light chain, more likely because of the appearance of both monomers and dimers)
  - ~10% of patients show only hypogammaglobulinemia
  - Immunofixation or immunosubtraction is indicated to characterize the M protein; urine should be screened for the presence of monoclonal free light chains; serum free light chain levels should be evaluated
  - M spike is most commonly the result of a plasma cell neoplasm, Waldenström macroglobulinemia (lymphoplasmacytic lymphoma), or chronic lymphocytic leukemia/small lymphocytic lymphoma
  - Pseudo-M spikes: Fibrinogen (incompletely clotted sample), hemoglobin (hemolyzed sample), elevated CRP, elevated transferrin, certain antibiotics and radiocontrast agents, and very high levels of serum tumor markers, such as CA19-9

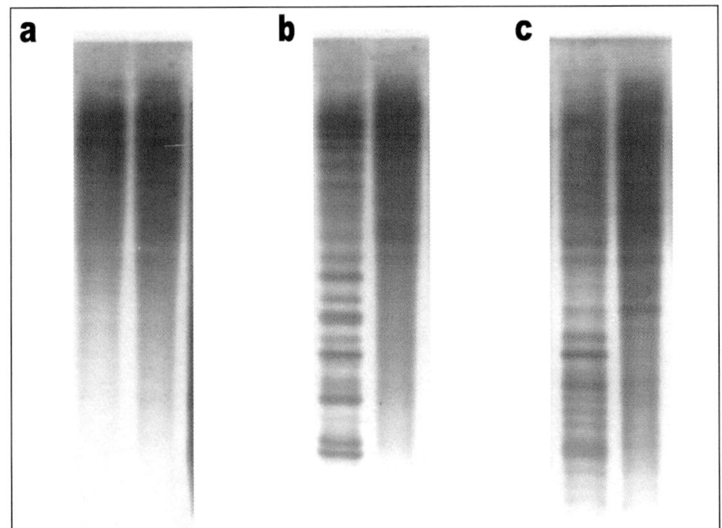

f2.11 Cerebrospinal fluid (CSF) protein electrophoresis
a CSF (left) & serum (right) from the same patient, neither demonstrating oligoclonal bands
b CSF (left) & serum (right) from the same patient, in which oligoclonal bands are present in the CSF but not in the serum, a result supportive of the diagnosis of MS
c CSF (left) & serum (right), both with oligoclonal bands, in which case the CSF bands would be discounted

- Cerebrospinal fluid (CSF) protein electrophoresis
  - CSF normally contains essentially all proteins present in serum, but in smaller quantities
  - Characteristic features of CSF are a prominent prealbumin band and a double β (transferrin) band also known as the τ protein
  - CSF electrophoresis used to support a diagnosis of multiple sclerosis by finding oligoclonal bands **f2.11**; these bands should be absent from the patient's serum
- Urine protein electrophoresis (UPEP) **f2.12**
  - Normal pattern: Faint bands from albumin, α_1, α_2, β and γ proteins
  - Glomerular proteinuria pattern: Strong albumin, α_1 and β bands; large proteins (persistence of some filtering function) and small proteins (tubular reabsorption) absent, leaving intermediate-sized proteins, notably albumin, AAT, and transferrin
  - Tubular proteinuria pattern: Weak albumin band, strong α_1 and β bands
  - Overflow proteinuria pattern: Most commonly this is a monoclonal light chain (Bence Jones proteinuria). Other possibilities include myoglobin and hemoglobin
- Immunoelectrophoresis (IEP) **f2.13**
  - This is no longer commonly used
  - Patient serum placed in every other well in a series of wells
  - An aliquot of normal serum is placed In the remaining wells
  - The gel is subjected to electrophoresis

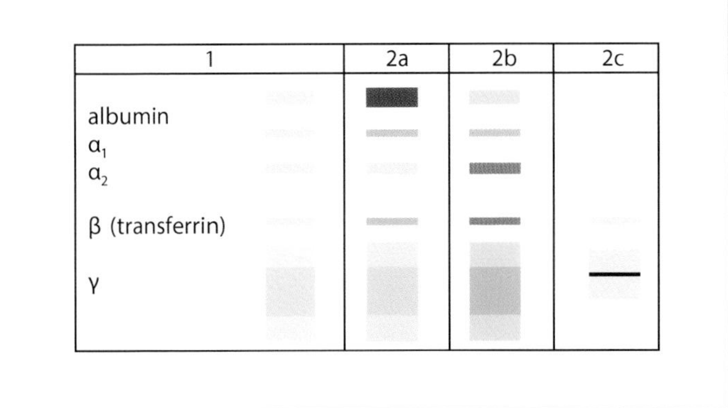

f2.12 Urine protein electrophoresis (UPEP); patterns representing normal (1), glomerular proteinuria (2a), tubular proteinuria (2b) & overflow proteinuria (2c) are shown

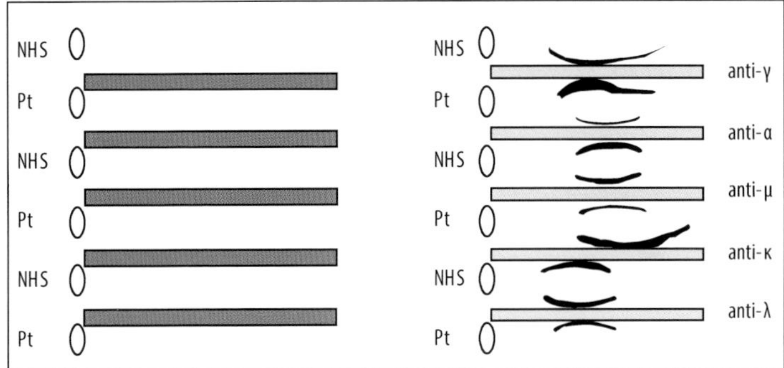

f2.13 Immunoelectrophoresis (IEP) with uninoculated wells (left) & a gel following electrophoresis, diffusion, fixation & staining (right) demonstrating an IgG κ monoclonal protein

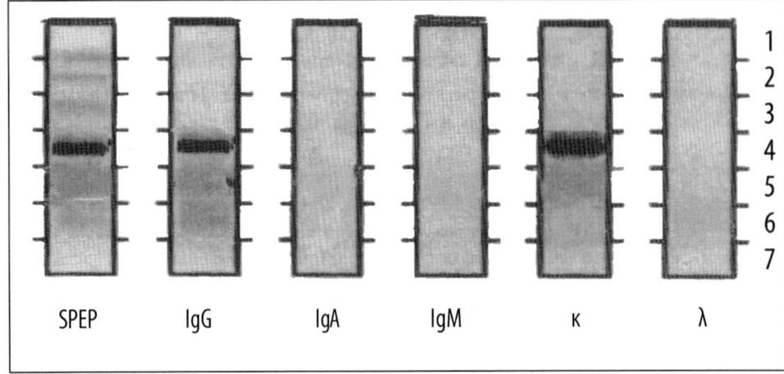

f2.14 Immunofixation electrophoresis (IFE) demonstrating an IgG κ monoclonal protein

  - Antiserum is added to each trough
  - Precipitation arcs form between the antisera in the troughs and the electrophoresed proteins in the gel. Interpretation depends on visual comparison of the arcs formed with patient serum
- Immunofixation electrophoresis (IFE) **f2.14**
  - IFE is used to characterize monoclonal proteins (M proteins) based on position in the gel and heavy and light chain composition
  - Look for bands in the IFE that comigrate with the M protein in the SPEP

ISBN 978-089189-6616

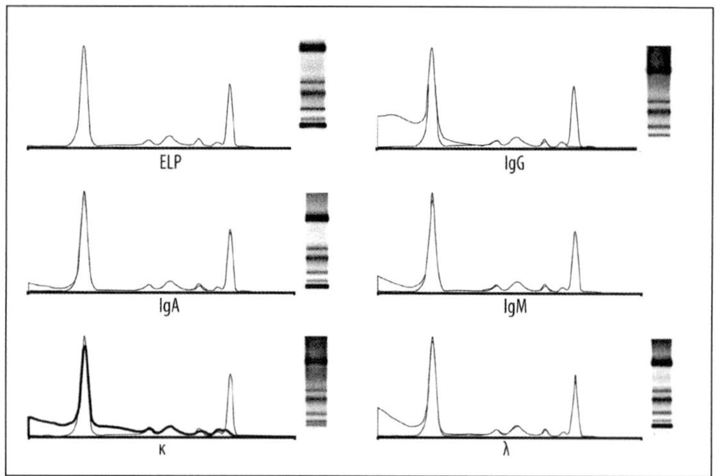

f2.15 Immunotyping (IT) or immunosubtraction demonstrating an IgG κ monoclonal protein

- Patient serum placed into each of 6 wells in an agarose gel
- The gel is subjected to electrophoresis
- 5 different antisera are applied to the gel: Anti-IgG, -IgA, -IgM, -κ, and -λ

- Immunotyping (immune subtraction) **f2.15**
  - Often used in conjunction with capillary electrophoresis
  - Serum sample is incubated with different solid-phase sepharose beads attached to antibodies against γ, α, μ, κ, or λ
  - Supernatants are subjected to electrophoresis to determine which of the reagents resulted in the removal of the abnormal spike

2.6 Enzymes

- Enzymes are organic molecules that accelerate biochemical reactions
- They act as catalyst and emerge from the reaction unchanged, in the same form and concentration as they were when entering the reaction
- The clinical laboratory usually measures enzymes that have leaked into the plasma from damaged cells to identify or monitor the presence of the site and amount of damaged tissue

2.6.1 Classification & nomenclature

- If the name ends in "ase" it is an enzyme
- "ose" is a carbohydrate
- "in" is often a protein
- Standard nomenclature uses
  - Substrate is used as the first name
  - Type of reaction is used as the last name
  - LD conducts a dehydrogenase (oxidation) reaction on lactate
    - Most dehydrogenases use NAD → NADH or NADP → NADPH as a cofactor for the reaction
    - NADH and NADPH both absorb at 340 nm
  - AST conducts a transamination (aminotransferase reaction) on aspartate
    - Most transaminases require pyridoxal phosphate (P5P; a derivative of vitamin B6) for full activity
  - Glucose oxidase conducts an oxidation reaction on glucose
    - Most oxidases use O_2 as the cofactor
  - CK conducts a kinase (phosphorylation) reaction on creatine
    - Most kinases use adenosine triphosphate (ATP) as the cofactor
  - ALP is an "old fashioned" enzyme whose name does not follow the rules
    - Conducts a phosphatase (remove Pi) reaction at alkaline pH
  - Amylase is an "old fashioned" enzyme whose name does not follow the rules
    - Conducts hydrolysis reaction (break a bond) on amylose (starch)

2.6.2 Enzyme kinetics

- Enzymes only make the reaction go faster, not farther
  - They act as a biological catalyst
  - They have an increased rate of reaction
  - No change in equilibrium constant is seen
  - They decrease activation energy of the reaction
- Enzymes make temporary intermediate bonds with substrate (chemical reacting with enzyme) to form ES complex, which has a lower activation energy

$$E + S \leftrightarrow ES \rightarrow E + P$$

- Enzymes are highly specific for the type of reaction they catalyze
  - Sequence of an enzymatic reaction
    - Enzyme (E) binds to substrate (S)

      $$E + S \leftrightarrow ES \text{ complex}$$

    - Bonds are rearranged forming product

      $$ES \rightarrow EP$$

    - Product (P) is released from enzyme

      $$EP \rightarrow E + P$$

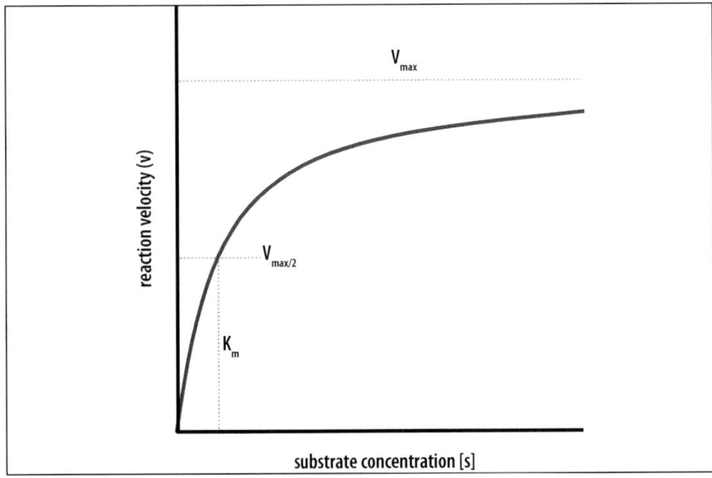

f2.16 Michaelis-Menten curve

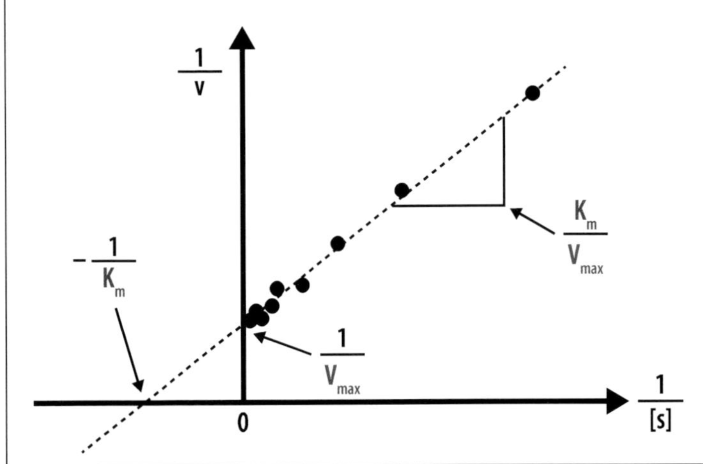

f2.17 Lineweaver-Burk plot

2.6.3 Factors influencing rate of reaction

2.6.3.1 Substrate concentration

2.6.3.1.1 Michaelis-Menten model

- Substrate readily binds to enzyme at low substrate concentration
- Rate of reaction increases as more substrate is added. Rate is directly proportional to substrate concentration—*first order kinetics*
- Eventually, substrate concentration is high enough to saturate all enzyme-binding sites and reaction velocity is at its maximum. Once the product is formed, free enzyme reacts with free substrate—*zero order kinetics*. The rate only depends on enzyme concentration
- Km is the Michaelis-Menten constant
- Michaelis-Menten curve **f2.16**
- Michaelis-Menten equation

$$V = \frac{V_{max}[S]}{K_m + [S]}$$

  - V = measured velocity of reaction
  - V_{max} = maximum velocity
  - [S] = Substrate concentration
  - K_m = Michaelis-Menten constant of enzyme for specific substrate

2.6.3.1.2 Lineweaver-Burk transformation f2.17

- Lineweaver-Burk equation

$$\frac{1}{V} = \frac{K_m}{V_{max}[S]} + \frac{1}{V_{max}}$$

  - This is a more accurate and convenient determination of V_{max} and K_m because it uses a linear plot
  - Y intercept = $1/V_{max}$
  - X intercept = $-1/K_m$

2.6.3.2 Enzyme concentration

- The higher the enzyme concentration, the faster the reaction will proceed because more enzyme is present to bind substrate
- Enzyme activity is extremely sensitive to its shape
- Any condition that changes the shape of a protein will change the shape of enzyme
- Change in enzyme shape is mostly because of its tertiary (3-dimensional) structure

2.6.3.3 Temperature

- ↑ temp → ↑ molecular movement → ↑ intermolecular collisions → ↑ rate of reaction
- Too high temp → irreversible denaturation → ↓ rate of reaction
- Rate of denaturation increases as temp. increases (usually 40°C - 50°C)
- For each 10° increase, the rate of reaction is doubled
- Optimal temperature is close to physiologic temperature (37°C [98.6°F])

2.6.3.4 pH

- Δ [H+] → change in ionizable groups on the enzyme → change in shape of protein → ↓ rate of reaction
- May denature enzyme or influence its ionic state
- Most enzyme reactions occur at pH 7.0-8.0

2.6.3.5 Ionic strength

- ionic strength = cumulative concentration of all solutes
- body enzymes are optimized for isotonic conditions (~300 mmol/L)
- Δ ionic strength changes polarity of the medium → change in shape of the enzyme → ↓ rate of reaction

ISBN 978-089189-6616

2.6.4 Calculating enzyme concentration

- The unit for reporting enzyme concentration is international unit/liter
- IU/L= micromoles (µmol) of substrate used up per minute of incubation per liter
- Using data when the reaction is in zero order:
  - calculate change in absorbance per minute
  - correct for dilution factor and serum volume
  - use molar absorptivity to convert from absorbance to micromoles

$$c = \frac{\Delta A}{\varepsilon b} \times 10^6 \frac{\mu mole}{mole} \times \text{dil factor (total vol/sample vol)}$$

- Example for calculating enzyme concentration:
  - LD reaction which produces NADH
  - Molar absorptivity of NADH at 340 nm = 6220 Abs per mol/L (in 1 cm cuvet)
  - Example: Assume that 10 µL of serum is added to 1 mL of substrate, and Absorbance readings are recorded every 10 seconds during a 1-minute incubation as follows

Time	Abs	∆Abs
10	0.015	
20	0.038	0.023
30	0.068	0.030
40	0.098	0.030
50	0.128	0.030
60	0.135	0.007

  - Use formula to calculate enzyme activity (concentration) in IU/L
- Kinetic vs single point assays
  - Kinetic assay = absorbance readings are measured continuously (or frequently) during incubation
  - One-point assay (also called end-point assay) measures absorbance once after a known incubation period and then calculates ∆Abs/min
  - Advantage of kinetic assay
    - Can inspect the data and use only the zero order reaction
    - Can detect and eliminate lag phase or substrate exhaustion
  - Advantage of one-point assay
    - Can run a big batch of samples all at once

2.6.5 Creatine kinase (CK)

2.6.5.1 Clinical significance

- CK shows highest activity in skeletal muscle, cardiac muscle & brain tissue but also present in intestinal tract, kidney, uterus, thyroid, liver & prostate
  - 3 isoenzymes by electrophoresis or immunoassay
    - CK-1 (BB)—brain and intestine
      - BB (CK1) is fast migrating: found primarily in the brain
    - CK-2 (MB)—mostly cardiac muscle (some skeletal)
      - MB (CK2): Found in skeletal muscle (1% MB) and cardiac muscle (30% MB)
      - Ratio of CK-MB to total CK (the "relative index") improves the specificity of CK-MB for MI; >5% is suggestive of a cardiac source
    - CK-3 (MM)—skeletal and cardiac muscle
      - MM (CK3): Found in skeletal muscle (99% MM) and cardiac muscle (70% MM)
- Total CK levels are always increased in acute MI and muscular dystrophy (50-100 × upper limit of normal)
- Not specific indicator of acute MI
- Macro CK (macro CK type 1) may be found in healthy elderly women
- Mitochondrial CK (macro CK type 2) may be found in patients with advanced malignancy
- Reference range = 25-170 U/L

2.6.5.2 Analytical measurement of CK

- Creatine + ATP ↔ creatine phosphate + ADP
- From adenosine diphosphate (ADP): (optimal pH = 9.0)
  - ADP + phophoenolpyruvate ↔ pyruvate + ATP
  - Pyruvate + NADH + H+ ↔ lactate + NAD+
- From creatine phosphate: (faster, optimal pH = 6.8)
  - Creatine phosphate + ADP ↔ creatine + ATP
  - ATP + glucose ↔ glucose-6-phosphate + ADP
  - Glucose-6-phosphate + $NADP^+$ ↔ 6-phosphogluconate + NADPH + H^+
  - Sample: Serum or heparinized plasma
  - Sources of error: Hemolysis, exercise
- CK isoenzyme electrophoresis **f2.18**
  - (–) CK-3, CK-2, (+) CK-1

2.6.6 Lactate dehydrogenase

2.6.6.1 Clinical significance

- Found in muscle (cardiac & skeletal), liver, kidney, erythrocytes, leukocytes, lungs, lymph nodes, spleen & brain

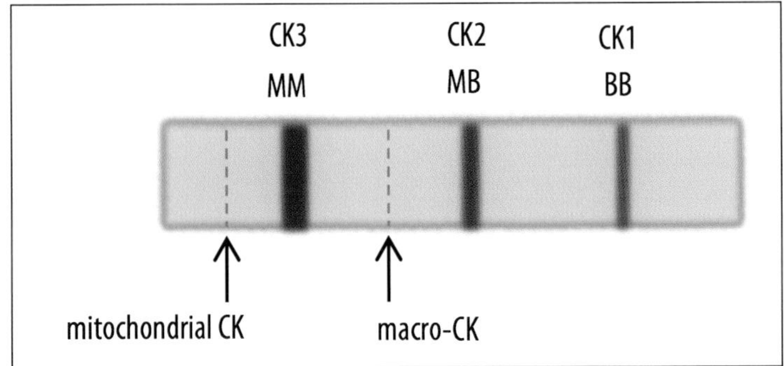

f2.18 Creatine phosphokinase electrophoresis

- Isoenzymes = LD_1(HHHH) to LD_5(MMMM)
  - LD_1 migrates fastest to anode; LD_5 migrates slowest
  - $LD_2 > LD_1$ = healthy
  - $LD_1 > LD_2$ "Flipped LD ratio": Acute MI, hemolysis, renal infarction
  - Increased LD_3 = lungs
  - Increased LD_4 and LD_5 = liver/skeletal muscle
  - Increased LD_5 = liver
  - Increased LD_6 = CAD with liver disease
  - LD isoenzymes rarely measured anymore; total LD elevation is a nonspecific marker of tissue injury or proliferation
- Reference range = 100-225 U/L

2.6.6.2 Analytical measurement of LD

lactate + NAD+ ↔ pyruvate + NADH + H^+

- LD activity is measured by monitoring absorbance at λ = 340 nm (NADH)
- Sources of error in measurement
  - Hemolysis (100-150× more in RBCs)
  - Refrigerated or subzero temperature (store at room temperature)

2.6.7 Aspartate aminotransferase (AST)

2.6.7.1 Clinical significance

- Found in highest concentration in liver (hepatocellular) and cardiac and skeletal muscle (small amounts in kidney, pancreas and RBCs)
- Increased levels in MI (peaks at 24 hours)
- Increase in pulmonary embolism
- Highest increase in acute hepatocellular disorders
- Viral hepatitis can cause values 100× the upper limit of normal
- Cirrhosis causes 4× the upper limit of normal
- Increased in skeletal muscle disorders (muscular dystrophy and inflammatory conditions – 4× the upper limit of normal)
- Reference range = 15-30 U/L

2.6.7.2 Analytical measurement of AST (coupled)

L-aspartate + α-ketoglutarate ←AST→ oxaloacetate + L-glutamate

oxaloacetate + $NADH^+$ + H^+←MDH→ malate + NAD

- Measures decrease in absorbance of NADH at 340 nm
- Must use nonhemolyzed serum

2.6.8 Alanine aminotransferase (ALT)

2.6.8.1 Clinical significance

- ALT is predominantly specific to the liver; it is hepatocellular and correlates well with hepatic release of AST
- Levels remain normal in acute MI
- Increased levels seen in hepatocellular disorders
- Levels increased to a lesser degree in obstructive hepatic disorders
- In acute inflammatory conditions of liver, ALT > AST and remains elevated for a longer period because of the longer half-life of ALT
- Hepatospecificity increases with higher level transaminase elevation; >3× the upper limit of normal rarely observed in nonhepatic disease (exception: rhabdomyolysis)
- AST and ALT has marked diurnal variation (highest in the afternoon)
- DeRitis ratio, the AST: ALT ratio, usually <1; may be >1 in alcohol abuse and cirrhosis
- Reference range = 6-37 U/L

2.6.8.2 Analytical measurement of ALT

- alanine + α-ketoglutarate ↔ pyruvate + glutamate
- pyruvate + NADH + H^+ ↔ lactate + NAD^+
- Measures decrease in absorbance of NADH at 340 nm
- Preferred sample is nonhemolyzed serum/lithium heparin plasma

2.6.9 Alkaline phosphatase (ALP)

2.6.9.1 Clinical significance

- Most significant in hepatobiliary and bone disorders
- Major isoenzymes—bone, liver, placenta & intestine
- Differ in heat stability (56°C for 10 minutes)

 ISBN 978-089189-6616

- Bone burns (<20%), liver lingers (~25%-55%), followed by intestine and placenta persists (>75%)
- Traditional methods for discovering the tissue source of elevated ALP t2.13; in current practice, one usually measures γ-glutamyl transferase (GGT) or 5'-nucleotidase to confirm hepatobiliary origin

t2.13 Characteristics of alkaline phosphatase isoenzyme

Source	Heat/urea inhibition	l-phe inhibition	Anodal mobility
Biliary	+	–	1
Bone	+++	–	2
Placenta	–	+++	3
Intestinal	+	+++	4

- Can be separated by electrophoresis
- Liver is fastest, followed by bone, placenta & intestine
- Selective chemical inhibition using phenylalanine (phe)
  - Inhibits intestinal and placental ALP more than bone and liver
- Regan (tumor) isoenzyme resembles placental ALP; observed in a small proportion of individuals with malignant disease; thought to be re-expression of placental ALP gene in tumor cells
- Specific location in tissue accounts for increases in certain disorders
- Liver: Lining of sinusoids and bile canaliculi, ie, biliary
- Bone: Osteoblasts (involved in production of bone matrix)
- In biliary tract obstruction: ALP is 3-10× the upper limit of normal
- In hepatocellular disorders: <3× the upper limit of normal
- Increased in bone disorders such as Paget disease, osteomalacia, rickets, osteogenic sarcoma
- ALP increased during childhood (bone growth) and pregnancy (placental ALP)
- Increase in healing bone fractures, during periods of physiologic bone growth, and in adults >50 years
- Pregnancy: ALP 1.5× the upper limit of normal (detected between 16 and 20 weeks)
- Can be increased in diseases of digestive tract because of intestinal fraction
- Postprandial ALP may be increased in certain individuals (intestinal ALP), particularly in Lewis positive group B or O secretors
- Medications (oral contraceptives, nonsteroidal anti-inflammatory drugs) may elevate ALP levels
- ALP is a sensitive marker of hepatic metastases
- Decreased ALP is found in hypophosphatasia (an inborn deficiency) and malnutrition; reported in hemolysis, Wilson disease, theophylline therapy, and estrogen therapy in postmenopausal women

2.6.9.2 Analytical measurement of ALP

- p-Nitrophenyl ↔ p-Nitrophenol + phosphate ion
- Increase in absorbance of p-nitrophenol is measured at 405 nm
- Sources of error
  - High fat meals (intestinal ALP)
  - Left at room temperature or refrigerated temperature for more than 8 hours (run ASAP)
- Reference range = 30-90 U/L

2.6.10 Acid phosphatase (AP)

2.6.10.1 Clinical significance

- Found mostly in the prostate
- Major significance in detection of prostatic carcinoma (particularly metastasized carcinoma)
- Also increased in benign prostatic hyperplasia and prostate surgery
- Used to monitor therapy

2.6.10.2 Analytical measurement of acid phosphatase

- Measured by the p-nitrophenol reaction (pH = 5)
- Sources of error: Hemolysis, room temperature (loss of CO_2 — pH change)

2.6.11 γ-glutamyl transferase (GGT)

2.6.11.1 Clinical significance

- Clinical applications in liver and biliary system disorders
- May be used to confirm that an elevated ALP is from the biliary tree
- Alcohol induces synthesis of GGT; used as indicator of alcohol abuse
- Increases also seen in pancreatitis, diabetes & MI
- Increased in patients exposed to warfarin, barbiturates, phenytoin, valproate, methotrexate & alcohol
- May be elevated in renal failure and pancreatic disease
- Reference range: Up to 45 U/L

2.6.11.2 Analytical measurement of GGT

λ-glutamyl-p-nitroaniline + glycylglycine ⟶ p-nitroaniline + λ-glutamylglycylglycine

- Increase in absorbance from p-nitroaniline is measured at 410 nm

2.6.12 Amylase

2.6.12.1 Clinical significance

- Catalyzes the breakdown of starch and glycogen
- Serum amylase consists primarily of salivary (S type) and pancreatic (P type) isoenzymes
- Diagnosis of acute pancreatitis
  - In uncomplicated acute pancreatitis, amylase rises within 2-24 hours and returns to normal in 2-3 days; persistence beyond 5 days suggests a complication such as pseudocyst
  - Higher amylase does not correlate with greater severity but is more specific for pancreatitis
  - Up to 10% of cases of acute pancreatitis are associated with normal levels of amylase; sensitivity lowest in chronic relapsing and alcoholic pancreatitis
- Up to 30% of amylase elevations are caused by nonpancreatic disorders (diabetic ketoacidosis, peptic ulcer disease, acute cholecystitis, ectopic pregnancy, salpingitis, bowel ischemia, intestinal obstruction, macroamylasemia & renal insufficiency)
- Sources of error: High TG suppress/inhibits amylase, EDTA, or citrate anticoagulant
- Reference range: 35-125 U/L

2.6.12.2 Analytical measurement of amylase

$$\text{maltoheptaose—nitrophenyl} \xleftarrow{} \text{amy} \rightarrow \text{4-nitrophenol + glucose fragments}$$
$$\xrightarrow{\text{alkaline pH}} \text{4-nitrophenoxide anion}$$

- Increase in abs is measured at 405 nm

2.6.13 Lipase

2.6.13.1 Clinical significance

- Hydrolyzes ester linkages of fats to produce alcohols and fatty acids
- Present in pancreas, stomach, leukocytes & adipose tissue
- Specific for diagnosis of acute pancreatitis
- More specific than amylase but remains elevated for up to 14 days
- Less dependent than amylase on renal clearance
- Reference range: 10-200 U/L

2.6.13.2 Analytical measurement of lipase

- Same as TG measurement except TG is in excess and lipase is limited

$$\text{triglycerides + lipase} \rightarrow \text{fatty acids + glycerol}$$
$$\text{glycerol + ATP}(Mg^{+2}) \text{ + glycerol kinase} \rightarrow \text{glycerol-1-phosphate + ADP}$$
$$\text{glycerol-1-phosphate} + O_2 + \text{glycerol oxidase} \rightarrow \text{DHAP} + H_2O_2$$
$$H_2O_2 + \text{4-AAP + dye-precursor} \rightarrow H_2O + \text{quinonimine dye (colored)}$$

- Confirming acute pancreatitis
  - Amylase: At a cutoff of 3× the upper limit of normal, the specificity is 95% and the sensitivity is 60%-80%
  - Lipase: At a cutoff of 3× upper limit of normal, the specificity and sensitivity approach 90% each

2.6.14 Cholinesterase

- Hydrolyzes esters of choline to destroy poisons or drugs
- Found in liver, heart, and white matter of brain
- Not specific but a sensitive marker for organophosphate poisoning
- Decrease seen in liver disease, starvation, burns & insecticide poisoning
- Two types
  - Acetylcholinesterase
  - Pseudocholinesterase
- Sources of error: Hemolysis (erythrocytes contain acetylcholinesterase)

2.6.15 5'-nucleotidase

- Biliary epithelium is the main source of 5'-nucleotidase

2.7 Renal & nonprotein nitrogen (NPN) compounds

2.7.1 Urinary system anatomy

- Kidney
  - Structure
    - Bean-shaped paired organs, located in the posterior part of the abdomen, each weighing ~150 g
    - Cortex: Outer layer, composed mostly of glomeruli, and proximal and distal convoluted tubules
    - Medulla: Inner layer, composed mostly of loops of Henle and collecting ducts
    - Renal pelvis: Collects urine
  - Function
    - Excretory: Serves to rid the body of the undesirable end-products of metabolism and excess inorganic substances ingested in the diet (urea, creatinine, uric acid)

ISBN 978-089189-6616

- Regulatory: The kidneys play a major role in homeostasis
  - Fluid & electrolyte balance
  - Acid-base balance
- Endocrine
  - Primary: Produces hormones (renin, prostaglandins, erythropoietin)
  - Secondary: Activation of hormones produced elsewhere (vitamin D)

- Ureter: Urine flows from the renal pelvis into the ureter and then to the bladder
- Bladder: Urine is stored in the bladder until voided
- Urethra: Urine is voided through the urethra to outside the body

2.7.1.1 Major components of the kidney (microanatomy)

- Nephron
- The nephron is the functional unit of the kidney. Each kidney contains approximately 1 million nephrons
- The nephron is composed of 3 main units:
  - Arterioles
  - Glomeruli
  - Tubules
- Afferent arteriole: Incoming blood supply to the glomerulus
- Efferent arteriole: Outgoing blood supply from the glomerulus
- Glomerulus
  - Located in the renal cortex
  - Tuft of porous capillaries that is formed from the afferent arteriole and drained by the efferent arteriole
  - Main function is filtration
- Bowman capsule: Surrounds the glomerulus and opens to the proximal convoluted tubule
- Proximal convoluted tubule
  - First segment of the tubule that runs through the renal cortex
  - Main function is reabsorption
- Loop of Henle
  - Extends into the renal medulla
  - Main function is urine concentration
- Distal convoluted tubule
  - Extends back into the renal cortex
  - Main function is homeostatic regulation
- Collecting duct
  - Extends into the renal medulla
  - Directs urine flow into the renal pelvis

2.7.2 Physiological mechanisms of urine formation

2.7.2.1 Renal blood flow

- Approximately 25% of cardiac output (1000-1500 mL) of blood pass through the kidney per minute
- The blood supply is crucial for optimal function of the kidney
- Glomerular filtration rate (GFR) is affected by the blood flow to the glomerulus
  - Afferent arterioles are larger in diameter than efferent arterioles. This provides a high hydrostatic pressure to achieve filtration
  - The size of afferent arterioles may increase or decrease, eg, if the blood pressure in the body is low and the GFR is decreased, the size increases. This increases the hydrostatic pressure and increases GFR
- Enzymes and hormones are released to control blood pressure and maintain GFR
  - Renin: Produced in the juxtaglomerular apparatus. This enzyme is released when blood pressure is decreased, blood volume is decreased, blood sodium is decreased, or blood K^+ is increased
  - Renin causes angiotensinogen to form angiotensin I, which forms angiotensin II, which stimulates the adrenal cortex to release aldosterone. Angiotensin II constricts arteries, which increases blood pressure and increases GFR
  - Aldosterone: Causes an increase in Na^+ reabsorption from tubule to blood, and an increase in K^+ and H^+ secretion in the urine
- Efferent arterioles flow into the peritubular capillaries, which supply blood to tubules. Low hydrostatic pressure here (small diameter) allows for reabsorption and secretion

2.7.2.2 Glomerular filtration

- Nonselective filtration across the semipermeable membrane of the capillary tuft occurs because of the high hydrostatic pressure
  - All substances of a molecular weight <70,000 are filtered into urine
  - The filtrate is almost identical to plasma, but contains no plasma proteins, any protein-bound substances, or cells
- Glomerular filtration rate
  - The volume of fluid that is filtered across the glomerular capillary per minute
  - Approximately 120 mL/min of ultrafiltrate is formed

  - Glomerular filtration rate depends on:
    - Blood pressure
    - Oncotic pressure
  - Because of the difference in proteins in plasma and the ultrafiltrate, the oncotic pressure difference opposes filtration

2.7.2.3 Tubular reabsorption

- Conservation of water & nutrients
- Returns substances to plasma from glomerular filtrate
- Passive transport: Requires no energy expenditure by the body, simple diffusion
- Substances reabsorbed by passive transport
  - Water
  - Urea
  - Chloride
- Active transport: Requires metabolic energy from transport cells to carry substances against a gradient. Active reabsorption depends on the concentration in the blood
- Substances requiring active transport to be reabsorbed include:
  - Glucose
  - Amino acids
  - Uric acid
  - Electrolytes (sodium, potassium, chloride)
  - Magnesium
  - Calcium
  - Bicarbonate
- Proximal convoluted tubule
  - Majority of reabsorption occurs here
  - 75% of the sodium, chloride & water of the ultrafiltrate is reabsorbed
  - Passive transport of chloride, potassium, water
  - Active transport of sodium, glucose
  - Most of the bicarbonate, phosphate, calcium & potassium is also reabsorbed
- Loop of Henle
  - Descending limb
    - Highly permeable to water
    - Passive reabsorption of water because of the hypertonic medulla environment
    - Concentration of urine occurs here
  - Ascending limb
    - Impermeable to water
    - Active reabsorption of sodium & chloride
    - Dilution of urine occurs here
  - Distal convoluted tubule
    - Hormonal control
    - Antidiuretic hormone (ADH) increases water permeability, more water absorbed
    - Aldosterone stimulates sodium reabsorption & potassium secretion
  - Collecting duct
    - ADH controls water reabsorption
    - Aldosterone stimulates sodium reabsorption

2.7.2.4 Tubular secretion

- Substances in the peritubular capillary blood are secreted into the filtrate
- Proximal convoluted tubules: Elimination of waste products not filtered by the glomerulus
  - Medications dissociate from their carrier proteins and are transported into the filtrate by the tubular cells
  - Organic waste is secreted: urea, uric acid
  - Tamm-Horsfall glycoprotein is secreted
- Distal convoluted tubules: Regulation of acid-base balance
  - H^+ secretion to conserve bicarbonate
  - H^+ secreted and exchanged for sodium (Na_2HPO_4)
  - H_+ secreted and NH_3 secreted to form NH_4^+ (excreted)

2.7.2.5 Renal threshold

- Substances are reabsorbed according to their concentration in the blood and the body's needs
- When the plasma concentration of a substance is high, reabsorption of the nutrient is no longer possible
- The nutrient is then spilled into the urine, eg, glucose renal threshold = 160 mg/dL

2.7.3 Nonprotein nitrogen compounds (NPN)

- An NPN compound is any nitrogen-containing compound that is not a protein
- NPN compounds are usually waste products from protein metabolism
- Azotemia: Any significant increase of NPN compounds (usually urea & creatinine) in the blood
- NPN compounds include:
  - Amino acids: Derived from the catabolism of either exogenous or endogenous proteins
  - Ammonia: Derived from the catabolism of amino acids

ISBN 978-089189-6616

- Urea: Derived from the catabolism of ammonia (75% of NPN compounds eventually excreted)
- Creatinine: Derived from the metabolism of creatine in muscle tissues
- Uric acid: Derived from the catabolism of nucleic acids

2.7.3.1 Urea

- Chemical structure of urea

$$NH_2-\overset{\overset{\displaystyle O}{\|}}{C}-NH_2$$

- Metabolism of urea
  - Urea is the end-product of protein catabolism and is synthesized in the liver
    Protein → amino acids → ammonia → urea
  - >90% of urea is excreted by the kidneys
- Urea vs blood urea nitrogen (BUN)
  - Results of a urea assay are usually reported in units of urea nitrogen (mg/dL) rather than units of urea (mmol/L)
  - Conversion of BUN values to urea concentrations
  - Atomic weight of nitrogen = 14 g/mol
  - Molecular weight of urea = 60 g/mol
- Urea contains 2 nitrogen atoms per molecule
  - 14 × 2 = 28 or 60/28 = 2.14
  - BUN (mg/L) × 2.14 = urea(mg/L)
  - BUN (mg/dL) × 0.357 = urea (mmol/L)
- Methods of BUN and urea measurement
  - Indirect methods: Based on the preliminary hydrolysis of urea with urease to liberate ammonium ions
    - Urease reaction

$$NH_2-\overset{\overset{\displaystyle O}{\|}}{C}-NH_2 + 2\,H_2O \xrightarrow{\text{urease}} 2\,NH_4^+ + CO_3^{2-}$$

    - The ammonium ion produced can then be quantitated by 1 of several methods
  - Glutamate dehydrogenase: Coupled enzyme system using an NAD/NADH indicator reaction. Ammonia reacts with 2-oxoglutarate in the presence of NADH and glutamate dehydrogenase to form glutamine and NAD. The decrease in absorbance at 340 nm is proportional to the ammonia concentration

$$NH_4^+ + \text{2-oxoglutarate} \xrightarrow[\text{NADH} \;\; \text{NAD}^+ + \text{H}^+]{\text{GLDH}} \text{glutamine}$$

GLDH = glutamate dehydrogenase

    - This is the most frequently used method and is very specific and rapid
  - Conductimetric: The urease reaction results in the conversion of the nonionic species (urea) to an ionic form (ammonium carbonate). The resultant change in conductivity is measured

$$\text{urea} \rightarrow (NH_4)_2CO_3 \xrightarrow{\text{urease}} 2NH_4^+ + CO_3^{2-}$$

    - This method is commonly used and is very specific and rapid
- Specimen collection and handling requirements
  - Specimen of choice: Serum or heparinized plasma
    - Ammonium heparin cannot be used as an anticoagulant for urease methods
    - Fluoride inhibits the urease reaction, therefore fluoride cannot be used as a preservative
    - Urea is stable in serum up to 24 hours at room temperature and several days when refrigerated
  - Urine samples
    - Urea is highly concentrated in urine, therefore urine samples are usually diluted 10-20 times before analysis
    - Urea is stable in urine at pH <5.0 for several days when refrigerated. Urine contaminated with bacteria that hydrolyze urea will cause a loss of urea and formation of ammonia
- Reference ranges
  - Serum (adults): 6-20 mg/dL (530-1768 μmol/L)
  - Urine:12-20 g/24 hours
- Clinical significance of BUN
  - Serum urea levels may vary with diet, synthesis in the liver & amount excreted by the kidneys
  - An increase in BUN is called azotemia, and uremia refers to high BUN and its toxic effects
  - Renal azotemia: A wide variety of renal diseases can cause an increase in plasma urea concentrations. The usefulness of urea as an independent indicator of renal function is limited by the variability of nonrenal factors
  - Prerenal azotemia: Increased amino acid metabolism in the liver (high protein diet, tissue breakdown, or decreased protein synthesis)
  - Postrenal azotemia: Obstruction of the urinary system
  - Decreased serum urea levels are seen with a low protein diet and severe liver disease

2.7.3.2 Creatinine

- Chemical structure of creatine & creatinine

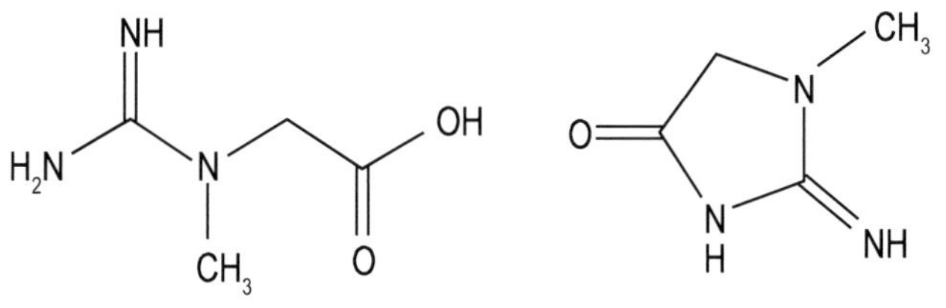

- Formation of creatinine
  - Creatinine is derived spontaneously from creatine in muscle tissue. Approximately 2% of muscle creatine is converted to creatinine daily. Because the amount of creatinine produced is proportional to muscle mass, the excretion rate is relatively constant
- Methods of creatinine measurement
  - Jaffe reaction: Reaction of creatinine with an alkaline solution of sodium picrate to form a red Janovski complex

    creatinine + picrate → Janovski complex

    - This reaction lacks specificity. Protein, ascorbic acid, pyruvate, acetone, acetoacetic acid, glucose, and uric acid will also give a positive reaction. Several modifications are available to increase the specificity of this method
    - Protein free filtrate: Tungstic acid is added to the specimen to precipitate out the protein. The supernatant is then made to react with the alkaline picrate solution
    - Absorbent material (Fuller earth, Lloyd reagent): Absorbs the creatinine present in the protein-free filtrate. The creatinine-adsorbent pellet then reacts with the alkaline picrate solution
    - Kinetic measurement: Measurement is made after fast-reacting interferents have reacted and before slow-reacting interferents have reacted with the alkaline picrate solution. Creatinine will react within this "window"
  - Enzymatic measurements
    - Creatinine amidohydrolase: This enzyme will convert creatinine to creatine. The creatine is then measured by a coupled indicator reaction
    - Creatinine iminohydrolase: This enzyme will convert creatinine to N-methylhydantoin and ammonia. The ammonia is then measured by a coupled indicator reaction
- Specimen collection and handling requirements
  - Specimen of choice: Serum or plasma
  - Ammonium heparin cannot be used for the creatinine iminohydrolase method
  - To minimize in vitro ammonia production, serum should be removed from red cells and analyzed promptly
  - Creatinine is stable for up to 7 days when refrigerated
  - Urine samples: Because creatinine is highly concentrated in the urine, urine samples are usually diluted before analysis
- Reference ranges
  - Serum: Male: 0.6-1.2 mg/dL (53-106 µmol/L); female: 0.5-1.1 mg/dL (44-97 µmol/L)
  - Urine: Male: 1400-2600 mg/24 h; female: 1100-2000 mg/24 h
- Clinical significance of creatinine
  - Serum creatinine levels are a direct reflection of muscle mass and show little or no response to dietary changes
  - Creatinine passes freely through the glomerulus
  - A small amount is secreted by the tubules, and the quantity of tubular secretion increases with increasing serum creatinine concentration
  - At all serum concentrations, creatinine slightly overestimates glomerular filtration rate (GFR)
  - The simplest way to calculate GFR is based on the creatinine clearance
  - Increased serum creatinine levels are seen with impaired renal function
  - Creatinine levels in amniotic fluid may be used to determine fetal muscle mass and thus fetal maturity
- BUN-creatinine reference range ratio: 10:1-20:1

 ISBN 978-089189-6616

2.7.3.3 Uric acid

- Chemical structure of uric acid
- Formation of uric acid
  - Uric acid is the end-product of purine (nucleic acid) metabolism. It is synthesized in the liver
  - Serum uric acid levels depend on several factors
    - Purine synthesis & metabolism
    - Dietary intake
    - Renal function
- Methods of uric acid measurement
  - Phosphotungstic acid reaction: Reduction of phosphotungstic acid by uric acid to form tungsten blue. Protein must be removed before the reaction. This method is of historical interest and lacks specificity. Many substances cause a false-positive interference (glucose, ascorbic acid, acetaminophen, caffeine)
  - Uricase methods: Uricase catalyzes the oxidation of uric acid to form allantoin and hydrogen peroxide

$$\text{uric acid} \xrightarrow{\text{uricase}} \text{allantoin} + H_2O_2$$

  - The decrease in absorbance as uric acid is converted may be monitored
  - The hydrogen peroxide produced may be measured by several different coupled reactions
  - Uricase methods have increased specificity and are widely used
- Specimen collection and handling requirements
  - Specimen of choice: Serum/plasma
  - Uric acid is stable in urine for 3-7 days when refrigerated
  - Uric acid in urine is stable several days at room temperature but should be refrigerated to avoid bacterial growth
- Reference ranges
  - Serum: Male: 3.5-7.2 mg/dL (0.21-0.43 mmol/L); female: 2.6-6.0 mg/dL (0.15-0.36 mmol/L)
  - Urine: 250-750 mg/24 h
- Clinical significance of uric acid: Increased uric acid levels are seen with:
  - gout
  - increased cell turnover
  - renal impairment
  - high protein diet or starvation
  - diabetes
- Uric acid is very insoluble and can form kidney stones

2.7.4 Renal clearance tests

- Renal clearance is a rate measurement that expresses the volume of blood cleared of the substance being measured per unit of time. Clearance tests are used to measure the GFR. Substances used to measure GFR should be filtered exclusively by the glomerulus but neither reabsorbed nor secreted by other regions of the nephron
- Inulin
  - Inulin clearance provides the most precise determination of GFR
  - The glomerular wall is freely permeable to inulin
  - Inulin is not reabsorbed, secreted, or metabolically altered by the renal tubules
  - Inulin is not an endogenous substance and requires intravenous administration thus limiting its practical use
- Creatinine
  - Glomerular function is most conveniently measured by the creatinine clearance test
  - Creatinine is freely filtered by the glomerulus and is not reabsorbed by the tubules
  - The amount of creatinine produced by endogenous metabolism is relatively constant and directly proportional to body surface area
- Urea
  - Urea clearance generally underestimates GFR
  - Urea is freely filtered and partially reabsorbed by the nephron; this reabsorption has the consequence that BUN always slightly underestimates GFR
  - Reabsorption increases with hypovolemia; BUN underestimates GFR even more in hypovolemic states
  - 90% of urea is excreted through the kidney
  - Approximately 40% of filtered urea is passively reabsorbed by the renal tubules
  - Urea production is too dependent on several nonrenal variables such as diet and hepatic synthesis to make it useful as a measure of GFR

2.7.4.1 Renal clearance test: Patient preparation & specimen requirements

- Patient preparation
  - Hydrate the patient with at least 600 mL of water
  - Withhold tea, coffee & medication on the day of the test
- Specimen requirements
  - Collect a 24-hour urine specimen
  - Collect a blood sample during the 24-hour period
  - Measure the volume of the 24-hour urine collection (in milliliters per minute)
  - Determine the plasma and urine creatinine levels (in milligrams per deciliter)
- Calculate a renal clearance
- Clearance formula:

$$C = \frac{U \times V}{P}$$

$$\text{clearance (mL/min)} = \frac{\text{urine level (mg/dL)} \times \text{urine volume (mL/min)}}{\text{plasma level (mg/dL)}}$$

- Corrected clearance formula:

$$\text{corrected clearance} = \text{clearance (mL/min)} \times 1.73/A$$

where A = body surface area (m^2)

- Relationship between GFR and creatinine is nonlinear; mild to moderate GFR impairment does not cause appreciable increase in creatinine. When GFR is about 1/2 normal, creatinine begins to linearly reflect changes in GFR
- Nonglomerular influences on creatinine; creatinine concentration is increased by muscle mass, muscle activity, muscle injury (trauma, surgery), and protein intake. It tends to decrease with age, and is influenced by race, sex, medications
- The Modification of Diet in Renal Disease (MDRD) Study equation is the most widely used formula, but it is being replaced by the Chronic Kidney Disease Epidemiologic Collaborative (CKD EPI) equation in many laboratories. The MDRD equation is invalid at high GFR (eGFR over 60 mL/min per 1.73 m^2 reported simply as ">60 mL/min per 1.73 m^2"), whereas the CKD EPI equation is valid over the whole eGFR range
- Reference ranges for creatinine clearance: Male: 97-137 mL/min; female: 88-128 mL/min
- Clinical significance of creatinine clearance
  - Creatinine clearance is used to measure glomerular function
  - As renal function fails, creatinine clearance decreases
- BUN/creatinine ratio

$$\frac{\text{serum urea nitrogen (mg/dL)}}{\text{serum creatinine (mg/dL)}}$$

  - Reference range: Normal is ~10:1
  - Decreased ratio: Acute tubular necrosis, low protein intake, starvation or severe liver disease
  - Increased ratio: Frequently to >20:1, in renal hypoperfusion (because of hypovolemia, hypotension, etc) termed prerenal azotemia, catabolic states of tissue breakdown, high protein intake, or postrenal azotemia
  - Ratio is maintained near normal in intrarenal causes of renal failure
- Estimated GFR (eGFR)
  - The national kidney foundation recommends that eGFR be reported each time with serum creatinine results
  - Does not require timed urine collection
  - Helpful in early detection of chronic kidney disease
  - Calculation:

$$\text{GFR (mL/min)} = \frac{(140 - \text{age}) \times \text{weight (kg)} \times K}{72 \times P \text{ (mg/dL)}}$$

$K = 0.85$ for women & 1.00 for men

2.7.4.2 Renal tubular function tests

- These are used to measure the absorption and secretion ability of the kidney
  - Osmolality
    - Measurement of the number of moles of particles per kilogram of water
    - Measures the concentrating and diluting ability of the renal tubules
    - Impairment of renal concentrating ability is a relatively early manifestation of chronic renal disease
  - Concentration tests: Withhold fluids overnight and then collect a urine specimen. An osmolality of 850 mOsm/kg indicates normal concentrating ability
  - Dilution tests: The patient is given a water load (1000-1200 mL). Urine specimens are collected every hour for the next 4 hours. An osmolality of <100 mOsm/kg indicates normal diluting ability
  - Specific gravity
    - The ratio of weight in grams per milliliter of a body fluid compared with water
    - Measures the concentrating and diluting ability of the renal tubules
    - Concentration tests: A specific gravity of 1.025 indicates normal concentrating ability
    - Dilution tests: A specific gravity of <1.005 indicates normal diluting ability

ISBN 978-089189-6616

- Phenolsulfonphthalein (PSP) dye test
  - Test the secretory function of the renal tubules
  - PSP dye is injected intravenously
  - This test is of historical interest and is not routinely used
- Para-aminohippurate (PAH) test
  - Test the secretory function of the renal tubules
  - PAH is injected intravenously
  - This test is not commonly performed

2.7.5 Pathological conditions of the kidney

- Acute renal failure: Rapid and severe reduction of GFR with oliguria
- Prerenal: Caused by reduced blood flow or cardiovascular failure
  - BUN ↑, creatinine N, Ratio ↑
  - Sodium & urea urine output ↓
- Renal: Caused by diseases affecting the glomerulus or tubule function (acute glomerulonephritis, acute tubular necrosis)
  - BUN ↑↑, creatinine ↑, ratio N or slightly ↑
  - Sodium and urea urine output ↑
- Postrenal: Caused by obstruction of urine flow
  - BUN ↑↑, creatinine ↑, ratio N or ↑

2.7.5.1 Glomerular diseases

- These are diseases that cause injury to the renal glomerulus without affecting tubular function. Eventually chronic progressive glomerular disease will affect the blood supply of tubules and result in complete loss of nephrons to produce chronic renal failure

2.7.5.1.1 Acute glomerulonephritis

- Rapid onset of hematuria (red cell cast), proteinuria, reduced GFR, oliguria, and hypertension
- Inflammatory response to immune complexes presents after a group A β-hemolytic streptococcal infection
- Other causes include reactions to drugs, acute infection of the kidney, systemic diseases with immune complexes (systemic lupus erythematosus [SLE], bacterial endocarditis)

2.7.5.1.2 Chronic glomerulonephritis

- Progressive loss of nephron mass
- Asymptomatic except for mild hematuria, proteinuria & reduced renal function
- Nephrotic syndrome: Glomerular injury with excessive permeability to plasma proteins
  - Massive proteinuria, hypoalbuminemia, hyperlipidemia & lipiduria (oval fat bodies)
  - Other laboratory findings include increased α_2 & β globulins, decreased binding proteins, and increased cholesterol and triglycerides (TG)
  - Nephrotic syndrome can be seen with several systemic diseases including diabetes mellitus, amyloidosis, and SLE

2.7.5.2 Tubular diseases

- Disorders of renal tubular function in which depressed renal function cannot be explained by decreased GFR

2.7.5.2.1 Tubular necrosis

- Ischemic or toxic damage to the tubules including bacterial, fungal, or viral infections; reactions to drugs; & rejection of kidney transplant
- Depressed secretion or reabsorption with impaired concentrating ability

2.7.5.2.2 Renal tubular acidosis

- Failure of the proximal tubule to reabsorb bicarbonate because of decreased secretion of H^+
- The loss of alkali in the urine causes the blood to become acidotic

2.7.5.3 Urinary tract obstruction

- Obstruction may be at any level in the urinary tract and may lead to chronic renal damage. Obstruction is frequently complicated by urinary tract infection. Causes may include:
  - Prostatic hypertrophy
  - Carcinoma of the prostate, bladder, or lymph nodes
  - Renal calculi
    - Crystallization of the following substances: Calcium oxalate, calcium phosphate, uric acid & cystine
    - Usually causes extreme pain

2.7.5.4 Chronic kidney disease

- The current recommendation of the National Kidney Foundation is annual testing for those at high risk for chronic kidney disease
- High-risk individuals are those who have diabetes mellitus, hypertension & family history of renal disease
- Recommended screening for high-risk groups includes eGFR and microalbuminuria screening (urine albumin-creatinine ratio)
- Chronic kidney disease is defined by
  - GFR <60 mL/min per 1.73 m^2 of body surface area
  - Albuminuria for ≥3 consecutive months

- The degree (or stage) of chronic kidney disease is categorized as follows:
  - Stage 1: Kidney damage (albuminuria) without decreased GFR (GFR >90 mL/min per 1.73 m^2)
  - Stage 2: Kidney damage with a mild decrease in GFR (60-89 mL/min per 1.73 m^2)
  - Stage 3: Moderate decrease in GFR (30-59 mL/min per 1.73 m^2)
  - Stage 4: Severe decrease in GFR (15-29 mL/min per 1.73 m^2)
  - Stage 5: Renal failure (GFR <15 mL/min per 1.73 m^2 or dialysis dependence)

2.7.5.5 Acute renal failure (ARF) t2.14, t2.15

- Prerenal ARF
  - Result of decreased renal perfusion
  - Sustained benefit by expansion of intravascular volume with colloid is characteristic
  - BUN-creatinine ratio usually elevated
  - Fractional excretion of sodium in urine (FENa) low (<1%)
  - "Inactive" urine sediment
- Postrenal ARF
  - Bilateral obstruction of the renal collecting system
  - BUN-creatinine ratio often elevated
- Intrarenal ARF
  - Injury to the nephron (glomeruli, tubules, vessels, or interstitium)
  - Most common cause of intrarenal ARF is acute tubular necrosis (ATN) & the most common causes of ATN are ischemia and nephrotoxins. Acute glomerulonephritis (AGN) may also cause intrarenal ARF
  - Usually normal BUN-creatinine ratio
  - FENa >1%
  - Urine may show "active" sediment: Dysmorphic red blood cells and red blood cell casts in glomerulonephritis; coarse granular casts in ATN, glomerulonephritis, or interstitial nephritis; white blood cell casts in pyelonephritis; eosinophils in acute allergic interstitial nephritis

t2.14 Prerenal vs renal ARF

Parameter	Prerenal ARF	Renal ARF
BUN/creatinine ratio	>20:1	<20:1
Urine specific gravity	High (>1.020)	Low (<1.010)
Urine osmolarity	High (>500 mOsm/kg)	Low (300 500)
FE Na	<1%	>1%
FE urea	<35%	>35%

ARF, acute renal failure; BUN, blood urea nitrogen; FENa, fractional excretion of sodium; Fe urea, fractional excretion of urea

t2.15 Causes of ARF

Prerenal	Renal	Postrenal
Acute tubulointerstitial nephritis (NSAIDs) Vasculitis Bilateral ureteral obstruction (tumor, retroperitoneal fibrosis)	Bladder outlet obstruction (prostatism)	

ACE, angiotensin converting enzyme; ARF, acute renal failure; CHF, congestive heart failure; NSAIDs, nonsteroidal anti-inflammatory drugs

2.8 Acid-base disorders

2.8.1 Metabolically produced acids

- Volatile acid = CO_2
  - ~20 mol produced each day by normal metabolism
- Nonvolatile acids are acids derived from sources other than CO_2, eg, uric acid, phosphoric acid, sulfuric acid
  - ~100 mmol/day produced by normal metabolism
- They cannot be removed through lungs and must be excreted through the kidney
- Present mainly as their conjugate base because their H^+ has been neutralized by body buffers

2.8.2 Body buffers

- Blood and tissues contain buffer systems to minimize changes in hydrogen ion concentration
- The bicarbonate buffer
- The CO_2 produced in tissues diffuses through the cell membranes and dissolves in plasma
- When acid (H^+) is added to HCO_3^-, it will combine with it to form H_2CO_3; excess CO_2 is eliminated through lungs and H^+ as water
$$H^+ + HCO_3^- \leftrightarrow H_2CO_3 \leftrightarrow CO_2 + H_2O$$
- When a base is added to the body, H_2CO_3 will combine with OH^- to form H_2O and HCO_3^- which is taken up by the kidneys
$$OH^- + H_2CO_3 \leftrightarrow H_2O + HCO_3^-$$
- The bicarbonate buffer
$$H^+ + HCO_3^- \leftrightarrow H_2CO_3 \leftrightarrow CO_2 + H_2O$$
- Henderson-Hasselbalch equation
$$K_{dissociation} = \frac{[H^+]\,[HCO_3^-]}{[H_2CO_3]}$$
$$pK = pH - \log \frac{[HCO_3^-]}{[H_2CO_3]}$$
Henderson-Hasselbalch equation
$$pH = pK + \log \frac{[HCO_3^-]}{[H_2CO_3]}$$
- Despite the variation of CO_2 and acids, blood pH remains between 7.35 and 7.45

ISBN 978-089189-6616

- $[H_2CO_3]$ is measured as dissolved CO_2, ie, PCO_2
  - PCO_2 mm Hg × 0.03 = H_2CO_3 mmol/L
  - Where PCO_2 is the partial pressure of CO_2, 0.03 is the solubility coefficient of CO_2
- Because of this equilibrium, acid component of bicarbonate buffer = dissolved CO_2 or PCO_2
- Base component is HCO_3^-

$$TCO_2 = H_2CO_3 + HCO_3^-$$

where TCO_2 is total carbon dioxide

- According to the Henderson-Hasselbalch equation, under normal conditions
  - Plasma PCO_2 is ~40 mm Hg
  - Plasma bicarbonate (HCO_3^-) concentration is ~24 mmol/L
  - pK of the bicarbonate buffer is 6.1
  - The acid, carbonic acid (H_2CO_3) = 0.03 × $PaCO_2$ = 0.03 × 40 mm Hg = 1.2 mol/L

$$pH = 6.1 + \log \frac{[24]}{[1.2]} = 7.4$$

  - The laboratory can assess acid-base status of a patient by measuring blood pH, PCO_2, and/or $[HCO_3^-]$
  - Measure any 2 of 3 and calculate the third using the Henderson-Hasselbalch equation

2.8.3 Classifying an acid-base disorder

- Determine the primary abnormality
  - Acidosis
    - Metabolic acidosis: pH and $[HCO_3^-]$ decreased from normal (bicarbonate usually <25 mEq/L [<25 mmol/L] and pH <7.35)
    - Respiratory acidosis: pH and $[HCO_3^-]$ abnormal in opposite directions (PCO_2 usually >44 mm Hg [5.8 kPa] and pH <7.35)
  - Alkalosis
    - Metabolic alkalosis: pH and $[HCO_3]$ increased from normal (bicarbonate usually >25 mEq/L [>25 mmol/L] and pH>7.45)
    - Respiratory alkalosis: pH and $[HCO_3]$ abnormal in opposite directions (PCO_2 usually <40 mm Hg [5.3 kPa] and pH >7.45)
- Determine if the compensation is appropriate
  - Metabolic acidosis: For each 1.3 mEq fall in $[HCO_3^-]$, the PCO_2 decreases by 1.0 mm Hg
  - Metabolic alkalosis: For each 0.6 mEq rise in $[HCO_3^-]$, the PCO_2 increases by 1.0 mm Hg
  - Respiratory alkalosis or acidosis
    - Acute: For each 1 mm Hg change in PCO_2, the $[HCO_3^-]$ changes by 0.1 in the same direction
    - Chronic: For each 1 mm Hg change in PCO_2, the $[HCO_3^-]$ changes by 0.4 in the same direction
- Differentiating the disorders
  - Metabolic acidosis: Disorders are categorized by presence or absence of anion gap **t2.16** and osmolal gap **t2.17**

t2.16 Metabolic acidosis

Increased anion gap (≥12)	Normal anion gap (<12)
Methanol	Diarrhea
Uremia	Recovery phase diabetic ketoacidosis
Ketoacidosis (diabetic, EtOH, starvation)	Ureterosigmoidostomy
Paraldehyde	NH_4Cl
Lactic acidosis	Carbonic anhydrase inhibitors
Ethylene glycol	Total parenteral nutrition
Salicylate	Renal tubular acidosis

t2.17 Increased osmolal gap

With metabolic acidosis	Without metabolic acidosis
Methanol	Isopropanol
Propylene glycol	Glycerol
Ethylene glycol	Sorbitol
Paraldehyde	Mannitol
Ethanol (sometimes)	Acetone
	Ethanol (sometimes)

- Calculate the anion gap

$$\text{Anion gap} = [Na]-[Cl]-[HCO_3]$$

- Normal is <12
  - In nonanion gap acidosis, the chloride level is often elevated (hyperchloremic metabolic acidosis)
  - Note that a low anion gap is uncommon, but may be caused by hypoalbuminemia and paraproteinemia, such as in multiple myeloma

- Calculate the osmolal gap

osmolal gap = $osm_{measured}$–(2[Na] + [glucose]/18 + [BUN]/2.8)

  - In this form of the calculation, Na is in mEq/L, glucose is in mg/dL, and BUN is in mg/dL. When international units (mmol/L) are used, the osmolality is calculated as follows

    $osm_{measured}$ – 2[Na] – [glucose] – [BUN]

- Normal osmolal gap is <10

- Metabolic alkalosis
  - Disorders are categorized by chloride responsiveness or resistance t2.18

t2.18 Metabolic alkalosis

Chloride responsive (UCl<10)	Chloride resistant (UCl>10)
Diuretic therapy	Hyperaldosteronism
Vomiting	Cushing syndrome
Nasogastric tube suction	Exogenous steroids
Villous adenoma	Licorice (glycyrrhizin)
Carbenicillin	Bartter syndrome
Contraction alkalosis	Milk-alkali syndrome

- Respiratory acidosis results from any impairment to ventilation
  - Causes include those directly affecting the lungs (airway obstruction, alveolar infiltrates, perfusion defects) and those affecting the neuromuscular support of breathing
- Respiratory alkalosis most often results from hypoxemia, in which compensatory hyperventilation leads to hypocapnea
  - A variety of other stimuli can lead to hyperventilation and hypercapnea, including anxiety, CNS insults, pregnancy, and a variety of medications

- Reference ranges for adult arterial blood gases
  - pH: 7.35-7.45
  - PCO_2: 35-45 mm Hg
  - PO_2: 80-100 mm Hg
  - HCO_3^-: 22-26 mmol/L
  - TCO_2: 23-27 mmol/L
  - O_2 saturation: 94%-100%
  - Base excess: –2 to +2
- Difference in CO_2 concentration between cytoplasm and plasma results in diffusion from tissues into cells and the formation of carbonic acid (H_2CO_3)
- Most CO_2 combines with H_2O to form carbonic acid which quickly dissociates into H^+ and HCO_3^-
- Dissociation in plasma is very slow (nonenzymatic) but is much faster in cells because of carbonic anhydrase
- Carbonic anhydrase is present in high concentrations in red cells and renal cells
- Dissociation causes increased HCO_3^- concentration in red cells, resulting in diffusion into plasma and circulates bound to Na
- In lungs
  - Oxygen diffuses from lungs to blood forming oxyhemoglobin
  - H^+ from deoxyhemoglobin in venous blood is released to recombine with HCO_3^- to form carbonic acid which dissociates into CO_2 and H_2O
  - CO_2 is exhaled and H+ is buffered resulting in minimal change in pH known as isohydric shift
  - Hemoglobin oxygen saturation
    - Oxygen saturation is the fraction (%) of hemoglobin that is saturated with oxygen
    - The degree of association or dissociation of oxygen with hemoglobin is determined by PO_2
    - P_{50} is PO_2 where hemoglobin is half saturated with oxygen
    - The affinity of hemoglobin for oxygen depends on temperature, pH, PCO_2 & concentration of 2,3-DPG
- In kidneys
  - Kidneys reabsorb HCO_3^- in the proximal convoluted tubule to restore it
  - Aldosterone causes Na reabsorption and exchanges it with either K or H ions (whichever is in excess)
  - Aldosterone takes bicarbonate along with Na to maintain electrical neutrality
  - Renal cells are rich in carbonic anhydrase, so the supply of bicarbonate is unlimited
  - H ions secreted in exchange with Na may react with phosphate (filtered through the glomerulus) to form phosphoric acid
  - Renal cells are rich in glutamate dehydrogenase which removes amino group from glutamic acid (derived from muscle and liver cells) and converts it into NH_3
  - NH_3 is a gas and can freely diffuse through cell membrane into filtrate
  - H ions react with $NH_3 \rightarrow NH_4^+$ which cannot diffuse through the cell membrane and is excreted with anions, such as phosphate, sulfate, or chloride
- Net effect
  - Sodium and bicarbonate are restored in plasma
  - Hydrogen ions, ammonia & nonvolatile acids are excreted in urine

 ISBN 978-089189-6616

- Isohydric shift
  - Isohydric = same H^+
    - The process by which blood manages to carry 20 mol of CO_2 from peripheral tissues to lungs without appreciable changing the blood pH
  - Normal arterial blood pH at 37°C (98.6°F) is 7.40 ± 0.05
  - Normal venous blood pH at 37°C (98.6°F) is 7.37 ± 0.05
- Both lungs and kidneys play a major role in maintaining blood pH
- Chloride shift
  - When the concentration of bicarbonate in RBC greater than in plasma during the buffering process, bicarbonate diffuses out
  - Chloride must diffuse into RBC to maintain electrical neutrality. This is the "chloride shift"
  - When CO_2 is expelled from the lungs, Cl again shifts out of the red cells into plasma
  - Plasma proteins and buffers combine with the free H^+
- Acid-base balance
  - Definitions
    - Acidemia: Arterial pH <7.35
    - Alkalemia: Arterial pH >7.45
    - Acidosis: A condition tending to lower the pH (the pH may not actually be lowered, because of compensation)
    - Alkalosis: A condition tending to raise the pH (the pH may not actually be raised, because of compensation)
    - Respiratory acidosis: Insufficient elimination of CO_2 by the lungs (hypoventilation). The primary change is in CO_2. Compensation involves altered renal handling of bicarbonate (HCO_3^-)
    - Respiratory alkalosis: Excessive elimination of CO_2 by the lungs (hyperventilation). The primary change is in CO_2. Compensation involves altered renal handling of bicarbonate (HCO_3^-)
    - Metabolic acidosis/alkalosis: Excessive intake of, excessive production of, or too little renal elimination of an acid or a base. The primary change is in bicarbonate (HCO_3^-). Compensation involves alterations in pulmonary handling of CO_2
    - Simple acid/base disorder: A primary acid-base disturbance and associated compensation
- Complex acid/base disorder: There is more than 1 primary acid-base disturbance
  - PCO_2 is the respiratory component and is controlled by lungs (rate of respiration)
  - HCO_3 is the metabolic component and is controlled by kidney and erythrocytes (nonvolatile acids produced in tissues)
  - Normally, ratio of base to acid is ~20:1
- Total CO_2 content

$$ctCO_2 \text{ content} = HCO_3^- + H_2CO_3$$
$$\text{where } HCO_3^- = \text{base}$$
$$\text{and}$$
$$H_2CO_3 = \text{acid } (PCO_2 \times 0.03)$$

- Base excess (BE)
  - Calculated perimeter which describes excess or deficit of base or bicarbonate
  - \+ BE = increased base
  - – BE = decreased base
  - Normal BE = 0 ± 2
  - Decreased base excess is an indicator of metabolic acidosis
  - Increased base excess is an indicator of metabolic alkalosis
- Compensation
  - No compensation
  - Partial compensation
  - Complete compensation
- Blood gas analysis – sample requirements
  - Arterial puncture is required if PO_2 is to be measured
  - Venous blood almost always has PO_2 = 40 mm Hg
  - No tourniquet and no fist clenching are required
  - Use glass syringe and do not pull on plunger; do not use vacutainer
  - Only heparin (liquid or dry); other anticoagulants alter the pH
  - Protect from air (anaerobic) to prevent equilibration with low PCO_2 and high PO_2 in the air
  - Immediately expel any small bubbles
  - Keep sample submerged in ice/water slush to impede WBC metabolism
  - pH decreases ~0.08 pH/h at 37°C (98.6°F) but 1/10th that much at 0°C (32°F)
  - PCO_2 increases and PO_2 decreases from metabolism
  - Results are stable from 1-2 hours at 0°C (32°F)
  - Volume of blood for most commercial electrodes is <1 mL

2.9 Water & electrolyte balance & disorders

2.9.1 Definition of terms

2.9.1.1 Electrolytes

- Essential components of all living matter. Major electrolytes occur as free ions. Trace elements occur in combination with proteins
- Cation: Positively charged ion. Includes major electrolytes Na^+, K^+, Ca^+, Mg^+ & trace elements Cu^{2+}, Zn^{2+}, Fe^{2+}, Co^{2+}, Mn^{2+}, Sr^{2+}, Li^+
- Anion: Negatively charged ion. Includes major electrolytes Cl^-, HCO_3^-, HPO_4^{2-}, SO_4^{2-}, and trace elements I^-, Br^-, F^-

2.9.1.2 Electrodes

- Components of an electrochemical cell in which an electrical field is established. Ions will migrate to oppositely charged electrode
- Cathode: Negatively charged, attracts positively charged cations. Reduction of ions occurs here (gain of electrons)
- Anode: Positively charged, attracts negatively charged anions. Oxidation occurs here (loss of electrons)

2.9.1.3 Fluids

- Total body water includes water both inside and outside of the cells and water normally present in the GI and genitourinary system
- Intracellular water
  - Includes all water within cell membranes (eg, RBC, WBC & tissues)
  - 66% of total body water in cell
  - Water and electrolytes can move freely across cell membranes, not proteins
- Extracellular water
  - All water external to cell membranes. Includes intravascular & extravascular
  - Proteins are main contributor to osmotic pressure in the plasma
  - Osmotic pressure keeps water in the capillaries and prevents edema, accumulation of water in the interstitial compartment
- Interstitial fluid
  - Part of extracellular water. Fluid that surrounds the cells and the capillaries
- The lymphatic system works to remove excess water from tissues and return it to the capillaries to prevent edema
  - Changes in blood pressure and protein levels can cause edema

2.9.1.4 Osmolality

- Measurement of the number of dissolved particles in a solution
- Osmolality: Moles of solute/kg of water
- Osmolarity: Moles of solute/L of water
- Major contributors: Na (50%), Cl
- Minor contributors: BUN, glucose, organic substances (ethanol, methanol when present)
- Osmolality is measured in biological fluids, high means more particles and low means less particles
- A small change in plasma osmolality will activate thirst receptors, and ADH secretions

2.9.2 Physiological functions of electrolytes

- Osmotic pressure
  - Pressure that would have to be exerted on a membrane to prevent the flow across that membrane from a dilute to a concentrated solution
  - Determines water distribution between compartments
  - Hypertonic solution has a greater osmotic pressure than that of plasma
  - Hypotonic solution has a lower osmotic pressure than that of plasma
- Conduction of neuromuscular impulses
  - Involves mostly magnesium, calcium & potassium
  - Increases or decreases causes hyperirritability, tetany, convulsions & heart arrhythmias
- Acid-base maintenance
  - Helps buffer pH
  - Chloride shift: Cl enters cell and HCO_3 leaves cell
  - Electrical neutrality: Number of anions equals number of cations in each compartment
- Enzyme activation
  - Needed as cofactor for enzymes in catalysis
  - Cofactors are Mg, Fe, Ca, Zn, K, Cl, Br
- Electron transfer
  - Involved in oxidation-reduction reactions

2.9.3 Sodium

- Na is major extracellular cation
- 30% in bones, 70% in fluids
- Source is dietary intake
- Renal control
  - Freely filtered by glomerulus
  - Majority actively reabsorbed by proximal convoluted tubule

ISBN 978-089189-6616

- Aldosterone increases reabsorption of Na
- Kidney can reabsorb 99% of Na if plasma low

- Also found in gastric fluid, intestinal fluid, cerebral spinal fluid & sweat
- Reference ranges
  - Serum: 136-145 mEq/L (136-145 mmol/L)
  - Urine: 40-220 mmol/24 h
  - Critical values: <115 to >160 mEq/L (<115 to >160 mmol/L)

2.9.3.1 Causes of abnormal sodium levels

2.9.3.1.1 Hyponatremia

- Caused by depletion of sodium
  - Renal loss from diuretics, hypoaldosteronism
  - Nonrenal loss: GI loss, skin loss, not enough in diet
- Caused by dilution of sodium in blood
  - Generalized edema: Congestive heart failure, cirrhosis, nephrotic syndrome
  - Syndrome of inappropriate antidiuretic hormone secretion (SIADH)
  - Hyperglycemia
- Pseudohyponatremia
  - Caused by artifact in measurement
  - Dilutional (indirect) method
  - May affect any instrument that uses "indirect" method of measurement, in which the sample is prediluted before analysis
    - Such analyzers calculate the plasma/serum sodium on the assumption that the water content of the plasma is 93%
    - This assumption may be incorrect in hypertriglyceridemia, hypercholesterolemia, and hyperproteinemia (water content in the original sample is lower)
  - Serum osmolarity is normal and an osmolal gap is present
  - Direct potentiometry, as performed on blood gas analyzers, not affected
- Spurious hyponatremia
  - Blood is drawn proximal to an intravenous infusion
- Hyperglycemia
  - The degree of change in sodium concentration attributable to glucose can be calculated by following formula (glucose expressed in mg/dL):

$$\frac{1.6 \times (\text{serum glucose} - 100)}{100}$$

  - True physiologic shift in sodium ions into extracellular space, producing hyponatremia that is real but unrelated to any intrinsic defect in sodium homeostasis
- Hypertonic (>295 mOsm/kg) hyponatremia
  - This suggests marked hyperglycemia, but may also be seen in patients given mannitol to reduce intracranial pressure
- True hypotonic hyponatremia (<280 mOsm/kg)
  - If the patient is hypovolemic: Sodium loss occurs through renal or extrarenal routes
  - Renal losses are suggested by elevated urine sodium (>30 mmol/L); this may be caused by diuretics, renal medullary disease, primary adrenal insufficiency (Addison disease), renal tubular acidosis type I & cerebral salt wasting syndrome
  - Extrarenal sodium losses may occur in the GI tract (vomiting, diarrhea) or result from 3rd spacing (eg, peritonitis or pleuritis). Extrarenal loss suggested by low urine sodium (<30 mmol/L)
  - If the patient is euvolemic: SIADH, psychogenic polydipsia, hypothyroidism, primary adrenal insufficiency (Addison disease) & drugs with ADH-like (vasopressin-like) effect, including desmopressin, serotonin reuptake inhibitors (SSRIs), tricyclic antidepressants & ecstasy (3,4-methylenedioxy-N-methylamphetamine or MDMA)
  - If Patient is hypervolemic: Congestive heart failure, cirrhosis, nephrotic syndrome

2.9.3.1.2 Hypernatremia

- Caused by increased sodium
  - Increased in diet
  - Infused intravenously
  - Hyperaldosteronism: Conn syndrome
- Caused by water depletion
  - Most commonly seen in an individual with excess water loss and inability to respond to a thirst response; infants, patients in intensive care units & debilitated adults
  - GI loss
  - Excessive sweating
  - Extrarenal water loss: Diarrhea, vomiting, burns
  - Renal water loss: Osmotic diuretics, loop diuretics, postobstructive diuresis, intrinsic medullary renal disease
- May be iatrogenic: Administration of sodium as part of intravenous fluid administration, sodium bicarbonate administration, or other intervention

- Diabetes insipidus (DI)
  - Central: damage to the hypothalamus or neurohypophysis related to surgery, space-occupying lesions in the region of the sella, head trauma, and infiltrative lesions such as eosinophilic granuloma and sarcoidosis
  - Nephrogenic: Diseases that affect the medullary space (sickle cell disease & tubulointerstitial nephritis), electrolyte disturbances (hypokalemia & hypercalcemia), renal tubular acidosis, Fanconi syndrome, drugs (lithium, demeclocycline, colchicine, amphotericin B, gentamicin, furosemide)

2.9.4 Potassium

2.9.4.1 Overall potassium balance

- Potassium is the major intracellular cation
- Mostly found in muscle cells
- Source is dietary intake
- Renal control
  - Freely filtered by glomerulus
  - Majority actively reabsorbed in the proximal tubule, then secreted in the distal tubule
- Also found in gastric fluid, intestinal fluid & cerebral spinal fluid
- Reference range
  - Serum: 3.5-5.0 mEq/L (3.5-5.0 mmol/L)
  - Urine: 25-150 mmol/24 h
  - Critical values: <2.5 to >6.5 mEq/L (<2.5 to >6.5 mmol/L); higher for infants

2.9.4.2 Causes of abnormal potassium

- Hypokalemia
  - Decreased blood potassium
  - Decrease in diet
  - Renal loss
    - Hyperaldosteronism with elevated urinary potassium (>30 mEq/d)
    - Diuretics
    - Hypomagnesemia, antibiotics (carbenicillin, amphotericin B), mineralocorticoid excess, renal tubular acidosis types I and II, severe Cushing syndrome, congenital adrenal hyperplasia, Bartter syndrome, Liddle syndrome, Gitelman syndrome, licorice (glycyrrhizin) consumption & hyper-reninism
- GI loss
  - Urinary potassium is low (<30 mEq/d)
  - Vomiting, nasogastric tube suction, diarrhea, large villous adenoma
- Transcellular shift (excess cellular uptake)
  - Metabolic alkalosis or correction of diabetic ketoacidosis (DKA)
  - Note that in DKA, there is an initial hyperkalemia (as in most acidotic states), but correction of DKA results in a profound hypokalemia unless supplemental potassium is given
- Hyperkalemia
  - Increased blood potassium
  - Increase in diet
  - Increased cellular release
  - Redistribution from extracellular to intracellular
    - Acidosis: H-K exchange
    - Insulin deficiency
  - Impaired renal excretion
    - Acute renal failure
    - Hypoaldosteronism
  - Pseudohyperkalemia
    - Elevated measured potassium in the absence of in vivo hyperkalemia
    - Causes
      - In vitro cellular leak of potassium from hemolysis, in vitro clot formation (release of potassium from platelets; especially in patients with hyperkalemia; serum has a higher potassium result than plasma for this reason), or leukocytosis
      - Prolonged tourniquet time, excessive fist clenching, traumatic draw, inappropriate order of tubes drawn, venipuncture proximal to intravenous infusion & small-gauge needles
    - Differential diagnosis includes acidosis, renal failure, potassium-sparing diuretics (spironolactone, triamterene, amiloride, eplerenone), adrenal insufficiency, iatrogenic & rhabdomyolysis. Nearly all cases of acidosis are associated with hyperkalemia. The main exception is renal tubular acidosis types I & II in which the potassium is low

2.9.4.3 Methods of measurement for sodium & potassium

- Ion selective electrode (ISE)
  - Principle
    - Ion exchange membrane, glass for Na, valinomycin for K
    - Measures ionic activity (mEq/L)
    - Can be direct (undiluted on whole blood or plasma) or indirect (diluted on plasma or urine)
  - Advantages
    - Sensitive method
    - Uses small sample volume
    - Direct method not affected by lipemia or altered protein levels

ISBN 978-089189-6616

- Disadvantages
  - May detect H^+ at pH <6.0 (never happens in blood)
  - Indirect method affected by lipemia
- Specimen collection
  - Serum, plasma, urine or other body fluids. Whole blood on direct method only
  - Serum or plasma must be separated from cells as soon as possible
  - Avoid hemolysis for K measurement
  - Stable for 1 week at 0-6°C (32°F-42.8°F), 1 year at –20°C (–4°F)
- Most commonly used method

- Atomic absorption spectroscopy
  - Principle: Light absorbed is proportional to concentration of sodium & potassium
  - Highly sensitive, reference method
  - Not used in clinical laboratories

2.9.5 Chloride

2.9.5.1 Overall chloride balance

- Chloride is the major extracellular anion
- Important in maintenance of anion-cation balance (Cl shift)
- Source is dietary intake
- Renal control
  - Freely filtered at glomerulus
  - Passively reabsorbed (along with Na) in the proximal convoluted tubule, actively reabsorbed in ascending loop of Henle
- Found in plasma, gastric fluid, intestinal fluid, sweat & CSF
- Chloride is measured in sweat, increase is diagnostic of cystic fibrosis
- Reference range
  - Serum: 99-109 mEq/L (99-109 mmol/L)
  - Urine: 110-250 mEq/L (110-250 mmol/L)
  - Cl <10 indicates gastric or diuretic-induced loss
  - Cl >10 indicates renal loss
  - Critical: <70 or >120 mEq/L (<70 or >120 mmol/L)

2.9.5.2 Causes of abnormal chloride

- Hypochloremia
  - Decreased blood chloride
  - Renal loss
    - Diuretics
    - Metabolic alkalosis
  - GI loss
    - Salt-losing nephritis (pyelonephritis)
    - Addisonian crisis
- Hyperchloremia
  - Increased blood chloride
  - Dehydration
  - Renal tubular acidosis
  - Metabolic acidosis
  - High salt intake

2.9.5.3 Methods of chloride analysis

- Ion selective electrode
  - Principle
    - AgCl electrode with silver sulfide sensing element
  - Direct (undiluted) & indirect (diluted)
  - Advantages
    - Small sample
    - Direct method not affected by lipemia
  - Disadvantages
    - Bromide (from medications) interferences
  - Specimen collection & handling
    - Serum, plasma, whole blood, urine, body fluids can be used
    - Separate serum from cells ASAP
    - Stable 1 week at 0°C-6°C (32°F-42.8°F), 1 year at –20°C (–4°F)
- Coulometric-amperometric (Cotlove titration)
  - Principle
    - Number of silver ions generated is proportional to the concentration of Cl
  - Indirect method
  - Advantages
    - Accurate & rapid
  - Disadvantages
    - Anode & cathode must be kept clean
    - Interferences from bromide
  - Specimen handling & collection
    - Serum, plasma, urine, body fluids
    - Separate serum from cells ASAP
    - Stable 1 week at 0°C-6°C (32°F-42.8°F), 1 year at –20°C (–4°F)

2.9.6 Carbon dioxide (bicarbonate)

2.9.6.1 Overall carbon dioxide balance

- Major component of total CO_2 in plasma is HCO_3^-
- HCO_3^- is part of bicarbonate-carbonic acid buffering system
- HCO_3^- is the transport form of CO_2 produced from metabolic processes in the tissues and delivered to the lungs for exhalation
- Renal control
  - reabsorbed in tubules
- Also contained in CSF
- Reference range
  - Serum: 22-28 mEq/L (22-28 mmol/L)

2.9.6.2 Causes of abnormal carbon dioxide levels

- Increased blood CO_2
  - Excess ingestion of antacids
  - Renal overcompensation for respiratory acidosis
- Decreased blood CO_2
  - Diarrhea
  - Metabolic acidosis
  - Renal overcompensation for respiratory alkalosis

2.9.6.3 Methods of total carbon dioxide measurement

- Modified pH
  - Principle: CO_2 from sample diffuses through a semipermeable membrane into an electrolyte solution. The change in pH is measured
  - Specimen collection & handling
    - Serum or plasma
    - Samples must remain in unopened tubes until measuring
    - Separate serum from cells ASAP
- Enzymatic method
  - Principle
    - HCO_3 + PEP (phosphoenolpyruvate) → oxaloacetate + P_i (inorganic phosphate)
    - Oxaloacetate + NADH + H^+ → maleate + NAD with decreased absorbance at 340 nm
  - Specimen collection & handling
    - Same as for modified pH method

2.9.7 Estimation of electrolyte balance

2.9.7.1 Anion gap

- Calculation of the difference between measured anions & cations
- Electrical neutrality still maintained
- Several possible ways to calculate
  - Na – (Cl + CO_2) (normal range 8-16)
  - Na + K = Cl + CO_2 + 17 (within 10)
  - Large anion gap arises from excess unmeasured anions such as PO_4, SO_4, organic acids, lactic acids, methanol poisoning, salicylate poisoning
- Measured electrolytes: Na, K, Cl, CO_2

2.9.7.2 Colligative properties

- Definition
  - Properties that are directly affected by number of solute particles per mass of solvent
    - Freezing point
    - Vapor pressure
    - Boiling point
    - Osmotic pressure
- As osmolality increases:
  - Freezing point decreases
  - Vapor pressure is lowered
  - Boiling point in increased
  - Osmotic pressure is increased
- All 4 properties can be used to estimate osmolality
- Freezing point depression is most commonly used in the laboratory

2.9.7.3 Methods of measuring osmolality

- Freezing point depression—osmometer (cryoscope)
  - Principle
    - Sample is supercooled to a temperature below its freezing point
    - Agitation with a stir bar causes crystals to form
    - The heat of fusion released warms the sample to its freezing point
    - The final reading is taken at equilibrium
  - Advantages
    - Easily automated, simple
    - Not affected by lipemia or hemolysis
    - Not affected by changes in room temperature
    - Volatile substances can be measured

ISBN 978-089189-6616

- Disadvantages
  - May require larger sample sizes (200-250 μL)
- Specimen collection & handling
  - Serum, plasma, or urine may be used
  - Avoid prolonged use of tourniquet causing stasis
  - Fasting specimen best
  - Specimen should remain stoppered, refrigerated, or analyzed ASAP
- Vapor pressure depression
  - Principle
    - Measurement of osmolality is related to the decrease in the dew point temperature of the pure solvent (water) caused by the decrease in vapor pressure of the solvent by the solutes
  - Advantages
    - Small sample size (7 μL)
    - Low maintenance
  - Disadvantages
    - Not as precise as freezing point depression
    - Volatile substances cannot be measured (alcohols)
    - Affected by dirty chamber
    - Lipemia gives false increase
  - Specimen collection & handling
    - Same as for freezing point depression method
- Reference ranges for osmolality
  - Serum: 275-295 mOsm/kg
  - Urine: 300-900 mOsm/kg

2.9.7.4 Causes of abnormal osmolality

- Increased serum osmolality
  - Diabetes mellitus
  - Renal disorders
  - Ethanol or methanol poisoning
- Decreased serum osmolality
  - Lymphomas
  - Shock
  - Myocardial infarction (MI)
- Increased urine osmolality
  - Fluid restrictions
  - Diabetes mellitus
- Decreased urine osmolality
  - Excess fluid intake
  - Diabetes insipidus
  - Chronic renal failure

- Calculated osmolality
  - Formula commonly used

    $1.86\times Na + Glu/18 + BUN/2.8 + 9$

  - Will be different from measured osmolality because only the common solutes are considered
- Osmolal gap
  - Measured osmolality minus calculated osmolality
  - Mean is 0 ± 6 mOsm
  - Gap is increased in
    - Ketoacidosis
    - Renal tubular acidosis
    - Lactic acidosis
    - Methanol, ethanol, ethylene glycol poisonings

2.9.7.5 Effect of protein on osmolality vs specific gravity

- Osmolality is directly dependent on the number of particles & concentration
  - Electrolytes dissociate into 2-3 ionized particles, so they contribute significantly
  - Proteins have low ionization & contribute only slightly
  - Glucose & BUN contribute when in high concentrations
- Specific gravity is dependent on the mass of dissolved particles (molecular weight, size) & number
  - Electrolytes have low molecular weight, so they contribute slightly
  - Proteins & glucose have high molecular weight, so they contribute greatly

2.10 Minerals

2.10.1 Calcium & phosphorus

- Present in bone in form of calcium phosphate crystals
- Functions of calcium
  - Bone & teeth formation
  - Membrane permeability
  - Neuromuscular excitability—regulates primary sensory neurons
  - Transmission of nerve impulses
  - Blood coagulation
  - Activities for enzymes including activation
- Functions of phosphorus
  - Bone & teeth
  - Intermediary metabolism of glucose
  - Phosphorus concentration ↓ after ingestion of meal

- ATP, ADP, nucleotides, nucleic acids, NADP, phospholipids: All contain phosphorus
- Buffering capacity

- Absorption
  - Absorbed in the upper part of small intestine
  - Factors that affect absorption
    - pH of intestine
    - Acid: Favors absorption
    - Alkaline: Form insoluble calcium-phosphorus compounds
  - Vitamin D
    - Enhances absorption
    - Deficiency of vitamin D causes rickets, some forms of cancer & heart disease
  - Parathormone
    - From parathyroid
    - Enhances absorption of Ca
- Reference ranges—serum values
  - Calcium: 9-11 mg/dL (2.25-2.75 mmol/L)
  - Phosphorus: Adults: 3.0-4.5 mg/dL (0.75-1.1 mmol/L); children: 4.5-6.5 mg/dL (1.1-1.6 mmol/L)
- Specimen collection
  - Phosphorus concentration is higher in RBC
  - Serum phosphorus should be measured when the patient is fasting
- Forms of calcium
  - Nondiffusable portion
    - Bound form
    - 45%-50% of serum calcium is bound to protein, mainly albumin, such that total calcium may be low in hypoalbuminemic patients, while free (ionized) calcium is normal; acidosis decreases the binding of calcium to albumin and thus increases the proportion of free calcium. Likewise, alkalosis decreases free calcium
  - Diffusable
    - Ionized form
    - Physiologically active form
    - Diffuses across CNS barrier
    - Measure Ca^{2+} in CSF for measure of ionized Ca^{2+}
- Factors that affect ionized calcium
  - Alkaline phosphatase
    - Decreased level
    - No change in total calcium
    - Tetany develops
  - Alteration in proteins
    - Decreased proteins, decreased total calcium
    - No change in ionized Ca^{2+}

2.10.1.1 Factors that affect calcium & phosphorus levels

- Parathormone
  - Causes bone resorption/ remodeling
    - Primary effect on osteoclasts
    - Increased serum Ca^{2+} (breaks down bone)
  - Affects renal tubules
    - Direct effect on the renal tubular epithelial cells
    - Increased reabsorption of calcium
    - Increased excretion of phosphorus by renal tubules
  - Increased calcium absorption by intestinal mucosa cells
  - Low level of serum ionized calcium is the primary stimulating factor for parathormone
  - Ionized Ca^{2+} levels are associated with hyperparathyroidism & hypoparathyroidism
- Vitamin D
  - Functions complementary to parathormone
  - Increased bone resorption
  - Increased Ca^{2+} and PO_4^{3+} absorption from GI tract
- Thyrocalcitonin
  - Hormone produced by thyroid gland
  - Immediate action
  - Antagonist to parathormone
  - Primary action: To block bone resorption
  - Stimulated by high levels serum ionized Ca^{2+}
  - Decreases calcium absorption from GI tract
  - Decreases calcium excretion in urine
  - Increases phosphorus excretion in urine
- Plasma protein level
  - Decreased in plasma proteins, ↓ total calcium
  - Increased in plasma proteins, increased total calcium
  - Ionized calcium will not change
  - Phosphorus not bound to protein, so protein level will not affect phosphorus level
- Bone structure: 2 groups
  - Organic matrix
    - 25% of weight
    - 97% collagen fibers
    - Gives bone tensile strength
    - Contains proline & hydroxyproline
    - 1/3 of total amino acid content

- 3% ground substance
- Mucoproteins
- Hyaluronic acid
- Chondroitin sulfate
- Extracellular fluid

- Inorganic mineral salts
  - 75% of weight
  - Hydroxyapatite crystals
- Crystals are embedded in an organic matrix composed largely of crystalline collagen

2.10.1.2 Cells responsible for bone tissue

- Osteoblasts
  - Main bone formation
  - Bone-forming cells
  - High alkaline phosphorus
  - Liberate inorganic phosphorus from organic esters
  - Osteoblasts surround the organic matrix (which has mineral salts deposited in it)
  - Ossification-calcification-osteogenesis
  - Responsive to fibroblast growth factor
- Osteoclasts
  - Responsible for bone resorption
  - Breakdown (dissolve) organic matrix which releases mineral salts
- Bone formation↔bone resorption takes place continuously
- 300 mg calcium are released & 300 mg are used each day

2.10.1.3 Bone disorders

- Rickets
- Osteomalacia—adult rickets
  - Loss (deficiency) of mineral salts
  - Caused by bone resorption (soft bones)
  - Decreased vitamin D causes decreased calcium absorption which causes bone resorption
- Osteoporosis
  - Involves loss of organic matrix
  - Bone mass decreased
  - Factors that cause osteoporosis
    - Old age, lack of weight-bearing exercise
    - Protein metabolism
    - Malnutrition
    - Malabsorption
- Cushing disease
  - Hyperaldosterone
  - Of the adrenal cortex
- Paget disease
  - Osteitis deformans
  - Increased alkaline phosphatase (ALP)
  - Destruction of bone
  - Bone resorption then replacement with poorly mineralized tissues
  - Bone tumors

2.10.1.4 Factors affecting calcium

- Hypercalcemia (Increased Ca in blood) **t2.19**
  - May present with nephrolithiasis, lethargy, hyporeflexia, slowed mentation, nausea, vomiting, constipation, depression & high peaked T waves on electrocardiography (ECG)
  - Hypercalcemia increases the risk of pancreatitis & peptic ulcer disease
  - Long-term hypercalcemia with concomitant hyperphosphatemia (increased calcium × phosphate product) may result in so-called "metastatic calcification of vessel walls & soft tissue" (calciphylaxis)

t2.19 Differential diagnosis of hypercalcemia

Etiology	Notes
Primary hyperparathyroidism	Parathyroid adenoma (most common), 4-gland hyperplasia, parathyroid carcinoma
Tertiary hyperparathyroidism	Post-renal transplantation
Malignancy	Squamous cell carcinoma, multiple myeloma, breast carcinoma, islet cell tumors, paraganglioma, renal cell carcinoma, hepatocellular carcinoma, T-acute lymphoblastic lymphoma, small cell carcinoma of ovary (hypercalcemic type)
Familial hypocalciuric hypercalcemia	*CASR* gene on 3q
Drugs	Thiazides, calcium-containing antacids or calcium supplements (milk-alkali syndrome), hypervitaminosis D
Other endocrine	Hyperthyroidism, Addison, acromegaly
Granulomatous disease	Sarcoidosis, primarily
Paget disease	Only if the patient is immobilized

- Hyperparathyroidism
  - Increased bone resorption
  - Excess parathyroid hormone (PTH) results in increased serum calcium with decreased serum phosphate, increased chloride/phosphate ratio, increased urinary cyclic adenosine monophosphate (cAMP)
  - Primary hyperparathyroidism
  - Secondary hyperparathyroidism: Excessive secretion of PTH in response to hypocalcemia of any cause (most commonly chronic renal failure)
  - Tertiary hyperparathyroidism: After long periods of secondary hyperparathyroidism, autonomous parathyroid function may develop
- Hypervitaminosis D
  - Increased vitamin D, increased calcium because of increased absorption & increased phosphorus
- Multiple myeloma
  - Often has bone involvement
  - Increased plasma ***c***alcium, ***r***enal problems, ***a***nemia & ***b***one lesions (CRAB)
- Neoplastic diseases of bone & other origins
  - Humoral hypercalcemia of malignancy not involving bone, most commonly mediated by PTH-related protein, most commonly seen in squamous cell carcinoma of lung, head and neck, skin, cervix & esophagus, breast carcinoma, T-cell lymphoma
  - Primary or secondary (metastasis) involvement of bone
- Hypocalcemia **t2.20**
  - Causes neurologic excitability, manifesting as perioral tingling (paresthesia), muscle spasm & hyperreflexia
  - Classic findings include Chvostek sign & Trousseau sign
  - ECG shows lengthening of the QT interval, low voltage T waves & dysrhythmias
  - Severe hypocalcemia may cause laryngeal spasm, tetany & respiratory arrest

t2.20 Differential diagnosis of hypocalcemia

Etiology	Notes
Hypoproteinemia	Due to low albumin; ionized calcium usually normal
Chronic renal failure	Hyperphosphatemia present
Drugs	Heparin, glucagon, osmotic diuretics, loop diuretics (eg, furosemide), aminoglycosides, mithramycin
Hypoparathyroidism	Postsurgical, hypomagnesemia, DiGeorge syndrome, autoimmune
Medullary thyroid carcinoma	Rarely affects serum calcium
Hyperphosphatemia	Calcium chelation
Vitamin D deficiency	Most patients with vitamin D deficiency have normal calcium levels
Pancreatitis	Extensive calcium deposition
Massive transfusion	Citrate

- Hypoparathyroidism
  - Primary hypoparathyroidism is most often iatrogenic
  - Prolonged or marked hypomagnesemia is capable of suppressing PTH secretion; mild transient hypomagnesemia may actually cause increased PTH secretion
  - Decreased absorption
    - Steatorrhea: Fat-soluble vitamins (vitamin D) are not absorbed
- Renal disorders
  - Nephrosis: Excess protein loss
  - Nephritis
  - Pancreatitis
  - Rickets

2.10.1.5 Factors affecting phosphorus levels

- Hyperphosphatemia
  - Hypervitaminosis D
  - Hypoparathyroidism
  - Renal failure
- Hypophosphatemia
  - Hyperparathyroidism
  - Rickets
  - Fanconi syndrome
  - Absorption problems (Sprue & celiac disease)
- Hyperparathyroidism
  - Primary—causes renal disorders
    - Get deposits in kidneys, renal tubules & other tissues
    - Irreversible kidney damage

- Secondary—caused by renal disorders
  - Renal disorder causes increased serum phosphorus and ↓ serum calcium, which in turn causes increased parathormone
- Hypoparathyroidism
  - Caused by decreased production of parathyroid hormone (PTH)
    - Decreased plasma calcium levels
    - Increased plasma phosphate levels
    - Decreased 1,25$(OH)_2$ vitamin D levels
  - Etiology
    - Iatrogenic
    - Thyroidectomy (most common cause)
  - Pathophysiology—decreased PTH levels cause
    - Decreased urinary excretion of phosphate at kidneys
    - Serum phosphate levels increase
    - Decreased conversion of inactive form of vitamin D to active form
    - 1,25$(OH)_2$ vitamin levels decrease
  - Laboratory findings
    - Decreased PTH
    - Decreased calcium
    - 1,25 vitamin D
    - Decreased urinary calcium
    - Increased serum phosphate
    - Normal ALP
    - pH alkalosis
      - Increases albumin binding to ionized calcium leads to hypocalcemia
    - Prolonged QT interval on ECG
  - Prognosis
    - No current hormone replacement therapy available
    - Treatment is aimed at supplementing vitamin D & calcium levels

2.10.1.6 Methods of determination

- Total calcium
  - Atomic absorption
    - Get chemical interference
    - Treat with lanthanum chloride (a chelating agent)
  - Titration with $KMnO_4$ (Clark-Collip)
    - $KMnO_4$ not a stable compound
  - Precipitation—colorimetric
    - Precipitate of calcium with chloranilic acid—Ca-chloranilate—dissolve in EDTA to liberate chloranilate—pink color
    - Titration with EDTA
  - Dye—calcein—colorimetric or fluorometric
    - Methyl thymolblue (MTB) MTB—deep blue complex
    - Cresolphthalein complexone
  - Flame photometry: Old and obsolete method
    - Calcium ions not very excitable
    - Sodium interferences
    - Protein interferences
  - Magnesium can interfere with all of the aforementioned methods
    - Use 8-hydroxyquinoline to remove magnesium before calcium testing
    - To measure ionized Ca^{2+} use special electrode
- Phosphorus
  - Fiske & Subbarow

molybdate reagent + phosphorus + ANSA (aminonaphalsufonic acid)

2.10.2 Trace elements

- Elements found in very small amounts in body, usually 1 µg/g of tissue
- The World Health Organization (WHO) establishes dietary requirements
- An element is considered essential if:
  - Deficiency impairs a biochemical or functional process and replacement of element corrects the impairment
- Excess concentrations of these elements are associated with toxicity
- They often function as enzyme cofactors
- Trace elements are vital to normal function & health
- If depleted secondarily to an illness, further complications may arise that may be also life-threatening
- Examples are zinc, copper, selenium, arsenic, cadmium, mercury, lead, iron, manganese, molybdenum & chromium

2.10.2.1 Iron

2.10.2.1.1 Iron distribution

- Reversible interaction of iron with oxygen makes iron physiologically important
- 3-5 g of iron in the body

- ~2-2.5 g in hemoglobin
- ~130 mg in myoglobin
- ~8 mg in tissues (bound to enzymes)
- ~3-5 mg found in plasma, bound to transferrin, albumin & free hemoglobin
- Also stored as ferritin and hemosiderin in bone marrow, liver & spleen

2.10.2.1.2 Iron intake

- Dietary intake
- Average of 1 mg loss per day in adults must be replaced
- Menstrual cycle removes ~30 mg of iron
- Pregnant and premenopausal women, children & patients with bleeding disorders have greater requirement

2.10.2.1.3 Iron absorption & transport

- Iron excretion
  - Small amounts are lost in epithelial and red cells excreted in urine and feces each day
  - Women lose 20-40 mg of iron with each menstrual cycle and 600-900 mg with each pregnancy
- Clinical significance
  - Iron (ferrous) allows hemoglobin to bind reversibly to oxygen & CO_2
- Iron-deficiency anemia
  - Reduction of iron stores
  - Reduction in circulating iron
  - Laboratory results
    - Decreased RBC, mean corpuscular hemoglobin (MCH), mean corpuscular hemoglobin concentration (MCHC) & mean cell volume (MCV)
    - Decreased serum iron & ferritin
    - Increased transferrin & total iron-binding capacity (TIBC)
- Iron overload (hemochromatosis or hemosiderosis)
  - Excess absorption of iron from normal diet
  - Leads to iron accumulation in tissues and altered liver function, and causes hyperpigmentation
  - Laboratory results:
    - Increased serum iron & ferritin
    - Decreased transferrin
  - Treatment
    - Therapeutic phlebotomy
    - Transferrin administration

2.10.2.1.4 Iron status determination

- Hemoglobin
- Serum iron
  - Measures Fe^{3+} bound to transferrin
  - Diurnal variation
  - Anticoagulants: Serum or heparinized plasma
- Total iron-binding capacity
  - Amount of iron that could be bound by transferrin and other proteins

    TIBC (µg/dL) = serum transferrin (mg/dL) × 1.25

    % saturation (transferrin saturation)

    ratio of serum iron to TIBC ≥ (total iron/TIBC) × 100%
- Transferrin & ferritin

2.10.2.2 Magnesium

- Significance
  - An essential dietary mineral
  - 35% of the body's magnesium is in cells, 64% in bones, and ~1% in extracellular fluid
  - An activator in the ATP phosphate transfer reactions and other physiological reactions
- Increased serum magnesium
  - After ingestion of magnesium sulfate, epsom salts
  - Impaired renal function (uremia)
- Decreased serum magnesium
  - Malabsorption or excessive loss (ie, chronic renal disease, pancreatitis, LE, hyperthyroidism)
  - May result in muscular weakness, tremor, vertigo, cardiac arrhythmia, tetany, and convulsive seizures
  - Is seen in alcoholic delirium tremors
- Measurement
  - Atomic absorption spectrophotometry
  - Colorimetry: Mg forms a colored complex with methylthymol blue (MTB)
    - Ca^{2+} chelators are added to reduce interference from Ca^{2+}
    - The amount of Mg-MTB complex formed is proportional to the Mg^{2+} concentration
    - Alternately, colored complexes may be formed with calmagite

2.10.2.3 Copper

- Copper is absorbed through the intestine from dietary substances
- It travels through blood bound to albumin or histidine for transport to the liver, brain, heart & kidneys

ISBN 978-089189-6616

- Half of the dietary copper is excreted through feces
- Most copper is incorporated as ceruloplasmin, an APR
- Deficiency is seen in premature infants, malnutrition, chronic diarrhea etc
- A deficiency of copper results in decreased hemoglobin & collagen production

2.10.2.4 Zinc

- It is second to iron in importance as an essential trace element
- Absorbed through the intestine from the dietary nutrients
- Transported in blood with albumin or α_2-macroglobulin carriers
- Excreted in feces or pancreatic secretions
- The concentration of zinc is higher in erythrocytes than in plasma or serum

2.10.2.5 Lead

- Heavy metal commonly found in the environment
- Present in batteries, ammunition, foil, patrol, household paints & recently in toys
- Exposure to lead is primarily respiratory or GI
- Transported to blood where 94% is transferred to erythrocytes (and is bound to hemoglobin) and 6% is in plasma
- Half-life in whole blood is 2-3 weeks
- Final storage of lead is in soft tissues (~5%) & bones (~95%)
- Excreted in urine, feces & others

2.10.2.6 Arsenic

- Has both metallic & nonmetallic properties
- Nonessential but can be toxic
- Currently, main use is as a wood preservative
- Main routes of exposure are ingestion from contaminated food, water, beverages, or inhalation of contaminated air

2.10.2.7 Selenium

- Component glutathione peroxidase & tetraiodinothyronine-5'-deiodinase
- Enters food chain via plants
- Organ meats and seafood, cereals, grains, dairy products, fruits & vegetables are sources of dietary selenium
- Low selenium content is seen in parts of China resulting in Keshan disease or Kashin-Beck disease

2.10.2.8 Mercury

- Heavy, silvery metal that is liquid at room temperature
- Mercury is a product of natural outgassing of rocks, a fungicide and is also used in electrical switches
- Extremely toxic
- Found in over-the-counter drugs, antiseptics, laxatives, diaper rash cream, eye drops & mascara
- Specimen considerations for analysis
  - Contamination must be avoided
  - All equipment used in analysis must be free of trace metals—cleaned with pure water
  - Methodology and equipment must have high sensitivity & specificity
  - Special royal blue tubes that are free of trace metals are used for blood collection
  - Elements are stable

2.10.2.9 Methods of analysis

- Atomic absorption spectroscopy is the most sensitive and precise method for trace metal analysis

2.11 Tumor markers

- Widespread screening with tumor markers is generally not cost effective
- Positive predictive value depends on the disease prevalence
- More effective if applied to a selected population
- Features of an effective screening test
  - Safe, highly sensitive, inexpensive & capable of detecting a disease for which early treatment improves survival
- The Hook effect
  - A very high concentration of an analyte gives a falsely low result
  - High concentration exceeds the binding capacity of both the binding capture antibodies and the signal bearing antibodies, preventing their association
  - If the sample is sufficiently diluted, the assay will give an appropriate result
- Heterophile antibodies can cause significant interference in any immunoassay; may cause false positives or false negatives

2.11.1 Prostate-specific antigen (PSA)

2.11.1.1 Prostate cancer screening

- Traditionally recommended for men >50 years
- Abnormal digital rectal examination findings or PSA >4 ng/mL (>4 µg/L) are considered indications for prostate needle biopsy

- PSA is organ specific but not cancer specific; may be elevated in benign prostatic hyperplasia, prostatitis, prostatic infarct & after a prostate needle biopsy
- Only ~30%-40% of men with elevated PSA (>4.0 ng/mL [>4 µg/L) have prostate cancer
- Significant intraindividual variation and varies with race, with levels being significantly higher in blacks
- Poor sensitivity; many men with prostate cancer have serum PSA <4.0 ng/mL (<4 µg/L)

2.11.1.2 Adjunctive PSA indices

- Age-specific cutoffs (PSA increases with age)
- PSA density (PSA divided by the estimated prostatic volume)
- PSA velocity (rate of change in successive PSA determinations)
- Free PSA (lower free PSA fraction correlates with the prostate cancer)

2.11.2 Carcinoembryonic antigen (CEA) & colorectal carcinoma screening

- Recommended colorectal cancer screening includes combination fecal occult blood testing, flexible sigmoidoscopy, barium enema, and/or colonoscopy
- Fecal occult blood testing
  - Guaiac-based testing: Hemoglobin has endogenous peroxidase activity that is capable of oxidizing guaiac in the presence of hydrogen peroxide to a blue product
  - Results can be false positive because of NSAID use, consumption of heme (in meat) & consumption of peroxidase (turnips & horseradish)
  - Results can be false negative because of excessive vitamin C consumption
- Immunochemical testing: No dietary restrictions
- CEA concentration is markedly increased in some patients with colorectal carcinoma
  - Not recommended for colon cancer screening
  - Plays a role in preoperative evaluation of patients with known colon cancer and in the postoperative monitoring of such patients
  - High preoperative CEA concentration implies a worse overall outcome
  - CEA is elevated in only 25% of tumors confined to the colon, 50% with nodal metastasis & 75% with distant metastases
- CEA may be elevated in gastric adenocarcinoma, breast cancer, lung cancer, pancreatic adenocarcinoma, medullary thyroid carcinoma, cervical adenocarcinoma & urothelial carcinoma
- Mild CEA elevation can be caused by smoking, peptic ulcer disease, inflammatory bowel disease, pancreatitis, hypothyroidism, biliary obstruction & cirrhosis

2.11.3 Thyroglobulin

- Detection of tumor recurrence in differentiated (follicular & papillary) thyroid carcinoma
- Antithyroglobulin antibodies are potential sources of interference

2.11.4 Cancer antigen (CA) 125

- Elevated in nonmucinous epithelial ovarian neoplasms
- May be elevated in pregnancy, leiomyomas, benign ovarian cysts, pelvic inflammation, ascites, endometriosis, and in some nonovarian neoplasms (endometrial, fallopian tube, pancreas, breast & colon)
- In postmenopausal women, levels tend to decrease

2.11.5 CA 27-29 & CA 15-3

- CA27.29 (also called BR 27-29) and CA15-3 measure different epitopes of a single antigen—the protein product of the breast cancer-associated *MUC1* gene
- Both are elevated in ~60%-70% of women with advanced stage breast cancer

2.11.6 CA 19-9

- CA19-9 is a marker for pancreatic adenocarcinoma; elevated in 80% at presentation
- It may be elevated in patients with other malignancies (hepatobiliary, gastric, colorectal & breast), pancreatitis, cholestasis, cholangitis & cirrhosis
- Not produced by Lewis antigen-negative patients

2.11.7 α_1-fetoprotein

- This is normally synthesized in the yolk sac, fetal liver & fetal GI tract
- It is elevated in normal pregnancy, cirrhosis & hepatitis
- Elevated in yolk sac tumors and most hepatocellular carcinomas

2.11.8 Human chorionic gonadotropin (HCG)

- Elevated in pregnancy, trophoblastic disease & choriocarcinoma
- Elevated in 15% of pure seminomas and in rare examples of tumors from numerous sites (GI tract, genitourinary tract)

ISBN 978-089189-6616

2.11.9 β_2-microglobulin (β_2M)

- Elevated whenever there is increased cell death
- An independent prognostic factor in multiple myeloma

2.11.10 Alkaline phosphatase

- An indication of osteoblastic activity
- Elevated in osteogenic sarcoma or bone metastases
- Sensitive test for hepatic metastases
- Regan isoenzyme may be elevated in a variety of advanced malignancies

2.11.11 Markers of neuroendocrine tumors

2.11.11.1 Carcinoid tumors

- Produce serotonin (5 hydroxytryptamine, 5-HT) that is eventually metabolized and excreted in urine as 5-hydroxyindoleacetic acid (5-HIAA)
- Foregut carcinoids often produce histamine, catecholamines & 5 hydroxytryptophan (5-HTP)
- Midgut carcinoids usually produce only serotonin
- Hindgut carcinoids are often nonsecretory
- Other peptides that may be produced in excess include synaptophysin, neuropeptide K, pancreatic polypeptide & chromogranin A (CGA)

2.11.11.2 Medullary thyroid carcinoma

- Plasma calcitonin, with or without provocative testing with calcium infusion
- Serum CEA commonly elevated
- Paraganglioma & pheochromocytoma
- Capable of producing norepinephrine with or without epinephrine; some are nonsecretory
    - Norepinephrine is metabolized to normetanephrine, which is metabolized to vanillylmandelic acid (VMA)
    - Epinephrine is metabolized to metanephrine, which is metabolized to VMA
- Available laboratory tests include urinary VMA, urinary metanephrines, urinary catecholamines, plasma metanephrines, or plasma catecholamines
- Certain antihypertensive and other medications can interfere with these assays including imipramine, reserpine, guanethidine, nitroglycerin & monoamine oxidase (MAO) inhibitors

2.11.11.3 Neuroblastoma

- Urine VMA and homovanillic acid (HVA) are elevated in most cases (HVA is the final metabolic product of DOPA & dopamine, whereas VMA is the final product of norepinephrine & epinephrine)
- Neuron-specific enolase, lactic dehydrogenase (LDH) & ferritin are nonspecific markers that may be used to follow disease activity

2.11.12 Urine markers for urothelial carcinoma

- The nuclear matrix protein 22 test detects a nuclear matrix protein called nuclear mitotic apparatus, which is released from the nuclei of tumor cells when they die
- The bladder tumor antigen test detects complement factor H and complement factor H-related proteins in the urine

2.12 Endocrinology

2.12.1 Thyroid gland

2.12.1.1 Anatomy of the thyroid gland

- Bilobular, butterfly shaped organ that is centered around the trachea
- Consists of 2 types of cells, follicular & parafollicular
- Follicles
    - Hollow balls formed by a single layer of follicular cells
    - Center of each follicle is filled with "colloid," which receives and stores thyroglobulin, a glycoprotein produced by follicular epithelial cells
    - Connective tissue between the follicles contains prefollicular or clear (C) cells

2.12.1.2 Function of thyroid hormones

- Stimulates general metabolism
- Energy expenditure
- Heat production
- Involved in growth, maturation & sexual development
- Stimulates protein synthesis and carbohydrate & lipid metabolism
- Increased lipolysis & fatty acid oxidation
- Affects heart rate & heart contraction
- Neurologic development

2.12.1.3 Synthesis of thyroid hormones

- The thyroid gland synthesizes and secretes thyroxine (T_4), triiodothyronine (T_3) & small amounts of reverse T_3 (rT_3)
- Requires dietary iodide (I^-)
- Iodine is the key to the synthesis of thyroid hormones and is normally ingested in the form of iodides

2.12.1.4 Thyroid hormones

2.12.1.4.1 Triiodothyronine

- T_3 is more physiologically active than T_4
- Circulating levels of T_3 & T_4 are not equal; the level of circulating T_4 is much higher
- T_3 is analyzed less frequently than other thyroid functions
- Ordered when a clinician suspects subclinical hyperthyroidism when free T_4 is normal
- Elevated in hyperthyroidism
- Decreased in situations of chronic illness because of stress and nonthyroid factors so T_3 levels are not useful in the differential diagnosis of hypothyroidism

2.12.1.4.2 Thyroid-stimulating hormone

- Glycoprotein hormone synthesized and secreted by the anterior pituitary
- Causes an increase in number and size of follicular cells (hyperplasia) so they can trap more iodide to synthesize more thyroid hormones
- Breaks down thyroglobulin to increase the release of thyroid hormones into circulation
- Reference range: 0.5-5.0 μU/mL

2.12.1.4.3 Thyroxine

- Steps in T_4 synthesis
  - Follicular cells synthesize protein called thyroglobulin which contains many tyrosine moieties
  - The initial step leading to thyroid hormone synthesis is the trapping of iodide form the circulating blood
  - Iodide trap is an energy-dependent, active transport mechanism that removes iodide from the blood and pumps it into the thyroid follicle
  - I^- enters follicular cell and undergoes enzymatic "activation"
  - Peroxidase enzyme attaches 2 iodides to tyrosine rings (1 by 1) → monoiodotyrosine (MIT) and diiodotyrosine (DIT)
  - MIT or DIT is then enzymatically coupled to form T_3 & T_4
  - The newly formed T_3 & T_4 remain attached to the thyroglobulin molecule and are stored in the colloid space until they are ready to be released into the blood (signal for secretion of thyroxine is received)
  - In response to stimulation by the pituitary (TSH), peptide bonds between tyrosine residues of thyroglobulin are enzymatically cleaved. Thyroglobulin is absorbed back into the follicular cells and hydrolyzed to release T_3 & T_4
- T_3 and T_4 are secreted in plasma
- Once T_4 enters the bloodstream and reaches peripheral tissue, a portion deiodinates enzymatically to become T_3
- The primary site of deiodination is the liver, and to a lesser extent, other tissues as well. Most of the T_3 is produced through this process
- Peripheral metabolism of T_4 can also remove an iodide to form rT_3, which is inactive
- Protein binding of thyroid hormone
  - Once released in circulation, thyroid hormones immediately bind to proteins:
    - Thyroxine-binding globulin (TBG)
      - Most of the T_3 & T_4 is bound to TBG
      - TBG is synthesized by liver
      - In severe liver disease→ ↓ TBG → ↓ total T_4 due to ↓ protein-bound T_4
      - ↑ estrogen (eg, pregnancy) → ↑ synthesis of TBG → ↑ total T_4 & T_3 due to ↑ protein-bound T_4 & T_3
    - Thyroxine-binding prealbumin (TBPA)
    - Albumin
  - >99% of thyroid hormones are carried in plasma bound to protein
  - <1% is free, biologically active (0.04% T_4 & 0.4% T_3)

2.12.1.4.4 Regulation of thyroid hormone secretion

- Hypothalamus and anterior pituitary (adenohypophysis) monitor the level of free, active T_4 using negative feedback
- ↓ free T_4 stimulates hypothalamus to secrete thyrotropin-releasing hormone (TRH)
- TRH stimulates pituitary to secrete thyrotropin (TSH)
- TSH stimulates the thyroid to increase the synthesis of T_4 and T_3 → depresses release of TSH (feedback)

2.12.1.5 Thyroid disorders

2.12.1.5.1 Primary hyperthyroidism

- An abnormality in the thyroid gland
- TRH, TSH, T_4, and T_3 concentrations reflect normal feedback response
- Thyroid gland secretes excess T_3 & T_4 without regard for feedback
- Graves disease is the most common condition
- Other causes: Toxic adenoma, toxic multinodular goiter (Plummer disease) or Graves disease, transient hyperthyroidism in various kinds of thyroiditis, exogenous thyroxine, and (rarely) pituitary adenoma and thyroid carcinoma

 ISBN 978-089189-6616

- Symptoms: Weight loss, sweat, anxiety & tremor
- Laboratory results:
  - Low TSH & high serum free T_4 (fT_4)
  - ↓↓ TSH (exponential decrease for modest decrease in thyroid hormones)
  - ↑ total T_4 and total T_3 (free and protein-bound)
  - ↑ fT_4 and free T_3 (fT_3)
  - When fT_4 is normal despite a low TSH, fT_3 should be measured to assess for T_3 thyrotoxicosis
  - ↓ TRH, but rarely measured

2.12.1.5.2 Graves disease

- Most common cause of thyrotoxicosis (excessive production of thyroid hormones)
- Graves disease is autoimmune production of an antibody that resembles TSH → inappropriate stimulation of thyroid gland → uncontrolled increase in secretion of T_4 and T_3 → hyperthyroidism
- TSH will be normal to ↓
- Thyroid receptor antibody and thyroid-stimulating antibody (TSI) ↑
- Thyroid-stimulating immunoglobulin (TSI), also called long-acting thyroid-stimulating antibodies
- Antimicrosomal antibodies are found in 60% of cases
- Antithyroglobulin antibodies in 30% of cases

2.12.1.5.3 Signs of hyperthyroidism

- Goiter (enlarged thyroid gland)
- Exophthalmos
- Muscle weakness
- Tachycardia
- Hyperthermia
- Weight loss

2.12.1.5.4 Primary hypothyroidism

- Thyroid gland secretes insufficient T_3 & T_4 without regard for feedback
- Destruction of the thyroid gland or congenital lack of development of thyroid gland
- Most common cause is Hashimoto thyroiditis
- Others include thyroidectomy, lymphocytic and granulomatous (de Quervain) thyroiditis, I-131 therapy, radiation, and drugs (iodine, lithium, interleukin 2, and α interferon)
- Laboratory results
  - Elevated TSH and low fT_4
  - ↓ total and free, active T_3 & T_4, ↑ TSH
- Symptoms
  - Slowdown of metabolic processes
  - Weight gain
  - Cold intolerance
  - Lethargy

2.12.1.5.5 Congenital hypothyroidism

- Defect in thyroid hormone synthesis or pituitary/hypothalamic hormone synthesis
- Causes mental & somatic restriction = cretinism
- Can cause hypothyroidism in newborns because of a deficiency of thyroid tissue (athyrosis)
- In many states, blood specimens of all newborn infants are sent to the health department for measurement of fT_4 to diagnose congenital hypothyroidism
  - If ↓ fT_4 then TSH is also measured
  - If congenital hypothyroidism is diagnosed, then the infant must receive oral T_4 for life to avoid intellectual disability
- Newborns normally have a higher level of T_4 than do adults

2.12.1.5.6 Myxedema

- Caused by severe hypothyroidism
- Results in enlarged thyroid (goiter), thickening of skin, hoarseness in speech & weight gain

2.12.1.5.7 Hashimoto thyroiditis

- Most common cause of primary hypothyroidism
- An autoimmune disease
- Characterized by antitissue peroxidase (TPO) and antithyroglobulin (>90%) antibodies
- TSI are not identified in Hashimoto thyroiditis
- Thyroglobulin autoantibodies are present in the early phase
- Involves massive infiltration of thyroid gland by lymphocytes
- Requires replacement thyroid hormone to inhibit TSH secretion

2.12.1.5.8 Secondary thyroid disease

- An abnormality in pituitary gland which causes error in the amount of TSH produced
- Uncommon
- Primary hypopituitarism → secondary hypothyroidism
- Same symptoms as primary hypothyroidism

- Laboratory results
  - ↓↓ TSH
  - ↓ total T_4 & total T_3
  - ↓ fFT_4 & fT_3

2.12.1.5.9 Tertiary thyroid disease

- Abnormality in hypothalamus causing an error in the amount of TRH produced

2.12.1.5.10 Euthyroid sick syndrome (the nonthyroidal illness syndrome)

- Euthyroid = normal thyroid function
- This occurs if an abnormal thyroid function result is found in a euthyroid individual who is suffering from a nonthyroidal illness
- Acute serious disease sometimes uses up thyroid hormones faster for tissue repair and to fight off the illness → faster turnover of fT_4 and fT_3 but both thyroid and pituitary glands are normal and feedback regulation is normal = "sick euthyroid"
- Laboratory tests: Decreased T_3 & T_4, increased rT3 & normal TSH
- Thyroid hormone-binding ratio can be used to differentiate between thyroid disease and euthyroid sick syndrome
- Thyroid function tests should never be performed on a patient who is experiencing a serious illness

2.12.1.6 Other thyroid diseases

2.12.1.6.1 Goiter

- Increased TSH for any reason such as insufficient iodine in diet → hyperplasia of thyroid cells (trying to trap more iodine) → goiter
- An enlargement of the thyroid gland causing a swelling in the front part of the neck

2.12.1.6.2 Thyroid cancer

- Atomic bombs and accidents at nuclear power plants release radioactive iodine into the air. Thyroid gland extracts the radioactive iodine → ↑ incidence of thyroid cancer
- Protection from radioactivity is oral dose of potassium iodide before and/or after (<3-4 hours') exposure to saturate the thyroid-uptake system and prevent uptake of radioactive iodine

2.12.1.7 Diagnosis of thyroid disorder

- Testing decision pathway (American Thyroid Association) for adults
  - Clear signs and symptoms of thyroid disorder
  - TSH is the first laboratory test to be ordered
  - Total T_4 levels should not be assessed in healthy or asymptomatic patients
  - Screening is recommended at age 35 and every 5 years thereafter
  - More frequent testing recommended with risk factors or symptoms: Goiter, family history, lithium use
  - If the results are abnormal compared to age-adjusted and sex-adjusted reference ranges, thyroid disease is likely present
  - For example, in adults with TSH values <0.1 mU/mL most likely have primary hyperthyroidism
  - fT_4 (or fT_4 index) can be analyzed if TSH results do not correlate with symptoms
  - Clinicians assess thyroid function using clinical signs and symptoms such as body temperature, respiratory rate, and pulse
  - High levels of thyroid hormones will increase body temperature, basal metabolic rate, cardiac output, cardiac rate, and respiratory rate, and influence mood and behavior

2.12.1.8 Diagnosis of neonatal thyroid disorders

- Most often caused by thyroid dysgenesis
- Other causes include familial thyroid dyshormonogenesis, peripheral hormone resistance (autosomal dominant Refetoff syndrome), hypopituitarism, and maternal factors (maternal autoantibodies, maternal medications)
- Because of the severe consequences of untreated thyroid disease in the neonate, particularly hypothyroidism, asymptomatic neonates are typically screened with fT4 and followed up with TSH if results are abnormal
- If untreated, there is a high risk of intellectual disability and growth restriction
- Most commonly, the TSH assay alone is used to screen for this condition

2.12.1.9 Other causes of abnormal thyroid tests

- Abnormal amount of thyroid-binding globulin (TBG) → abnormal total T_4 & T_3 but normal TSH
- Pregnancy → ↑ estrogen level → ↑ TBG → ↑ protein-bound T_4 & T_3 but normal fT_4 & fT_3 → normal TSH
- Severe liver disease → ↓ TBG → ↓ protein-bound T_4 & T_3 but normal FT_4 & FT_3 → normal TSH

 ISBN 978-089189-6616

2.12.1.10 Laboratory diagnosis of thyroid disease

- Thyroid function tests
  - TSH (thyrotropin)
    - Best first-line test for diagnosing hypo- and hyperthyroidism; in nearly all instances elevated in true hypothyroidism and elevated in hypothyroidism
    - The single best screening test for thyroid dysfunction in all contexts except in potential hypothalamic or pituitary dysfunction and perhaps in neonatal screening
    - In these latter populations, a broader panel including fT4 may be indicated
  - Total T_4 (thyroxine)
    - Bound mainly to prealbumin (transthyretin) and TBG
    - Elevated in most hyperthyroid patients and decreased in hypothyroidism
    - <5% of hyperthyroid patients have normal T_4 but elevated T_3 ("T_3 toxicosis")
    - Because they are highly bound, fluctuations in serum proteins somewhat limit the value of total T_4 and total T_3
  - Thyroid-binding globulin
    - Increased by pregnancy, oral contraceptives, estrogen therapy, active hepatitis & hypothyroidism
    - When circulating thyroid-binding globulin (TBG) is increased, it elevates total thyroxine (T_3 & T_4). The fT_4 and TSH remain normal
    - Decreased by hypoproteinemic states, androgen therapy & cortisol
    - T_3 resin uptake is a conceptually confusing test that is no longer commonly used
      - Hyperthyroidism: High T_3 resin uptake
      - Hypothyroidism: Low T_3 resin uptake
      - fT_4 & fT_3 measurement correlates well with clinical thyroid status
  - Reverse T_3
    - Metabolic product of T_4
    - rT_3 is elevated in so-called euthyroid sick syndrome
  - TRH stimulation test
    - Used sometimes in the evaluation of hypothyroidism
    - Measures pituitary TSH stores
    - TRH is injected and blood samples are collected for TSH analysis
    - TSH levels rapidly rise in normal patients but will have no response in a hyperthyroid patient
    - An exaggerated secretion of TSH in response to TRH in primary hypothyroidism (hypothyroidism caused by intrinsic thyroid hypofunction)
    - An inappropriate TSH response to TRH stimulation suggests hypopituitarism
  - Anti-TSH receptor antibody
    - Detects TSH receptor antibodies for diagnosis of autoimmune hyperthyroidism (such as Graves disease)

2.12.1.11 Laboratory methods of analysis

- Thyroxine
  - Enzyme immunoassay or fluorescent immunoassay of plasma & serum samples
  - For total T_4 assays, because >99% of the hormone is bound to protein, the first step in the reaction involves displacing T_4 from the binding proteins
  - Monoclonal or polyclonal antibody that is highly specific to thyroxine, binds with the hormone
  - Enzyme labeled hormone competes with the endogenous thyroxine
  - Substances that did not bind to antibody are removed from the system
  - Specific substrate is then added, which reacts with the enzyme label and the product formed can be measured on a spectrophotometer
- fT_4 analysis
  - fT_4 is more difficult to measure because of the small amount of it in the presence of increased TBG-bound T_4 and the slightest error releases so much T_4 from TBG that the amount of fT_4 is ↑↑↑

2.12.1.12 Medications

- Amiodarone effect is largely unpredictable, but a general rule of thumb is that in developed (iodine rich) parts of the world, amiodarone causes hypothyroidism, and in underdeveloped (iodine poor) places, amiodarone causes hyperthyroidism
- Lithium inhibits the release of thyroxine from the thyroid gland; results in hypothyroidism

2.12.2 Adrenal cortex

2.12.2.1 Disorders

2.12.2.1.1 Cushing syndrome (hypercortisolism)

- Diagnosis
  - Requires demonstration of persistent hypercortisolism. The recommended screening tests are the low-dose dexamethasone suppression test (DST), 24-hour urinary free cortisol, or midnight salivary or serum cortisol. A positive screening result should be confirmed with repeat testing
  - The underlying cause of Cushing syndrome must then be determined, first by measuring adrenocorticotropic hormone (ACTH) to distinguish ACTH-dependent from ACTH-independent Cushing syndrome
  - ACTH-dependent Cushing syndrome is further evaluated with bilateral inferior petrosal sinus sampling, if available, or the high-dose DST and/or cortisol-releasing hormone (CRH) stimulation tests. Imaging of the pituitary provides corroborative information, but it lacks sensitivity and specificity for Cushing disease when used in isolation
  - ACTH-independent Cushing syndrome requires, after the exclusion of surreptitious glucocorticoid administration, adrenal imaging
- Iatrogenic Cushing syndrome
  - Administration of corticosteroids for the treatment of inflammatory disease, The most common cause in the developed world
- Noniatrogenic (spontaneous) Cushing syndrome
  - May be caused by pituitary adenoma (Cushing disease), adrenal gland abnormalities, or ectopic ACTH production
  - Usually found in association with a pituitary microadenoma (<1.0 cm) of basophilic cells (corticotrophs)
  - Ectopic ACTH is associated with small cell lung carcinoma, lung carcinoid, pancreatic endocrine tumors, non-small cell lung carcinoma, thymic tumors, medullary thyroid carcinoma & breast carcinoma
  - Primary adrenal hypercortisolism may be caused by adenoma, carcinoma, or bilateral adrenal hyperplasia
    - The effects include hyperglycemia, hypokalemia, protein catabolism, osteoporosis, centripetal fat deposition & skin thinning with striae
  - Patients with major depression often exhibit biochemical findings indistinguishable from Cushing syndrome, as may patients with anorexia nervosa, alcoholism & pregnancy (pseudo-Cushing)

2.12.2.1.2 Addison disease (primary adrenal insufficiency)

- Diagnosis
  - Depends on demonstration of a low 8 am serum cortisol and/or a blunted increase in cortisol following cosyntropin stimulation
  - The ACTH level is used to guide further evaluation
  - Elevated ACTH indicates primary adrenal insufficiency, which may be further evaluated with autoantibody studies and/or adrenal imaging
  - Normal or low ACTH suggests secondary adrenal insufficiency, most likely related to pituitary pathology or exogenous glucocorticoid administration
- Causes
  - Historically, most cases were related to primary destruction of the adrenal gland by granulomatous disease (tuberculosis)
  - Presently, the most common cause in developed nations is autoimmunity
  - Other causes are metastatic tumor, amyloid, or bilateral adrenal hemorrhage (Waterhouse-Friderichsen syndrome), congenital diseases (congenital adrenal hyperplasia & adrenoleukodystrophy), and drugs (ketoconazole etomidate & mitotane)
  - Addisonian crisis is characterized by altered mental status, with hypotension, hypoglycemia, hyponatremia, hyperkalemia & metabolic acidosis
  - May present insidiously as fatigue, weakness, weight loss, mood alteration, postural hypotension, skin hyperpigmentation & hypoglycemia

2.12.2.1.3 Secondary adrenal insufficiency

- Most cases are related to the administration of exogenous glucocorticoid that can lead to irreversible (or slowly reversible) suppression of endogenous ACTH production
- Not as severe as Addison disease, because mineralocorticoid production is maintained by the renin angiotensin system; hyperkalemia is absent and hyponatremia mild; hyperpigmentation is not a feature

2.12.2.1.4 Conn syndrome (hyperaldosteronism)

- Usually caused by an adrenal adenoma or bilateral adrenal hyperplasia; secondary hyperaldosteronism is seen in hyperreninemic states such as renal artery stenosis or the rare renin-producing juxtaglomerular cell tumor of the kidney
- Causes hypertension, hypokalemia & metabolic alkalosis

ISBN 978-089189-6616

- Ratio of the plasma aldosterone concentration to plasma renin activity is considered the best screening test; must be confirmed by a 24-hour urinary aldosterone level

2.12.2.1.5 Congenital adrenal hyperplasia t2.21

- 21-hydroxylase deficiency is the most common cause, followed by 11-hydroxylase deficiency
- Particularly common in Native Americans and Yupik Eskimos
- The gene for 21-hydroxylase is found on 6p21.3, within the HLA complex
- Compensatory increase in ACTH by the pituitary leads to increased production of steroid hormone precursors in the adrenal cortex; resulting adrenal hyperplasia leads to some degree of salt wasting, hypertension & virilization
- Affected individuals have increased 17-hydroxyprogesterone, decreased cortisol, increased ACTH, increased androgens, increased 17-ketosteroids & decreased aldosterone

t2.21 Congenital adrenal hyperplasia (CAH)

Enzyme deficiency	Adrenal hyperplasia	Virilization	Salt wasting	Hypertension
21-hydroxylase	+	+	+	–
11-hydroxylase	+	+	–	+

2.12.2.2 Tests

- Serum cortisol secretion undergoes diurnal variation (trough around midnight and peak ~8 am); also depends on levels of cortisol binding globulin. Timed draws are essential for interpretation
- Cushing syndrome is characterized by not only elevated serum cortisol but also loss of diurnal variation
- Elevated midnight serum cortisol is highly suggestive of Cushing syndrome
- Low 8 am serum cortisol is highly suggestive of adrenal insufficiency
- Urine free cortisol test requires a 24-hour urine collection but reflects free (unbound) serum cortisol and is independent of time of day considerations
- Dexamethasone suppression test (DST): With normal endocrine function, a dose of dexamethasone will suppress both ACTH and cortisol; suppression patterns are abnormal in Cushing syndrome
- Low-dose DST may be administered in 2 forms: The rapid (overnight) DST and the standard (2-day) DST. Both are meant to answer the question: "Does the patient have Cushing syndrome (hypercortisolism)?" Healthy individuals experience suppression of plasma cortisol in both tests. Impaired suppression confirms the diagnosis of Cushing syndrome; however, abnormal suppression can also be seen in severe stress, alcohol abuse & major depression (so-called pseudo-Cushing)
- High-dose DST is used to answer the question: "Is the Cushing syndrome caused by a pituitary adenoma (Cushing disease)?" Suppression implies pituitary adenoma. Nonsuppression points to either ectopic ACTH production by tumor or primary adrenal hypercortisolism. The latter 2 possibilities can be distinguished by plasma ACTH measurement
- CRH stimulation test, like the high-dose DST, is aimed at determining the cause of Cushing syndrome; exaggerated elevation in ACTH and cortisol suggests Cushing disease (pituitary adenoma); no response is seen with adrenal tumors or ectopic ACTH

2.12.3 Adrenal medulla

- Principal site of the conversion of the amino acid tyrosine into the catecholamines; epinephrine, norepinephrine, and dopamine
- Produces catecholamines by hydroxylation of amino acid tyrosine
  - In the blood, catecholamines circulate 50% bound to albumin
  - Norepinephrine—predominantly synthesized in CNS 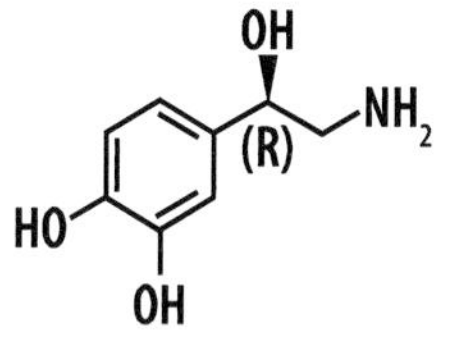
  - Epinephrine—predominantly synthesized by adrenal medulla
    - 80% of the catecholamine secretion of the medulla is in the form of epinephrine 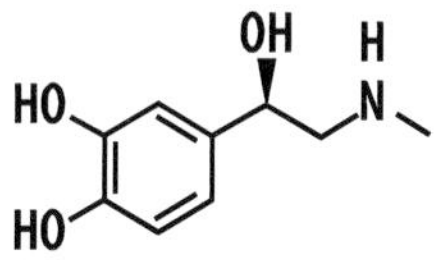
  - Dopamine
    - Small amount produced by medulla
    - Neurotransmitter—sometimes called the "reward" hormone

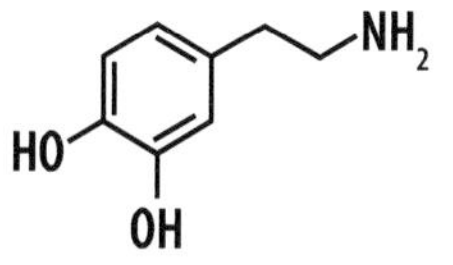

OH
NH2
(R)
HO
OH

OH H
HO
N
HO

NH2
HO
OH

- Functions:
  - Neurotransmitter actions
  - Released in response to pain and emotional disturbance and slows digestion
  - Increase blood pressure, heart rate, and blood sugar and dilates arteries
- The major effects mediated by epinephrine and norepinephrine are:
  - Vasoconstriction, which results in increased resistance and increased arterial blood pressure
  - Dilation of bronchioles
  - Increased glycogenolysis for energy production
  - Stimulation of lipolysis in fat cells, which more sustained energy production in many tissues than glycolysis
  - Increased metabolic rate, resulting in increased oxygen consumption and heat production
- Catecholamines are transported free in blood and regulated by feedback inhibition synthesis
  - Metabolites—metanephrine and normetanephrine → vanillylmandelic acid (VMA) (enzyme is monoamine oxidase)—passed in the urine
  - The medullary hormones have the same effects on target organs as direct stimulation by sympathetic nerves, although their effects are longer lasting and circulating hormones may cause effects in cells and tissues that are not directly innervated
  - Catecholamines are synthesized from the amino acid tyrosine through reactions that are catalyzed by the enzymes, catechol-O-methyl transferase (COMT) and monoamine oxidase (MAO)
- Laboratory testing: Urinary metanephrines, VMA
  - Vanillylmandelic acid (VMA) is the oxidation metabolite of epinephrine, norepinephrine, metanephrine, and normetanephrine
  - Homovanillic acid (HVA) is the metabolite of dopamine (measured in acidified 24 hr urine by HPLC)
- Disorders: pheochromacytoma
  - Extreme hypertension
  - Increased metanephrines & VMA
- Neuroblastoma
  - Increased HVA & VMA

2.12.4 Pituitary

- Hypersecretion of any of the anterior pituitary hormones is nearly always the result of a pituitary adenoma; prolactinomas are the most common secretory tumors of the pituitary
- In contrast, pituitary hypofunction rarely involves a single hormone, instead manifesting as panhypopituitarism; causes include tumors impinging on the pituitary gland (nonsecretory pituitary adenomas, craniopharyngiomas), infarction (Sheehan syndrome, sickle cell anemia), sarcoidosis, histiocytosis X, hemochromatosis, irradiation & autoimmune destruction
- Hypothalamic disorders and interruption of the pituitary stalk may produce a distinct pattern in which all anterior pituitary hormones except prolactin are suppressed. This pattern of prolactin-sparing hypopituitarism is called the "stalk effect"
- Growth hormone (GH)
  - Hyposecretion
    - In children, GH deficiency causes dwarfism
    - In adults, it is relatively asymptomatic
    - GH levels frequently are undetectable in healthy subjects and are not diagnostic of hyposecretion; provocative testing is required, performed by measuring GH in the fasting state, during sleep, following exercise, or following insulin or arginine administration
  - Hypersecretion
    - Causes gigantism in children
    - Causes acromegaly in adults
    - Insulinlike growth factor 1 (IGF-1) consistently elevated in GH hypersecretion; normal IGF-1 excludes GH excess
    - Markedly elevated GH from a random blood sample or a relatively normal level that fails to be suppressed with glucose administration can diagnose GH excess
- Follicle-stimulating hormone (FSH)
  - FSH assays can be useful in younger women (eg, 45 years) presenting with possible early menopause; persistently elevated FSH suggests ovarian failure
- Prolactin
  - Unique in that it does not have a dedicated stimulator for its release; instead, the hypothalamus produces a potent inhibitor, dopamine
  - If connections between the hypothalamus and pituitary are severed, all anterior pituitary hormones decrease (because of lack of stimulation) except prolactin, which markedly increases (because of lack of inhibition)

ISBN 978-089189-6616

- Hyperprolactinemia
  - In women, amenorrhea galactorrhea syndrome
  - In men, testicular atrophy, impotence & gynecomastia
  - Usually caused by a prolactin-secreting pituitary adenoma
  - Other causes include pregnancy, lactation, stalk compression, macroprolactinemia & phenothiazine therapy
- Antidiuretic hormone
  - Diabetes insipidus (DI)
    - Results from inadequate antidiuretic hormone (ADH) activity
    - Symptoms include polyuria and polydipsia with low urine osmolarity and hypernatremia
    - Central DI (inadequate ADH secretion) caused by head trauma, mass lesions involving the pituitary & an X-linked recessive familial form
    - Nephrogenic DI (renal tubules unresponsive to ADH) caused by hypercalcemia, hypokalemia, a very low protein diet, demeclocycline therapy, lithium therapy, relief of longstanding obstruction, and familial causes. Normal aging may by itself be associated with partial nephrogenic DI
    - Confirmed with an overnight water deprivation test followed by administration of ADH (vasopressin)
      - In healthy individuals, urine osmolarity progressively increases during water deprivation, and administration of exogenous ADH has no additional effect on urine concentration
      - In central DI, there is failure to appropriately concentrate the urine in response to dehydration and a rise in urine osmolarity in response to administered ADH
      - In nephrogenic DI, urine cannot be concentrated in either case
  - Syndrome of inappropriate ADH
    - Hyponatremia with normovolemia
    - Urine sodium >20 mEq/L (>20 mmol/L), urine osmolarity >100 mOsm/kg
    - Caused by tumors (especially small cell carcinoma of the lung, pancreatic adenocarcinoma & intracranial tumors), interstitial lung disease, cerebral trauma & the drug chlorpropamide

2.12.5 Reproductive hormones

2.12.5.1 Female reproductive hormones

- Estradiol

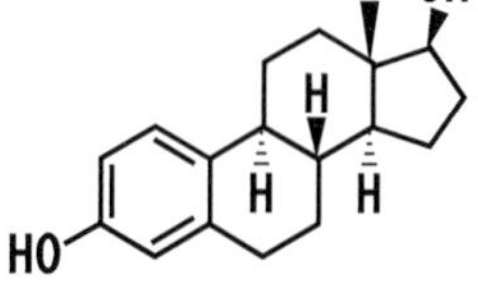

  - Chief circulatory product of maturing follicle
  - Is derived by degradation from the cholesterol molecule
  - Formed by aromatization of androgens
  - Promotes increased numbers of granulosa cells & follicle stimulating hormone (FSH) receptors on them
  - Drives events leading to dominant follicle selection
  - Peak production from pre-ovulatory follicles
  - Typical pre-ovulatory level is 250 pg/mL
  - Lowest concentrations at the time of menses
  - Low concentrations in many pathologic states
  - Concentrations normally low in pre-pubertal girls and menopausal women
- Progesterone

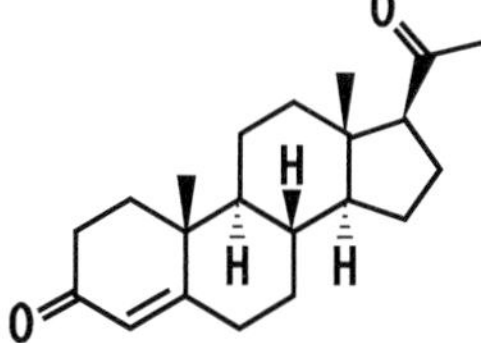

  - Chief secretory product of corpus luteum
  - Prepares the endometrium for implantation (promotes gestation)
  - If pregnancy fails to occur, the corpus luteum regresses and menses ensues
- Menstrual cycle—changes are due to luteinizing hormone (LH) and follicle stimulating hormone (FSH) release at the appropriate time
  - Day 1: Start of menses
  - Day 5-7: Follicle selected, begins prostaglandin E2 (PGE2) secretion
  - Day 13: LH Surge
  - Day 14: Ovulation
  - Day 18-23: ↑ PGE2 and progesterone
  - Day 25: ↓ PGE2 and progesterone demise, Endometrium breakdown
- Female hypogonadism and hypergonadism
  - Hypergonadotropic hypogonadism
    - Primary ovarian dysfunction
    - Turner syndrome
    - Chromosomal defect
    - Female with partly or completely missing an X chromosome (45 XO, OO)
  - Premature ovarian failure (POF): Genetic defects, Autoimmune disease, environmental insults, idiopathic

- Hypogonadotropic hypogonadism
    - Pituitary or hypothalamic dysfunction
    - Pituitary surgery, prolactinoma, empty sella syndrome
    - Functional hypothalamic amenorrhea (exercise, eating disorders)
  - Hypothyroidism
- Female reproductive hormones in diagnosis
  - LH, FSH, estrogens, progesterone, testosterone, prolactin
    - Measured by immunoassay
  - Pregnancy hormones
    - Progesterone
    - Human chorionic gonadotrophin (hCG)
    - Inhibin
  - Gonad functional tests
    - hCG stimulation test: assay for primary disease
      - hCG is structurally similar to LH and can mimic LH
      - hCG injection should stimulate the testes to produce testosterone or the ovaries to produce progesterone
      - Failure to see the increase indicates a primary disease
    - Gonadotropin releasing hormone (GnRH) test: assay for secondary disease
      - Synthetic GnRH is administered
      - If the pituitary is responsive, LH & FSH should rise
  - Infertility tests
    - Basal body temperature to establish time of ovulation
    - LH and FSH
    - Estrogen, progesterone, prolactin
    - Thyroid stimulating hormone (TSH): abnormal thyroid function inhibits fertility
    - Malnutrition or chronic illness may influence fertility
  - Hirsutism
    - Male pattern hair growth
    - Usually caused by hyperactivity of adrenal gland
    - Work up includes adrenocorticotropic hormone (ACTH), androgens, testosterone, LH, FSH
  - Amenorrhea
    - Absence of menstruation
    - Work up includes: LH, FSH, estradiol, testosterone, thyroid function, prolactin

2.12.5.2 Male reproductive hormones (androgens)

- Responsible for masculine differentiation of the fetal genital tract and the development and maintenance of male secondary sex characteristics
- Strong androgens—synthesized in the testes
  - Testosterone, dihydrotestosterone (DHT)
  - Weak androgens—made in the adrenal glands
    - Androstenedione, dehydroepiandrosterone (DHEA) and DHEAS
- Testosterone 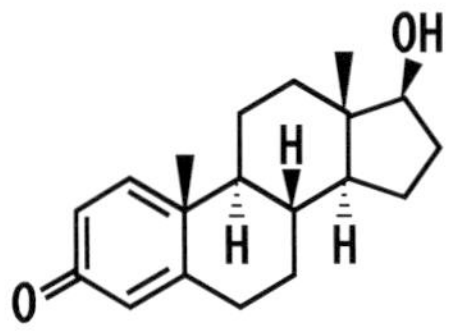
  - Essential for sperm development
  - Serum concentrations (morning sample)
    - Normal = 250-1000 ng/dL
    - Hypogonadotropic ≤200 ng/dL
  - If testosterone is low, need FSH for etiology
    - FSH: Normal ≤15 mIU/mL
    - Hypogonadotropic ≤10
    - Hypergonadotropic ≥20
  - hCG Stimulation
    - Stimulates LH receptors which increases testosterone
    - Measure baseline testosterone
    - Give intramuscular hCG (5000 IU)
    - Measure testosterone 48-96 hr later
    - <150 ng/dL indicates primary hypogonadism
- Male hypo- and hypergonadism
  - Hypogonadotropic hypogonadism
    - Secondary—pituitary or hypothalamic hypofunction
    - Causes: panhypopituitarism hypothalamic, syndrome, GnRH deficiency, hyperprolactinemia, malnutrition and anorexia, drugs
    - Test results: ↓ LH, ↓ FSH, ↓ testosterone
  - Hypergonadotropic hypogonadism
    - Primary testicular hypofunction
      - Causes
        - Acquired
        - Chromosomal defects (Klinefelter XXY-left, Defective androgen biosynthesis)
        - Testicular agenesis, Leydig cell failure in older men
        - Acute and chronic disease
      - Test results: ↑ LH, ↑ FSH, ↓ testosterone

ISBN 978-089189-6616

- Male reproductive hormones in diagnosis
  - Infertility
    - Sperm Evaluation
    - Testosterone
    - LH and FSH levels

2.13 Toxicology

2.13.1 Drugs of abuse screening (forensic toxicology)

- Refers to testing in the workplace, in a drug treatment program, or in legal settings
- Urine is the usual specimen
- Screening drug tests are usually based on immunoassay
- Specificity is fairly low
- Cross-reacting substances causing false positives are common
- Positive test results often require confirmation (gas chromatography/mass spectrometry usually)
- Witnessed collection often required to ensure that the urine sample has not been altered
- Often the specimen is divided into 2 aliquots so that retesting can be performed if a positive result is obtained
- To detect adulterants it is routine to check the specimen color, odor (eg, for bleach), temperature (suspicious if cool), pH (suspicious if <4.5 or >8.0), specific gravity (suspicious for dilution if <1.005), creatinine (suspicious if <20 mg/dL) and/or nitrite (suspicious if >500 µg/mL)
- Chain of custody precautions are a requirement for any test that may have implications in criminal proceedings
- The duration that an agent may be detected (window of detection) depends upon a range of variables including dose, methodology & sample type; general guidelines are provided in t2.22

t2.22 Approximate detection periods for urine drugs of abuse screening tests

Drug	Window of detection (in urine)
Cannabinoids (THC)	3 (single use) to 30 (chronic user) days
Benzodiazepines	2-10 days, depending on agent
Amphetamines, methamphetamines, opiates, cocaine	2-3 days
Barbiturates	3-15 days, depending on agent
Alcohol	1 day

2.13.1.1 General aspects of laboratory evaluation

- Toxidromes are constellations of findings that suggest a particular agent or group of agents t2.23 & t2.24

t2.23 Common toxidromes

Class	Signs	Agents
Anticholinergic	Hyperthermia, dry skin, flushing, altered mental status, psychosis ("hot as a hare, dry as a bone, red as a beet, mad as a hatter"), mydriasis, constipation	Atropine, antihistamines, tricyclic antidepressants, scopolamine
Cholinergic	Salivation, lacrimation, urination, diarrhea, GI cramps, emesis ("SLUDGE"); diaphoresis, miosis & wheezing	Organophosphates, pilocarpine, carbamate
Adrenergic	Hypertension, tachycardia, mydriasis, anxiety, hyperthermia	Amphetamines, cocaine, pseudoephedrine ephedrine, PCP
Sedative	Altered mental status, slurred speech, hypopnea/apnea	Barbiturates, alcohols, opiates
Narcotic	Altered mental status, hypopnea/apnea	Opiates
Hallucinogenic	Hallucinations, anxiety, hyperthermia	LSD, PCP, amphetamines, cocaine

GI, gastrointestinal; LSD, lysergic acid diethylamide; PCP, phencyclidine

t2.24 Signs or symptoms associated with toxic agents

Sign or symptom	Associated agents
Pinpoint pupils (miosis)	Cholinergics (organophosphates, pilocarpine, carbamate) Opiates Benzodiazepines
Dilated pupils (mydriasis)*	Anticholinergics (atropine, antihistamines, tricyclics, scopolamine) Sympathomimetics (cocaine, amphetamines) Carbon monoxide
Diaphoresis	Sympathomimetics (cocaine, amphetamines) Organophosphates
Red skin	Carbon monoxide Cyanide Anticholinergics
Tremor	Lithium vs withdrawal
Dystonia	Neuroleptics (antipsychotics)
Bitter almond odor	Cyanide
Mothball odor	Camphor
Garlic odor	Organophosphates, arsenic

**A unilateral dilated pupil is indicative of an anatomic defect such as brain stem herniation, glaucoma, or cranial nerve palsy. It also may be caused by topical atropine*

- The National Academy of Clinical Biochemistry (NACB) guidelines advise tier 1 testing for all laboratories that support emergency medicine departments see **t2.25**

t2.25 National Academy of Clinical Biochemistry tier 1 test recommendations

Testing category	Specific agents
Stat quantitative serum assays	Acetaminophen (paracetamol) Lithium Salicylate Theophylline Valproic acid Carbamazepine Digoxin Phenobarbital Iron Transferrin (or UIBC) Ethanol Methanol Ethylene glycol Co-oximetry
Stat qualitative urine assays	Cocaine Opiates Barbiturates Amphetamines Propoxyphene Tricyclics Phencyclidine

2.13.1.2 Laboratory evaluation of the apparently intoxicated patient

- May include urine toxicology screening, serum/plasma toxicology tests & assessment of the anion gap, osmolar gap & oxygen gap
- Anion gap over 20 mEq/L is significant (note that hypoalbuminemia may falsely lower the anion gap); toxins that cause an increased anion gap metabolic acidosis include acetaminophen, salicylates, ascorbate, hydrogen sulfide, ethylene glycol, methanol, ethanol, formaldehyde, carbon monoxide, nitroprusside, epinephrine & paraldehyde
- Osmolal gap >10 mOsm is significant; osmolal gap is the difference between the measured osmolarity and the calculated osmolarity by the following formula:

  $$(2 \times Na) + (BUN \div 2.8) + (glucose \div 18)$$

- Oxygen saturation gap is the difference between the saturation given by co-oximetry and the saturation given by the pulse oximeter; normally, this difference should be <5%. Causes of an increased oxygen saturation gap include carbon monoxide poisoning (carboxyhemoglobin), methemoglobin, hydrogen sulfide poisoning (sulfmethemoglobin) & cyanide poisoning. Abnormally high venous oxygen content (arterialization of venous blood) is seen in cyanide and hydrogen sulfide poisoning

2.13.2 Ethanol

- Metabolized by hepatic alcohol dehydrogenase to acetaldehyde, which is converted by aldehyde dehydrogenase to acetic acid
- Specimen
  - In an overdose evaluation, usually serum or plasma is measured
  - In forensic testing, whole blood or breath alcohol is measured (ratio of blood-breath alcohol is 2100:1)
- Limits
  - Most states define the legal limit for operation of a motor vehicle as 80-100 mg/dL (0.08%-0.1%) in whole blood **t2.26**. Whole blood ethanol tends to run lower than serum or plasma ethanol concentration, and legal definitions are usually in terms of whole blood

t2.26 Clinical effects of blood alcohol

Blood alcohol concentration (%)	Clinical findings
<0.05	Sobriety
0.05-0.1	Euphoria
0.1-0.2	Excitement
0.2-0.3	Confusion
0.3-0.4	Stupor
>0.4	Coma & death

- Markers of alcohol consumption
  - γ-glutamyl transferase (GGT) concentration is increased in heavy consumers of alcohol; 4 weeks of abstinence usually required for normalization of GGT
  - Carbohydrate-deficient transferrin is at least as sensitive and probably more specific than GGT

2.13.3 Toxic alcohol poisoning t2.27

- Ethylene glycol (antifreeze), methanol (windshield washer fluid, paint removers, wood alcohol), or isopropyl alcohol (rubbing alcohol)
- Ingestion suspected if the osmolal gap exceeds 10 mOsm

t2.27 Toxic alcohol poisoning

Alcohol	Source	Anion gap acidosis	Osmolal gap	Increased ketones	Metabolite
Ethanol		–/+	+	–/+	
Ethylene glycol	Antifreeze	+	+	–	Oxalate & glycolate
Isopropanol	Rubbing alcohol	–	+	–	Acetone
Methanol	Windshield washer fluid	+	+	–	Formate & formaldehyde

ISBN 978-089189-6616

- Ethanol is often present in conjunction with toxic alcohol ingestion, and ethanol can itself widen the osmolal gap. To calculate this effect:

  calculated osmolality = 2[Na mEq/L] + [BUN mg/dL]/2.8 + [glucose mg/dL]/18 + [ethanol mg/dL]/4.6

- Ethylene glycol and methanol cause both increased anion gap and increased osmolal gap
- Isopropyl alcohol, like ethanol, does not cause acidosis but does cause an osmolal gap
- Ethylene glycol is metabolized to oxalate; oxalate crystals can be found in the urine, where they appear envelope shaped, translucent & birefringent
- Methanol is metabolized to formaldehyde and then to formic acid
- Isopropyl alcohol is metabolized to acetone
- Treatment of methanol or ethylene glycol poisoning consists of inhibiting the activity of alcohol dehydrogenase, because metabolites cause toxicity; traditionally, ethanol was given for this effect, and more recently fomepizole

2.13.4 Lead poisoning (plumbism)

- Sources include lead paint, lead pipes, lead gasoline, contaminated soil, and the manufacture of lead batteries & lead smelters
- Enters the body through inhalation and ingestion; distributed mainly into erythrocytes, bone, and kidney
- Toxicity derives from 2 mechanisms: Nonspecifically binds to and inhibits enzymes having sulfhydryl groups, and is directly toxic to mitochondria
- Inhibits key enzymes in heme synthesis, δ-ALA-dehydratase and ferrochelatase, leading to accumulation of the precursor protoporphyrin (free erythrocyte protoporphyrin or FEP) which binds to available zinc, yielding zinc protoporphyrin (ZPP); both FEP and ZPP are increased in lead toxicity (and in iron deficiency)
- Inhibits sodium channel ATPases, leading to increased osmotic fragility and shortened red cell survival
- Basophilic stippling results from the inhibition of 5'-nucleotidase, an enzyme whose function is to break down RNA
- The effect of coexistent iron deficiency is to enhance the toxic effects of lead
- Manifestations
  - Microcytic, hypochromic anemia with basophilic stippling
  - Neurologic impairment, central & peripheral (bilateral wrist drop)
  - Renal insufficiency, especially aminoaciduria, glycosuria, and phosphaturia (similar to Fanconi renal syndrome)
  - Abdominal pain
- Laboratory testing
  - Nonspecific: Hemoglobin, hematocrit, FEP, ZPP, urinalysis (proteinuria & glycosuria), iron studies
  - Specific: Venous blood lead level by atomic absorption spectrophotometry; the Centers for Disease Control and Prevention (CDC) considers ≥10 μg/dL (≥0.48 μmol/L) to be elevated
- Treatment: Environmental interventions to address source; chelation therapy

2.13.5 Carbon monoxide (CO) poisoning

- Sources: Incomplete combustion of fossil fuels; produced endogenously from the breakdown of heme, resulting in normal hemoglobin-CO ≤1%
- CO binds (with 200× the affinity of oxygen) to hemoglobin, forming carboxyhemoglobin (hemoglobin-CO); has even greater avidity for fetal hemoglobin; also directly toxic to intracellular oxidative mechanisms
- Laboratory testing
  - Nonspecific: Lactate, anion gap, cardiac markers, cyanide levels (may be coexistent toxicity following smoke inhalation)
  - Specific: Co-oximetry, with levels correlating with clinical effect **t2.28**; pulse oximetry may give a falsely reassuring oxygen saturation
- Treatment: 100% O_2

t2.28 Clinical effects of carbon monoxide poisoning

Level of CO	Clinical findings
0.4%-2%	Normal nonsmoker
2%-6%	Normal smoker
10%-20%	Mild symptoms: dyspnea on exertion
20%-50%	Severe symptoms: intoxication, with headache, lethargy, loss of consciousness
>50%	Coma & death

2.13.6 Acetaminophen poisoning

- Manifestations are polyphasic
  - Phase I: Mild nausea & abdominal discomfort; abates within hours
  - Phase II: Usually after 24 hours, progressive liver injury
  - Phase III: Fulminant hepatic failure

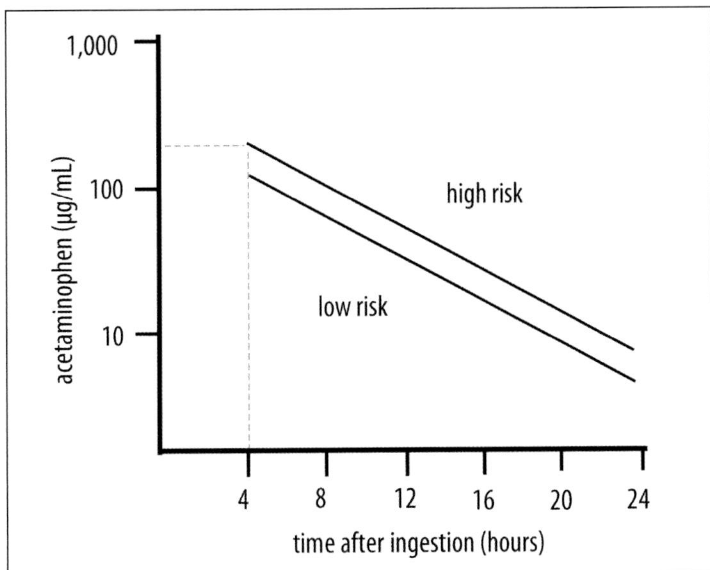

f2.19 Acetaminophen (Rumack-Matthew) nomogram for determination of toxicity severity; if the time of ingestion is known, plotting a single serum acetaminophen level, drawn >4 hours after ingestion, can triage the patient as being at high or low risk for toxicity

- Phase IV: Resolution in the form of recovery, liver transplantation, or death

- Rumack-Matthew nomogram
  - Most poisonings do not result in significant hepatic necrosis
  - Rumack-Matthew nomogram **f2.19** may be used to predict risk
  - Approximate time of ingestion must be known; initial blood sample is drawn ≥4 hours after ingestion
  - Stratifies patients into probable hepatic toxicity, possible hepatic toxicity, and no hepatic toxicity
  - In healthy individuals, any dose over ~150 mg/kg is potentially toxic
  - Most acetaminophen is conjugated with glucuronide or sulfate to form nontoxic metabolites; some is metabolized by the P450 system into the toxic metabolite N-acetyl-P-benzoquinone imine (NAPQI) which induces centrilobular (zone 3) hepatic necrosis
  - Treatment: N-acetylcysteine

2.13.7 Cyanide poisoning

- Sources: Inhalation of smoke from a fire (burning insulation), exposure to pesticides and other industrial materials, accidental or intentional ingestion
- Inhibits cytochrome a3, thus uncoupling the electron transport system; results in diminished oxygen-dependent metabolism & severe anion gap metabolic (lactic) acidosis; oxygen accumulates in the blood, giving rise to the typical bright cherry red skin color
- Hydrogen cyanide gas imparts a bitter almond odor (only ~50% of people are capable of detecting this odor)
- Laboratory testing
  - Nonspecific tests: Lactate, blood gases, anion gap. Normal lactate essentially excludes the diagnosis. Poisoned patients usually have elevated serum glucose. Arteriovenous oxygen gap is decreased
  - Specific tests: Not usually available; cyanide is rapidly metabolized to thiocyanate, which is a better analyte if testing is available
  - Treatment: Sodium nitrite and amyl nitrite (formation of methemoglobin, which binds available cyanide) and sodium thiosulfate (enhances the conversion of cyanide to thiocyanate)

2.13.8 Salicylate (aspirin)

- Affects acid-base balance
- First directly stimulates the respiratory center within the medulla, promoting respiratory alkalosis (3-8 hours after ingestion)
- Second, there is physiologic compensation with metabolic acidosis
- Third, it uncouples oxidative phosphorylation and inhibits the Krebs cycle, leading to anaerobic metabolism with the development of a metabolic acidosis
- Fourth, CNS depression may result in respiratory acidosis
- Mortality is best correlated with the 6-hour plasma salicylate concentration, with values of >130 mg/dL having a high fatality rate

2.13.9 Arsenic

- Sources: Intentional poisoning through ingestion, accidental poisoning through exposure to pesticides, wood preservatives, leather tanning, contaminated water supplies, or arsine gas in certain industries
- Largely excreted in urine, with some distributed into skin, nails, and hair
- Inhibits oxidative production of ATP
- Initial toxicity is manifested in dividing tissue such as GI mucosa, with nausea, vomiting, bloody diarrhea, and abdominal pain. The marrow is affected, causing cytopenias (with erythrocyte basophilic stippling similar to that seen in lead toxicity). Chronic toxicity results in peripheral neuropathy, nephropathy, skin hyperpigmentation and hyperkeratosis (particularly palms & soles), and transverse Mees lines in the nails
- Samples for the diagnosis of chronic intoxication may include fingernails, hair, or urine; most reliable test is a quantitative 24-hour urinary arsenic excretion; blood arsenic level is highly unreliable

ISBN 978-089189-6616

2.13.10 Tricyclic antidepressants (TCAs)

- Anticholinergic effects (dry mouth, constipation, urinary retention, pupillary dilation, hyperthermia, lethargy, confusion) & cardiac conduction effects (QRS prolongation & ventricular arrhythmias) lead to toxic manifestations

2.13.11 Organophosphates & carbamates

- Source: Insecticides
- Inhibit acetylcholinesterase, leading to cholinergic effects (miosis, or pinpoint pupils), diaphoresis, excess salivation, lacrimation, GI hypermotility, bradycardia, and bronchospasm (muscarinic toxidrome)
- Laboratory testing shows increased erythrocyte or plasma cholinesterase activity

2.13.12 Mercury

- Source: Occupational ("mad hatter's disease"), mainly from inhalation of vapor
- Acute toxicity manifests as respiratory distress and renal failure; chronic toxicity takes the form of acrodynia or erethism
- Acrodynia (Feer syndrome): Autonomic manifestations (sweating, hemodynamic instability) and a desquamative erythematous rash on the palms and soles
- Erethism: Personality changes, irritability, and fine motor disturbances
- Laboratory testing: 24-hour urine collection for elemental mercury; whole blood or hair analysis for organic

2.14 Therapeutic drug testing

2.14.1 Pharmacokinetics

- Half-life
  - Half-life (t½) is the time it takes for the concentration of drug to reach 1/2 of the starting concentration
  - Drug is usually dosed according to its t½; that is, if a drug's half-life is 12 hours, then doses are given every 12 hours
  - Elimination of most agents follows so-called 1st order kinetics, meaning that the rate of loss is exponential, with a graph that is asymptotic to zero
  - The steady state exists when the amount of drug leaving the body equals the amount entering; in most instances, this point is reached after 5 half-lives (ie, after 5 doses given at intervals of 1 half-life each)
  - In the steady state, drug concentration is lowest right before a dose (trough), and highest after (peak)
- Free vs bound
  - A variable fraction of drug is usually bound to protein (such as albumin)
  - The free drug is the therapeutically (and toxicologically) active component
  - Small molecules compete for binding spots, and a 2nd drug may displace the 1st, leading to increased free drug concentrations
- Volume of distribution (Vd)
  - Drug size and solubility influence how widely the drug is distributed in the body
  - Drugs that are hydrophilic remain confined within the vascular space
  - Others are capable of distributing within the vascular and extravascular aqueous (interstitial) spaces, and others (hydrophobic) are primarily sequestered into adipose tissue
  - The volume of distribution is defined as the theoretical volume in which drug is distributed
  - Hydrophilic drugs have low Vd, whereas hydrophobic drugs have high Vd
  - Vd is usually expressed in L/kg of body weight
  - If D is the administered intravenous dose and C is the plasma concentration, then

$$Vd = (D \div C) \div (\text{body weight in kg})$$

2.14.2 Drugs

2.14.2.1 Digoxin

- Monitoring may be indicated when dosing is adjusted, or when changes occur in renal function or a change is made in concomitantly administered medications
- Half-life ~36 hours; samples should be drawn ~8-12 hours after the last dose
- Factors that increase digoxin toxicity: Hypokalemia, hypercalcemia, hypomagnesemia, hypoxia, hypothyroidism, quinidine, and calcium channel blockers
- Endogenous substances that cross-react with digoxin, termed "digoxinlike immunoreactive substances," are found in the blood of some individuals who are not taking digoxin. This finding is particularly common in neonates, pregnant women, and those with liver failure and kidney failure

2.14.2.2 Procainamide

- Cleared predominantly by the liver; metabolized to N-acetylprocainamide (NAPA), which also has pharmacologic activity, and is renally cleared
- Rate of conversion to NAPA depends on genetically determined concentration of hepatic acetyltransferase, which is genetically determined; rate of clearance of NAPA depends on renal function

2.14.2.3 Aminoglycosides (eg, gentamicin)

- Cleared by the kidneys; monitoring is advisable to ensure efficacy and to prevent toxicity
- Toxicity manifested primarily as nephrotoxicity & ototoxicity
- Peaks are considered most useful for assessing efficacy, whereas troughs reflect the likelihood of toxicity

2.14.2.4 Vancomycin

- Only troughs are routinely measured

2.14.2.5 Lithium

- The margin between therapeutic effect and toxicity is narrow for lithium. The therapeutic range is from 0.4-1.2 mmol/L. At levels >1.5 mmol/L, the risk of adverse effects is high
- Several guidelines have been proposed for the routine monitoring of lithium therapy (patients who are stable on therapy), with a range of recommended monitoring intervals of 1-3 months. For routine monitoring, a sample should be measured 12 hours following the last dose
- The half-life of lithium varies from 8-40 hours, depending largely on age and renal function. Thus, following initiation of lithium or a change in dose steady state conditions would be expected in 2-8 days. Checking levels after a period of 3 days to 1 week is recommended

2.14.2.6 Carbamazepine

- The therapeutic range is 4-12 µg/mL, with toxicity occurring at >15 µg/mL
- Because of the long half-life (15-24 hours), trough specimen is usually measured
- If toxicity is suspected, peak specimen is measured (4-8 hours after dose)

2.14.2.7 Ethosuximide

- Therapeutic range is 40-100 µg/mL
- Toxicity is rare

2.15 Vitamins & nutrition

2.15.1 Biochemical theory & physiology

- Properties
  - Fat-soluble vitamins include vitamins A, D, E, and K
  - Water-soluble vitamins include the B vitamins (B_{12}/folate) and vitamin C
  - Trace minerals are elemental metals found in low concentration in plasma and include chromium, copper, manganese, molybdenum, selenium, and zinc and require carrier proteins for transport. APRs may be analyzed simultaneously to assess negative effect on trace mineral circulating level
- Metabolism and action of vitamins and trace minerals are often as antioxidants, cofactors (minerals), or coenzymes (water-soluble vitamins) to enzymes. Fat-soluble vitamins have diverse action including as a precursor. See **t2.29** for action of vitamins and minerals

t2.29 Role of vitamins & minerals

A	Vision, reproduction & growth
D	Calcium metabolism for bone & teeth; many other organs
K	Blood clotting factors; osteocalcins
B_{12}	Metabolism of amino acids & keto acids
Folic acid	Amino acid & nucleic acid synthesis
Niacin	Oxidation-reduction actions
Copper	Antioxidant; formation of collagen, chitin & structural proteins
Selenium	Assists vitamin E; cofactor to enzymes
Zinc	Cell division & growth as metalloenzyme

- Normal states of intracellular enzyme activity, affecting metabolism and gene expression and regulation are maintained with optional levels of vitamins and minerals. Abnormal states including free radical damage to DNA and cell membranes, fatigue, lack of stamina, poor immune and cognitive function arise with depletion of vitamins and minerals

2.15.2 Test procedures

- Principles of analysis
  - Vitamins are measured by competitive protein binding immunoassays, fluorometric and HPLC methods. Vitamin K is more commonly assessed indirectly through prothrombin time/international normalized ratio (INR). Trace metals are measured by inductively coupled plasma mass spectrometry (ICP-MS) or optical emission spectrometry **t2.30**

t2.30 Assay method of vitamins & minerals

A	HPLC, immunoassay
D	HPLC/MS/MS
K	HPLC
B_{12}	CPB immunoassay
Folic acid	CPB immunoassay
Niacin	HPLC, fluorometric
Copper	ICP-MS
Selenium	ICP-MS, AAS
Zinc	ICP-MS, ICP-OES, AAS

AAS, atomic absorption spectroscopy; CPB, competitive protein binding; HPLC, high-pressure liquid chromatography; ICP, inductively coupled plasma; MS, mass spectrometry; OES, optical emission spectrometry

ISBN 978-089189-6616

- Special precautions, specimen collection and processing, troubleshooting, and interfering substances
  - Vitamins may be measured in serum, and in the case of vitamins A and K, may also be measured in heparinized or EDTA plasma. Vitamin A and niacin are light sensitive; plasma should be separated within 1 hour after collection and kept refrigerated or frozen until analyzed
  - Trace metals may be analyzed in a variety of body fluids, hair, or nail samples. Urine is the preferred specimen for selenium. Blood specimen must be collected in acid-washed, trace metal-free containers and may require silanized needles, must be refrigerated and analyzed within a few days. Long-term storage causes analytical errors
- Test result interpretation compared to reference ranges
  - Vitamin reference levels are age adjusted. Plasma levels of vitamin A levels provide only an estimate of clinical status because hepatic storage plays a major influence
- Disease state correlation **t2.31**

t2.31 Deficiencies of vitamins & trace minerals

A	Nyctalopia, xeropthalmia
D	Rickets, osteomalacia
K	Hemorrhagic disease, prolonged clotting time
B12	Pernicious anemia & megaloblastic anemia
Folic Acid	Megaloblastic anemia
Niacin	Pellagra
Copper	Anemia, neuropathy & cardiac damage
Selenium	Cardiomyopathy & arthritis
Zinc	Depressed growth & immune function

2.16 Measurement techniques

2.16.1 Spectrophotometry

- Principle
  - Routine absorption photometry is the measurement of light intensity at a specific wavelength as it passes through a solution compared to a reference solution. Absorbance of light is proportional to concentration of the solute in solution

$$A = abc$$

$$C\ unk = A\ unk \times C\ std / A\ std$$

- Components of a spectrophotometer:
  - Light source (tungsten or mercury vapor lamp or LASER)
  - Monochromator (filters, prism or diffraction grating) with entrance & exit slits
  - Cuvet
  - Photodetector
  - Readout device/meter
- Wavelength calibration, photodetector linearity, and elimination of stray light are important quality assurance factors
- Reflectance photometry is similar to routine spectrophotometry but light intensity is measured that is reflected from a solid surface such as in dry-film chemistry
- Nephelometry is the measurement of scattered light at a specific wavelength as it passes through a turbid solution compared to a reference solution. The light measured is not in a direct path from the incidence or transmitted light
  - Forward scatter
  - Right-angle scatter
- Fluorometry is the measurement of light by atoms or molecules in solution that, when excited by short wavelength high-energy light, emit longer-wavelength lower-energy light
  - Components
    - Light source is often mercury arc or xenon lamp
    - Two monochromators: Excitation monochromator and emission monochromator at a right angle to the light source
  - Types
    - Spectrofluorometry
    - Fluorescence polarization
- Atomic absorption spectrophotometry is the measurement of light of a specific wavelength produced when an element is returning from an excited state to an unexcited state
  - Components
    - Excitation source is usually a hollow cathode lamp composed of the same element to be measured
    - Sample is atomized into a low-energy flame that is used to dissociate the molecules into atoms
    - Reference method, for mineral analysis

2.16.2 Kinetic measurement

- Enzyme activity is the measure of the chemical reaction rate as substrate is consumed and product is formed in µmole of substrate per minute/L
- Often a coenzyme is measured at 340 nm to minimize interference from other substances which may absorb at higher wavelengths
  - NADP to NADPH
  - NAD to NADH

2.16.3 Electrophoresis

- Principle
  - Separation technique in which ionized molecules in a buffer solution migrate often to a specific zone, based on their isoelectric point on a support medium within an electrical field created between an anode & cathode
  - Zones of separated molecules can be stained, media cleared, and quantified using densitometry
- Routine zone electrophoresis
  - Cellulose acetate
  - Agarose gel
  - Polyacrylamide gel
- Isoelectric focusing electrophoresis has higher resolution than routine zone electrophoresis because higher voltages are used; the medium has carrier ampholytes which allow for stable narrow pH gradients to occur

2.16.4 Immunoassays (see chapter 8 Immunology)

- Principle
  - Immunochemical methods are qualitative (such as western blotting) or more commonly quantitative methods that use antibody-antigen reactions to detect the analyte of interest
  - Analyte may be antigen/hapten or antibody. Homogeneous immunoassays do not require a separation step of free versus antibody-bound labeled antigen or antibody and are usually noncompetitive assays
- Nonlabeled assays
  - Turbidimetric use spectrophotometry to measure the change in light intensity caused by large particles forming from Ag-Ab complexes
  - Nephelometric measure forward or right-angle scatter of light resulting from complexes are formed as antibody binds antigen
- Labeled assays include the use of radioisotopic, fluorometric, enzyme-mediated & chemiluminescent labels
  - Competitive assays have labeled antigen and unlabeled patient antigen/hapten competing for limited amount of antibody causing an inverse relationship between the concentration of antibody-bound labeled antigen and patient unlabeled antigen. This is a very sensitive method
  - Radioimmunoassay
  - Chemiluminescent immunoassay
  - Noncompetitive/sandwich techniques
  - Enzyme-linked immunosorbent assay
  - Enzyme-multiplied immunoassay technique
  - Cloned enzyme donor
  - Fluorescent polarization
  - Electrochemiluminescence

2.16.5 Electrochemistry

- Potentiometry is the measurement of change in electrical potential between 2 half-cell electrodes connected with an electrolyte solution and often with a selective membrane, known as ion selective electrodes. Useful in measuring electrolyte activity
  - Glass membrane electrodes with unique composition measure pH, Na, and PCO_2 with Ag/AgCl reference electrodes
    - PCO_2 is measured with a polymeric membrane selective for CO_2 gas that diffuses into weak bicarbonate solution and produces H+ which are detected by a pH electrode and Ag/Ag/Cl reference electrode both in contact with the buffer solution
  - Polymer membrane electrodes may facilitate charged, dissociated ion exchange (aka liquid membrane ion selective electrode [ISE]), charged with a carrier or neutral ion carrier (such as valinomycin in PVC membrane for K^+)
- Amperometry/voltammetry
  - Current is measured because of ionic activity when external voltage is applied to a polarizable working electrode vs a reference electrode. Oxidation or reduction occurs at the polarized working electrode because of ionic activity
    - PO_2 is measured as oxygen diffuses through a polymeric membrane to an internal electrolyte solution and is reduced at the platinum cathode vs the Ag/AgCl reference electrode
    - Electrochemical detection on high pressure liquid chromatography (HPLC) such as for homocysteine measurement
- Coulometry measures electrical charge passing between 2 half-cell electrodes with oxidation and reduction occurring at the electrodes. Chloride can be measured using coulometric titration with silver ions

2.16.6 Blood gas analyzer

- Components
  - pH, PCO_2, and PO_2 electrodes
  - May include co-oximetry to measure oxygen saturation using spectrophotometry to measure different forms of hemoglobin including oxyhemoglobin
  - Several calculations are also made including HCO_3^-/total CO_2 with the Henderson-Hasselbalch equation

ISBN 978-089189-6616

2.16.7 Chromatography

- This is a technique in which diverse solutes separate based on their different solubility in a stationary phase vs a mobile phase. A detector is used to qualitatively identify and quantify each solute
- Planar chromatography takes place on a flat surface with Rf (ratio of solute migration to solvent migration in centimeters)
  - Paper is used in the stationary phase and liquid mobile phase. Detection is by measuring distance migrated
- Thin-layer chromatography has a solid surface bound to a plastic or glass plate. Detection is often quantified with densitometry in addition to identification by Rf
- Column chromatography takes place with beads packed into a column and a liquid or gas mobile phase
  - HPLC uses small-diameter beads packed with liquid pumped at high pressure. Detection is based on retention time in the column using spectrofluorometry, electrochemical or mass spectrometry
    - Normal phase uses a nonpolar liquid mobile phase & polar stationary phase
    - Reverse phase uses a polar liquid mobile phase & nonpolar stationary phase
- Gas chromatography uses a nitrogen or helium carrier gas mobile phase and coated particles in the column as the stationary phase. Samples are heated in an oven to vaporize the solutes. Detection is based on retention time in the column or mass spectrometry
- Ion exchange uses charged stationary and opposite charged mobile phases to enhance separation of ionized solutes and is commonly used for separation of hemoglobin variants or glycated hemoglobin quantification

2.17 Quality assurance/total quality management (TQM) (see chapter 7 Laboratory Operations)

- Quality assurance is part of TQM's quality control of processes and outcomes, quality leadership and continuous quality improvement with a focus on customer service, management commitment, training, process control, and measurement of quality improvement
- TQM requirements
  - Requirements include quality planning, quality laboratory processes, quality control, quality assessment, and quality improvement
    - Quality manual, approved policies, and standard operating procedures
    - Quality control includes statistical control procedures, linearity checks, reagent and standard checks, instrument/analyzer function checks & temperature checks
    - Quality assessment monitors laboratory processes through turnaround time, specimen identification, patient identification & test utility
- Method validation for precision & accuracy
  - Daily monitoring of preanalytical, analytical & postanalytical quality
- Categorization of Clinical Laboratory Improvement Amendments (CLIA) testing complexity
  - Waived
  - Nonwaived moderate complexity
  - Nonwaived high complexity
- Quality control
  - Three major roles:
    - Management elements, including controls, control rules to monitor for changes in precision and accuracy, shift and trend, compared to control intervals, work process control, internal audit, and job management
    - Personnel technical competence, skills, experience & qualifications
    - Personnel professional behaviors & organizational culture

2.18 Selected readings

Bishop M. *Clinical Chemistry: Principles, Techniques, Correlations*. 8th ed. Jones & Bartlett Learning. 2017. ISBN 978-1496335586

Campbell J, Campbell J. *Laboratory Mathematics: Medical and Biological Applications*. 5th ed. Mosby. 1997. ISBN 978-0815113973

Doucette LJ. *Mathematics for the Clinical Laboratory*. 4th Edition. Saunders. 2020. ISBN 978-0323554824

Larson D. *Clinical Chemistry: Fundamentals and Laboratory Techniques*. Saunders. 2016. ISBN 978-1455742141

McPherson RA, McPherson RI, Matthew RP. *Henry's Clinical Diagnosis and Management by Laboratory Methods*. 23rd ed. Elsevier. 2016. ISBN 978-0323295680

Rifai N, Horvath AR, Wittwer CT. *Tietz Fundamentals of Clinical Chemistry and Molecular Diagnostics*. 8th Edition. Saunders. 2018. ISBN 978-0323350446

Rifai N. Tietz *Textbook of Clinical Chemistry and Molecular Diagnostics*. 6th ed. Saunders. 2017. ISBN 978-0323359214

Chapter 3

Body Fluids

ISBN 978-089189-6616

3.1 Urine

- See Chemistry 2.7.1 for an overview of renal anatomy and 2.7.2 for discussion of the synthesis and composition of urine

3.1.1 Specimen collection & handling

3.1.1.1 Handling & preservation

- Examine within 1 hour if kept at room temperature
- Refrigerate if longer delay expected; must be examined within 2-4 hours
- Aseptic technique is used when sample is shared with the microbiology laboratory

3.1.1.2 Methods of specimen collection

- The midstream or clean-catch method is used when a urinary tract infection is suspected as it minimizes bacterial contamination from the skin and genital region; patients self-collect after receiving instructions on how to cleanse and collect the mid-portion of the void
- A random or non-clean catch method may be used if bacteriological testing is not anticipated; patients self-collect with no special instruction or preparation
- A pediatric collection bag may be used for infants and small children; care-giver applies the bag over the genital region after cleansing the area
- A catheter may be used for patients that cannot void on their own; a healthcare professional inserts a thin, flexible tube up through the urethra and into the bladder, allowing urine to flow through it into a collection bag
- Suprapubic aspiration may be used for patients with a urinary obstruction or to obtain a sterile sample from infants or small children; a clinician inserts a needle into the bladder and aspirates urine into a sterile syringe

3.1.1.3 Time of collection

- A random or routine collection is performed when timing is not important
- A first morning collection is performed to obtain a concentrated sample; patient collects their first void after waking
- A timed collection is performed to obtain sample during a set time frame (eg, 2 hour or 24 hours); patient collects all voids during the specified time and the total volume is recorded

3.1.2 Physical examination

3.1.2.1 Color & clarity t3.1

- Normal fresh urine is pale-yellow to dark-yellow and clear
- Red/red brown coloration may indicate presence of hemoglobin, blood (fresh/old), methemoglobin, myoglobin, porphyrins, rifampin, L-dopa or beets
- Amber or brown coloration may indicate presence of bilirubin
- Green or blue-green coloration may indicate presence of biliverdin, medications containing a dye or infection with *Pseudomonas*
- Bright orange coloration may indicate presence of pyridium
- Dark-brown or black coloration may indicate presence of homogentisic acid (alkaptonuria) or melanin
- Cloudy and turbid specimens contain formed and cellular elements (eg, crystals, bacteria, cells)

t3.1 Macroscopic analysis of urine

Color	Possible pathologic etiologies
Colorless	Diabetes insipidus
Hazy	Casts, crystals, microorganisms, cells
White	Pyuria, lipids, chyle
Amber	Bilirubin and its metabolic derivatives
Pink-red	Hemoglobin, RBCs, myoglobin, porphyrins, beeturia (not a pathologic cause)
Red/red brown	Methemoglobin, myoglobin, porphyrins

3.1.2.2 Odor

- Normal fresh urine has a mild odor
- Urines containing asparagus metabolites have a sulfur odor
- A musty or mousy smell is associated with phenylketonuria (PKU) and some liver diseases
- Old samples and samples associated with a UTI smell of ammonia
- A sweet smell is associated with maple syrup urine disease (MSUD)
- A pungent odor may be associated with the presence of ketones

3.1.3 Chemical examination

3.1.3.1 Dipstick procedure

- Mix urine by inversion
- Moisten strip completely but briefly in urine
- Tap off excess urine and begin timing
- Compare the color of each test pad with the color blocks on the dipstick container at the specified times
- Record results
  - Most reactions are reported semi-quantitatively as 1+, 2+, 3+, 4+ or trace, small, moderate, large
  - A few are reported as a percent concentration such as mg/dL

3.1.3.2 Specific gravity

- Density of urine compared to density of pure water
  - Correlates with urine osmolality

- Not always correlated with darker color or turbidity
- Methods of analysis
  - Refractometer
    - Indirect measurement based on the refractive index of light
    - Affected by high concentrations of protein, glucose, radiographic contrast dyes
  - Dipstick
    - Color reaction from deep blue-green to yellow-green based on pKa change of polyelectrolytes in relation to solution's ionic concentration
    - Reference interval: 1.003-1.040
    - Not affected by presence of radiographic contrast dyes or high concentrations of protein or glucose

3.1.3.3 pH

- Dipstick reaction based on color change from orange (acid) to blue (alkaline) due to double indicator system
- Reference interval: 4.8-7.5
- Urine becomes more alkaline upon standing because of bacteria that produce urease
- Urinary pH affected by acid-base disorders
- Fixed urine pH >6.5 may indicate renal disorders such as renal tubular acidosis (see Chemistry 2.7.5.2.2)

3.1.3.4 Glucose

- Dipstick
  - Color reaction generally from blue to green to brown based on a double sequential enzyme reaction
  - Manufacturers may vary in dye used and color may turn from pale yellow to darker green
  - Specific for glucose
  - Detects at 100 mg/dL
  - Reference interval: negative
  - False positive due to contamination with peroxide, bleach or other strong oxidizer
  - False negative due to presence of reducing substances such as ascorbic acid and salicylates
  - Predominate method for screening for glucosuria in pediatric and adult patients
  - Glucosuria does not correlate well with blood glucose <180 mg/dL
- Clinitest tablets
  - Copper reduction test
  - Color change from blue to green to orange due to presence and amount of reducing substances

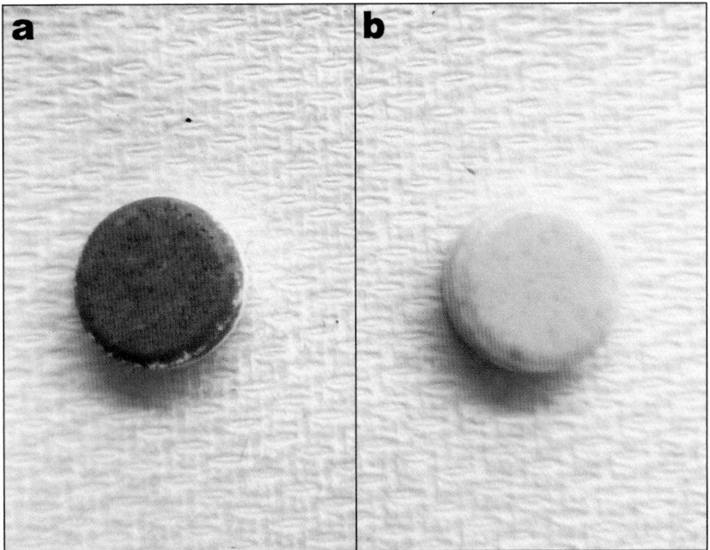

i3.1 Acetest controls: a positive, b negative

  - Specific for reducing substances, eg, galactose, lactose, ascorbic acid, and homogentisic acid
  - Detects at 250 mg/dL
  - Reference interval: negative
  - Historically used as a screening test for inborn errors of metabolism in newborns or small children (eg, galactosemia)

3.1.3.5 Ketones

- Ketone bodies (acetoacetic acid, acetone, and β-hydroxybutyric acid) are by-products of excess acetyl-CoA production in fat catabolism
- Dipstick
  - Purple color of increasing intensity when acetoacetic acid reacts with sodium nitroprusside
  - Specific for acetoacetic acid
  - Detects at 5-10 mg/dL
  - Reference interval: negative
  - False positives occur in highly pigmented urine or in presence of levodopa metabolites or sulfhydryl compounds
- Acetest tablets i3.1
  - Development of lavender to purple color when urinary ketones react with sodium nitroprusside in the tablet
  - Lactose and disodium phosphate in tablet enhance reaction
  - Specific for acetoacetic acid and acetone
  - Detects at approximately 5-10 mg/dL
  - Reference interval: negative

ISBN 978-089189-6616

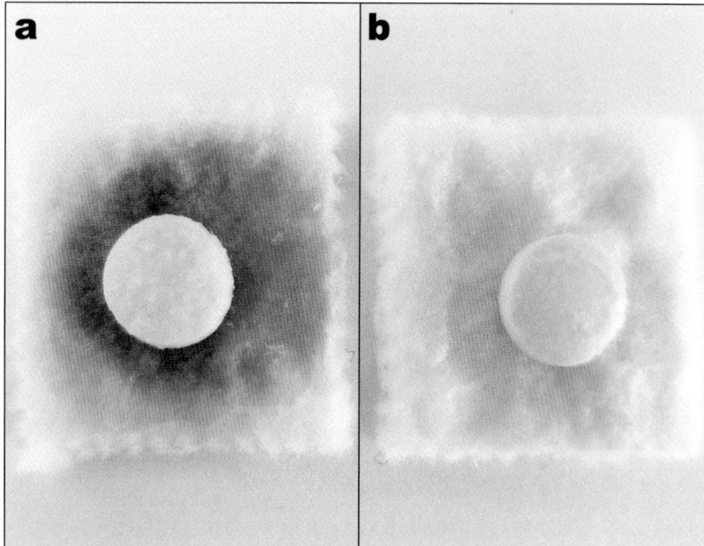

i3.2 Ictotest controls: a positive, b negative

3.1.3.6 Protein

- Dipstick
  - Reaction is based on protein error of indicators using tetrabromophenol blue buffered to pH 3
  - Color changes range from yellow-green to blue-green as more protein is detected
  - More sensitive to albumin than globulins, hemoglobin or mucoproteins
  - Detects albumin at 15-30 mg/dL
  - Reference interval: negative
- Screening for proteinuria due to infections or kidney disease such as nephritis
- Transitory or intermittent benign proteinuria seen after stress or exercise
- Early stages of diabetic nephropathy may not yield a positive reaction; microalbumin test strips available
- Nephrotic syndrome associated with significant proteinuria

3.1.3.7 Occult blood

- Means hidden blood; not obvious by direct observation
- Dipstick
  - Test pad contains a chromagen and a peroxide, which reacts with the pseudoperoxidase activity of the heme moiety to produce a color change
  - Greenish blue color develops in the presence of RBCs, hemoglobin or myoglobin
  - More sensitive to hemoglobin than intact RBCs
  - Detects 5-10 RBCs/μL or hemoglobin at 0.015-0.062 mg/dL
  - Small numbers of RBCs produce a spotted reaction
  - Reference interval: negative
  - False positives due to presence of oxidizing agents (eg, bleach), povidone-iodine, and some bacterial infections
  - False negatives due to presence of ascorbic acid, Captopril, formalin, and high levels of protein and/or nitrites
- Associated with hematuria, hemoglobinuria, myoglobinuria

3.1.3.8 Bilirubin

- By-products of heme catabolism; conjugated form is water-soluble and can be excreted in urine
  - Conjugated forms are water-soluble, found in urine
- Dipstick
  - Color change from tan to purple based on reaction of diazonium salt with bilirubin
  - Specific for conjugated bilirubin; unconjugated bilirubin not present in urine
  - Detects at 0.2-0.4 mg/dL
  - False positives due to presence of indican, chlorpromazine, and pyridine
  - False negatives due to presence of ascorbic acid and exposure to light
  - Bilirubinuria seen in liver disease and conjugated hyperbilirubinemia
- Ictotest tablets i3.2
  - Development of blue or purple color on test mat following reaction of diazo salts and urinary bilirubin
  - More sensitive than dipstick method
  - Used as a confirmatory test for positive dipstick results
  - Reference interval: negative

3.1.3.9 Urobilinogen

- Colorless by-product of conjugated bilirubin hydrolysis by intestinal bacteria
- Dipstick
  - Color change from light pink to red based on reaction of urobilinogen with Ehrlich reagent
  - Detects at 0.2 mg/dL
  - Will not detect the absence of urobilinogen
  - Reference interval: <1.0 mg/dL
  - False positives due to presence of salicylates, pyridine and sulfonamides
  - False negatives due to presence of formalin, high concentration of nitrites, or exposure to light
  - Urobilinogen is increased in liver disease
  - Not detectable in biliary obstruction

3.1.3.10 Nitrites

- Detects presence of nitrate-reducing bacteria in the urine such as *Escherichia coli*
- Dipstick
  - Color change from white to pink based on reaction of nitrite with p-arsanilic acid to form a diazonium product which then reacts with quinoline
  - Detects at 0.06-0.10 mg/dL
  - Reference interval: negative
  - False positives due to presence of pyridine; may also occur if the sample is not tested in a timely fashion or allowed to sit at room temperature
  - False negatives due to high specific gravity, presence of ascorbic acid or high levels of urobilinogen
- Not all bacteria reduce nitrates to nitrite
- Poor correlation between nitrite test and positive cultures on random samples
- Best to use first morning sample since nitrites form after 4 hour incubation in the bladder

3.1.3.11 Leukocyte esterase

- Dipstick
  - Purple color develops as a result of hydrolysis reaction of esters and diazonium salt catalyzed by esterases from granulocytic leukocytes
  - False positives due to presence of strong oxidizing agents (eg, bleach), formalin, vaginal fluid, eosinophils, and *Trichomonas*
  - False negatives due to high specific gravity, presence of ascorbic acid, some antibiotics and high concentrations of protein or glucose
  - Detects esterase from >10 leukocytes/mL
  - Reference interval: negative
- Screening test for WBCs, particularly neutrophils

3.1.4 Microscopic examination

3.1.4.1 General considerations

- The results of the microscopic should correlate with physical and chemical test results
- Contamination is common, especially in voided specimens when no effort is made to obtain a "clean catch" specimen
- Cellular elements tend to lyse in dilute (hypotonic) or alkaline urines
- Reference intervals vary due to variation in methods used to concentrate the sediment by centrifugation (eg, sample volume, speed, time)

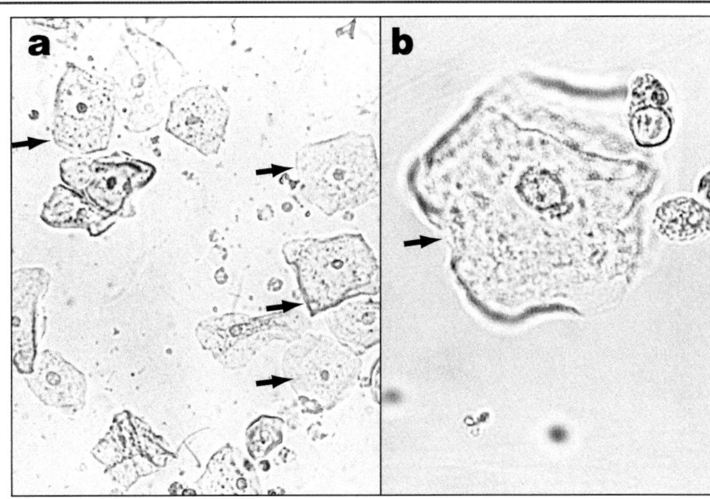

i3.3 Squamous epithelial cells (arrows)

- Unpreserved urine results in cell degradation, bacterial proliferation, glycolysis, pH changes and if exposed to light, decrease in bilirubin and urobilinogen

3.1.4.2 Sediment preparation & examination

- Centrifuge 12 mL of well-mixed urine (1500-2000 rpm) for 5 minutes
- Suction or pour off all but 1 mL of urine
- Resuspend sediment in remaining 1 mL and place 50 µL on a glass slide; add coverslip
- Examine under low power with dimmed light or with phase contrast microscopy for casts and crystals; report as number per low power field (LPF)
- Examine under high dry power for RBCs, WBCs, bacteria, yeast, and epithelial cells; report as number per high power field (HPF)

3.1.4.3 Epithelial cells

3.1.4.3.1 Squamous epithelial cells i3.3

- Large (30-50 µm), flagstone-shaped cells with small central nuclei
- Appear flat with abundant cytoplasm
- Originate from the superficial lining (skin cells) of the urethra and vagina
- Contaminant commonly seen in non-clean catch specimens; significant numbers may be associated with a UTI

ISBN 978-089189-6616

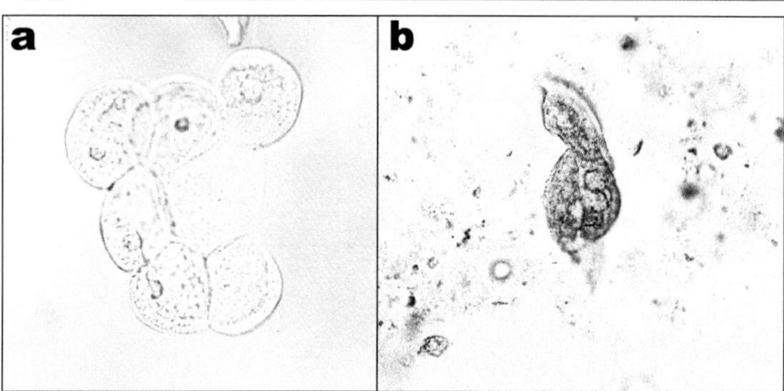

i3.4 a Urothelial cells; b clumped urothelial cells

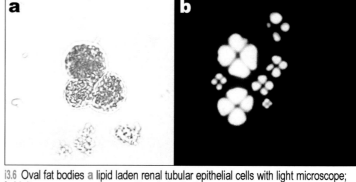

i3.6 Oval fat bodies a lipid laden renal tubular epithelial cells with light microscope; b Maltese cross appearance with polarized microscope

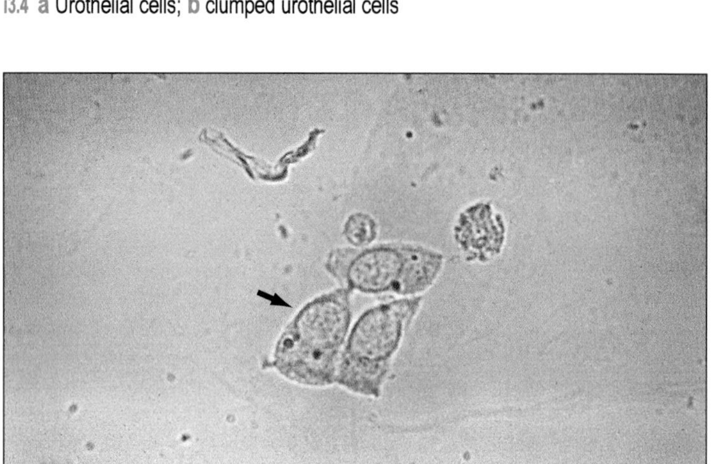

i3.5 Renal tubular epithelial cells (arrow) (brightfield microscopy)

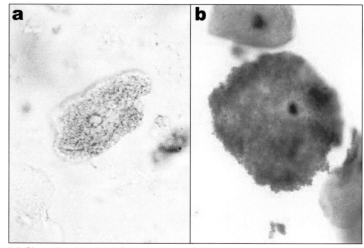

i3.7 Clue cells with a brightfield microscopy, b Papanicolaou stain

3.1.4.3.2 Transitional (urothelial) epithelial cells i3.4

- Medium (20-30 μm), polyhedral-shaped cells with small central nuclei (may be bi-nucleated)
- Appear as having round or pear-shaped contours and moderate cytoplasm; may swell to spheroidal shape
- Originate from transitional epithelial lining of the renal pelvis, ureter, urinary bladder and proximal urethra
- A few are seen in normal urine; elevated amounts may be associated with a UTI and large clumps suggest possible carcinoma

3.1.4.3.3 Renal tubular epithelial cells i3.5

- Small (14-60 μm), oblong or egg-shaped cells with large nuclei may be centric or eccentric
- Appear to have coarsely granular eosinophillic cytoplasm
- Originate from proximal and distal convoluted tubules
- Presence may be associated with acute tubular necrosis, kidney infection, or drug/heavy metal toxicity

3.1.4.3.4 Oval fat bodies i3.6

- Renal tubular cells or WBCs that have absorbed lipids
- Highly refractile and produce a characteristic Maltese cross appearance with polarized light i3.6b
- Extremely significant finding; seen in lipid nephrosis and terminal kidney disease

3.1.4.3.5 Clue cells

- Squamous epithelial cells covered with coccobacilli; most common pathogen is *Gardnerella vaginalis* i3.7
- Associated with bacterial vaginosis

3.1.4.4 Blood cells

3.1.4.4.1 Red blood cells

- Small (6-8 μm), biconcave discs with central pallor i3.8
- May appear swollen in hypertonic urine and crenated in hypertonic urine i3.9
- Empty RBC membranes, referred to as "ghost cells," may be seen from lysed cells in alkaline urine i3.10
- Elements that may be confused with RBCs include oil droplets, crystals (eg, urates), and yeast
  - Correlate with occult blood test pad

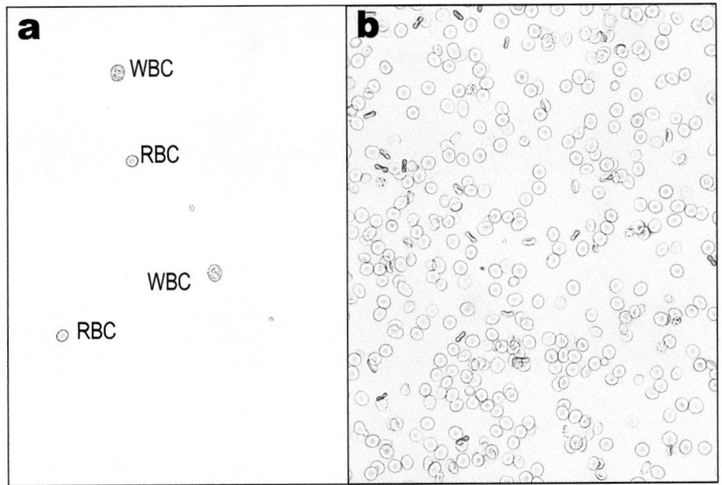

i3.8 a A mixed population of RBCs & WBCs, b Primarily RBCs

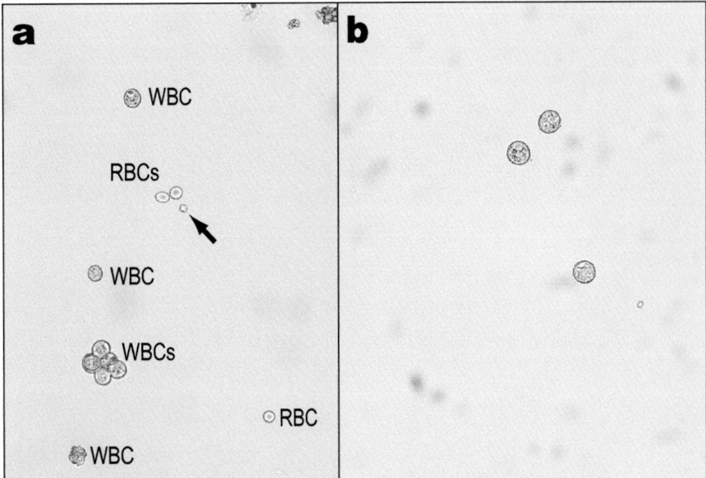

i3.11 a WBCs, RBCs & dihydrate calcium oxalate crystal (arrow); b WBCs

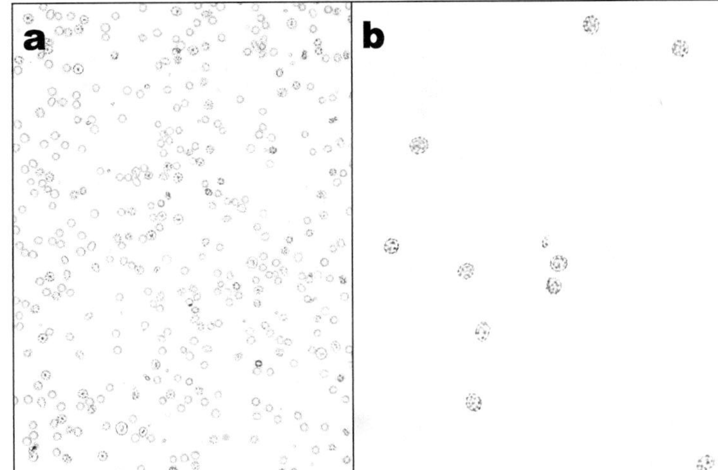

i3.9 a, b Crenated RBCs in hypertonic solution

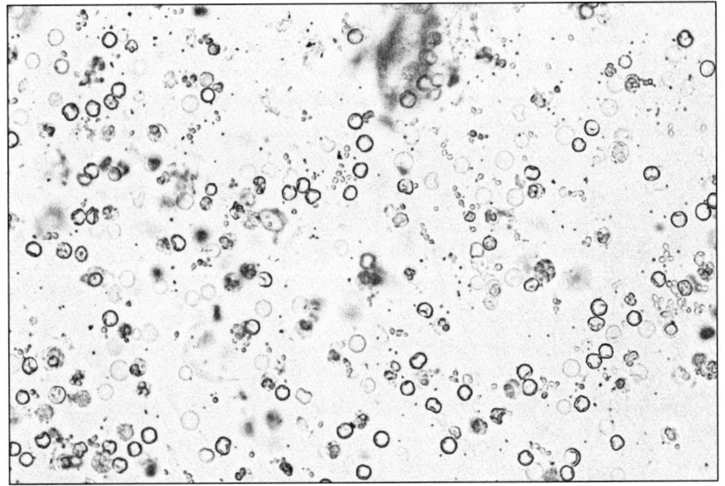
i3.10 Ghost cells

- The addition of glacial acetic acid may assist in differentiation as RBC will lyse
- Reference interval: 0-5 RBCs/HPF
- Increased presence may be associated with:
  - Renal disease such as glomerulonephritis, lupus nephritis, kidney stones, tumors and trauma
  - Lower urinary tract disease such as acute and chronic infection, tumors and strictures
  - Extrarenal disease such as acute appendicitis

3.1.4.4.2 White blood cells i3.11

- Small (10-12 µm), spherical cells; appearance of nuclei, cytoplasm, and granules dependent on type
- May swell in alkaline or hypotonic urine; referred to as "glitter cells" due to Brownian movement of granules in the cytoplasm
- Differentiate from renal tubular epithelial cells which have larger nuclei; correlate with leukocyte esterase
- Reference interval: 0-8 WBCs/HPF
- Increased presence may be associated with lower and upper UTIs or prostatitis

3.1.4.5 Urine casts

- Cylindrical structures primarily composed of uromodulin (Tamm-Horsfall mucoprotein) that form in the lumen of the renal tubules
- When present, albumin and globulins may contribute to cast formation by combining with uromodulin
- Conditions that increase urine cast formation include:
  - Dehydration or increased concentration of the urine
  - Increased acidity of the urine
  - High protein concentration

ISBN 978-089189-6616

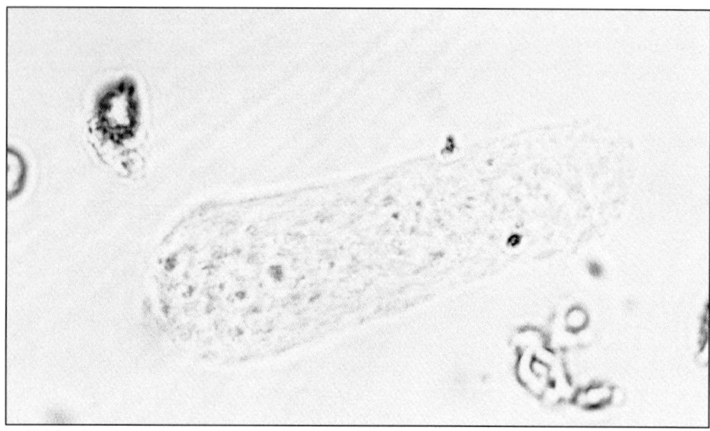

i3.12 Hyaline cast

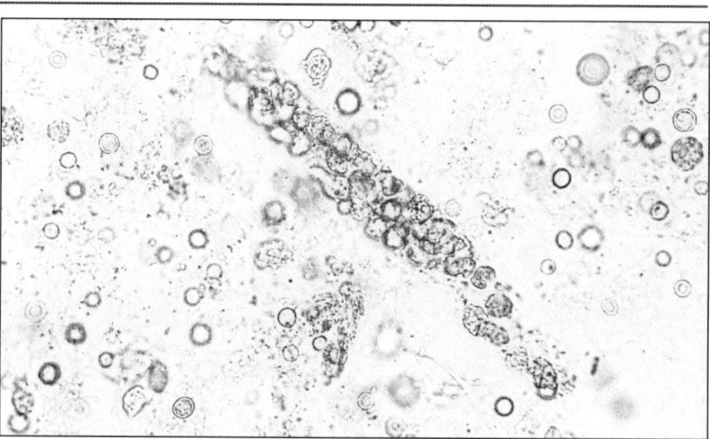

i3.14 White blood cell casts

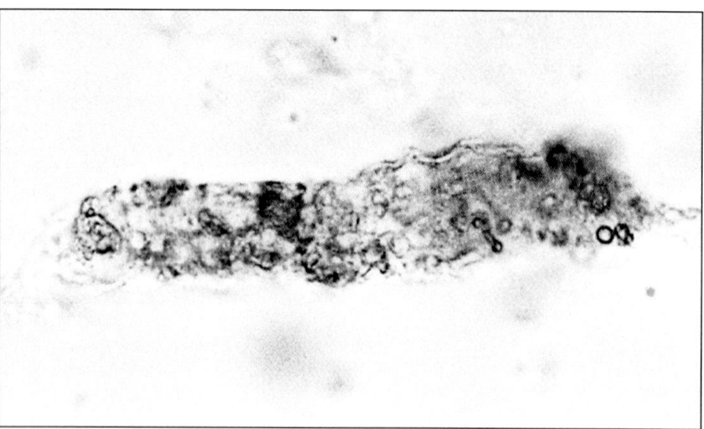

i3.13 Red blood cell cast

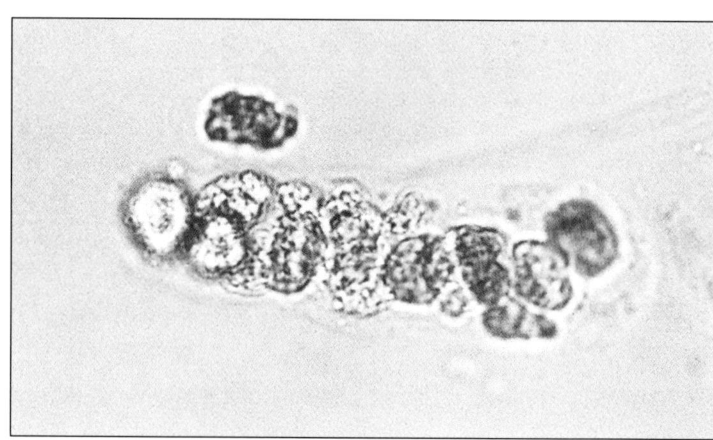

i3.15 Renal tubular epithelial cell cast

- Urinary stasis or obstruction
- Classified by their appearance and presence of inclusions

3.1.4.5.1 Hyaline casts i3.12

- Formed in the lumen of the distal convoluted tubules or collecting ducts; serve as the matrix of all casts
- Appear as pale, smooth cylinders with rounded ends and low refractive index
- Narrow casts form in the convoluted tubules while broad casts form in the collecting ducts
- A few hyaline casts may be present in urine sediment from normal, healthy adults
- Increased numbers may be associated with renal disease

3.1.4.5.2 Red blood cell casts i3.13

- Hyaline cast with RBCs embedded in the matrix; RBCs must be clearly identifiable
- Presence is clinically significant and associated with glomerular disease or damage (eg, acute glomerulonephritis)

3.1.4.5.3 Hemoglobin casts

- RBC cast in which the red cells have ruptured; appears reddish-brown due to acid hematin formation
- Presence is clinically significant and associated with glomerular disease or damage (eg, acute glomerulonephritis)

3.1.4.5.4 White blood cell casts i3.14

- Hyaline cast with WBCs embedded in the matrix
- Presence is clinically significant and associated with renal inflammation or infection (eg, acute pyelonephritis)

3.1.4.5.5 Renal tubular epithelial cell casts i3.15

- Hyaline cast with renal tubular epithelial cells embedded in the matrix
- Form as a result of stasis and necrosis of the tubules

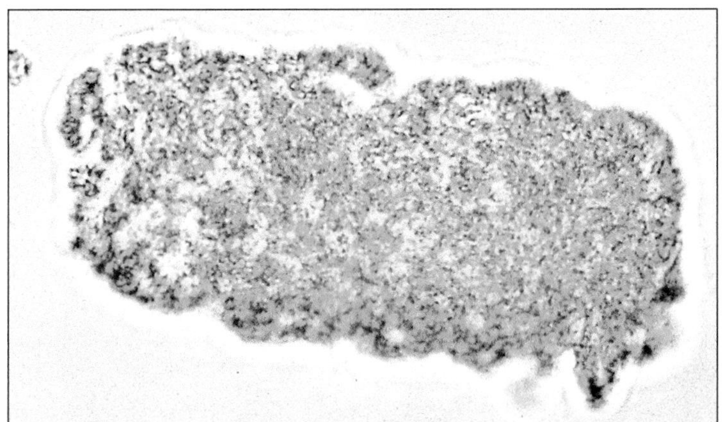

i3.16 Granular cast

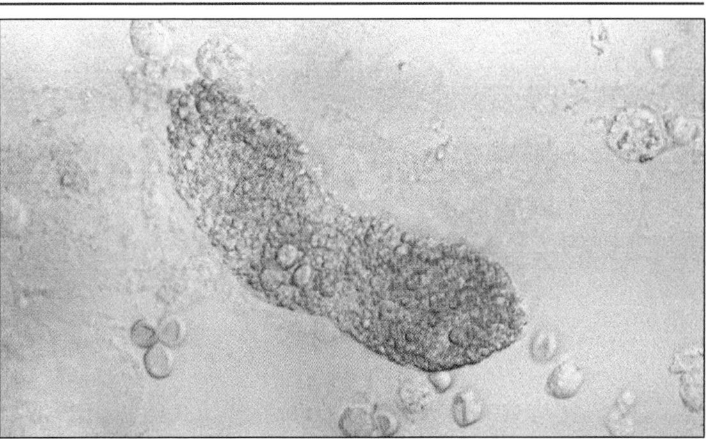

i3.18 Fatty cast

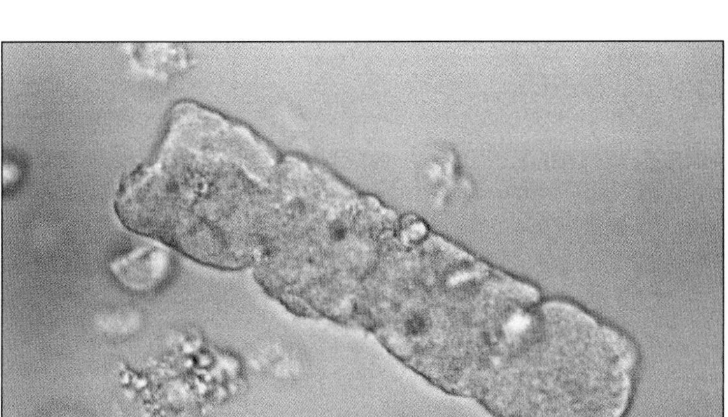

i3.17 Waxy cast

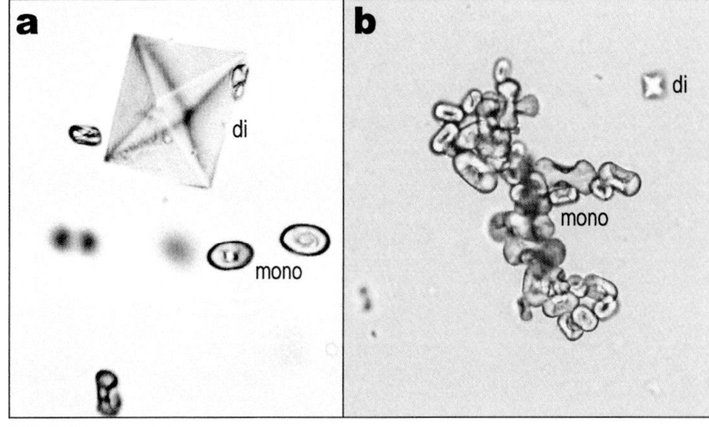

i3.19 Calcium oxalate:
a large octahedral dihydrate crystal (di) with a few smaller monohydrate forms (mono);
b cluster of monohydrate forms (mono) with a single dihydrate crystal (di)

- Presence is clinically significant; seen in severe chronic renal disease, exposure to nephrotoxic agents or viruses and rejection in kidney transplants

3.1.4.5.6 Granular casts i3.16

- Thought to be the result of degeneration of cellular cast components (eg, RBCs, WBCs)
- Progressive cellular deterioration leads to the appearance of coarse granules which transition into fine granules
- Presence is clinically significant and associated with prolonged renal disease

3.1.4.5.7 Waxy casts i3.17

- Appear as smooth, homogenous cylinders with blunt, broken ends and cracked or serrated edges; highly refractive
- Presence is clinically significant and associated with severe chronic renal failure, malignant hypertension, diabetic nephropathy, acute renal disease, and renal transplant rejection

3.1.4.5.8 Fatty casts i3.18

- Casts that have incorporated either free fat droplets or oval fat bodies
- If cholesterol is present, the droplets will demonstrate a "Maltese cross" appearance under polarized light
- Droplets which consist of triglycerides or neutral fat will not polarize light but will stain with Sudan III or Oil Red O

3.1.4.6 Crystals seen in acidic urine

3.1.4.6.1 Calcium oxalate

- Dihydrate form i3.19a
  - Colorless octahedrons that are described as "envelopes" and do not polarize light
  - Predominate in urine from patients with diets rich in oxalic acid; most common cause of kidney stones
- Monohydrate form i3.19b
  - Described as dumbbells or rings
  - Predominate in urine from patients who have ingested ethylene glycol (anti-freeze)

ISBN 978-089189-6616

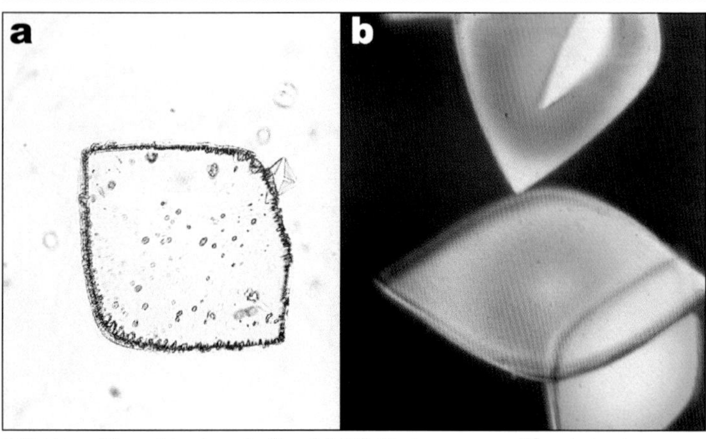

i3.20 Uric acid crystals viewed with a brightfield microscopy and b polarized microscope

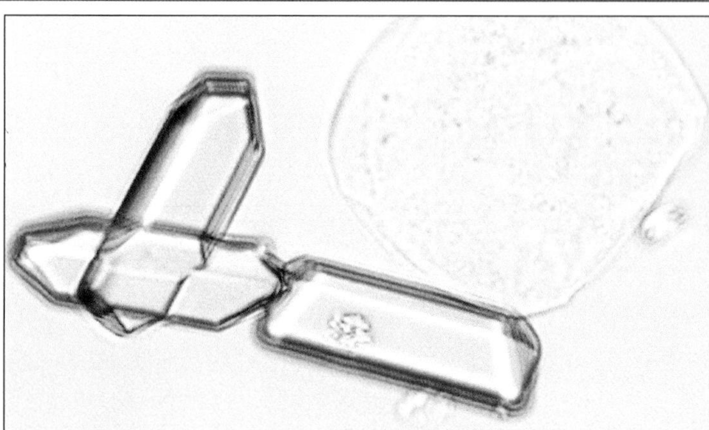
i3.22 Triple phosphate crystals

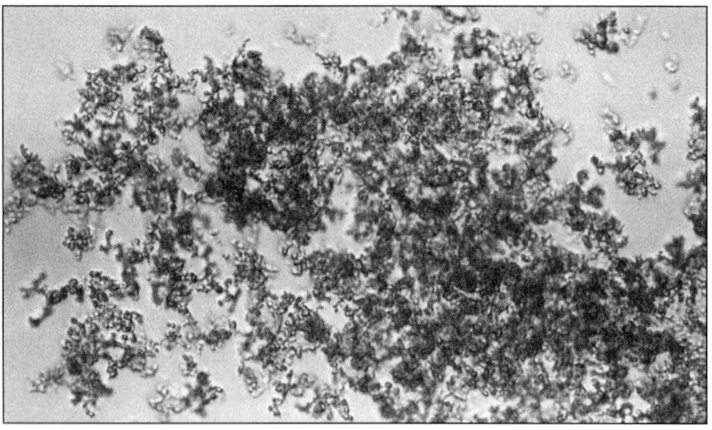
i3.21 Amorphous urate crystals

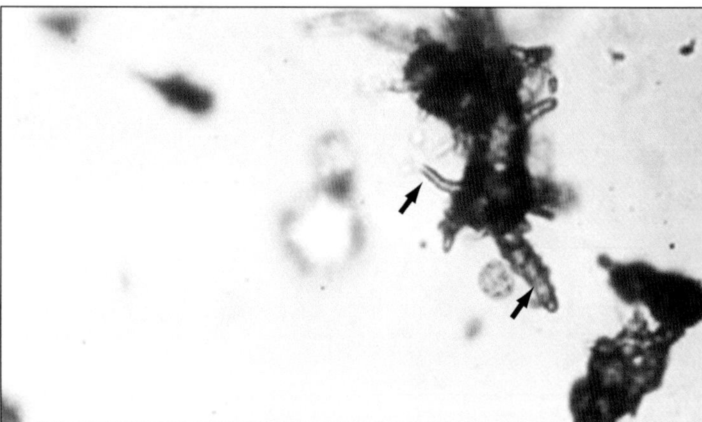
i3.23 Ammonium biurate crystals showing spicules (arrows)

3.1.4.6.2 Uric acid

- Colorless, rhombic plates that also appear as rosettes, wedges, and needles; appear as multicolored under polarized light i3.20
- Presence associated with gout or treatment with chemotherapy

3.1.4.6.3 Amorphous urates

- Brown-yellow granules that resemble sand i3.21
- Presence in urine is considered clinically insignificant and generally associated with old specimens

3.1.4.7 Crystals seen in alkaline urine

3.1.4.7.1 Triple phosphate

- Colorless, prisms that are described as "coffin lids" and demonstrate birefringence under polarized light i3.22
- Presence in urine is considered clinically insignificant

3.1.4.7.2 Ammonium biurate

- Yellow-brown, spicule-covered spheres that are described as "thorny-apples" i3.23
- Presence may be clinically significant if formed in vivo (dehydration)

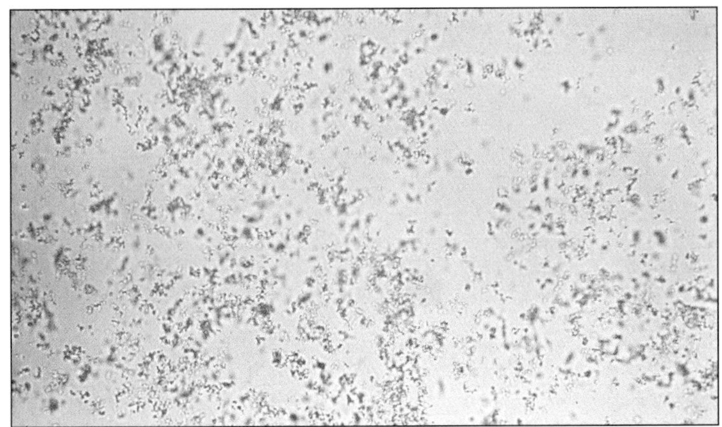

i3.24 Amorphous phosphate crystals

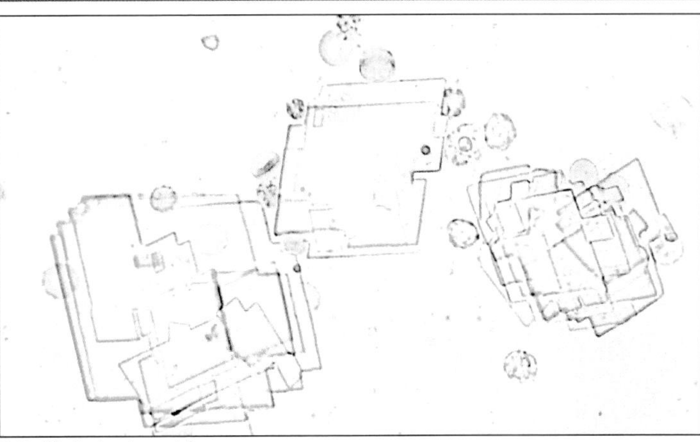

i3.26 Cholesterol crystals

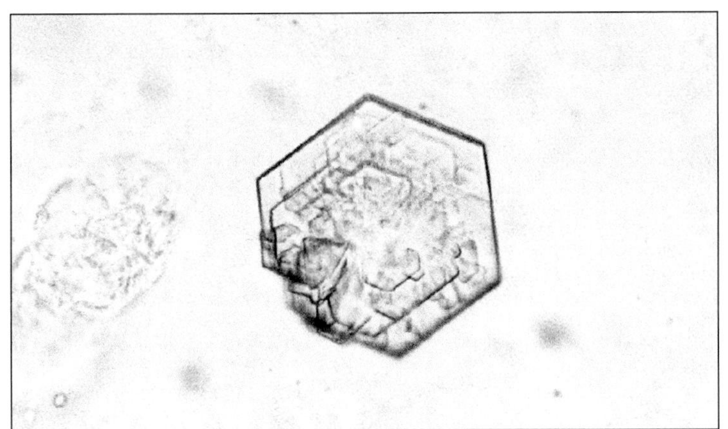

i3.25 Cystine crystal

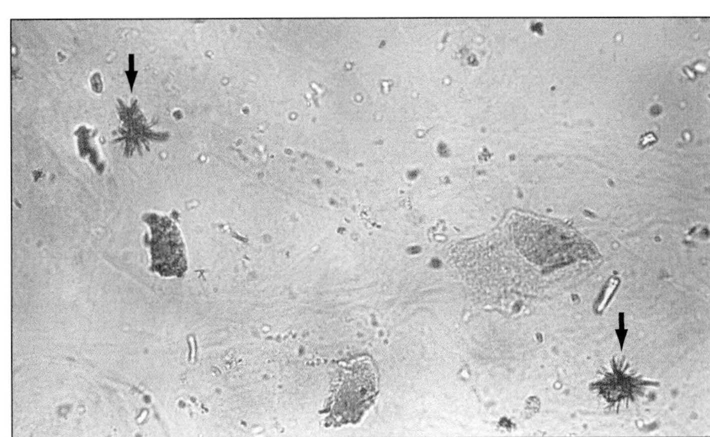

i3.27 Bilirubin crystals (arrows)

3.1.4.7.3 Amorphous phosphates i3.24

- Fine, colorless granules that resemble sand
- Presence in urine is considered clinically insignificant and generally associated with refrigeration

3.1.4.7.4 Cystine

- Colorless, hexagonal plates that do not polarize light; may be layered or laminated i3.25
- Associated with inborn errors of metabolism such as hereditary cystinosis or cystinuria

3.1.4.7.5 Cholesterol

- Colorless, rectangular plates with notched corners that often appear layered; demonstrate weak birefringence i3.26
- Associated with nephritic and nephrotic conditions or lymphatic damage
- Differentiate from radiographic contrast media based on specific gravity

3.1.4.7.6 Bilirubin i3.27

- Most commonly appear as small clusters of fine, yellow-brown needles, but may also form granules
- Associated with hepatic disorders

ISBN 978-089189-6616

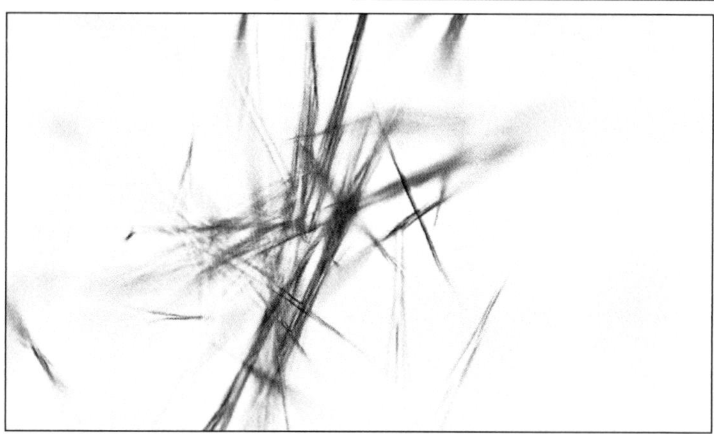

i3.28 Tyrosine crystals

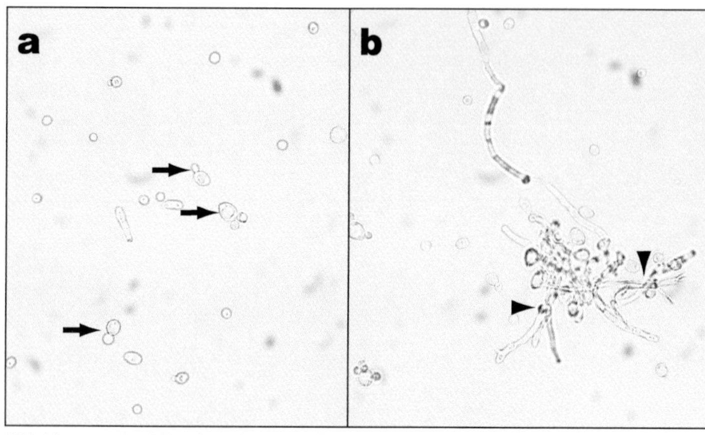

i3.30 Yeast: a budding form (arrows), b branching form (arrowheads)

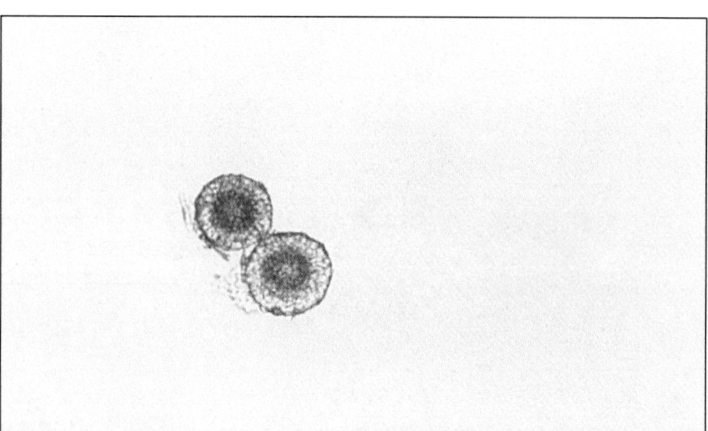

i3.29 Leucine crystals

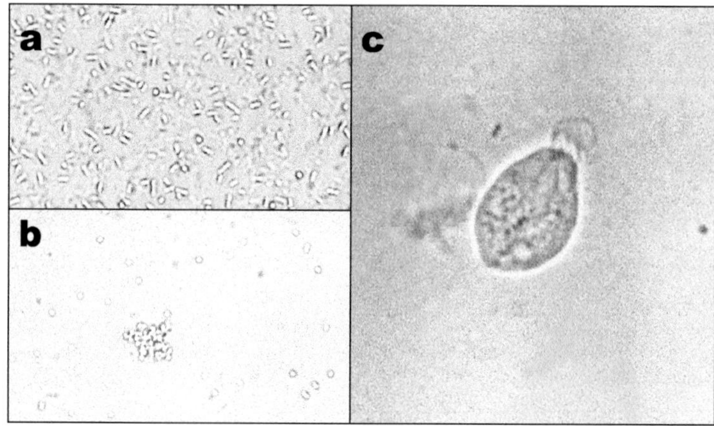

i3.31 Infectious agents: a rods, b cocci, c *Trichomonas*

3.1.4.7.7 Tyrosine

- Colorless, fine needles that often appear in clusters or sheaves i3.28
- Associated with inborn errors of metabolism such as tyrosinemia and in certain liver disorders in which amino acid metabolism is impaired

3.1.4.7.8 Leucine i3.29

- Yellow-brown spheres with concentric circles that are birefringent under polarized microscopy
- Presence is associated with inborn errors of metabolism such as maple syrup urine disease

3.1.4.8 Other urinary elements

3.1.4.8.1 Yeast

- Colorless, ovoid cells that may show budding i3.30a or development of pseudohyphae i3.30b; refractile when viewed with brightfield microscopy
- May be confused with RBCs; correlate with occult blood test pad result and look for budding
- Presence may indicate a UTI, but is most commonly the result of contamination with vaginal secretions

3.1.4.8.2 Bacteria

- Rod-shaped bacilli are most frequently observed (eg, *E coli*) i3.31a, but cocci may also be encountered (eg, *Staphylococcus* spp) i3.31b
- Bacteria are reported semi-quantitatively (1+, 2+, 3+, 4+); the presence of >100,000 organisms/mL indicates significant bacteriuria
- Bacteria may be present due to a UTI or contamination during collection; correlate with the nitrite test pad result

3.1.4.8.3 *Trichomonas*

- Colorless, turnip-shaped flagellates with 4 anterior flagella, a posterior axostyle, and an undulating membrane i3.31c
- May be confused with WBCs or RTEs; compare with leukocyte esterase and look for undulating membrane movement

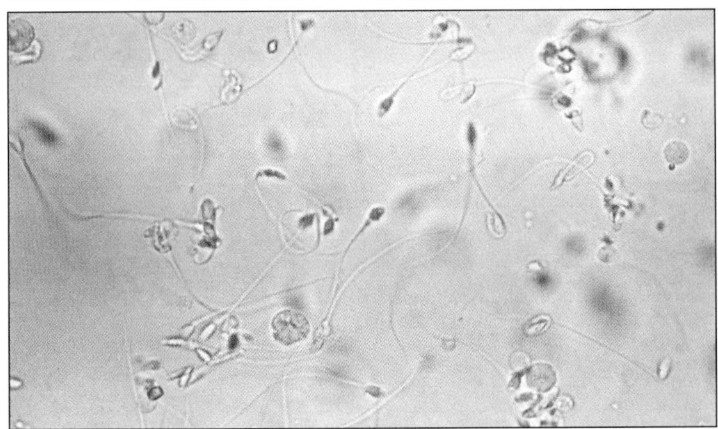

i3.32 Spermatozoa

- Presence indicates contamination with vaginal fluid but is still considered clinically significant

3.1.4.8.4 Sperm

- Male reproductive cells with oval heads and long, thin tails i3.32
- Presence in urine is considered clinically insignificant unless patient is considered part of a vulnerable population (eg, pediatric, geriatric)

3.1.5 Clinical significance

- See Chemistry 2.7.5 for discussion of renal diseases and 2.5.2 for aminoacidopathies

3.1.5.1 Diabetes insipidus (DI)

- Due to lack of antidiuretic hormone (ADH) (neurogenic/central DI) or decreased renal response to ADH (nephrogenic DI) (see Chemistry 2.9.3.1.2 and 2.12.4)
- Characterized by polyuria, polydipsia, pale-yellow urine, and a low (fixed) specific gravity

3.1.5.2 Diabetes mellitus (DM)

- Due to lack of insulin or poor response to insulin (see Chemistry 2.1.5)
- Characterized by hyperglycemia, polyuria, polydipsia, pale-yellow urine, glucosuria, and high specific gravity; proteinuria may occur as renal disease progesses

3.1.5.3 Renal glycosuria

- Characterized by glucosuria despite a normal or decreased fasting blood glucose concentration
- Due to poor renal tubular reabsorption of glucose

3.1.5.4 Galactosemia

- Due to inability to metabolize galactose (see Chemistry 2.1.7.3)
- Characterized by positive Clinitest t3.2

t3.2 Urine glucose screening scenarios

Reducing substance	Clinitest	Dipstick
Reducing substance present, not glucose, eg, galactose	+	–
Glucose in urine and/or another reducing substance in addition to glucose	+	+
Glucose in urine below sensitivity of Clinitest	–	+

3.1.5.5 Jaundice

- Due to increased heme catabolism (eg, hemolytic anemia, transfusion reaction), impaired liver function (eg, acute hepatitis), or hepatobiliary obstruction (eg, gallstones or tumor) (see Chemistry 2.4)
- Characterized by increased concentrations of bilirubin (unconjugated or conjugated) and/or urobilinogen; bilirubin crystals may be present t3.3
- Differential diagnosis of jaundice is presented in t3.3

t3.3 Differential diagnosis of jaundice

Condition	Urine bilirubin	Urobilinogen
Hemolytic disease	Negative	Positive 3+
Liver damage	Negative or 1+	Positive 2+
Obstructive jaundice	Positive 3+	Negative

3.1.5.6 Urinary tract infections (UTIs)

- Result of infection of the urethra (urethritis), bladder (cystitis), or kidney (pyelonephritis); most common pathogen is *Escherichia coli*
- Characterized by frequent, painful urination (dysuria); fever and flank pain associated with a kidney infection
- Chemical examination may be positive for occult blood, nitrites, and leukocyte esterase
- Microscopic examination may reveal presence of RBCs, WBCs, and bacteria; epithelial cells may also be present

ISBN 978-089189-6616

3.2 Amniotic fluid

3.2.1 Synthesis & composition

- Produced early in gestation by the amnion and placenta and is a dialysate of fetal and maternal plasma
- As the fetus develops, composition is primarily determined by fetal swallowing and intestinal absorption, capillary exchange in the fetal lungs, and fetal urination

3.2.2 Function

- Cushions the fetus throughout pregnancy while still allowing fetal movement
- Facilitates transport of nutrients and waste products between the fetus and maternal plasma

3.2.3 Volume

- In early pregnancy (12 weeks), the total volume is 25-50 mL, rising to 800-1,200 mL by 37 weeks and is replenished every 2-3 hours
- Oligohydramnios, characterized by abnormally low volumes of amniotic fluid (<800 mL), is associated with congenital malformations and intrauterine infection
- Polyhydramnios, characterized by abnormally high volumes of amniotic fluid (>1,200 mL), is associated with congenital malformations and decreased fetal swallowing

3.2.4 Specimen collection & handling

3.2.4.1 Amniocentesis

- Sample obtained transabdominally by passing a needle through the mother's abdomen, through the uterine wall, and into the amniotic sac

3.2.4.2 Transport & storage requirements

- Protect from light during transport to prevent photo-oxidation of bilirubin
- Maintain specimens for cell culture, genetic studies, and microbial or viral culture at body temperature (37°C) or room temperature (20°C-25°C)
- Assay specimens for fetal lung maturity (FLM) testing immediately or store refrigerated (2°C-5°C)

3.2.5 Physical examination

3.2.5.1 Color

- Normally appears colorless, pale yellow, or yellow
- A dark yellow or amber color may indicate an increased bilirubin concentration
- A green color suggests fetal distress and the passage of meconium in utero
    - Meconium is a mucus-like substance that forms in the fetal intestinal tract from swallowed amniotic fluid and intestinal secretions
    - Normally excreted as the infant's first bowel movement after delivery
- A pink or red color indicates the presence of intact red blood cells (RBCs) or hemoglobin, which may be the result of contamination during collection. Specimens that may contain blood should be centrifuged immediately to remove intact red cells because oxyhemoglobin can interfere with biochemical tests such as bilirubin
- A dark red-brown color may indicate fetal death

3.2.5.2 Clarity

- Naturally decreases as gestation progresses because of the accumulation of cellular and particulate matter (fetal hair, cells, and vernix)

3.2.6 Chemical examination

3.2.6.1 Differentiation from maternal urine

- It may be necessary to determine if fluid collected during amniocentesis is amniotic fluid or maternal urine because of the close proximity of the bladder and uterus and similar appearance of these fluids.
- Biochemical tests performed to aid in this determination may include creatinine, urea, total protein, and glucose
    - Creatinine and urea are non-protein nitrogen compounds produced at fairly constant rates that are excreted solely by the kidneys (see Chemistry 2.7.3)
        - Both compounds have a much higher concentration in urine compared to plasma (×50-×100)
        - Amniotic fluid concentrations are similar to that of maternal plasma until late pregnancy when fetal kidneys filter creatinine and urea for excretion into amniotic fluid
    - Total protein is found in significant amounts in amniotic fluid, whereas maternal urine should have essentially none unless maternal renal disease is present (see also Chemistry 2.7.5)
    - Glucose, which is found in amniotic fluid, should not be present in maternal urine unless the mother has diabetes or renal disease
- See chapter 2 Chemistry for discussion of common test methods used to measure these substances in the clinical laboratory

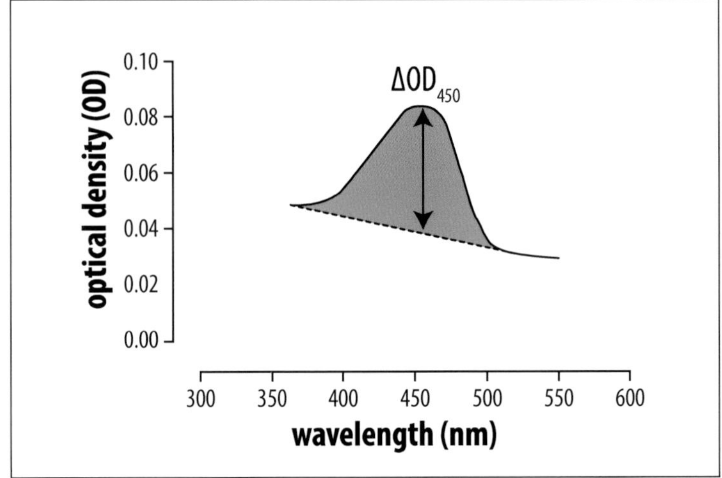

f3.1 Absorption spectrophotometry scan of amniotic fluid for determining the ΔOD450. The dashed line represents the baseline drawn between 350-550 nm. The difference between the optical density of the curve and the dashed line at 450 nm is the ΔOD450 value.

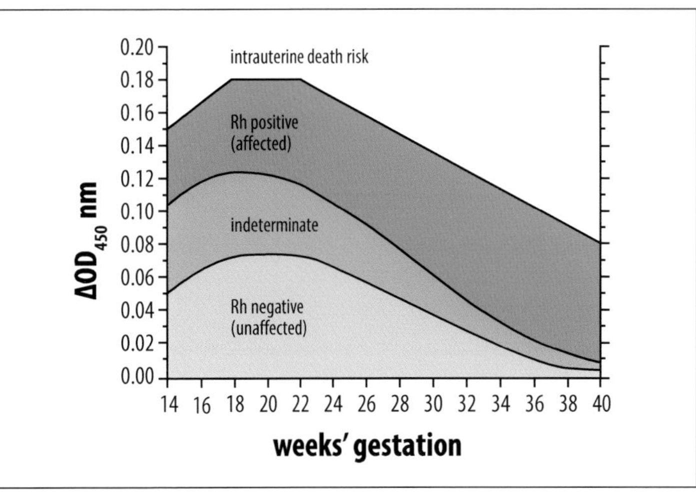

f3.2 The Queenan chart for interpreting the ΔOD450

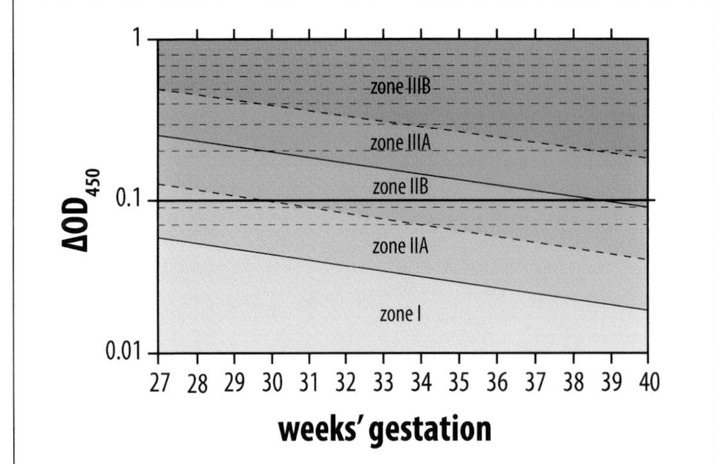

f3.3 The Liley chart for interpreting the ΔOD450

3.2.6.2 Amniotic fluid bilirubin or ΔA_{450}

- Increased destruction of fetal RBCs, as occurs with hemolytic disease of the fetus, leads to an increased amount of unconjugated bilirubin, which enters the amniotic fluid and can be detected spectrophotometrically
  - Bilirubin concentration is directly related to the severity of RBC hemolysis
  - Serial measurement of bilirubin concentrations through the ΔA_{450} test may be used to monitor progression of the disease
- The ΔA_{450} test is performed by spectrophotometrically scanning the specimen from 350 to 580 nm and graphing absorbance vs wavelength **f3.1**
  - Bilirubin has an optimal absorbance at 450 nm
  - In healthy individuals, the spectral curve is essentially a straight line with decreasing absorbances between 365 nm and 550 nm
  - As the bilirubin concentration increases, the absorbance at 450 nm will also increase yielding a larger ΔA_{450}
- Interpretation is based on gestational age, using either the Queenan (<27 weeks) **f3.2** or Liley (≥27 weeks) chart **f3.3**

3.2.6.3 Fetal lung maturity (FLM) testing

- Performed to evaluate if the fetus will be viable outside the mother's womb if premature delivery is expected or necessary because of fetal distress
- Not performed before 32 weeks' gestation because all tests will indicate fetal immaturity
- Starting at weeks 20-24 of gestation, lamellar bodies are secreted by fetal type II pneumocytes
  - Lamellar bodies contain pulmonary surfactants, such as lecithin and sphingomyelin, which alter the surface tension of the alveoli, preventing their collapse during expiration and reducing the pressure needed to reopen the alveoli during inspiration
  - Phospholipids such as phosphatidylglycerol (PG) enhance the spread of pulmonary surfactants across the alveoli
- A cascade of testing is performed, and a single "mature" value indicates low risk for respiratory distress syndrome
  - Lecithin and sphingomyelin are produced in equal concentrations until 34-36 weeks' gestation when the production of lecithin significantly increases

- Both phospholipids can be measured using thin-layer chromatography and are reported as the ratio of lecithin to sphingomyelin (L/S)
- An L/S ratio ≥2.0 is associated with fetal lung maturity

- PG is undetectable until 35 weeks' gestation
    - PG can be measured using thin-layer chromatography or an agglutination slide test using polyclonal anti-PG antibodies
    - A positive result is associated with fetal lung maturity
- The lamellar body count (LBC) can be measured using the platelet channel of an automated hematology analyzer
- In uncentrifuged specimens, an LBC >5.0×10^4/μL indicates fetal lung maturity whereas a value <1.5×10^4/μL indicates fetal lung immaturity

3.2.6.4 α-fetoprotein (AFP)

- AFP is a glycoprotein secreted in fetal serum, with concentrations reaching a peak during the 13th week of gestation and then declining until the fetus is full term
- AFP is transferred to maternal circulation through diffusion across the placenta
- High concentrations are associated with open neural tube defects, fetal abnormalities, fetal distress, and other conditions

3.2.6.5 Acetylcholinesterase (AChE)

- AChE is an enzyme found in the CNS, RBCs, skeletal muscle tissue, and fetal serum
- Analysis performed as a confirmatory test when a positive AFP value is obtained
- Normal amniotic fluid does not contain AChE and a positive result is generally associated with an open neural tube defect

3.2.7 Genetic studies (see chapter 9)

- An extensive array of molecular testing is available for use with amniotic fluid to enable early detection and diagnosis of many congenital disorders

3.2.8 Clinical significance

3.2.8.1 Hemolytic disease of the fetus (see also chapter 1 Blood Banking 1.4.1)

- Increased hemolysis of fetal RBCs leads to an elevated bilirubin concentration in amniotic fluid which can be measured spectrophotometrically with the ΔA_{450} test

3.2.8.2 Neural tube defects (NTDs)

- Birth defects affecting the brain, spine, or spinal cord; the 2 most common open NTDs are spina bifida and anencephaly
    - In spina bifida, the spinal column does not completely close, which leads to nerve damage and paralysis
    - In anencephaly, the brain and skull do not fully develop, leading to stillbirth or death shortly after birth
- NTDs can be diagnosed through imaging studies and prenatal testing of amniotic fluid for AFP and AChE
- Maternal blood may also be screened in the second trimester for AFP, human chorionic gonadotropin, and estriol in what is referred to as a "triple screen"

3.2.8.3 Respiratory distress syndrome

- Primarily occurs in neonates with immature lungs that do not have a sufficient amount of pulmonary surfactants
- When surfactants are deficient, the neonate may show symptoms such as cyanosis, apnea, and rapid or shallow breathing
- If premature delivery is necessary, fetal lung maturity testing is performed to evaluate if the lungs are mature enough to survive outside the uterus and to determine the fetus' risk of developing respiratory distress syndrome

3.3 Cerebrospinal fluid

3.3.1 Synthesis & composition

- Approximately 70% of cerebrospinal fluid (CSF) is produced by choroidal cells lining the choroid plexus into the 4 ventricles of the brain
- The remaining 30% is produced by ependymal cells lining the brain and spinal cord
- CSF is formed through selective secretion of plasma

3.3.2 Function

- CSF is found in the subarachnoid space between the pia mater and arachnoid mater
- It serves to protect and cushion the brain and spinal cord while facilitating transport of nutrients and waste products through the CNS

3.3.3 Specimen collection & handling

- CSF is obtained by passing a needle between the 3rd and 4th or 4th and 5th lumbar vertebra and into the subarachnoid space

3.3.3.1 Specimen labeling

- As CSF is collected, the tubes should be labeled numerically in the order in which they are filled
  - The 1st tube is usually used for chemical and immunologic testing because any cellular or bacterial contamination from the collection procedure will not interfere with these tests
  - The 2nd tube is typically used for microbiological testing such as Gram stain and culture
  - The 3rd tube is generally reserved for cellular studies because it is the least likely to be contaminated with peripheral blood

3.3.3.2 Transport & storage requirements

- Testing should be performed as soon as possible
- If testing is delayed, the specimen should be stored according to site-specific procedures
  - Specimens for chemical or immunologic testing should be frozen (−15°C to −30°C)
  - Specimens for microbiological testing should be maintained at room temperature (20°C-25°C)
  - Specimens for cellular studies should be stored refrigerated (2°C-5°C)

3.3.4 Physical examination

3.3.4.1 Color

- In healthy individuals, the CSF specimen is colorless i3.33
- The presence of a small amount of blood from a traumatic collection may give the first tube a pink/red coloration, but this should decrease in subsequent tubes, with the final tube appearing colorless
  - Disease states may result in a CSF specimen with pink, orange, or yellow coloration consistent across all tubes (referred to as xanthochromia)
  - A pink coloration suggests the presence of hemoglobin, which may be associated with a subarachnoid or intracerebral hemorrhage i3.33
  - A yellow coloration suggests the presence of bilirubin associated with hyperbilirubinemia i3.34
  - Specimens with an orange coloration may contain both hemoglobin and bilirubin

3.3.4.2 Clarity

- In healthy individuals, the CSF specimen is clear
- Fluids that are hazy, cloudy, or turbid may contain an increased presence of white blood cells (WBCs), RBCs, microorganisms, proteins, or other constituents

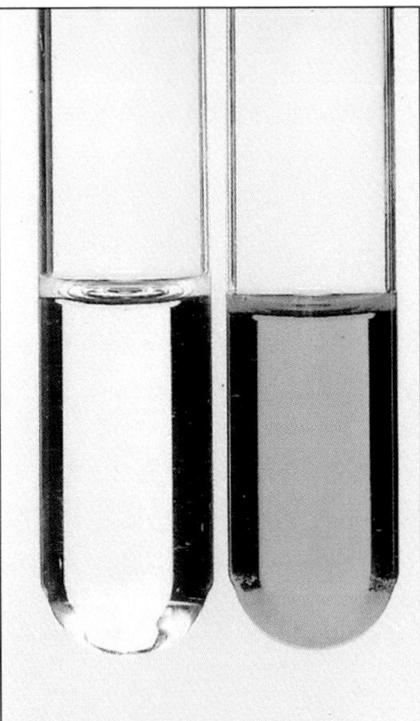

i3.33 The left tube shows normal, clear & colorless CSF. The right tube shows pigmentation of CSF following a recent subarachnoid hemorrhage (6 hours) imparting a pink to orange color

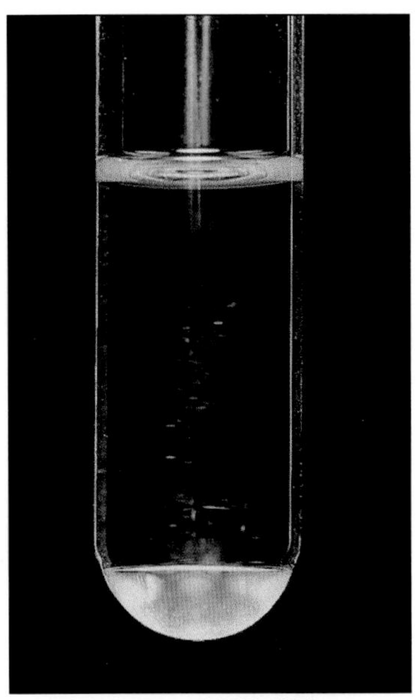

i3.34 Appearance of CSF >36 hours after a subarachnoid hemorrhage demonstrating pigmentation of the CSF imparting a yellow color due to breakdown of blood components

- A milky appearance may indicate a high lipid concentration
- Radiographic contrast media may give specimens an oily appearance

3.3.5 Chemical examination

3.3.5.1 Glucose

- Concentrations are dependent on active transport by endothelial cells and simple diffusion across the blood-brain barrier
- In healthy individuals, concentrations are approximately 60%-70% of the plasma concentration
- To accurately interpret CSF glucose determinations, a paired plasma specimen should be collected 0-2 hours before the lumbar puncture and analyzed simultaneously with the CSF using the same test method
- Elevated concentrations are considered clinically insignificant but may occur as a result of hyperglycemia or contamination with peripheral blood
- Decreased concentrations are considered clinically significant and may be associated with hypoglycemia, impaired glucose transport, increased CNS glycolysis, meningitis, metastatic carcinoma, or other conditions
- Quantitation performed using an enzymatic reaction and photometry (see also Chemistry 2.1.8.2)

ISBN 978-089189-6616

3.3.5.2 Protein

- Concentrations are dependent on the transport of low-molecular-weight plasma proteins through the endothelium of the choroid plexus and meninges and as a result of intrathecal synthesis
- Total protein
  - In healthy individuals, concentrations are generally 15-45 mg/dL (0.15-0.45 g/L), but may vary slightly according to patient age and collection site
  - Elevated concentrations may be the result of contamination with peripheral blood, damage to the blood-brain barrier, increased intrathecal synthesis, or decreased reabsorption
  - Decreased concentrations may be the result of fluid loss from damage to the dura mater or increased reabsorption because of increased intracranial pressure
  - Quantitation performed using spectrophotometry (see also Chemistry 2.5.8)
- Albumin
  - Not synthesized in the CNS, therefore any albumin present in CSF is the result of transport across the blood-brain barrier or, less commonly, contamination with peripheral blood
  - To assess the integrity of the blood-brain barrier, a paired serum specimen is collected, and the CSF/serum albumin index is determined as follows:

$$\text{CSF/serum albumin index} = \frac{\text{CSF albumin (mg/dL)}}{\text{serum albumin (g/L)}}$$

  - A normal CSF/serum albumin index is considered <9; values >9 suggest damage to the blood-brain barrier and increased permeability
  - Quantitation performed by nepholometry or reflectance spectrophotometry (see also Chemistry 2.5.9.2)
- Immunoglobulin G (IgG)
  - In healthy individuals, CSF contains a small amount of IgG from intrathecal synthesis
  - Elevated IgG may be the result of increased synthesis in the CNS or increased transport across the blood-brain barrier
  - To distinguish the cause of an elevated IgG concentration, a paired serum specimen is collected and both specimens are analyzed for IgG and albumin
  - The CSF IgG index is calculated as follows:

$$\text{CSF IgG index} = \frac{\text{serum albumin (g/dL)}}{\text{CSF albumin (mg/L)}} \times \frac{\text{CSF IgG (mg/dL)}}{\text{serum IgG (g/dL)}}$$

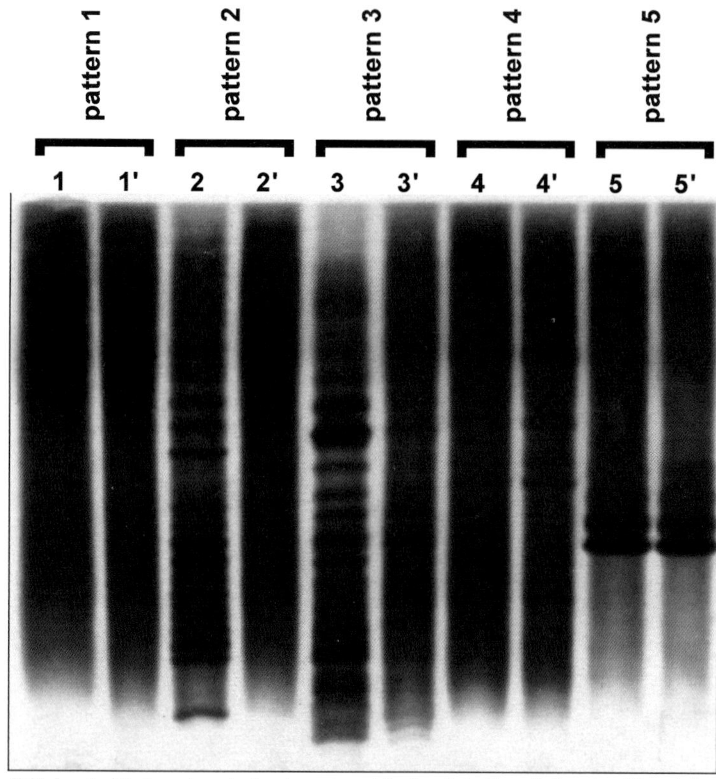

i3.35 Isoelectric focusing electrophoresis gel for the detection of oligoclonal bands in CSF. Note the 5 classic patterns that can be observed:
pattern 1: no bands in the CSF or serum, negative result
pattern 2: oligoclonal IgG bands in the CSF but not the serum, positive result and indicative of intrathecal IgG synthesis
pattern 3: oligoclonal IgG bands in the CSF and additional identical bands in the CSF and serum, positive result and indicative of intrathecal IgG synthesis
pattern 4: identical bands in the CSF and serum, negative result, indicative of a systemic immune reaction
pattern 5: monoclonal bands in the CSF and serum, negative result and indicative of the presence of a monoclonal IgG

  - Elevated CSF IgG indices indicate increased intrathecal synthesis as seen in multiple sclerosis or inflammatory disorders
  - Decreased indices may be associated with damage to the blood-brain barrier
- Protein electrophoresis i3.35 (see also Chemistry 2.5.11)
  - Performed on concentrated CSF and a paired serum specimen
  - In healthy individuals, CSF yields 4 distinct bands: transthyretin (prealbumin), albumin, and 2 transferrin bands in the β region, transferrin and τ transferrin (β_1 and β_2, respectively)
  - τ transferrin confirms the presence of CSF which may assist in the diagnosis of CSF rhinorrhea or otorrhea when present in nasal or middle ear fluids, respectively

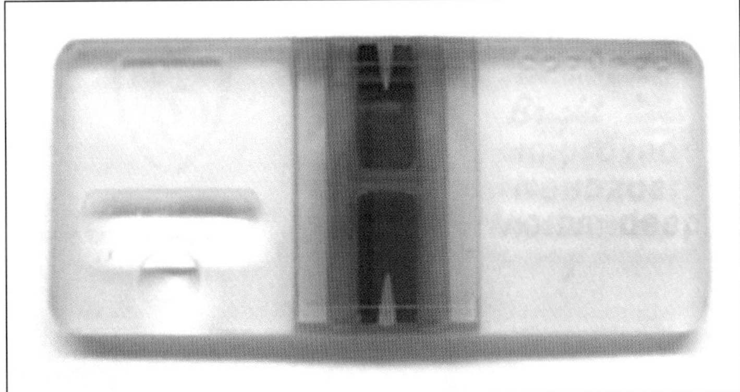

i3.36 Neubauer hemacytometer with coverslip

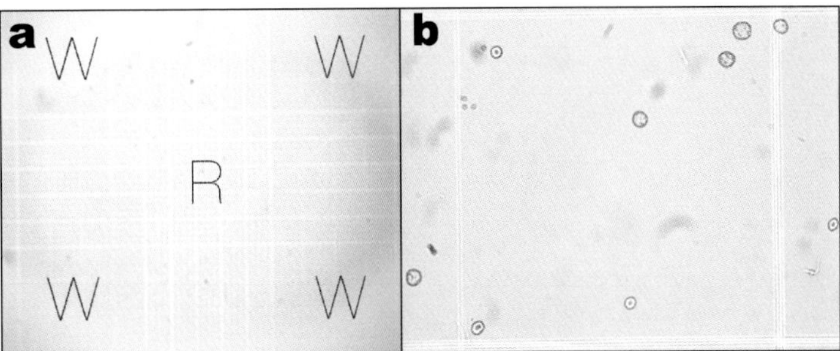

i3.37 a Neubauer hemacytometer with gridlines (×4 objective); b Neubauer hemacytometer loaded with positive control (×40 objective)

- Multiple sclerosis is highly indicated when oligoclonal bands are present in the γ region of the CSF pattern, but absent in the serum electrophoretic pattern
- Myelin basic protein (MBP)
  - Found in the myelin sheath surrounding the axons of nerves
  - In multiple sclerosis and other demyelinating disorders, the myelin sheath is degraded releasing MBP which can be measured and used to follow the course of disease progression

3.3.5.3 Lactate

- Present in CSF as a result of anaerobic metabolism in the CNS
- In healthy individuals, concentrations are approximately 10-22 mg/dL (1.1-2.4 mmol/L)
- Elevated concentrations associated with decreased oxygenation of CNS tissues as may occur with intracranial hemorrhage, cerebral infarction, cerebral arteriosclerosis, traumatic brain injury, or other conditions
- Determinations may aid in differentiating causes of meningitis
  - Viral meningitis results in a mildly elevated concentration (25-30 mg/dL [2.7-3.3 mmol/L])
  - Bacterial, fungal, or tuberculous meningitis result in values >35 mg/dL (3.9 mmol/L)

3.3.6 Microscopic examination

3.3.6.1 Manual cell count

- The concentration of nucleated cells per microliter of CSF or total cell count is determined on a well-mixed undiluted CSF specimen
- Adult CSF normally contains 0-5 WBCs/μL, whereas CSF from neonates may have up to 30 WBCs/μL
- Increased WBC concentrations may be associated with infection (meningitis), inflammation, tumor, or other diseases of the CNS
- RBC counts provide little diagnostic value aside from aiding in the differentiation of a traumatic lumbar puncture (see i3.39) and a hemorrhage
- High cell concentrations may require dilution with saline
- Counts should be performed as soon as possible to minimize cellular degeneration
- The manual cell count is performed by loading the well-mixed specimen onto a cover-slipped Neubauer hemacytometer, taking care not to overfill the chamber i3.36
- The etched lines on the hemacytometer delineate 9 quadrants (W) arranged in a 3×3 grid. Each W quadrant is 1×1 mm; with a coverslip, the depth is 0.1 mm, resulting in a 0.1 μL volume for each W quadrant i3.37a
  - The center quadrant is further divided into 0.2×0.2 mm quadrants (R); with a coverslip, the volume of each R quadrant is 0.004 μL
  - A total cell count or WBC count may be performed by counting all 9 large W quadrants on each side of the hemacytometer
  - Counts from both sides of the hemacytometer should match within the laboratory's predefined acceptance criteria
  - The average from both sides of the hemacytomer is used to determine the cell concentration using the following calculation:

$$\text{cell concentration} = \frac{(\text{average number of cells}) \times (\text{dilution factor})}{(\text{number of quadrants counted}) \times (\text{quadrant volume [μL]})}$$

ISBN 978-089189-6616

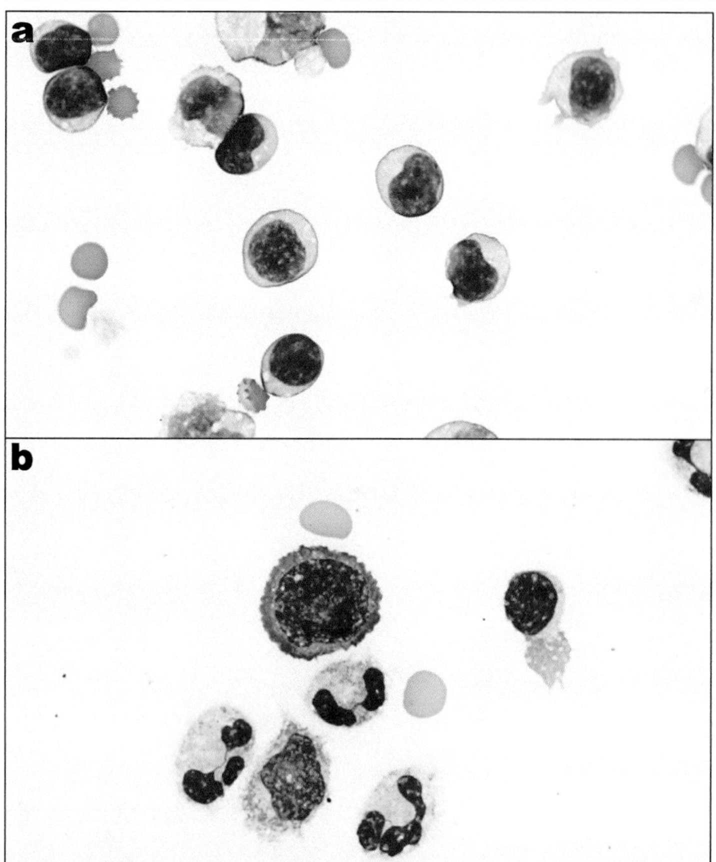

i3.38 a Lymphocytic & monocytic pleocytosis in a patient with viral meningitis showing increased numbers of small & reactive lymphocytes & monocytes
b Neutrophilic pleocytosis in a patient with bacterial meningitis showing increased numbers of neutrophils with monocytes & lymphocytes

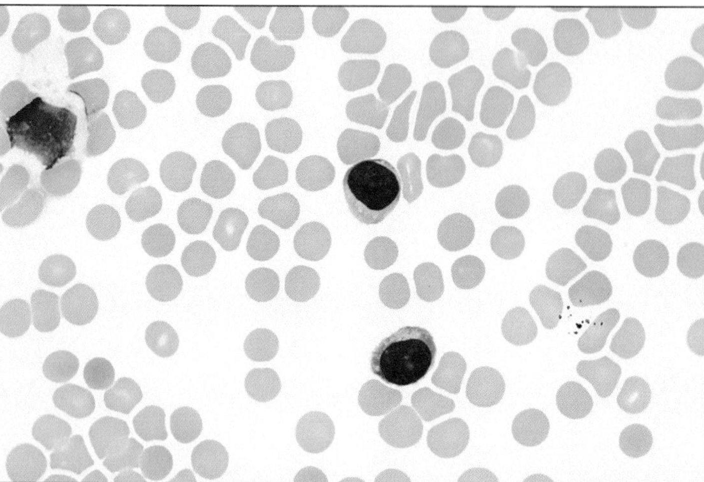

i3.39 Normal CSF usually shows very few cells; however, small lymphocytes & occasional monocytes may be seen. The large numbers of red cells in the background indicate the possibility of a traumatic tap

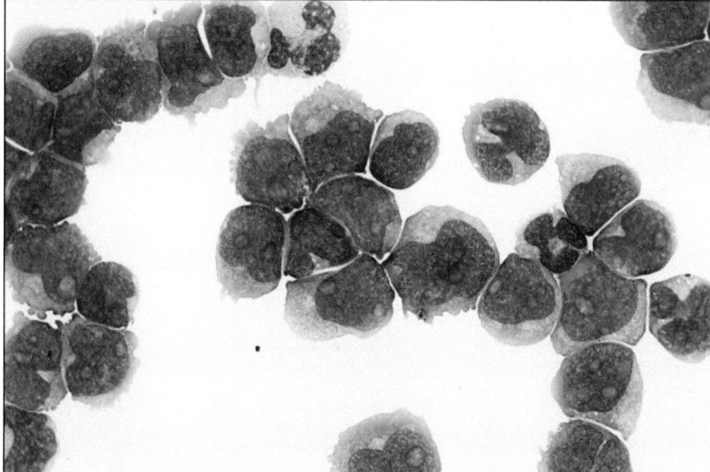

i3.40 CSF from a patient with AML & central nervous system involvement showing increased numbers of large blasts with fine chromatin, relatively prominent nucleoli, irregular nuclear contours & moderate amounts of cytoplasm

3.3.6.2 WBC differential (see Hematology 4.10)

- A cytocentrifuged, stained smear is used to perform the WBC differential
- Lymphocytes and monocytes are the predominant white cells normally seen in CSF t3.4

t3.4 Normal cerebrospinal fluid differential counts

Cell type	Adults	Neonates
lymphocytes	30%-90%	10%-40%
monocytes	10%-50%	50%-90%
neutrophils	0%-6%	0%-10%
ependymal	rare	rare
eosinophils	rare	rare

- Pleocytosis or an increased WBC count may be the result of infection, inflammation, or other noninfectious condition i3.38, i3.39
  - Neutrophilic pleocytosis is most commonly associated with bacterial meningitis but may also occur in early viral, fungal, tubercular, and parasitic infections
  - Lymphocytic pleocytosis generally occurs in later stages of viral, tubercular, and fungal infections; lymphocytes may also predominate in syphilitic meningitis
  - Monocytic pleocytosis is uncommon, but monocytes may be elevated in mixed pleocytosis associated with tubercular, fungal, or bacterial infections
  - Eosinophil pleocytosis may be associated with parasitic or fungal infections or allergic reactions
  - The presence of macrophages is suggestive of a subarachnoid or cerebral hemorrhage
  - Plasma cells are abnormal in CSF and may be seen in acute viral or chronic inflammatory conditions and these cells are often associated with multiple sclerosis
  - Malignant cells may be present as a result of a primary tumor, metastases, or leukemia i3.40

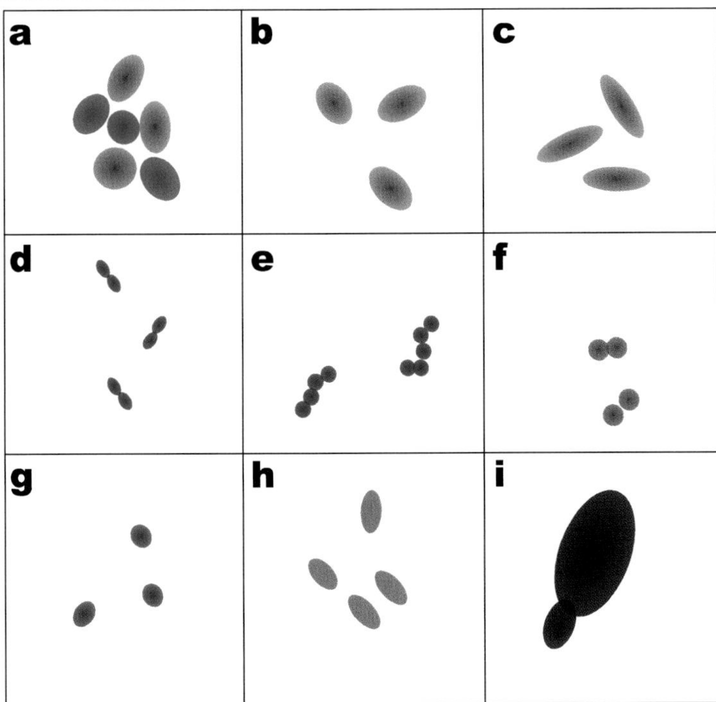

f3.4 Diagramatic representation characteristic of Gram stain morphologies of potential CSF pathogens; the following organisms are represented:
a *Acinetobacter* spp
b *Escherichia coli*
c *Pseudomonas aeruginosa*
d *Streptococcus pneumoniae*
e *Streptococcus agalactiae (GBS)*
f *Neisseria meningitidis*
g *Listeria monocytogenes*
h *Haemophilus influenzae*
i *Candida* spp, budding form (may be very large, up to 8 μm in size)

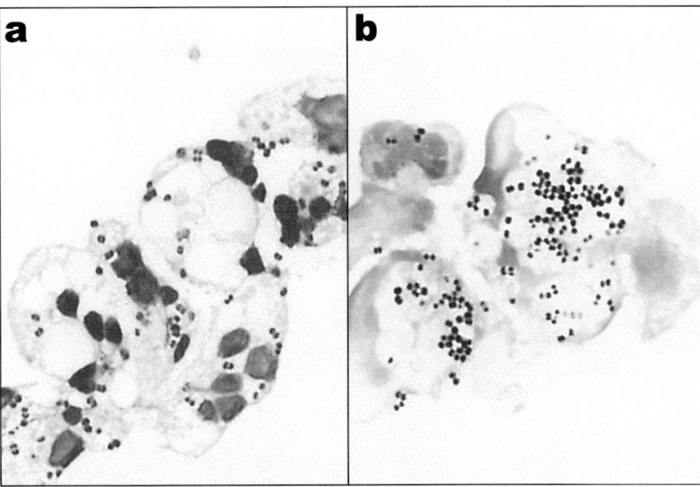

i3.41 a Many gram-negative bacteria in CSF in a case of meningitis due to *Neisseria meningitidis*
b Many gram-positive bacteria in CSF in a case of meningitis due to *Streptococcus pneumoniae*

3.3.6.3 Gram stain & culture

- A Gram stain is performed to aid in the rapid (presumptive) diagnosis of bacterial meningitis **f3.4**, i3.41, **t3.6** (see also Microbiology 6.1.3)
- Aerobic culture may be performed to isolate the causative organism

t3.5 Most common causes of bacterial meningitis

Haemophilus influenza
Neisseria meningitides
Streptococcus pneumoniae

3.3.7 Clinical significance

3.3.7.1 Meningitis

- Inflammation of the meninges, which are the membranes surrounding the brain and spinal cord
- Causes include, but are not limited to, bacterial, viral, parasitic, and fungal infections (see also Microbiology 6.7.6.4)
- Chemical, microscopic, and microbiological studies on CSF allow for diagnosis and appropriate treatment **t3.6**

t3.6 Cerebrospinal fluid differential counts in meningitis

Type of infection	Leukocyte count	Protein	Leukocyte differential	Glucose	Comment
bacterial	1,000-10,000	>100	polys predominate	<40	partially treated infections may be lymphocyte predominant
viral	50-500	20-100	polys early, lymphs late	normal	decreased glucose is characteristic of HSV encephalitis
fungal & mycobacterial	50-500	20-100	lymphs predominate	<50	

HSV = herpes simplex virus

3.3.7.2 Multiple sclerosis (MS)

- Autoimmune disease in which the myelin sheaths surrounding nerve fibers is deteriorated, leading to nerve damage
- Chemical studies on CSF, such as electrophoresis, may aid in the diagnosis of multiple sclerosis

3.4 Serous fluids

3.4.1 Synthesis & composition

- Formed through ultrafiltration of the plasma in the parietal membranes and absorption by the visceral membranes
- As ultrafiltrates of the blood, the composition of these fluids reflects that of the serum

3.4.2 Function

- Pleural, pericardial, and peritoneal fluids are named respective to the body cavity in which they are formed
- Serous fluids serve as a cushion, lubricant, and transport media between the visceral and parietal membranes

3.4.3 Effusions

- An excess amount of fluid within a body cavity is referred to as an effusion; an effusion in the peritoneal cavity is referred to as ascites
- Effusions are categorized as either a transudate or exudate based on the cause of the fluid accumulation
  - Transudates are the result of a noninflammatory process leading to an increase in hydrostatic pressure or a decrease in oncotic pressure
  - Exudates are the result of an inflammatory process causing an increase in endothelial permeability or a decrease in lymphatic absorption

3.4.4 Specimen collection & handling

- The effusion is collected by paracentesis in which a sterile needle is inserted into the body cavity and the fluid is aspirated into a sterile syringe; referred to as a thoracentesis, pericardiocentesis, or peritoneocentesis with respect to the specific body cavity
- Serous fluids should be transported at room temperature and tested immediately to prevent cellular degradation, chemical changes, and bacterial growth
- Bronchioalveolar lavage may be performed by inserting a bronchoscope through the mouth/nose into the lungs to dispense a small amount of fluid which is recollected for analysis

3.4.5 Physical examination

3.4.5.1 Color

- Transudates are clear, pale-yellow to yellow fluids with viscosity similar to that of serum
- Exudates are cloudy and may be yellow, green, pink, or red

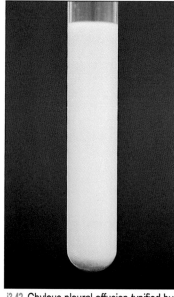

i3.42 Chylous pleural effusion typified by milky white fluid

3.4.5.2 Clarity

- Chylous fluids appear milky after centrifugation because of the presence of chyle and may be the result of an obstruction or damage to the lymphatic system i3.42
- Pseudochylous fluids are visually similar to chylous effusions but are the result of a chronic effusion and cellular breakdown
- Chylous and pseudochylous fluids can be differentiated based on several characteristics t3.7

t3.7 Chylous vs pseudochylous effusions

	Chylous	Pseudochylous
gross appearance	milky	milky
microscopic appearance	lymphocytes	mixed leukocytes, cholesterol crystals
triglycerides	>110 mg/dL	<50 mg/dL
chylomicrons (by electrophoresis)	+	–

3.4.6 Chemical examination

3.4.6.1 Total protein & lactate dehydrogenase

- Simultaneous measurements of serum and serous total protein and lactate dehydrogenase are performed to identify the effusion as a transudate or an exudate using the following ratios and criteria t3.8
- Exudates require additional testing whereas transudates generally do not merit further analysis

$$\text{total protein ratio} = \frac{\text{serous TP (g/dL)}}{\text{serum TP (g/dL)}}$$

$$\text{lactate dehydrogenase ratio} = \frac{\text{serous LD (U/L)}}{\text{serum LD (U/L)}}$$

t3.8 Light criteria for exudative effusions

Pleural fluid:serum protein ratio >0.5
Pleural fluid:serum LD ratio >0.6
Pleural fluid LD >2/3 of the upper limit of normal for serum LD

The presence of any criterion is indicative of exudate
LD = lactate dehydrogenase

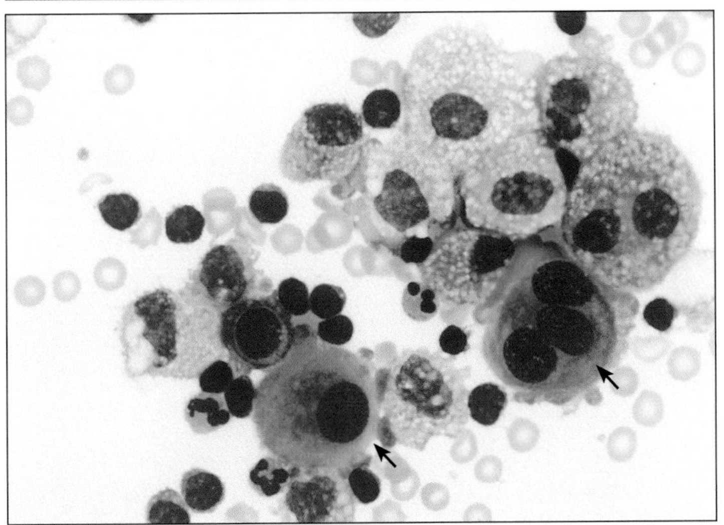

i3.43 Mesothelial cells (arrows) & macrophages

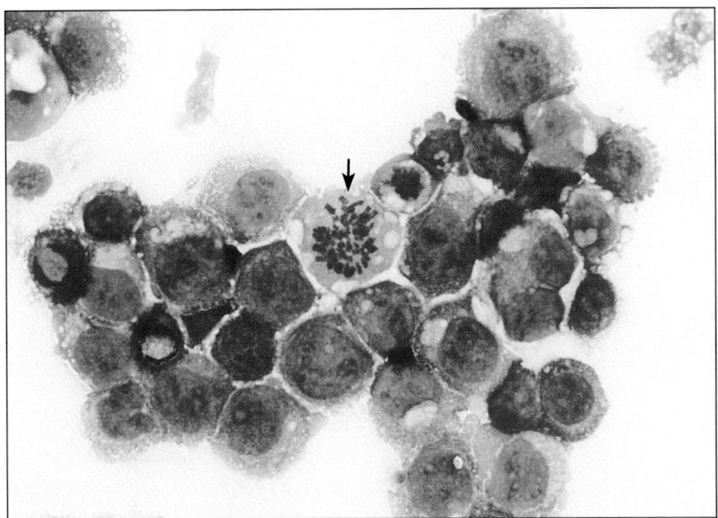

i3.44 Metastatic breast carcinoma with an abnormal mitotic figure (arrow)

3.4.6.2 Glucose

- Simultaneous measurements of serum and serous glucose may be performed on exudates
- Serous fluids with glucose concentrations <60 mg/dL (<3.3 mmol/L) or a difference between the serous and serum glucose concentrations of >30 mg/dL (>1.6 mmol/L) identify an exudative process
- Conditions associated with low serous glucose concentrations include bacterial infection, malignancy, and rheumatoid arthritis

3.4.6.3 Lipids

- Lipid concentrations can aid in differentiating between chylous and pseudochylous fluids
- Triglycerides
  - Concentrations >110 mg/dL (>6.1 mmol/L) are indicative of a chylous effusion; whereas, values <50 mg/dL (<2.7 mmol/L) indicate a pseudochylous effusion
  - Lipoprotein electrophoresis may be performed for effusions with triglyceride concentrations between 50 mg/dL (0.56 mmol/L) and 110 mg/dL (1.2 mmol/L); the presence of chylomicrons indicates a chylous effusion
- Cholesterol ratio
  - In pleural fluids, simultaneous measurement of serum and serous cholesterol may aid in differentiating chylous from pseudochylous effusions
  - Effusions with values <1.0 would be categorized as chylous, whereas ratios >1.0 indicate a pseudochylous fluid rich in cholesterol

3.4.6.4 Amylase

- Simultaneous measurements of serum and serous amylase may be performed on pleural and peritoneal fluids
- Conditions associated with elevated serous amylase values include pancreatitis, esophageal damage, or gastrointestinal damage

3.4.6.5 pH

- Pleural fluid pH can aid in deciding treatment options for patients with parapneumonic effusions
- Effusions with pH >7.3 generally prompt for treatment with antibiotics only whereas those with pH <7.3 require placement of a drainage tube in addition to antibiotics

3.4.6.6 Carcinoembryonic antigen (CEA)

- This marker is used in the evaluation of pleural and peritoneal fluids from patients with possible carcinoembryonic antigen-producing tumors

3.4.7 Microscopic examination

3.4.7.1 Cell count & WBC differential (see Hematology 4.10)

- In general, transudates have <1,000 WBCs/μL and exudates have more than 1,000 WBCs/μL
- A cytocentrifuged, stained smear is used to perform the WBC differential
- All nucleated cells are included in the count and each type is reported as a percentage
- A variety of cell types may be seen in serous fluids including neutrophils, lymphocytes, monocytes, eosinophils, plasma cells, mesothelial cells, and cells associated with malignancy i3.43, i3.44

ISBN 978-089189-6616

3.4.7.2 Gram stain & culture

- Performed to aid in the identification of microbes (see also Microbiology 6.7.7)

3.5 Synovial fluid

3.5.1 Synthesis & composition

- Formed by secretions of the synoviocytes (enzymes and hyaluronic acid) and ultrafiltration of the plasma across the synovial membrane
- The concentration of some analytes, like glucose and uric acid, in synovial fluid mirrors that of the plasma, whereas the concentration of other analytes, like total protein and antibodies, are only a fraction of that seen in plasma

3.5.2 Function

- Serves as a lubricant and source of nutrients for the articular cartilage

3.5.3 Specimen collection & handling

- Collected by arthrocentesis in which a sterile needle is inserted into the joint and fluid is aspirated into a sterile syringe
- A paired, fasting blood specimen should be collected at the same time into a tube with no anticoagulant if the plasma-synovial fluid glucose difference is to be determined

3.5.4 Physical examination

3.5.4.1 Color

- Normal synovial fluid is pale yellow or colorless
- Fluids with a pink or red coloration may indicate the presence of blood because of a traumatic collection
- Fluids that are yellow are typically associated with a noninflammatory process
- Yellow-white fluids are suggestive of an inflammatory process
- Infection or sepsis can result in a yellow-green fluid
- Red or brown fluids may indicate a hemorrhagic condition

3.5.4.2 Clarity

- Normal synovial fluid is clear
- Hazy, cloudy, or turbid fluids are associated with inflammation or infection
- The presence of rice bodies, composed of collagen and fibrinous tissue, are most commonly seen in patients with rheumatoid arthritis
- Ochronotic shards, which are pieces of pigmented cartilage, may be seen in the synovial fluid of patients with alkaptonuria

3.5.4.3 Viscosity

- Normally extremely viscous because of its high concentration of hyaluronic acid which is secreted by synoviocytes to lubricate the joints
- In inflammatory conditions or infection, the viscosity may be decreased because of the activity of hyaluronidase produced by neutrophils and some bacteria
- Assessed using the string test, in which a drop of fluid is expelled from the syringe and the resultant string length is measured; normal fluid forms a string at least 4 cm in length before breaking

3.5.5 Chemical examination

3.5.5.1 Mucin clot test

- Performed by adding a few drops of acetic acid to an aliquot of synovial fluid to promote clot formation
- Poor clot formation is associated with inflammatory conditions such as rheumatoid arthritis

3.5.5.2 Glucose

- Simultaneous measurements of plasma and synovial glucose may be performed
- Normally, the difference between plasma and synovial glucose is less than 10 mg/dL (0.5 mmol/L)
- Noninflammatory and hemorrhagic joint disorders are associated with a difference of 10-20 mg/dL (0.5-1.1 mmol/L)
- Inflammatory conditions yield a difference of 20-40 mg/dL (1.1-2.2 mmol/L)
- Septic conditions demonstrate differences >40 mg/dL (>2.2 mmol/L)

3.5.5.3 Uric acid

- Plasma and synovial uric acid concentrations are normally equivalent; therefore, plasma is generally used for uric acid determinations because the sample collection is less invasive

3.5.6 Microscopic examination

3.5.6.1 WBC differential

- A cytocentrifuged, stained smear is used to perform the WBC differential
- A variety of cell types may be seen including monocytes/macrophages, lymphocytes, neutrophils, eosinophils, and cells associated with malignancy

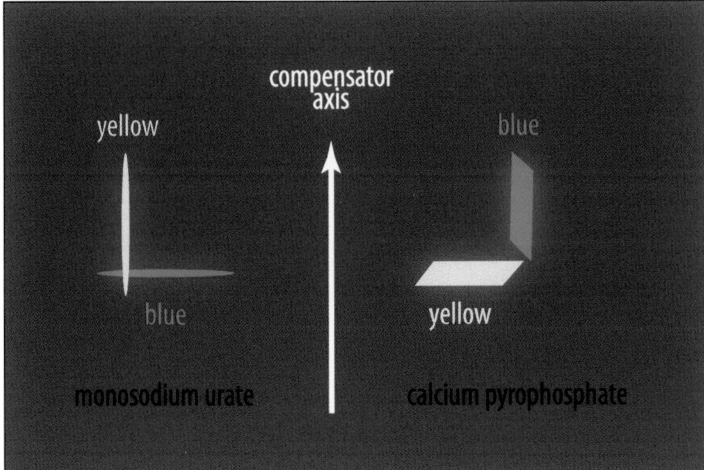

f3.5 2-dimensional schematic representation of MSU & CPPD crystals when viewed under a compensated polarized light microscope. MSU crystals appear yellow when parallel to the compensator, while CPPD crystals appear blue when parallel to the compensator

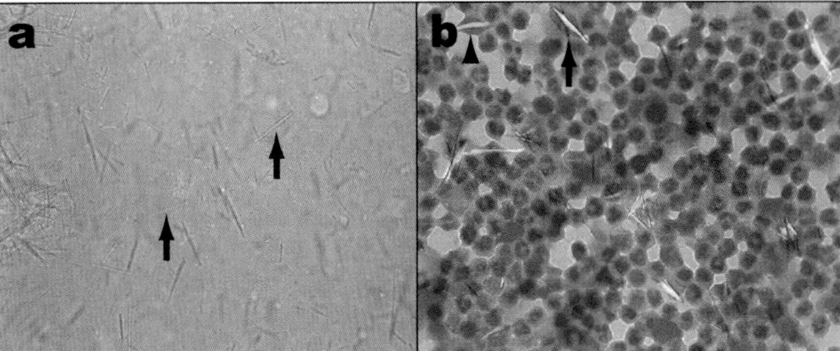

i3.45 Fluid monosodium urate (MSU) crystals
a MSU crystals in direct light, in which they appear as translucent needle shaped crystals (arrows)
b MSU crystals in polarized light, in which they appear as negatively birefringent crystals, those parallel to the compensator being yellow (arrow), and those perpendicular being blue (arrowhead); note the abundance of neutrophils

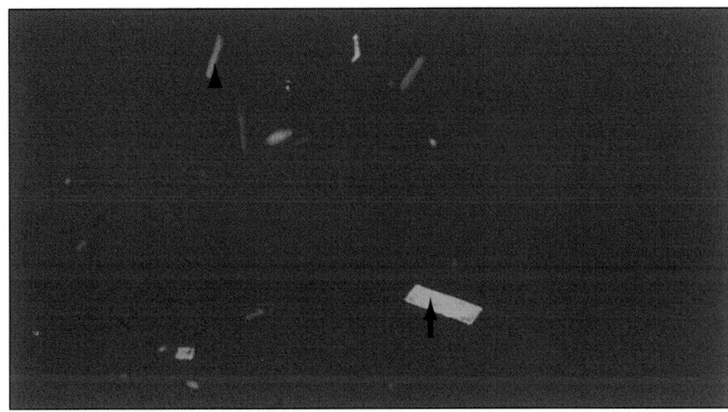

i3.46 Several calcium pyrophosphate dihydrate (CPPD) crystals as seen with polarized light & red compensator, with those parallel to the compensator being yellow (arrow), and those perpendicular being blue (arrowhead)

3.5.6.2 Gram stain & culture

- A Gram stain is performed to aid in the identification of microbes (see also Microbiology 6.7.7)
- Aerobic and anaerobic cultures may be prepared

3.5.6.3 Polarizing microscopy f3.5,

- A cytocentrifuged smear and/or wet prep may be used to evaluate the presence of crystals
- Using a polarizing microscope, birefringent substances appear as bright objects on a dark background
- Using a compensating polarizing microscope with a red compensator allows for differentiation of positive and negative birefringent substances
- Monosodium urate (MSU) crystals
  - MSU crystals have a needle-like shape and strong negative birefringence i3.45a
  - Using a red compensator they appear yellow when their longitudinal axis is parallel to the plate and blue when it is perpendicular to the plate i3.45b
  - MSU crystals are associated with increased purine metabolism as occurs in gout
- Calcium pyrophosphate dihydrate (CPPD) crystals
  - CPPD crystals have a rodlike or rhomboid shape and weak positive birefringence
  - Using a red compensator, they appear blue when their longitudinal axis is parallel to the plate and yellow when it is perpendicular to the plate i3.46
  - CPPD crystals are associated with a group of diseases known as pseudogout

3.5.7 Clinical significance

3.5.7.1 Gout

- Result of increased purine metabolism leading to elevated blood and synovial concentrations of uric acid
- Causes pain and swelling in the joints, predominantly affecting the great toe
- Elevated plasma uric acid concentrations and the presence of MSU crystals aid in the diagnosis of this disease

3.5.7.2 Pseudogout

- Causes pain and swelling in the joints, predominantly affecting the knee
- The presence of CPPD crystals aid in the diagnosis of this disease

3.5.7.3 Arthritis

- Classified as noninflammatory, inflammatory, septic, or hemorrhagic
- The color, clarity, viscosity, WBC concentration, WBC distribution, plasma-to-fluid glucose difference and gram stain/culture aid in differentiation

ISBN 978-089189-6616

3.6 Seminal fluid

3.6.1 Fertility evaluations

- Seminal fluid is commonly evaluated to aid in assessment of male fertility; post-vasectomy samples are also evaluated to determine the success of the surgical procedure

3.6.2 Synthesis & composition

- Semen is a complex fluid composed of spermatozoa and secretions from the testes, epididymis, seminal vesicles, and prostate gland

3.6.3 Function

- Serves as a transport medium and source of nutrients for spermatozoa

3.6.4 Specimen collection & handling

- Collected by the patient at home or within a private room located near the laboratory. The specimen should be labeled with the date and time of collection and transported to the laboratory within 1 hour of collection

3.6.5 Physical examination

3.6.5.1 Color & clarity

- In healthy adults, seminal fluid is gray-white and translucent
- Yellow coloration may be the result of certain medications or infection
- A red or brown coloration may indicate the presence of blood
- Clear fluid is generally associated with a low sperm concentration and infertility

3.6.5.2 Liquefaction time

- Semen from a healthy adult should rapidly coagulate after ejaculation then liquefy within 30 minutes
- The time between collection and liquefaction is recorded as the liquefaction time
- Samples that do not liquefy by 60 minutes are considered abnormal and must be chemically treated to allow additional testing to be performed

3.6.5.3 Volume

- In healthy individuals, a complete collection yields a volume of 2-5 mL
- Volumes <2 mL or >5 mL have been associated with infertility

3.6.5.4 Viscosity

- Seminal fluid is normally watery and forms discrete droplets when allowed to fall by gravity
- Viscosity is assessed by aspirating the fluid into a Pasteur pipette and observing the droplets that form
- Abnormal viscosity would be indicated if the fluid formed a string >2 cm in length and may be associated with the presence of antisperm antibodies

3.6.6 Chemical examination

3.6.6.1 pH

- Fresh semen is slightly alkaline (7.2-7.8)
- A pH <7.2 may be associated with an abnormality of the epididymis, vas deferens, or seminal vesicles
- A pH >7.8 may indicate an infection
- It is critical to test the specimen's pH within 1 hour of collection to avoid a falsely alkaline pH caused by loss of carbon dioxide or a falsely acidic pH caused by accumulation of lactic acid

3.6.6.2 Fructose

- Produced and secreted by the seminal vesicles, making it useful as a marker for their secretory function
- Low fructose concentrations are associated with azoospermia or an obstruction of the male reproductive tract
- Fructose levels may be measured using spectrophotometric methods

3.6.6.3 Citric acid & zinc

- Produced and secreted by the prostate, making them potentially useful markers for its secretory function

3.6.6.4 Acid phosphatase

- Secreted by the prostate gland in high concentrations
- Used to confirm the presence of seminal fluid

3.6.6.5 α-glucosidase

- Enzyme produced by the epididymis
- Its activity in seminal fluid represents the secretory function of the epididymis and may be useful in identifying an obstruction as the cause of azoospermia

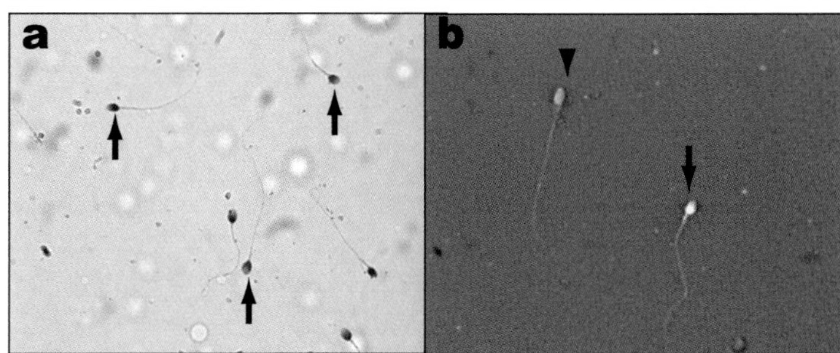

i3.47 a Seminal fluid stained with Papanicolaou stain (×100 objective) with normal sperm (arrow)
b Seminal fluid stained with eosin-nigrosin stain (×100 objective) distinguishing white viable sperm (arrow) from pink non-viable sperm (arrowhead)

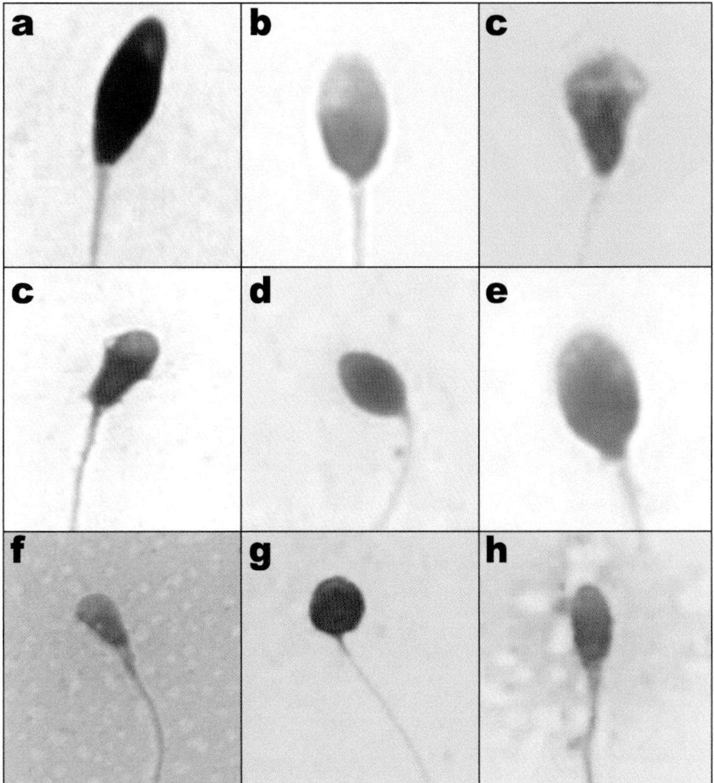

i3.48 Examples of abnormal sperm head morphology. Abnormal morphologies include: a tapered, b amorphous with irregular membrane, c amorphous abnormal head shape, d pyriform, e no acrosome, f increased acrosomal vacuoles (enlarged for better viewing of vacuoles), g postacrosomal vacuole, h round

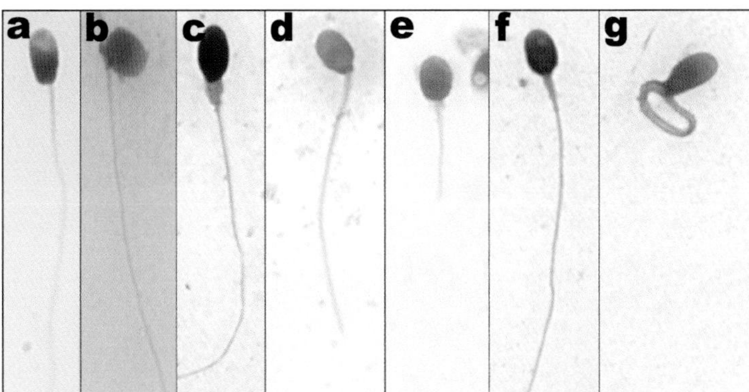

i3.49 Abnormal sperm midpiece & tail morphology. Abnormal morphologies include a asymmetrical tail insertion, b bent neck, c excess residual cytoplasm, d, e short tail, f thick insertion, g coiled tail

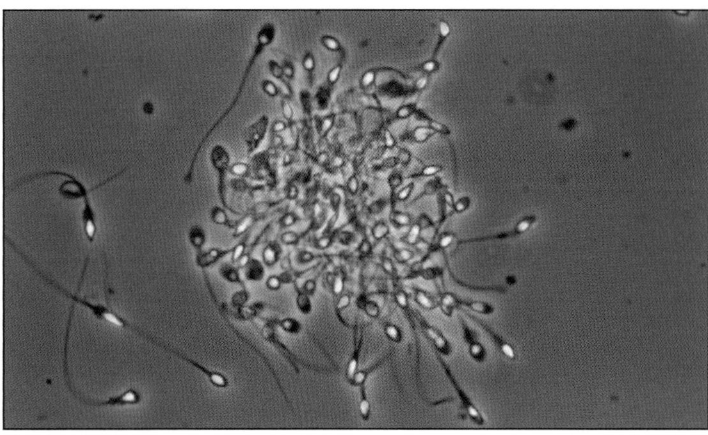

i3.50 Sperm agglutination observed during the initial microscopic evaluation of semen

3.6.7 Microscopic examination

3.6.7.1 Motility

- Evaluated microscopically by preparing a wet mount and observing the slide under high dry power; often 2 slides are prepared and evaluated for better accuracy
- Normal semen evaluated within 60 minutes of collection should show moderate to strong linear forward progression of at least 50% of the sperm

3.6.7.2 Morphology

- Evaluated by preparing a stained smear using the Giemsa, Wright, or Papanicolaou stains and observing the slide using oil immersion i3.47a
- Normal sperm have 3 distinct components: a head, midpiece, and tail; abnormalities may occur in any of these components i3.48, i3.49
- Specimens with <14% of sperm demonstrating normal morphology may be associated with infertility

3.6.7.3 Vitality/viability

- Evaluated by preparing a stained smear using eosin or eosin-nigrosin stain and observing the slide using oil immersion i3.47b
- Dead or damaged sperm do not have an intact plasma membrane and readily take up stain, whereas living sperm do not
- Specimens with <58% vitality may be associated with infertility

3.6.7.4 Agglutination

- Observed on the wet mount during evaluation of other parameters and can be confirmed using a macroscopic agglutination test or immunobead methods i3.50

ISBN 978-089189-6616

- The presence of antisperm IgG or IgA antibodies can lead to head-to-head, head-to-tail, or tail-to-tail agglutination
- The presence of these antibodies has been correlated with reduced fertility

3.6.7.5 Cell counts

- The concentration of sperm or round cells such as germ cells or WBCs, per microliter of seminal fluid or sperm count, can be determined by performing a manual count on a well-mixed specimen
- Because of the high concentration of sperm, an initial dilution of 1:20 is performed using an approved diluent; additional dilutions may be required
- A manual cell count is performed by loading the well-mixed, diluted specimen onto a cover-slipped Neubauer hemacytometer, being careful not to overfill the chamber
- The sperm count is performed by counting the 0.2×0.2 mm quadrants (R) on both sides of the hemacytometer
- A WBC count may also be performed by counting the 1.0×1.0 mm quadrants (W) on both sides of the hemacytometer
- The count from both sides of the hemacytometer should match within the laboratory's predefined acceptance criteria. Failure to meet this criterion should prompt for the hemacytometer to be reloaded with well-mixed specimen
- The average from both sides of the hemacytometer is used to calculate the cell concentration using the following calculation:

$$\text{cell concentration} = \frac{(\text{average number of cells})\times(\text{dilution factor})}{(\text{number of quadrants counted})\times(\text{quadrant volume [µL]})}$$

- Sperm concentrations of 20-250 million per milliliter are considered normal and associated with fertility (note that a unit conversion is required to change the above calculation from cells/µL to cells/mL)
- A WBC count less than 1×10^6/mL is considered normal

3.7 Feces

3.7.1 Synthesis & composition

- Feces are the end waste product of digestion and absorption in the small and large intestines
- They are composed of undigested food, intestinal normal flora, sloughed intestinal cells, and secretions such as digestive enzymes, pigments, electrolytes and water

3.7.2 Specimen collection & handling

- The type and volume of sample to be collected is determined by the test(s) to be performed but random and timed collections are common
- Specimens should be collected in a clean, nonbreakable container with a sealable lid. Urine cups are often used for random collections; larger containers are required for multiday collections
- Patients should be provided with clear instructions on how to perform the collection to avoid contamination
- Some foods and medications can interfere with testing therefore patients should receive detailed instructions on what to omit from their diet before collection

3.7.3 Physical examination

3.7.3.1 Color

- In healthy individuals, feces have an orange-brown color because of the presence of urobilins
- Pale or clay-colored specimens are referred to as "acholic" and are most commonly the result of a posthepatic obstruction that inhibits urobilin production
- Red specimens generally indicate the presence of blood from the lower gastrointestinal tract, but may also be the result of some foods, dyes, or drugs
- Black specimens (melena) may indicate the presence of blood from the upper gastrointestinal tract, but may also be the result of iron therapy, charcoal ingestion, or certain medications
- Green specimens may point to the presence of biliverdin following antibiotic therapy but may also be the result of ingestion of green vegetables

3.7.3.2 Consistency & form

- Normally, stools are formed, cylindrical masses
- Small, round, and hard stools (scybala) generally indicate low water volume associated with dehydration or constipation
- Soft, loose, ribbonlike stools are associated with increased water consumption or decreased water absorption
- Watery stools are associated with diarrhea and/or steatorrhea

3.7.4 Chemical examination

3.7.4.1 Occult blood

- Testing for fecal occult or "hidden" blood is largely performed to screen for colorectal cancer but will yield a positive result because of the presence of blood from anywhere in the gastrointestinal tract

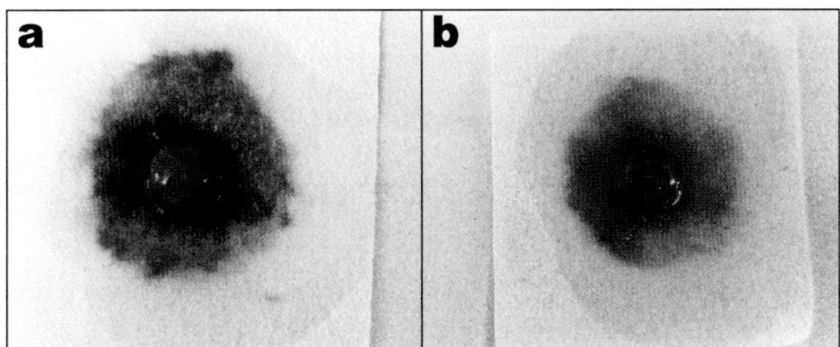

i3.51 a Positive & b negative fecal controls for guaiac-based fecal occult blood

- Guaiac-based fecal occult blood (gFOBT) methods are most commonly used
  - The guaiac method is based on the pseudoperoxidase activity of the heme moiety of hemoglobin. In the presence of hydrogen peroxide and hemoglobin, an indicator is oxidized resulting in a color formation i3.51
  - Patients may be instructed to avoid foods or medications containing high concentrations of ascorbic acid (vitamin C) or those having peroxidase/ pseudoperoxidase activity to prevent false-negative or -positive results, respectively
- Immunochemical-based fecal occult blood (iFOBT) methods
  - These methods use polyclonal antihuman antibodies specific to the globin chain of intact hemoglobin molecules, thereby reducing dietary interferences encountered when using gFOBTs
  - As hemoglobin passes through the digestive tract, it is degraded and cannot be detected by iFOBT, therefore this test method is more specific for a lower gastrointestinal bleed
- Porphyrin-based fecal occult blood methods
  - These methods are based on the conversion of heme to porphyrins and their resulting fluorescence
  - The test measures total hemoglobin and is not influenced by peroxidase or pseudoperoxidase activity of foods or medication but it can yield a false-positive result because of the presence of animal hemoglobin from ingested meats

3.7.4.2 Fetal hemoglobin

- The presence of fresh blood in the stool of a newborn may indicate that the infant has gastrointestinal bleeding or ingested maternal blood during delivery
- The alkali denaturation test or "Apt test" may be used to differentiate adult hemoglobin (HbA) from fetal hemoglobin (HbF)
  - HbA is denatured in an alkali solution but HbF resists denaturation
  - A suspension is mixed with sodium hydroxide and the color observed for 2 minutes. If the pink color persists, HbF is identified but if the color changes to yellow or brown, maternal HbA is confirmed

3.7.4.3 Fecal carbohydrates

- Maldigestion or malabsorption of carbohydrates can lead to characteristic symptoms of osmotic diarrhea, bloating, and flatulence
- A semi-quantitative pH may be used to screen for abnormally acidic stool specimens because intestinal normal flora ferment undigested disaccharides, leading to a decrease in pH

3.7.4.4 Fecal leukocytes

- Lactoferrin, a glycoprotein expressed in activated neutrophils, may be qualitatively measured using immunochemical methods to determine inflammation associated with chronic inflammatory bowel disease
- Calprotectin, a calcium-binding protein found in neutrophils, monocytes, and macrophages, may be qualitatively measured using immunochemical methods to differentiate inflammatory bowel disease and inflammatory bowel syndrome

3.7.5 Microscopic examination

3.7.5.1 Fecal fat

- Increased fecal fats, or steatorrhea, may indicate maldigestion or a malabsorption syndrome
- Qualitative determination is performed by microscopically examining 2 wet preparations
  - The first slide is treated with ethanol and stained with Oil Red O, Sudan III, Sudan IV, or other acceptable stain. Neutral fat globules take up the stain and are enumerated using high dry power
  - The second slide is treated with acetic acid and heated to hydrolyze the fatty acid salts then stained. The stained droplets are enumerated on high dry power and represent the total fecal fat content
  - Malabsorption is indicated when a normal amount of neutral fats is present despite an elevated total fat, whereas maldigestion is associated with an increase in neutral fats
- Quantitative determination is performed by analyzing a multiday collection using gravimetric, titrimetric, or nuclear magnetic resonance methods

3.7.5.2 Fecal leukocytes

- Microscopic evaluation of the quantity and type of fecal WBCs in a wet preparation allows for differentiation of various causes of diarrhea

ISBN 978-089189-6616

   - Neutrophils indicate an invasive or inflammatory condition such as ulcerative colitis or Crohn disease, whereas, noninflammatory conditions such as malabsorption do not result in an increased amount of fecal neutrophils
   - The presence of lymphocytes is associated with conditions such as celiac disease and sprue

3.8 Sweat

3.8.1 Synthesis & function

- Sweat is an ultrafiltrate produced by eccrine glands in the forehead, cheeks, hands, palms, and soles of the feet
- Secretions from the eccrine glands are clear and odorless and aid in the regulation of body temperature through evaporative cooling

3.8.2 Sweat chloride test

- Considered the "gold standard" for diagnosis of cystic fibrosis
- Specimens are collected using pilocarpine nitrate iontophoresis
- The specimen is then analyzed with chloridometry to determine the chloride concentration

3.8.3 Cystic fibrosis

- Autosomal recessive disease caused by mutations in the *CFTR* gene
- Causes abnormal electrolyte and mucous secretion, leading to an elevated sweat chloride and abnormally viscous secretions throughout the body
- Mortality is most commonly the result of pneumonia

3.9 Vaginal secretions

- See also Microbiology 6.7.9
- These may be collected to evaluate for risk of premature delivery in pregnancy

3.9.1 Fetal fibronectin

- Glycoprotein found in the cells joining the placenta to the uterine wall
- Between the 24th and 35th weeks of pregnancy, fetal fibronectin (fFN) concentrations should be undetectable in vaginal secretions
- During labor, fFN is released and can be detected in cervicovaginal secretions
- Pregnant women with an elevated fFN concentration have a higher risk of premature delivery
- fFN levels may be measured using a lateral-flow, solid-phase immunochromatographic assay

3.9.2 Placental α-microglobulin-1 (PAMG-1)

- Glycoprotein found in high concentrations in amniotic fluid
- Presence in cervicovaginal secretions is associated with premature rupture of membranes and risk of premature delivery
- PAMG-1 levels may be measured using a lateral-flow, solid-phase immunochromatographic assay

3.10 Selected readings

3.10.1 Books

Bishop M. *Clinical Chemistry: Principles, Techniques, Correlations.* 8th ed. Jones & Bartlett Learning. 2017. ISBN 978-1496335586

Brunzel NA. *Fundamentals of Urine & Body Fluid Analysis.* 4th ed. Elsevier. 2018. ISBN 978-0323374798

Kjeldsberg C, Hussong J. *Kjeldsberg's Body Fluid Analysis.* ASCP Press. 2024. ISBN 978-0891895824

Kjeldsberg C, Hussong J. *Body Fluids: Morphology Bench Guide.* ASCP Press. 2014. ISBN 978-0891896296

Mundt L. *Graff's Textbook of Urinalysis & Body Fluids.* 3rd ed. Jones & Bartlett Learning. 2015. ISBN 978-1496320162

Nader R, Horvath AR, Wittwer CT. *Tietz Fundamentals of Clinical Chemistry and Molecular Diagnostics.* 8th Edition. Saunders. 2018. ISBN 978-0323350446

Strasinger SK, Di Lorenzo MS. *Urinalysis & Body Fluids.* 7th ed. FA Davis. 2020. ISBN 978-0803675827

3.10.2 Journals & online

Online Urinalysis Tutorial. https://library.med.utah.edu/WebPath/TUTORIAL/URINE/URINE.html

Chapter 4

Hematology

ISBN 978-089189-6616

4.1 Hematopoiesis

- The production & development of all blood cells

4.1.1 Stem cell & progenitor cell development

- Types of stem cells & progenitor cells
  - Hematopoietic precursor cells (HPCs) are stem cells, progenitor cells & maturing cells
- Proliferation and differentiation potential
  - Stem cells constitute about 0.5% of total HPCs
  - Stem cells are capable of self-renewal and have multilineage differentiation potential
  - Progenitor cells represent about 3% of all HPCs
  - Progenitor cells have no capability of self-renewal and have limited differentiation potential
  - Maturing cells constitute the majority of HPCs at 95%
  - Maturing cells proliferate before fully matured
  - Maturing cells are committed to one cell line
- Morphology and phenotypic features
  - Stem cells are not morphologically recognizable
  - Important markers for stem cells include CD34, CD38, CD49, and HLA-DR
  - Progenitor cells are not morphologically recognizable
  - Progenitor cells may also express CD34 as well as lineage-specific markers (such as CD13 and CD33 for myeloid progenitors)
  - Maturing cells are morphologically recognizable by lineage and subtype
  - Phenotypes vary depending on lineage and subtype
- Key regulatory cytokines
  - Cytokines (growth factors, interleukins) regulate differentiation and proliferation of HPCs **t4.1**

t4.1 Key cytokines & their major targets

Cytokine	Target
Erythropoietin (EPO)	Erythroid cells
Granulocyte macrophage-colony-stimulating factor (GM-CSF)	Granulocytes, monocytes, eosinophils, erythroid cells
Interleukin 3 (IL-3)	HPCs
Granulocyte-colony-stimulating factor (G-CSF)	Granulocytes, early HPCs
Macrophage-colony-stimulating factor (M-CSF)	Monocytes & macrophages
Stem cell factor (SCF)	Stem cells, early HPCs, basophils & mast cells
Flt3 ligand (FL)	Stem cells, HPCs, B & T lymphocytic precursors
Thrombopoietin (TPO)	Megakaryocytes

4.1.2 Sites of hematopoiesis

4.1.2.1 Embryo & fetus

- Hematopoiesis initially begins in the yolk sac as erythropoiesis
- Then (at 4 weeks' gestation), lymphopoiesis and continued erythropoiesis occur in the aorta-gonad-mesonephros
- The liver becomes the site of hematopoiesis at about the 3rd month of gestation and includes the production of erythroid, myeloid, and lymphoid cells
- From approximately 3-6 months of fetal life, the spleen becomes a site of erythroid, myeloid, and lymphoid cell development
- The bone marrow assumes its primary role in hematopoiesis at about the 6th month of gestation. Granulocyte, erythrocyte, and megakaryocyte production all occur in the bone marrow. In addition, the thymus functions as the major site of T-lymphocyte development and the lymph nodes produce B lymphocytes

4.1.2.2 Infants & children

- Hematopoiesis occurs in bone cavities to include the flat bones of the skull, clavicle, sternum, ribs, vertebrae, and pelvis, and long bones of the arms and legs

4.1.2.3 Adults

- Only the flat bones and ends of long bones are sites for hematopoiesis

4.1.2.4 Extramedullary

- The formation and development of blood cells at sites other than the bone marrow, usually the liver and spleen
- Associated with certain hematologic disorders, such as primary myelofibrosis

4.1.3 Erythropoiesis

- The production & development of erythrocytes
- Key regulatory factors include:
  - Erythropoietin (EPO)
  - Granulocyte macrophage-colony-stimulating factor (GM-CSF)
- Bone marrow location of developing cells
  - Immature red blood cell (RBC) development within erythroblastic islands located in the bone marrow. These islands consist of a macrophage surrounded by maturing erythrocytes (nucleated RBCs)
- Characteristics of developing cells
  - Several morphologic changes occur in blood cells as they mature

- Cell size
  - Decreases as cells mature
- Nucleus
  - Nuclear-to-cytoplasmic (N:C) ratio decreases as cells mature
  - Nuclear chromatin pattern becomes clumped and condensed
  - Nucleoli disappear
- Cytoplasm
  - Color changes from dark blue to gray-blue to pink (depending on the amount of hemoglobin synthesized by each cell)
  - Relative amount of cytoplasm increases
  - Nucleus is expelled from the cell

- Maturation sequence
  - Pronormoblast (rubriblast)
  - Basophilic normoblast (prorubricyte)
  - Polychromatic normoblast (rubricyte)
  - Orthochromatic normoblast (metarubricyte)
  - Polychromatophilic erythrocyte (reticulocyte)
  - Mature erythrocyte

4.1.4 Leukopoiesis

- The production and development of leukocytes

4.1.4.1 Characteristics of developing cells

- Several morphologic changes occur in blood cells as they mature
  - Cell size
    - Decreases as cells mature
  - Nucleus
    - Size
      - N:C ratio decreases, resulting in smaller nucleus
    - Shape
      - Nucleus may change shape, becoming lobulated or segmented
  - Chromatin pattern
    - Chromatin becomes clumped and condensed
  - Presence of nucleoli
    - Nucleoli disappear
  - Cytoplasm
    - Color changes from dark blue to lighter blue-gray to blue depending on cell type
    - Azurophilic (primary, nonspecific) granules seen in some cell types
    - Secondary (specific) granules develop in granulocytes

4.1.4.2 Granulopoiesis

- The production & development of granulocytes
- Key regulatory factors
  - Granulocyte macrophage-colony-stimulating factor (GM-CSF)
  - Granulocyte-colony-stimulating factor (G-CSF)
  - Eosinophils: IL-5
  - Basophils: IL-3/4
- Bone marrow location of developing cells
  - Produced close to trabeculae & arterioles in the bone marrow
- Maturation sequence
  - Neutrophils
    - Myeloblast
    - Promyelocyte
    - Myelocyte
    - Metamyelocyte (juvenile)
    - Band (stab)
    - Segmented (polymorphonuclear) neutrophil
  - Eosinophils
    - Maturation stages same as neutrophils
    - Morphologically recognizable at myelocyte stage
    - Last stage is mature eosinophil
  - Basophils
    - Maturation stages same as neutrophils
    - Morphologically recognizable at myelocyte stage
    - Last stage is mature basophil

4.1.4.3 Lymphopoiesis

- The production & development of lymphocytes
- Key regulatory factors
  - IL-2, IL-4, IL-7, IL-10, IL-12, IL-15
- Location of developing cells
  - Bone marrow, thymus, lymph nodes & spleen all serve as locations for lymphoid development
    - Primary lymphoid tissues
      - Fetal liver
      - Bone marrow for B lymphocytes
      - Thymus for T lymphocytes
    - Secondary lymphoid tissues
      - Spleen
      - Lymph nodes
      - Gut-associated lymphoid tissue

ISBN 978-089189-6616

- Maturation sequence
  - Lymphoblast
  - Prolymphocyte
  - Lymphocyte

4.1.4.4 Monopoiesis

- The production & development of monocytes
- Key regulatory factors
  - Granulocyte macrophage-colony-stimulating factor (GM-CSF)
  - IL-3
  - M-CSF
- Locations of developing cells
  - Monocytes
    - Mature & develop in the bone marrow
  - Macrophages
    - Monocytes migrate to tissues and become macrophages (histiocytes)
- Maturation sequence for monocytes
  - Monoblast
  - Promonocyte
  - Monocyte

4.1.5 Megakaryopoiesis

- The production & development of platelets
- Key regulatory factors
  - TPO
  - IL-11
- Location of developing cells
  - Bone marrow, near sinusoidal endothelial cells
- Maturation sequence
  - Megakaryoblast
  - Promegakaryocyte
  - Megakaryocyte with granules
  - Megakaryocyte (releases individual platelets)

4.1.6 Collection & evaluation of bone marrow samples

- Aspiration
  - Approximately 1.0-1.5 μL of aspirate needed to evaluate bone marrow morphology
  - Assessed for marrow spicules
  - Used to make smears for differential cell count (500 cell count)
- Core biopsy
  - Used to make touch preparations (preps)
  - Assesses marrow cellularity & architecture
- Myeloid-to-erythroid (M:E) ratio
  - May be determined from the bone marrow differential count
  - 2:1-4:1 in a normal adult

4.2 Role of the spleen

- Culling/filtration
  - Destruction of erythrocytes lacking proper deformability
  - Erythrocytes (6-8 μm) must stretch 117% of their capability throughout some of the circulatory vessels
  - Destruction of erythrocytes that lack functioning membrane proteins (spectrin, actin)
  - Destruction of normal aging red cells
- Pitting
  - Cytoplasmic inclusion removed
  - Antibody sheared from antibody-coated red cells (spherocytes created)
  - Intracellular parasites removed
- Immunologic (see chapter 8 Immunology)
  - Spleen is the largest secondary lymphoid organ
  - Opsonizing antibodies produced by spleen
  - Encapsulated organisms (*Haemophilus influenza, Neisseria meningitidis, Streptococcus pneumoniae*) are vulnerable to opsonizing antibodies
  - Capsule is stripped from bacterial surface by phagocytosis
  - Unencapsulated bacteria are susceptible to destruction by the reticuloendothelial system
- Storage
  - Spleen harbors 1/3 of platelet & granulocyte volume
  - Splenectomy may precipitate unwanted thrombotic complications as excess platelets pour into vessels as a result of splenic removal

4.3 Erythrocyte structure & function

4.3.1 Membrane composition

- RBC membrane is composed of 50% protein, 40% phospholipid & 10% cholesterol

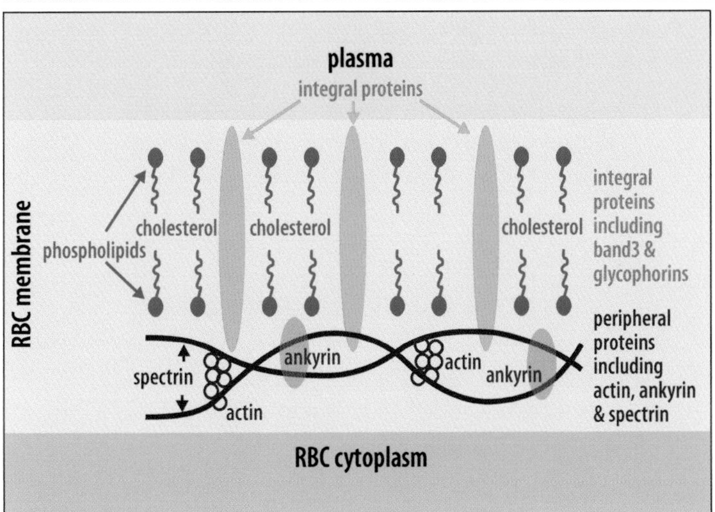

f4.1 RBC membrane structure

- Protein matrix has 2 types of protein: integral & peripheral **f4.1**
- Integral proteins expand through membrane and support active and passive transport of electrolytes as well as positioning 30 red cell antigens on glycophorin A, B & C
- Peripheral proteins are located on internal (cytoplasmic) side of the membrane and manage red cell deformability through spectrin, ankyrin & actin

4.3.2 Function

- The primary function of red cells is oxygen delivery to tissues through hemoglobin
- Passive process requiring no energy
- Red cells originate through pluripotent stem cells under the influence of the human cytokine, erythropoietin (EPO), secreted by the kidneys
- Six red cell stages are recognized
- The reticulocyte & mature red cells are anucleated
- Hemoglobin formation begins at the basophilic normoblast stage in the bone marrow and the RBC is fully hemogobinized at the reticulocyte stage
- In Wright-stained smears, reticuloctyes are recognized as polychromatic macrocytes
- The reticulocyte count is an excellent indicator of the bone marrow response to anemic conditions

4.3.3 Metabolic pathways

- Embden-Meyerhof
  - 90% of adenosine triphosphate (ATP) generated anaerobically
- Hexose monophosphate shunt
  - Produces NADPH from NAD so that red cells are protected from degradation
- Methemoglobin reductase
  - Maintains iron in the Fe+2 state for effective iron delivery
- Luebering-Rapaport
  - Causes 2,3-DPG to be stored for oxygen affinity (2,3-DPG decreases oxygen affinity)

4.4 Hemoglobin synthesis

4.4.1 Heme synthesis

- Iron absorption & transport
  - Four iron atoms in each hemoglobin molecule
  - Iron in the +2 state to bind oxygen
- Protoporphyrin formation
  - Final product in hemoglobin synthesis
- Insertion of iron
  - Transferrin receptors in the pronormoblast bind iron for incorporation during erythropoiesis

4.4.2 Globin synthesis

- Genetic control
  - Chromosome 11 has 1 gene each for the production of ε, β, γ, and δ chains
  - Chromosome 16 has 3 genes for the production of α (2) and ζ (1) chains
- Globin chain structure
  - Primary
    - α chains have 141 amino acids
    - β chains have 146 amino acids

4.4.3 Normal hemoglobins

- Molecular structure
  - Embryonic
    - Hemoglobin Gower: $\zeta_2\varepsilon_2$
    - Hemoglobin Portland: $\gamma_2\zeta_2$
  - Adult
    - Hemoglobin A: $\alpha_2\beta_2$
    - Hemoglobin A_2: $\alpha_2\delta_2$
    - Hemoglobin F: $\alpha_2\gamma_2$ (after 6 months)
- Reference values
  - Newborns
    - Hemoglobin F ≥60%
  - Adults
    - Hemoglobin A: 95%-98%
    - Hemoglobin A_2: 3%-5%
    - Hemoglobin F: ≤2%

4.4.4 Abnormal hemoglobin derivatives

- Etiology
  - Formation of physiologic abnormal hemoglobin may arise from inherited defects, unhealthy working or home conditions, or toxicity
- Carboxyhemoglobin
  - Affinity for oxygen is 200 times higher than normal
  - Oxygen not delivered
  - Can be fatal
- Methemoglobin
  - Iron in ferric state (Fe^{+3}), individuals are cyanotic
  - Hemoglobin M is inherited condition
- Sulfhemoglobin
  - Affinity for oxygen is 100 times more than normal
  - Toxic to humans

4.5 Leukocyte function

4.5.1 Granulocytes

- Phagocytosis (neutrophils)
  - Important in host defense
  - Occurs primarily in tissues
  - Neutrophils activated by chemokines migrate through tissue (chemotaxis)
  - Neutrophils recognize & attach to foreign bacteria
  - Killing and/or degranulation occurs after bacteria are ingested
- Allergic response & defense against parasites (eosinophils)
  - Eosinophils downregulate allergic responses by neutralizing products from basophils & mast cells
  - Several proteins released from eosinophils are toxic for larval parasites (like major basic protein
- Hypersensitivity mediators (eosinophils & basophils)
  - Both eosinophils & basophils have receptors for IgE
  - Cell activation and resulting degranulation release enzymes important in hypersensitivity reactions
  - Basophils especially are mediators of immediate hypersensitivity reactions

4.5.2 Lymphocytes

- Humoral immunity
  - Antigen-activated B lymphocytes (10%-20%) differentiate and mature into memory B cells and antibody-producing plasma cells
  - Antibodies assist in defense against microorganisms
- Cellular immunity
  - T lymphocytes (60%-80%) protect against microorganisms which evade contact with antibodies
  - This function depends on interaction with various antigen-presenting cells which activate T cells (such as macrophages & dendritic cells)
  - T cells can also secrete cytokines which can stimulate other cells like B cells & macrophages
- Cytotoxicity
  - A function of natural killer (NK) cells
  - NK cells (<20%) directly attack other cells infected with microorganisms and sometimes tumor cells
  - NK cells activated by various cytokines and also produce many cytokines

4.5.3 Monocytes

- Phagocytosis
  - Ingestion & killing of microorganisms
- Antigen presenting
  - Process & display antigens to T lymphocytes

4.6 Erythrocyte destruction

4.6.1 Extravascular hemolysis

- Represents majority (90%) of normal erythrocyte destruction (senescence is the term describing RBC aging)
- Location
  - Lysis of RBCs by macrophages in the spleen (and sometimes liver or bone marrow)
- Process
  - Often results when antibodies directed against RBCs (and sometimes activated complement) adhere to erythrocytes and then are removed by splenic macrophages
  - Another mechanism is the removal by macrophages of erythrocytes with inherited or acquired defects
- Key breakdown products
  - Hemoglobin in macrophages dissociates into heme, iron & globin
  - Amino acids in globin recycled to amino acid pool

    - Protoporphyrin ring broken
    - Iron in heme transported by transferrin to developing nucleated RBCs in bone marrow
    - Carbon monoxide excreted by lungs
    - Enzymes process biliverdin to bilirubin in liver and finally to urobilinogen (in urine & feces)

4.6.2 Intravascular hemolysis

- This represents only about 10% of normal erythrocyte destruction
- Location
    - Lysis of RBCs within the circulation
- Process
    - Results when complement is activated on the RBC membrane and lyses the erythrocytes
    - May also occur when RBCs experience physical or mechanical trauma that causes their destruction
    - Erythrocytes may encounter toxic substances in their environment, which results in lysis (such as bacteria or heat)
- Transport proteins
    - Free hemoglobin is released into plasma and is bound by various transport proteins
    - Hemoglobin-haptoglobin complex is transported to the liver for processing as occurs in extravascular hemolysis
    - When haptoglobin is depleted, hemopexin complexes with heme and transports it to the liver
    - Some heme is also bound by albumin to form methemalbumin, which stores heme until more haptoglobin or hemopexin are available
    - Some hemoglobin dissociates into α and β dimers that are filtered in the kidney as methemoglobin or stored as hemosiderin
    - Amino acids in globin are recycled to the amino acid pool

4.6.3 Laboratory findings in hemolysis

- t4.2 summarizes laboratory findings associated with intravascular & extravascular hemolysis

t4.2 Intravascular vs extravascular hemolysis

Intravascular hemolysis	Extravascular hemolysis
schistocytes ↑ LD ↓ haptoglobin ↑ free Hb, ↑ urine Hb hemosiderinuria	microspherocytes ↑ LD normal to ↓ haptoglobin ↑ indirect bilirubin ↑ urine & fecal urobilinogen

4.7 Diseases of erythrocytes

4.7.1 Anemia

4.7.1.1 Microcytic

- This is characterized by a decreased mean corpuscular volume (MCV)

4.7.1.1.1 Iron deficiency

- Etiology
    - Excessive loss
    - Increased requirements
    - Deficient intake
    - Defective absorption
- Pathophysiology
    - Iron major constituent of hemoglobin & many enzymes
    - Deficiency develops in stages & ranges in severity
- Laboratory findings t4.3

t4.3 Manifestations of iron deficiency

blood	microcytosis (↓ MCV) hypochromia (↓ MCH) anemia anisocytosis (↑ RDW) poikilocytosis (pencil cells) thrombocytosis
marrow	↓ iron stores mild erythroid hyperplasia
chemistries	↑ zinc protoporphyrin (ZPP) ↓ iron ↑ total iron binding capacity (TIBC) ↓ iron saturation ↓ ferritin iron deficiency anemia

MCH = mean corpuscular hemoglobin; MCV = mean corpuscular volume; RDW = red blood cell distribution width

    - Peripheral blood i4.1
        - Microcytic, hypochromic RBCs (decreased MCV & mean corpuscular hemoglobin [MCH])
        - Anisocytosis (increased red cell distribution width [RDW])
        - Abnormal RBC shapes (pencil cells/elliptocytes) & some target cells
            - Sometimes thrombocytosis
        - Abnormal chemistry & whole blood findings
            - Increased zinc protoporphyrin (ZPP) & free erythrocyte protoporphyrin (FEP; not routinely performed)
            - Decreased serum iron
            - Increased total iron-binding capacity (TIBC)
            - Decreased iron saturation
            - Decreased ferritin
            - Decreased reticulocytes (relative & absolute)
            - Decreased immature reticulocyte fraction (IRF)
            - Decreased reticulocyte hemoglobin content (CHr/RetHe)

ISBN 978-089189-6616

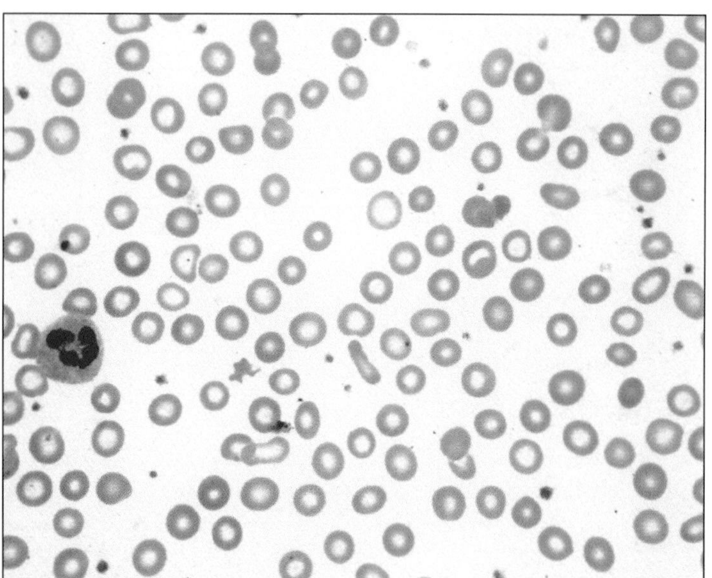

i4.1 Iron deficiency anemia; higher magnification image, showing hypochromic red cells & frequent thin elliptocytes (pencil cells)

- Bone marrow
  - Decreased iron stores
  - Slight erythroid hyperplasia

4.7.1.1.2 Thalassemia

- Etiology
  - Genetic
  - Quantitative decrease in production of globin chains needed for hemoglobin synthesis (hemoglobin molecule structurally normal)
  - Common in the Mediterranean area, Africa & Southeast Asia
  - Incidence parallels malaria belt
  - Classified according to specific globin chain with reduced production
  - Two α genes are located on each chromosome 16 (total 4 α genes inherited)
  - Four clinical conditions possible depending on how many α genes affected (1-4)
  - α^0 genes produce no α-globin chain and α^+ genes produce decreased amounts of α-globin chains
  - One β gene is located on each chromosome 11 (total 2 β genes inherited)
  - β^0 genes result in no production of any β globin chains
  - β^+ genes result in decreased production of β globin chains
- Heterozygous vs homozygous
  - α thalassemia (4 clinical conditions)
    - α^+/α (α-thal-2 or –α/αα) is a heterozygous condition also called the silent carrier; only 1 α gene deleted and patients are asymptomatic
    - α^+/α^+ (α-thal-2, –α/–α or α-thal-minor) is a homozygous condition; 2 of 4 α genes affected and produce decreased α-globin chain; patients are asymptomatic with a mild anemia to include microcytic, hypochromic RBCs
    - α^0/α (α-thal-1, ––/αα or α-thal-minor) is a heterozygous condition; 2 of 4 α genes affected; patients are asymptomatic with a mild anemia to include microcytic, hypochromic RBCs
    - α^0/α^+ (α-thal-1/α-thal-2 or ––/–α) is a heterozygous condition also called hemoglobin H (HbH) disease; 3 of 4 α genes are deleted; patients have a moderately severe hemolytic anemia with microcytic, hypochromic RBCs
    - α^0/α^0 (α-thal-1 or ––/––) is a homozygous condition also called hydrops fetalis, a fatal hemolytic anemia of fetuses & newborns
  - β thalassemia (major & minor)
    - β^0/β^0 or β^+/β^+ is a homozygous condition resulting in no production or marked decreased production of β chains; patients have severe microcytic, hypochromic anemia
    - β^0/β^+, β^0/β, or β^+/β is a heterozygous condition in which some β chain is produced; patients have no or variable anemia depending on the level of β chain production
- Pathophysiology
  - α thalassemia
    - Decreased production of α chains results in formation of hemoglobin tetramers
    - β_4 is HbH (5%-40%)
    - HbH inclusions may be seen and represent denatured hemoglobin
    - Visualized using supravital stain
    - γ_4 is hemoglobin Bart
    - HbH and HbBart ineffective as oxygen carriers
  - β thalassemia
    - Decreased production of β chains results in increased hemoglobin A_2 (HbA_2) & hemoglobin F (HbF) levels
    - Excess free α chains still exist and precipitate in RBCs, causing hemolysis and ineffective erythropoiesis

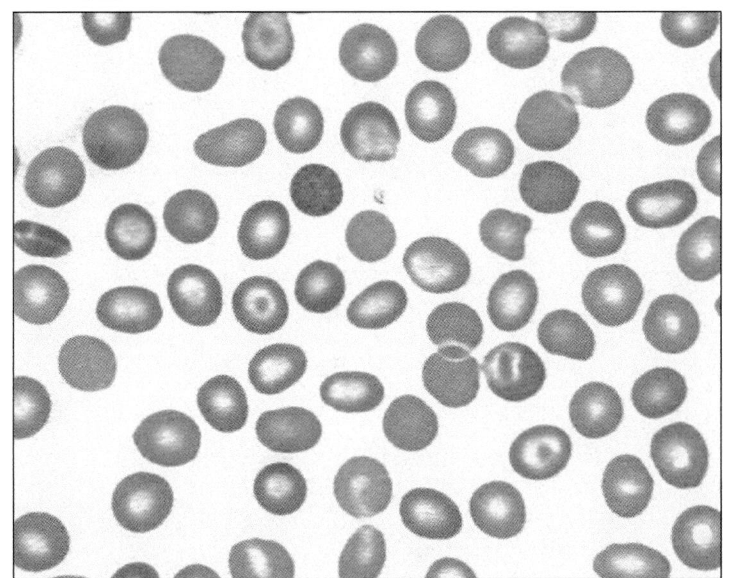

i4.2 Thalassemia blood smear; red cells are microcytic & there are numerous target cells

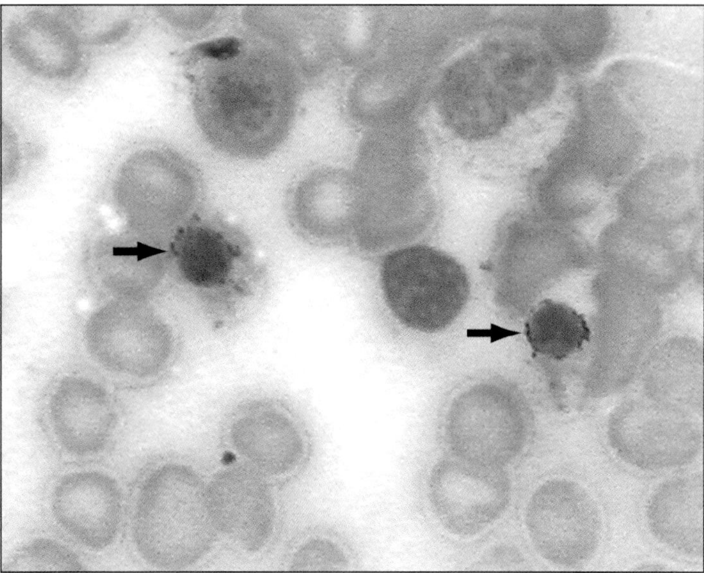

i4.3 Ringed sideroblasts (arrows)

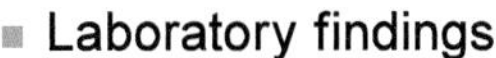

- Laboratory findings
  - Increased RBC count
  - Decreased MCV (65-75 fL in α thalassemia, 55-65 fL in β thalassemia)
  - Decreased hemoglobin & hematocrit (depending on classification)
  - Peripheral blood RBC changes may include anisocytosis, poikilocytosis, nucleated RBCs, basophilic stippling, polychromasia, target cells, microcytosis & hypochromia i4.2
  - Abnormal hemoglobin electrophoresis (often increased HbA_2 and HbF in β thalassemia and HbH and HbBart in α thalassemia)
  - Increased reticulocyte count
- Other findings
  - Massive bone marrow expansion results in bone changes & skeletal deformities
  - Splenomegaly & hypersplenism common
  - Transfusion-dependent patients can develop iron overload & iron chelators must be used in treatment

4.7.1.1.3 Sideroblastic

- Etiology
  - May be inherited or acquired and caused by either mutations in heme synthetic enzymes or impaired activity of heme
  - Inherited forms rare with X-linked inheritance
  - Acquired forms include myelodysplastic syndromes (MDSs), medications (isoniazid, chloramphenicol, chemotherapy), irradiation, copper deficiency, and alcohol abuse
- Pathophysiology
  - Enzymatic defect in heme synthesis results in excess iron accumulation in mitochondria & developing RBCs
- Laboratory findings
  - Peripheral blood
    - Hypochromic RBCs that may be microcytic (usually inherited forms), normocytic, or macrocytic (usually acquired forms)
    - Dimorphic (bimodal) population of RBCs commonly seen in inherited forms
    - Basophilic stippling & Pappenheimer bodies
    - Moderate to severe anemia (hemoglobin 6-10 g/dL [60-100 g/L])
    - Increased serum iron, elevated transferrin saturation, increased ferritin, decreased TIBC
  - Bone marrow
    - Increased ringed sideroblasts i4.3
    - Increased iron stores
    - Erythroid hyperplasia with mild dyserythropoiesis possible
  - Lead poisoning
    - Lead inhibits several enzymes in hemoglobin synthetic pathway
    - Laboratory findings similar to sideroblastic anemia
    - Mild to moderate anemia (hemoglobin 8-13 g/dL [80-130 g/L])
    - Microcytic, hypochromic RBCs
    - Basophilic stippling (coarse)
    - Erythroid hyperplasia & ringed sideroblasts in bone marrow

ISBN 978-089189-6616

4.7.1.1.4 Chronic inflammation (anemia of chronic disease)

- Etiology
  - Common cause of anemia in hospitalized patients
  - Associated with infections, inflammatory or malignant conditions (rheumatoid arthritis, collagen vascular diseases, osteomyelitis & chronic kidney disease)
- Pathophysiology
  - Defective iron utilization (iron is trapped in macrophages and is unavailable to developing RBCs) mediated by hepcidin
  - Ineffective erythropoietin production results in inadequate RBC response
  - Direct suppression of erythropoiesis by cytokines
  - Possible decreased erythrocyte survival because of overactive macrophages or hemolytic factors released from tumors
  - RBC sensitivity to erythropoietin suppressed
- Laboratory findings **t4.4**
  - Normocytic or microcytic anemia (hemoglobin usually only 1-2 g/dL [10-20 g/L] below normal)
  - Anisocytosis
  - Serum iron is normal to decreased with normal to decreased TIBC, transferrin saturation is >15%, serum soluble transferrin receptor is normal, ferritin is normal to increased
  - Decreased reticulocyte count
  - Increased iron stores in bone marrow
  - Must be distinguished from iron-deficiency anemia

t4.4 Anemia of chronic disease vs iron deficiency anemia

	Serum iron	TIBC	% transferrin saturation	SSTR	Ferritin
IDA	↓	↑	<10%	↑	↓
ACD	Normal to ↓	Normal to ↓	>15%	Normal	Normal to ↑

ACD = anemia of chronic disease; IDA = iron deficiency anemia; SSTR = serum soluble transferrin receptor; TIBC = total iron binding capacity

4.7.1.2 Macrocytic

- This is characterized by an elevated MCV

4.7.1.2.1 Megaloblastic

- Common causes of macrocytosis are the megaloblastic anemias, of which vitamin B_{12} and folate are both needed for normal DNA synthesis
- Megaloblasts are large RBC precursors with basophilic cytoplasm and fine, particulate chromatin; a nuclear-to-cytoplasmic asynchrony is often present
- Vitamin B_{12} & folate deficiencies **t4.5, t4.6**
  - Etiology
    - The etiologies of vitamin B_{12} & folate deficiencies are summarized in **t4.5**

t4.5 Causes of folate & vitamin B_{12} deficiency

	Folate deficiency	B_{12} deficiency
diet	common (alcoholics)	rare (strict vegetarians)
malabsorption	sprue	pernicious anemia postgastrectomy pancreatic insufficiency Crohn disease *Diphyllobothrium latum* infestation
increased demand	pregnancy hemolysis	pregnancy hemolysis
drugs	methotrexate	dilantin
inherited	none	transcobalamin II deficiency

t4.6 Manifestations of folate & vitamin B_{12} deficiency

peripheral blood		oval macrocytosis hypersegmented neutrophils pancytopenia (when severe) anisopoikilocytosis (variable)
bone marrow		hypercellularity megaloblastic changes erythroid hyperplasia with left shift
chemistry	folate deficiency	↑ LD & indirect bilirubin ↓ serum & RBC folate ↑ urinary FIGLU (formiminoglutamic acid)
	B_{12} deficiency	↑ LD & indirect bilirubin ↓ serum B_{12} ↑ urinary methylmalonic acid ↓ RBC folate (2/3 of cases)

LD = lactate dehydrogenase; RBC = red blood cell

  - Pathophysiology: Vitamin B_{12}
    - Ingested in animal products, transported to the stomach and then duodenum, where bound to gastric derived intrinsic factor (IF)
    - IF-bound B_{12} is absorbed in the ileum and is exported to the bloodstream
    - B_{12} is a cofactor for conversion of methyl folate to the active form tetrahydrofolate (THF); in B_{12} deficiency, methyl folate accumulates (the "methyl folate trap"); DNA synthesis & nuclear maturation impaired

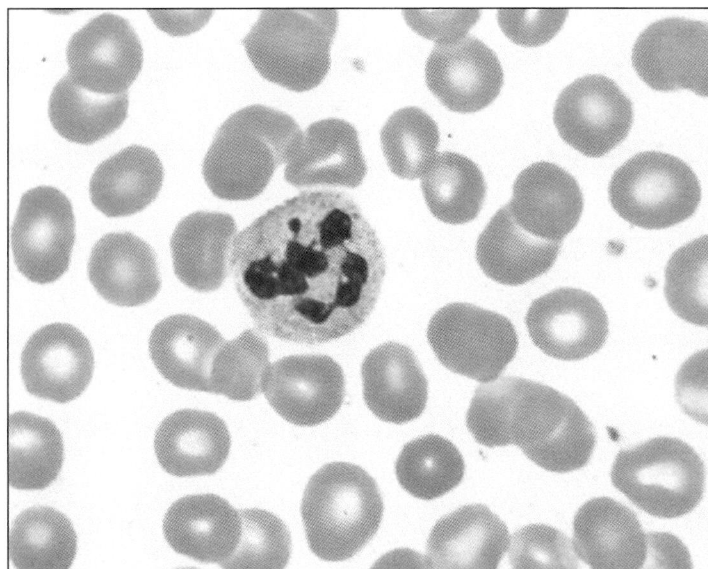

i4.4 Megaloblastic anemia; note hypersegmented neutrophil & numerous oval macrocytes

- B_{12} is also a cofactor for methylmalonyl coenzyme A (CoA) mutase, which converts methylmalonyl CoA to succinyl CoA; in B_{12} deficiency, methylmalonyl CoA accumulates

- Pathophysiology: Folate
  - Ingested in green vegetables, absorbed in jejunum, and released from enterocytes as methyl folate
  - Converted in cells to THF by a B_{12}-dependent methyltransferase
  - THF acts as a cofactor in methyl transfer reactions like conversion of deoxyuridilate (dUMP) to deoxythymidylate (dTMP)
  - Folate deficiency leads to impaired DNA synthesis & impaired nuclear maturation
- Laboratory findings **t4.6**
  - Peripheral blood i4.4
    - Increased MCV(>115 fL in fully developed megaloblastic anemia)
    - Decreased hemoglobin, hematocrit, RBC
    - Pancytopenia
    - Decreased reticulocyte count
    - Macro-ovalocytes
    - Anisocytosis & poikilocytosis
    - RBC inclusions to include Howell-Jolly bodies & basophilic stippling
    - Hypersegmented neutrophils
    - Decrease in vitamin B_{12}, increase in methylmalonic acid & plasma total homocysteine in vitamin B_{12} deficiency
    - Decrease in serum & RBC folate, increase in formiminoglutamic acid associated with folate deficiency
    - Increase in lactate dehydrogenase (LD) & indirect bilirubin levels
  - Bone marrow
    - Megaloblasts
    - Hypercellularity
    - Giant leukocyte precursors

4.7.1.2.2 Nonmegaloblastic

- Etiology
  - Macrocytosis may occur unrelated to a vitamin B_{12} or folate deficiency (nonmegaloblastic) in alcoholism, liver disease, and hemolytic anemia
- Pathophysiology
  - Mechanisms include:
    - Alcoholism that causes direct damage to erythroid precursors
    - Liver disease in which RBC membrane lipids are increased and accumulate on RBCs, increasing their surface area relative to volume
    - Hemolytic anemia that stimulates increased erythropoietin and the early release of reticulocytes from the bone marrow; reticulocytes are larger than mature RBCs
- Laboratory findings
  - Mild macrocytosis
  - Polychromasia
  - RBCs are round, not oval
  - No hypersegmented neutrophils are seen and no other megaloblastic changes in peripheral blood or bone marrow

4.7.1.3 Normocytic

- Characterized by a normal mean corpuscular volume (MCV)

4.7.1.3.1 Hereditary hemolytic

- Inherited defects intrinsic to the RBC result in shortened survival

4.7.1.3.1.1 Membrane disorders

- Inherited abnormalities in the erythrocyte membrane
- Hereditary spherocytosis
  - Etiology
    - Most commonly autosomal dominant inheritance pattern but sometimes autosomal recessive
    - Defects in RBC membrane composition most often affecting ankyrin (*ANK1* gene), band 3 (*SLC4A1* gene), and spectrin (*SPTB* gene)
  - Pathophysiology
    - Defects diminish the elasticity & deformability of the RBC membrane

ISBN 978-089189-6616

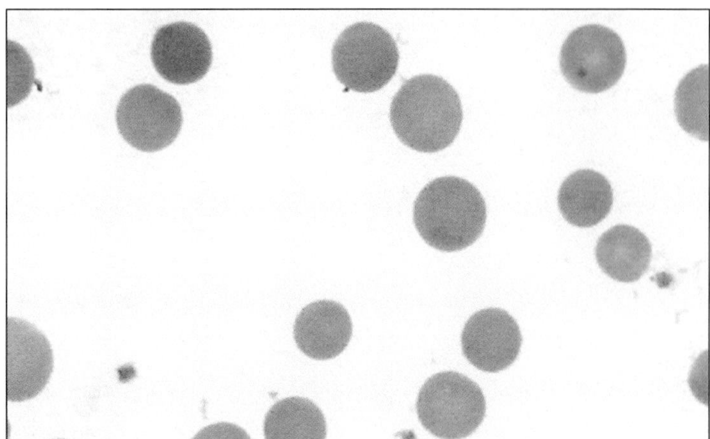

i4.5 Spherocytes are red cells lacking central pallor; artifact is a common cause, but true spherocytes are most often seen in autoimmune hemolytic anemia & hereditary spherocytosis

- RBCs have decreased surface to volume ratio, become more rigid, have decreased survival, and are trapped and removed by the spleen (splenomegaly classic symptom)
- Laboratory findings
  - Increased mean corpuscular hemoglobin concentration (MCHC) in 50% of patients
  - Spherocytes & polychromasia on peripheral blood smear i4.5
  - Increased lactate dehydrogenase (LD) & bilirubin
  - Decreased eosin-5-maleimide (EMA) binding test (band 3 reduction test)
  - Increased osmotic fragility
  - Negative result on the direct antiglobulin test (DAT) (spherocytes not caused by immune-mediated process)
- Hereditary elliptocytosis (HE) i4.6a
  - Etiology
    - Autosomal dominant disorder caused by mutations in the spectrin α chain, affecting RBC membrane
    - Diagnosed when >25% of circulating RBCs are elliptocytes (elliptocytes are twice as long as they are wide)
    - Several morphologic subtypes
      - Common HE has elliptocytes; clinical severity from patients who are asymptomatic to severe hemolytic anemia
      - Spherocytic HE is characterized by the presence of not only elliptocytes, but spherocytes; rare form but results in hemolysis
      - Stomatocytic HE (Southeast Asian ovalocytosis) results in either no hemolysis or only mild hemolysis; elliptocytes may appear more roundish and stomatocytic; associated with protection against malaria (primarily *Plasmodium vivax*)

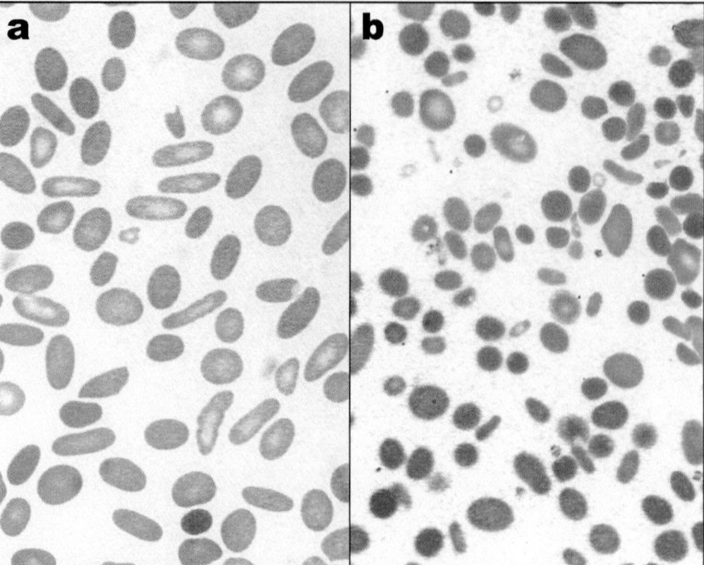

i4.6 Elliptocytes are red cells that are twice as long as they are wide
a While they are the hallmark of hereditary elliptocytosis, they are usually seen (in small numbers) in iron deficiency anemia & myelodysplasia
b Hereditary pyropoikilocytosis

  - Pathophysiology
    - Several protein abnormalities disrupt normal membrane structure, especially in horizontal interactions between the proteins & membrane cytoskeleton
      - Spectrin dimers have decreased ability to associate into tetramers because of defective spectrin
      - Band 4.1 is abnormal and impairs spectrin binding to actin within the membrane
    - Vertical defects in the membrane as related to glycophorin, ankyrin, and band 3 may also occur
  - Laboratory findings
    - Elliptocytosis >25%
    - Slightly elevated reticulocyte count
    - Spherocytes in spherocytic HE
    - Some stomatocytes in stomatocytic HE
- Hereditary pyropoikilocytosis i4.6b
  - Etiology
    - Autosomal recessive disorder associated with both a deficiency of and defects in spectrin
    - Severe subtype of HE
  - Pathophysiology
    - Spectrin deficiency and defects in spectrin destabilize the RBC membrane
    - RBCs fragment & crenate
  - Laboratory findings
    - Marked RBC morphologic abnormalities to include fragments, budding, microspherocytes, elliptocytes & other bizarre poikilocytes

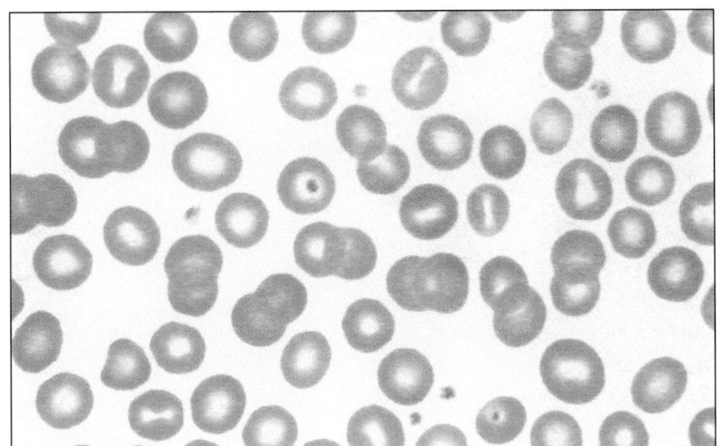

i4.7 Stomatocytes

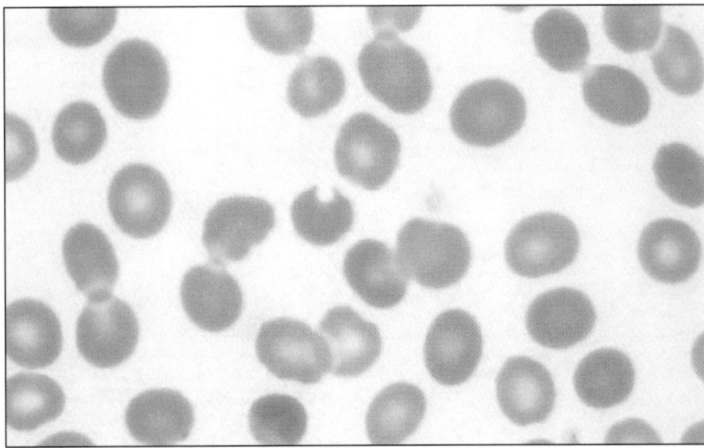

i4.8 Bite cells

- Markedly decreased MCV
- RBCs have increased and unusual sensitivity to heat
- Hereditary stomatocytosis i4.7
  - Etiology
    - Autosomal dominant disorder associated with impaired production of stomatin in the RBC membrane
  - Pathophysiology
    - Decreased stomatin causes the RBC to have abnormal cation (sodium/potassium) permeability
    - Increased intracellular cations allow water influx into cell, with formation of stomatocytes
    - Two main types
      - Severe hydrocytotic (overhydrated)
      - Xerocytotic
  - Laboratory findings
    - Both types associated with decreased hemoglobin & hematocrit, increase in reticulocytes, and stomatocytes
    - Severe hydrocytotic
      - Macrocytosis
      - Increased MCV
      - Decreased MCHC
    - Xerocytotic
      - RBCs with hemoglobin puddled at cell's periphery
      - Target cells
      - Increased MCV
      - Increased MCHC
- Paroxysmal nocturnal hemoglobinuria (PNH)
  - Acquired clonal hematopoietic stem cell disorder
  - Blood cell membranes lack glycosylphosphatidyl inositol (GPI)–anchored proteins
  - Missing GPI-anchored proteins (CD55, CD59) on RBCs results in increased susceptibility to complement lysis and intravascular hemolysis occurs
  - Flow cytometry typically used to detect absence of GPI-anchored proteins on WBCs
  - Methods include a fluorescein-labeled proaerolysin variant (FLAER) as well as monoclonal antibodies to GPI-anchored lineage-specific antigens
  - Combined methods sensitive for diagnosis of PNH

4.7.1.3.1.2 Enzyme disorders

- Glucose-6-phosphate dehydrogenase (G6PD) deficiency
  - Etiology
    - Sex-linked disorder seen primarily in boys & men
    - Associated with African Americans & individuals of Mediterranean descent
    - Hundreds of variants, but 4 major genotypes
  - Pathophysiology
    - G6PD-deficient RBCs sensitive to oxidant stress (induced by medications like methylene blue, sulfa drugs, nitrofurantoin, primaquine, as well as fava beans & infection)
    - Oxidized hemoglobin precipitates as Heinz bodies (visualized with supravital stains)
    - Heinz bodies are pitted by splenic macrophages, producing blister & bite cells i4.8
  - Laboratory findings
    - Peripheral blood changes include poikilocytosis with bite cells
    - Polychromasia
    - Possibly spherocytes
    - Heinz bodies (supravital stain)
    - Positive fluorescent spot screening test
      - NADPH produced & fluoresces

ISBN 978-089189-6616

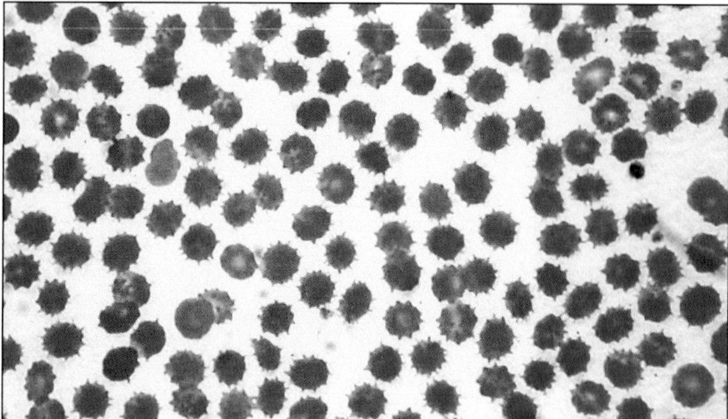

i4.9 Burr cells

- Confirm with G6PD quantitative assay
  - Note that fluorescent spot test & enzyme assay may be falsely normal immediately after a hemolytic crisis
  - Young RBCs (reticulocytes) have higher enzyme levels
- Pyruvate kinase deficiency
  - Etiology
    - Autosomal recessive inheritance
    - High frequency in northern Europe & Pennsylvania Amish
  - Pathophysiology
    - Pyruvate kinase (PK) catalyzes rate limiting step in the Embden-Meyerhof pathway to produce adenosine triphosphate for RBCs
    - PK deficient RBCs lack energy (ATP) for normal processes
  - Laboratory findings
    - Echinocytes (burr cells) on peripheral blood smear i4.9
    - Screen with fluorescent spot test which determines conversion of NADPH to NAD
    - NAD does not fluoresce and indicates PK is deficient
    - Confirm with PK quantitative assay

4.7.1.3.2 Immune hemolytic

- Increased RBC destruction by an antibody
- RBCs intrinsically normal
- Acquired condition
- Alloimmune
  - Etiology
    - Antibodies produced after exposure to foreign antigens from an individual of the same species
    - Donor RBCs have antigens recipient lacks
    - Antibodies produced against donor cells
    - Characteristically seen in:
      - Transfusion reactions
      - Pregnancy
      - Organ transplantation
        - Not common
        - Recipient exposed to foreign antigens on "passenger" RBCs that may be associated with organ transplant
  - Pathophysiology
    - Transfusion reactions: Immediate
      - Patient antibody to transfused cells activates complement
      - Intravascular hemolysis results
      - Most often seen in ABO blood group incompatibilities
      - IgM antibody produced
    - Transfusion reactions: Delayed
      - Patient previously sensitized to antigen
      - Transfused RBCs have antigen
      - Usually blood groups other than ABO
      - IgG antibody produced
      - Extravascular hemolysis results
    - Pregnancy (hemolytic disease of the newborn [HDN]) t4.7

t4.7 Selected characteristics of Rh vs ABO hemolytic disease of the newborn

	Rh	ABO
Blood group		
Mother	Rh negative	O
Infant	Rh positive	A or B
Severity	Severe	Mild
Spherocytes	Rare	Present
Anemia	Severe	Mild if present at all
Direct antiglobulin test (DAT)	Positive	Negative/weakly positive

- Rh incompatibility occurs when the mother is Rh negative and newborn (or fetus) is Rh positive
- The mother has prior sensitization and produces IgG antibodies
- Severe disorder
- Also occurs in ABO incompatibility
- The mother does not need prior sensitization
- Group O mother has a child with blood type A or B
- The mother "naturally" produces anti-A or anti-B
- Mild disorder

- Transfusion reactions: Laboratory findings
  - Immediate
    - Decreased hemoglobin & hematocrit
    - Normal RBC indices
    - Decreased haptoglobin

- Hemoglobinemia
- Hemoglobinuria
- Hemosiderinuria
- Increased LDH
- Increased bilirubin

- Delayed
  - Decreased hemoglobin & hematocrit
  - Normal RBC indices
  - Spherocytes
  - Increased bilirubin
  - Increased urobilinogen
  - Positive antibody screen
  - Positive DAT
- Pregnancy (HDN)
  - Rh:
    - Decreased hemoglobin & hematocrit
    - Erythroblastosis
    - Increased reticulocytes
    - Increased bilirubin
    - Positive DAT
    - Maternal antibodies present
    - Polychromasia
  - ABO:
    - Spherocytes
    - Polychromasia
    - Possibly schistocytes
    - Variable DAT
    - Increased reticulocytes

4.7.1.3.3 Autoimmune

- Failure to recognize individuals' red cell antigens
- Etiology
  - Autoantibodies are produced and may have serologic activity at body temperature (98.6°F [37°C]) (warm reacting) or less than body temperature (cold reacting)
  - Warm autoimmune hemolytic anemia (WAIHA) is the most common autoimmune hemolytic anemia (AIHA) and may be primary (or idiopathic) or secondary (70% of cases)
  - Secondary WAIHA may be associated with lymphoma, underlying systemic autoimmune disorders, or collagen vascular diseases, thymoma, and stem cell transplantation
  - Mechanism of antibody formation is unknown, but most antibodies are IgG
  - There are 3 types of cold AIHA (CAIHA)
    - Idiopathic cold AIHA (cold agglutinin syndrome) in which IgM antibodies with ant-I, anti-i, anti-H, anti-IH, or anti-Pr specificity are formed

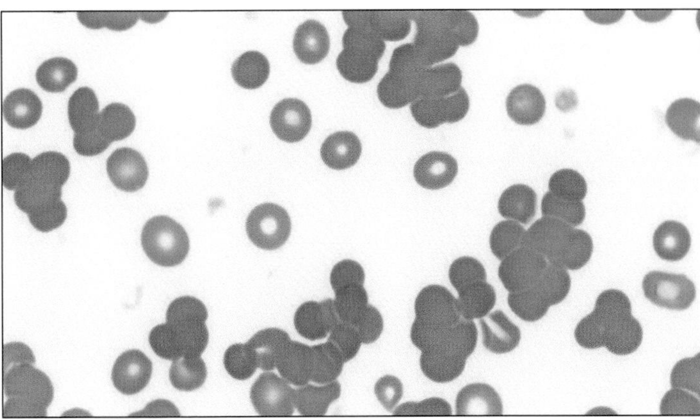

i4.10 Cold agglutinin syndrome; red cell clumps are the morphologic hallmark

    - Secondary cold AIHA is associated with *Mycoplasma pneumoniae* infection (anti-I) or Epstein-Barr virus-related infectious mononucleosis (anti-i)
    - Paroxysmal cold hemoglobinuria (PCH)
      - Uncommon and primarily affects children with viral illnesses such as measles, mumps, chickenpox & infectious mononucleosis
      - Mediated by the biphasic IgG Donath-Landsteiner antibody that has anti-P specificity
- Pathophysiology
  - Warm autoimmune hemolytic anemia
    - Antibodies bind to RBCs and act as opsonins that result in erythrocyte destruction by splenic macrophages
    - Hemolysis is extravascular
  - Cold autoimmune hemolytic anemia: Cold agglutinin syndrome i4.10
    - Agglutination & complement fixation occur in the extremities causing intravascular hemolysis
  - Cold autoimmune hemolytic anemia: Secondary
    - Immunologic response to antigen expressed by a microorganism that produces a cross-reacting antibody
    - Transient condition
  - Paroxysmal cold hemoglobinuria
    - The Donath-Landsteiner antibody reacts with RBCs at cold temperatures (39.2°F [4°C]), but hemolysis occurs when blood is subsequently warmed to 98.6°F (37°C)
- Laboratory findings
  - Warm autoimmune hemolytic anemia
    - Decreased hemoglobin & hematocrit
    - Positive DAT

- Spherocytes, polychromasia, possibly some schistocytes & nucleated RBCs on the peripheral blood smear
- Elevated reticulocyte count

- Cold autoimmune hemolytic anemia
  - Positive DAT if reagent contains anticomplement activity
  - Polychromasia, RBC agglutination on peripheral blood smear
- Paroxysmal cold hemoglobinuria
  - DAT positive with polyspecific antihuman globulin
  - Positive Donath-Landsteiner test

4.7.1.3.4 Nonimmune hemolytic anemia

- Premature destruction of intrinsically normal RBCs by infectious agents & mechanical factors
- Etiology
  - Infectious agents (see Microbiology 6.4.3.3)
    - Malarial parasites of *Plasmodium* spp
  - Mechanical factors
    - Microangiopathic hemolytic anemia (MAHA) resulting from deposition of fibrin in small vessels as seen in hemolytic uremic syndrome, thrombotic thrombocytopenic purpura, and disseminated intravascular coagulation
- Pathophysiology
  - Malaria
    - Hemolysis caused by the intracellular asexual multiplication of the parasite, action of splenic macrophages to remove parasites, and immune-mediated processes whereby antimalarial antibodies and complement attach to erythrocyte membranes with exposed malarial antigens
    - Hemolysis can be intravascular or extravascular
  - Microangiopathic hemolytic anemia
    - Lesions or microthrombi form in small vessels because of an abnormal activation of the coagulation system
    - Lesions impede blood flow through the microcirculation, producing enough traumatic stress to lyse RBCs
- Laboratory findings
  - Malaria
    - Normocytic, normochromic anemia
    - Intracellular parasites in RBCs
    - Signs of intravascular & extravascular hemolysis to include hemoglobinemia, hemoglobinuria, and increased bilirubin

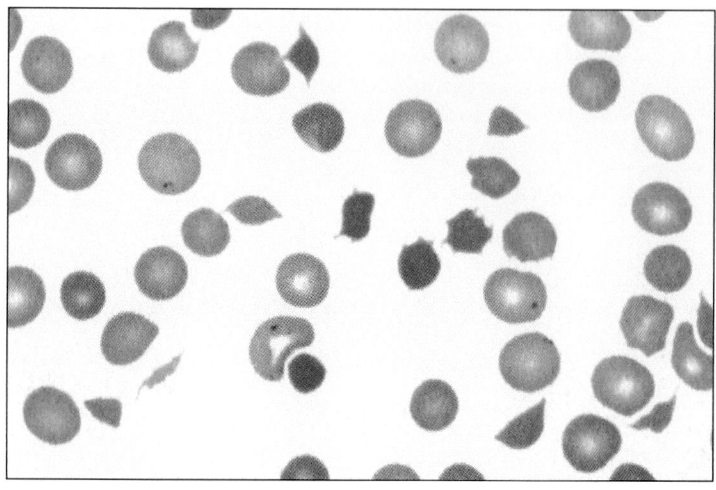

i4.11 Schistocytes

  - Microangiopathic hemolytic anemia
    - Normocytic, normochromic anemia
    - Thrombocytopenia
    - Schistocytes i4.11 & polychromasia on peripheral blood smear
    - Increase in reticulocytes

4.7.1.3.5 Hypoproliferative

- Disorder of blood cell production by the bone marrow resulting from hypoproliferation and failure of hematopoietic stem cell growth
- Major condition is aplastic anemia
- Etiology
  - Congenital
  - Acquired idiopathic
  - Acquired secondary to drugs, chemicals, radiation, or infectious agents
- Pathophysiology
  - Autoimmune process
    - Antibodies to hematopoietic precursor cells or stem cell modification stimulates autoantibody production
  - Direct damage to stem cells
  - Altered marrow microenvironment
  - T-cell suppression of hematopoiesis
  - Defects in DNA or DNA repair
- Laboratory findings
  - Bone marrow
    - Aspiration often results in dry tap
    - Hypocellular
  - Peripheral blood
    - Pancytopenia

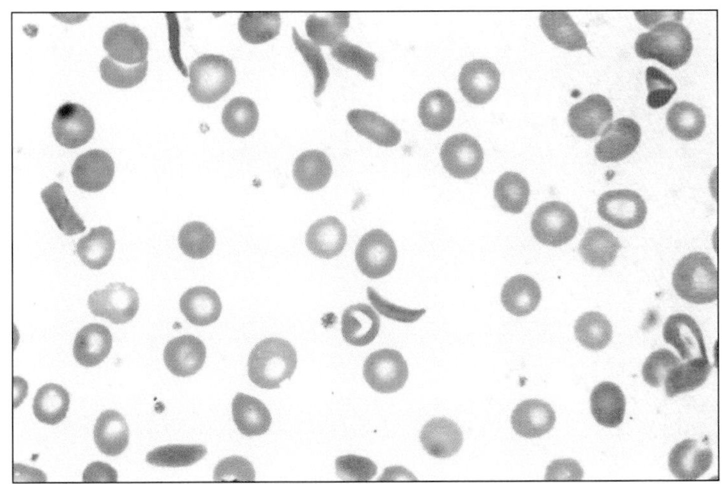

i4.12 Sickle cells

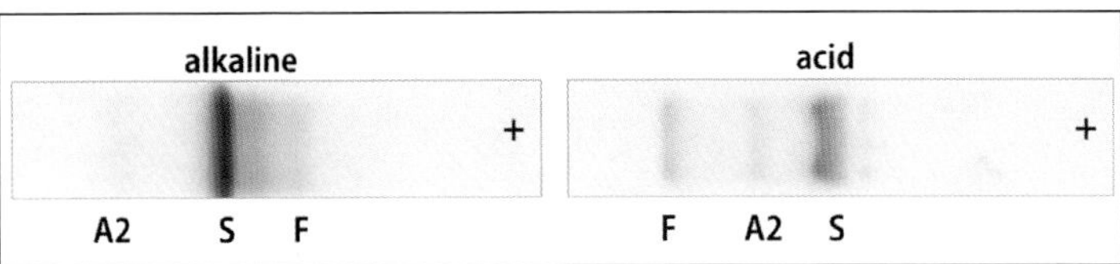

f4.2 Sickle cell disease as seen on alkaline gel in hemoglobin electrophoresis (left) & acid gel (right)

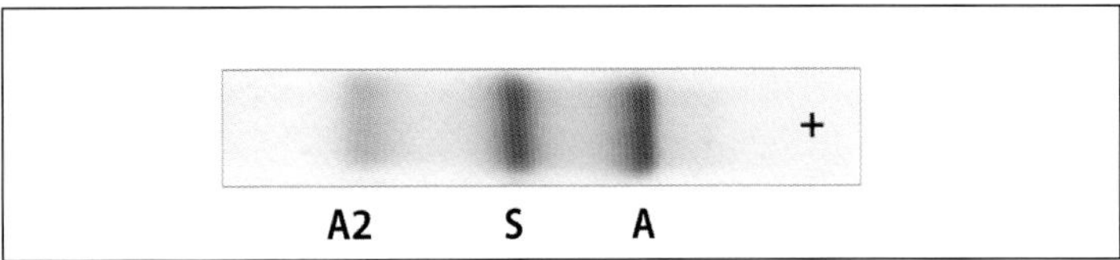

f4.3 Sickle cell trait as seen on alkaline gel

- Decreased hemoglobin & hematocrit
- Decreased corrected & absolute reticulocyte counts
- Sometimes immature granulocytes & macrocytes

4.7.1.3.6 Acute hemorrhage

- Etiology
  - Most common cause is blood loss through such conditions as traumatic injury, massive gastrointestinal bleeding, or ruptured ectopic pregnancy
- Pathophysiology
  - Sudden loss of RBCs reduces oxygen carrying capacity of blood
- Laboratory findings
  - Acute decrease in hemoglobin to ~7-8 g/dL (~70-80 g/L)
  - Decreased hematocrit to ~21%-24%

4.7.1.3.7 Hemoglobinopathies

4.7.1.3.7.1 Sickle cell anemia

- Genotype
  - Sickle cell disease is HbSS
- Pathophysiology
  - S allele has valine instead of glutamic acid at position 6 of the hemoglobin β chain (β6 glu→val)
  - Hemoglobin S abnormally polymerizes when deoxygenated and sufficiently concentrated (over 50%)
  - RBCs become rigid and less deformable, obstructing vessels & inhibiting oxygen delivery to tissues
  - RBCs have shortened survival with an average lifespan of 17 days
- Laboratory findings
  - Severe anemia (hemoglobin 5-9 g/dL [50-90 g/L])
  - Peripheral blood findings include:
    - Sickle cells i4.12
    - Anisocytosis
    - Target cells
    - Howell-Jolly bodies
    - Pappenheimer bodies
    - Polychromasia
    - Nucleated RBCs
  - Increased reticulocytes
  - Elevated white blood cells (WBCs) possible (leukocyte redistribution from marginating to circulating pool)
  - HbSS on electrophoresis (80%-95%) **f4.2**

4.7.1.3.7.2 Sickle cell trait

- Genotype
  - Sickle cell trait is expressed as HbAS
- Pathophysiology
  - Sickle cell trait is generally asymptomatic
- Laboratory findings
  - Normal complete blood cell count (CBC) and peripheral blood smear and patients are asymptomatic
  - Electrophoresis shows 35%-45% HbS **f4.3**

4.7.1.3.7.3 Hemoglobin C

- Genotype
  - Hemoglobin C disease is expressed as HbCC
- Pathophysiology
  - C allele has lysine instead of glutamic acid at position 6 of the hemoglobin β chain (β6 glu→lys)

ISBN 978-089189-6616

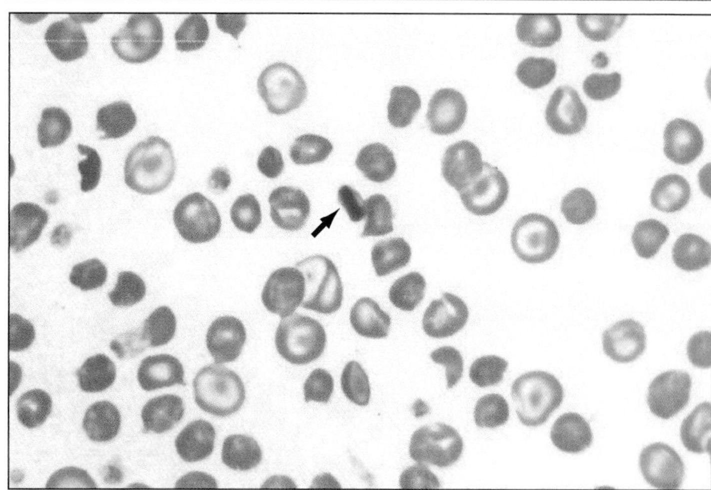

i4.13 Hemoglobin C disease (homozygous CC) peripheral blood smear, showing hemoglobin C crystal (arrow) & numerous target cells

- Hemoglobin C has decreased solubility
- Intracellular crystals form when RBCs are dehydrated or in hypertonic solutions
- RBCs with crystals are rigid and are trapped and removed by splenic macrophages

- Laboratory findings
  - Mild anemia (hemoglobin 8-12 g/dL [80-120 g/L])
  - Target cells i4.13
  - Hexagonal or rod-shaped crystals (hemoglobin C crystals) in RBCs, especially after splenectomy
  - Electrophoresis shows 90% hemoglobin C
    - Note that HbA_2, HbE & HbO_{Arab} migrate with HbC at alkaline pH)

4.7.1.3.7.4 Hemoglobin C trait

- Genotype
  - Hemoglobin C trait is expressed as HbAC
- Pathophysiology
  - Normal complete blood cell count (CBC) and patients are asymptomatic
- Laboratory findings
  - Some target cells on peripheral blood smear
  - Electrophoresis shows about 30%-40% hemoglobin C

4.7.1.3.7.5 Hemoglobin E

- Genotype
  - Hemoglobin E is expressed as HbEE
- Pathophysiology
  - E allele has lysine for glutamic acid at position 26 on the hemoglobin β chain
  - (β26 glu→lys)
  - Instability of hemoglobin E occurs under oxidant stress
  - Decreased hemoglobin E β chains also produced as a result of impaired messenger RNA processing related to the amino acid substitution
- Laboratory findings
  - Mild anemia
  - Mild microcytosis & hypochromia
    - Note that patients are usually asymptomatic
  - Target cells
  - Electrophoresis shows 90% hemoglobin E
    - Note that hemoglobin E migrates with HbA_2, HbC & HbO_{Arab} on alkaline electrophoresis

4.7.1.3.7.6 Hemoglobin E trait

- Genotype
  - Hemoglobin E trait is expressed as HbAE
- Pathophysiology
  - Hemoglobin E trait is asymptomatic
- Laboratory findings
  - Microcytic RBCs
  - Few target cells
  - Electrophoresis shows 30%-35% hemoglobin E

4.7.1.3.7.7 Hemoglobin SC disease

- Genotype
  - Both hemoglobin S & hemoglobin C present (patient is doubly heterozygous)
- Pathophysiology
  - Both β chains are abnormal but are substituted with 2 different amino acids
  - No hemoglobin A produced
  - Both hemoglobin polymerization & crystal formation occur
  - RBCs become rigid with shortened survival
- Laboratory findings
  - Moderate anemia (hemoglobin >8 g/dL [>80 g/L])
  - Peripheral blood smear i4.14
    - Target cells
    - Possible microcytic hypochromic RBCs, spherocytes and fragmented cells
    - "SC" cells (folded cells, cells with fingerlike projections, crystalloids & misshapen cells, all with hemoglobin precipitated in the cell)
    - Anisocytosis & poikilocytosis
    - Rare sickle cell & boat cell

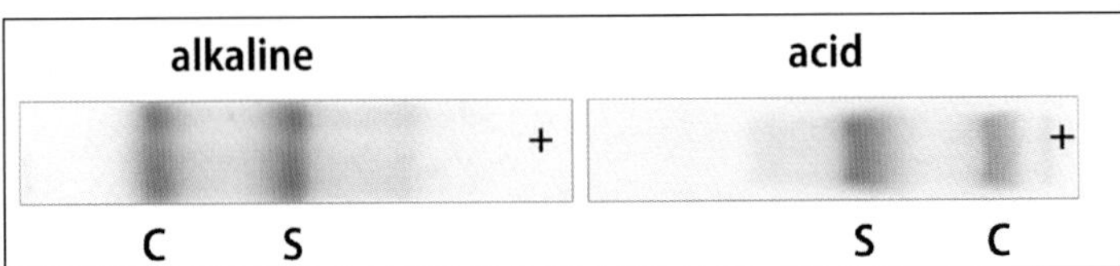

f4.4 Hemoglobin SC disease as seen in hemoglobin electrophoresis on alkaline gel (left) & acid gel (right)

- Electrophoresis shows 50%-55% HbS and 45%-50% HbC f4.4

4.7.1.3.7.8 Hemoglobin SC/β-thalassemia

- Genotype
  - Hemoglobin S can be combined with either β^0 or β^+ genes
  - Patient is doubly heterozygous for a quantitative & qualitative defect
- Pathophysiology
  - Hemoglobin S with β^o gene produces no β chain & no hemoglobin A
  - Hemoglobin S with β^+ gene produces some β chains (decreased amounts) and therefore some hemoglobin A
- Laboratory findings
  - S/β^0 thalassemia is a severe disease similar to sickle cell anemia
  - Peripheral blood findings
    - Sickle cells
    - Target cells
    - May see microcytosis & hypochromia
    - Pappenheimer bodies, Howell-Jolly bodies & basophilic stippling
    - Polychromasia
    - Nucleated RBCs
  - Hemoglobin decreased (5-10 g/dL)
  - Electrophoresis shows 80%-90% HbS, 1%-15% HbF, 4%-8% HbA_2
  - S/β^+ thalassemia may be more moderate in severity or asymptomatic depending on amount of hemoglobin A produced
    - Moderate anemia with hemoglobin 7-11 g/dL (70-110 g/L)
    - Peripheral blood smear displays possible microcytosis, hypochromia, sickle cells, target cells, polychromasia, nucleated RBCs & inclusions as seen in S/β^0 thalassemia i4.15
  - Electrophoresis shows 60%-80% HbS, 10%-30% HbA, 4%-8% HbA_2, 1%-15% HbF

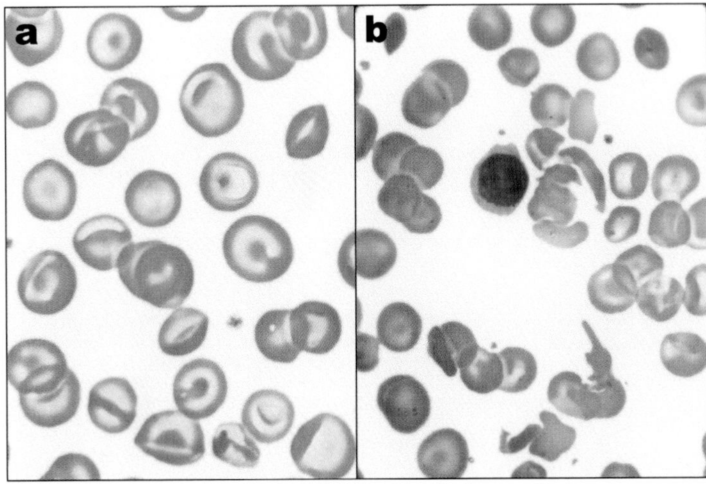

i4.14 a Anisocytosis, microcytic red cells, hypochromia, target cells b sickle cells, blisterlike cells, spherocytes, microspherocytes, schistocytes & hemoglobin SC precipitate/crystalloids

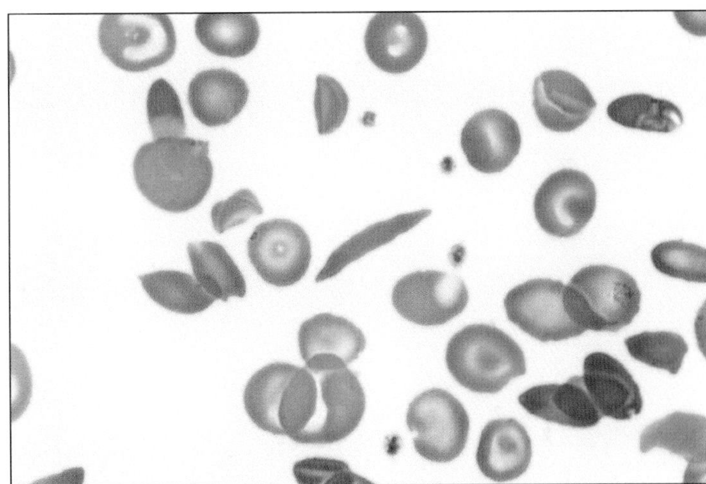

i4.15 Anisocytosis, poikilocytosis, microcytic red cells, target cells, sickle cells, polychromasia & schistocytes

4.7.1.3.7.9 Hereditary persistence of fetal hemoglobin

- Etiology
  - Either deletion or inactivation of the β and δ gene complex or mutations of proteins inhibiting gene expression or in the γ gene promoter region
  - Delayed switch from γ to β or δ production
  - No hemoglobin A synthesized
- Pathophysiology
  - Hemoglobin F production persists into adulthood
  - Hemoglobin F synthesis effectively compensates for lack of hemoglobin A
- Laboratory findings
  - Increased hemoglobin (15-18 g/dL [150-180 g/L])
  - Electrophoresis shows 100% HbF
  - Cell-wide (pancellular) distribution of hemoglobin F in RBCs

ISBN 978-089189-6616

4.7.1.3.7.10 Hemoglobin Lepore

- Etiology
  - Fusion of δ and β genes resulting from abnormal crossing-over during meiosis
- Pathophysiology
  - The δ/β fusion gene produces δ/β chains, 2 of which combine with 2 α chains to synthesize hemoglobin Lepore
  - No normal hemoglobin A and excess α chains with ineffective erythropoiesis results
- Laboratory findings
  - Decreased hemoglobin (4-11 g/dL [40-110 g/L])
  - Peripheral blood smear
    - Anisocytosis & poikilocytosis
    - Microcytosis & hypochromia
    - Target cells
    - Basophilic stippling
  - Electrophoresis shows 20%-30% hemoglobin Lepore, 70%-80% HbF, and normal HbA_2 levels
    - Note that hemoglobin Lepore migrates with HbS on alkaline electrophoresis

4.7.1.3.7.11 Unstable hemoglobins

- Group of disorders characterized by precipitation of denatured abnormal hemoglobin as inclusions (Heinz bodies)
- Etiology
  - Amino acid substitutions or deletions affect the stability of the hemoglobin molecule, resulting in hemoglobin variants with unusual sensitivity to oxidative stress
  - Inherited conditions
- Pathophysiology
  - Unstable hemoglobins denature & precipitate as Heinz bodies
  - Heinz bodies attach to inner side of RBC membrane, affecting permeability & decreasing deformability
  - Heinz bodies pitted by splenic macrophages but result in a cell with decreased membrane and less hemoglobin, causing eventual RBC destruction (and anemia)
- Laboratory findings
  - Decreased hemoglobin & hematocrit
  - Increased reticulocyte count
  - Peripheral blood smear
    - Basophilic stippling
    - Bite cells (smear can appear like G6PD deficiency)
  - Heinz bodies may be seen with supravital stains
  - Positive screening results with 17% isopropanol & heat instability tests
  - Most unstable hemoglobins migrate with HbA on electrophoresis

4.7.1.3.7.12 Hemoglobin D ($HbD_{Los\ Angeles}$, HbD_{Punjab})

- Etiology
  - Inherited amino acid substitution in the 121st position of the β hemoglobin chain
  - Glutamine replaces glutamic acid
- Pathophysiology
  - Hemoglobin solubility affected and RBCs have shortened survival
- Laboratory findings
  - Mildly decreased hemoglobin & hematocrit
  - Possibly target cells on peripheral blood smear
  - Electrophoresis shows 95% HbD
    - Note that HbD migrates with HbS on alkaline electrophoresis and with HbA on acid electrophoresis

4.7.1.3.7.13 Hemoglobin Constant Spring (HbCS)

- Etiology
  - Inherited condition
  - Type of α-thalassemia
  - 31 extra amino acids on α chains
  - Chromosome with Constant Spring gene still has 1 normal α gene
    - Homozygotes have 2 normal α genes
    - Heterozygotes have 3 normal α genes
- Pathophysiology
  - Ineffective alpha chain synthesis occurs because the long α chain is unstable
- Laboratory findings (homozygotes)
  - Similar to α thalassemia
    - Hemoglobin decreased (9-11 g/dL [90-110 g/L])
    - Increased reticulocyte count
    - Microcytic, hypochromic RBCs
    - Target cells
    - Anisocytosis & poikilocytosis
  - Electrophoresis shows HbBart at birth; in adults, 5%-7% HbCS, normal levels of Hb A_2 & HbF, and the remaining hemoglobin as HbA

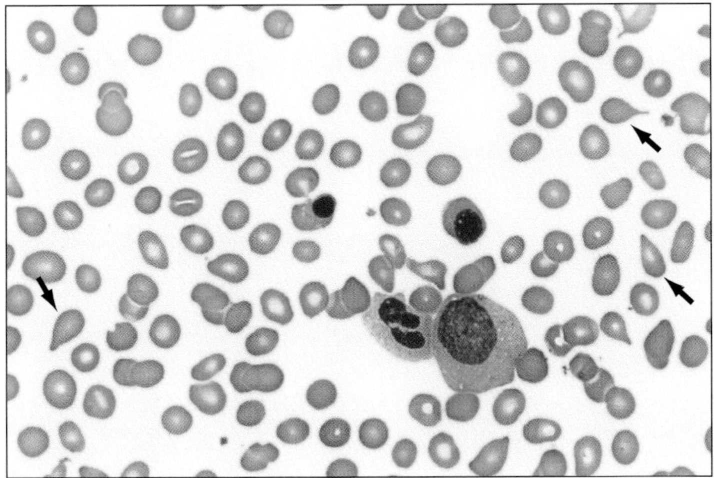

i4.16 Myelophthisic anemia associated with primary myelofibrosis: leukoerythroblastosis & teardrop cells (arrows)

4.7.1.3.8 Anemias associated with systemic disorders

4.7.1.3.8.1 Nonhematologic disorders

- Etiology
  - Anemias may arise as a secondary consequence in patients with a primary malignancy or who have chronic renal disease
- Pathophysiology
  - Malignancy
    - Normal bone marrow cells replaced or infiltrated by malignant cells or fibrosis and results in ineffective hematopoiesis, to include decreased production of RBCs (myelophthisic anemia)
  - Chronic renal disease
    - Major mechanism is the decreased production of erythropoietin or synthesis of nonfunctional erythropoietin that reduces erythropoiesis
- Laboratory findings
  - Malignancy
    - Overall pancytopenia may be present in addition to anemia
    - Leukoerythrobastosis & dacryocytes (teardrop cells) on a peripheral blood smear as well as anisocytosis & poikilocytosis i4.16
    - Decreased absolute reticulocyte count
  - Chronic renal disease
    - Decreased hemoglobin (5-8 g/dL [50-80 g/L])
    - Peripheral blood smear shows anisocytosis, poikilocytosis, echinocytes & schistocytes
    - Increased blood urea nitrogen (BUN) (>30 mg/dL [10.7 mmol/L]) & creatinine
    - Abnormal electrolyte levels
    - Microcytes may be associated with developing iron-deficiency anemia if blood loss occurs or macrocytes if folate deficiency is associated with hemodialysis

4.7.2 Erythrocytosis

- Secondary polycythemia & relative erythrocytosis are benign conditions, although RBC, hemoglobin, and hematocrit values will be elevated
- These conditions must sometimes be distinguished from primary polycythemia vera, a malignant disorder (see 4.9.3.1.2.2)

4.7.2.1 Secondary polycythemia

- Etiology
  - Normal increase in erythropoietin (EPO) due to tissue hypoxia
  - Abnormal increase in erythropoietin without tissue hypoxia
- Pathophysiology
  - Decreased oxygen saturation at high altitude and with lung disease result in tissue hypoxia because RBCs have less oxygen to deliver as they circulate
  - Erythropoietin levels can be inappropriately increased when tumors secrete erythropoietin or erythropoietinlike substances
    - Most often associated with renal disease
    - Can be seen with other tumors such as in liver, cerebellum & uterus
- Laboratory findings
  - Elevated RBC, hemoglobin, hematocrit, RBC mass, erythropoietin
  - Normal values
    - Leukocytes & basophils
    - Leukocyte alkaline phosphatase (LAP) score
    - Serum iron
    - Platelet count & platelet function tests
    - Serum B_{12}

4.7.2.2 Relative erythrocytosis

- Etiology
  - Dehydration & Gaisböck syndrome
- Pathophysiology
  - Low plasma volume results because of loss of body fluid (dehydration) or in stress erythrocytosis (Gaisböck) possibly associated with changes in hormone levels

ISBN 978-089189-6616

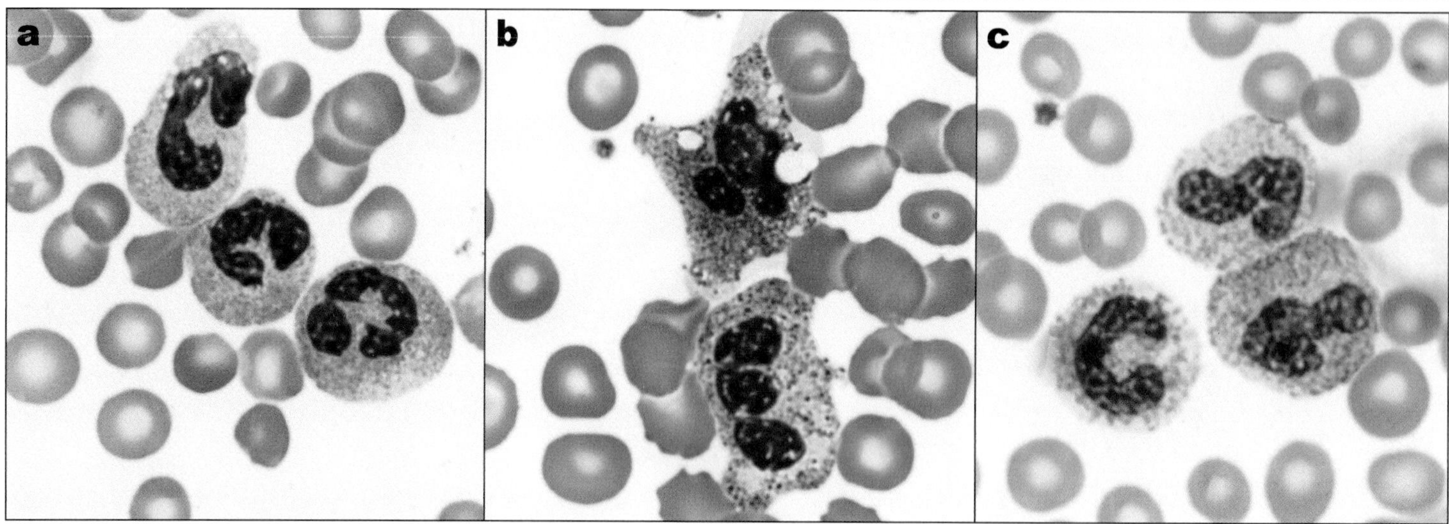

i4.17 a Increased number of mature neutrophils associated with inflammation. b Toxic granules & toxic vacuoles in neutrophils associated with infection (bacterial). c Left shift of neutrophils (bandemia) with toxic granules associated with granulocytic growth factor therapy

- Laboratory findings
  - Elevated RBC, hemoglobin & hematocrit
  - Normal values
    - RBC mass
    - Erythropoietin
    - Leukocytes & basophils
    - Leukocyte alkaline phosphatase (LAP)
    - Serum iron
    - Platelet count & platelet function tests
    - Serum B_{12}

4.8 Nonmalignant disorders of leukocytes

4.8.1 Quantitative granulocytic

4.8.1.1 Neutrophilia

- Definition
  - Increase in circulating neutrophils (adults) >7500/µL (>7.5×10^9/L; but usually not >3000/µL [>3.0×10^9/L])
- Etiology
  - Associated with infection (especially bacterial), trauma, burns, systemic inflammation (collagen vascular diseases, gout), seizures, exercise, post-splenectomy, leukocyte adhesion defect, pregnancy, juvenile rheumatoid arthritis & medications (such as granulocyte-colony-stimulating factor)
- Peripheral blood findings i4.17
  - Neutropilic left shift (bands, metamyelocytes, myelocytes)
  - Toxic changes to neutrophils
    - Toxic granulation
    - Döhle bodies
    - Vacuolation
    - Elevated leukocyte alkaline phosphatase (LAP)

4.8.1.2 Neutropenia

- Definition
  - Decrease in circulating neutrophils to <2500/µL (<2.5×10^9/L) in infants and <1500/µL (<1.5×10^9/L) in adults
- Etiology
  - Associated with Kostmann syndrome (congenital neutropenia); other neutropenias to include cyclic, familial, immune & idiopathic; systemic lupus erythromatosus; hypersensitivity reactions; systemic infections; hypersplenism; megaloblastic anemia; aplastic anemia; malignancy infiltrating the bone marrow; chemotherapy & radiation treatment; & drug reactions
- Peripheral blood findings
  - Toxic changes to neutrophils may or may not be present
  - Neutrophilic left shift
  - Possible increase in monocytes

4.8.1.3 Eosinophilia

- Definition
  - Increase in circulating eosinophils >500/µL (>0.5×10^9/L)

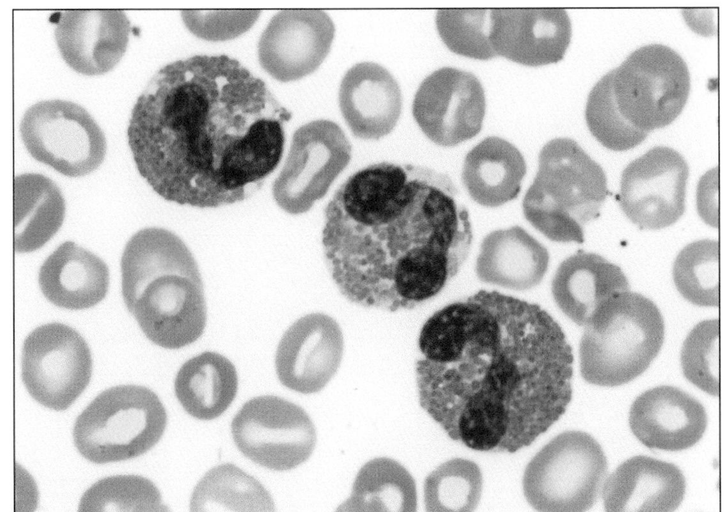

i4.18 Increased number of mature eosinophils associated with asthma

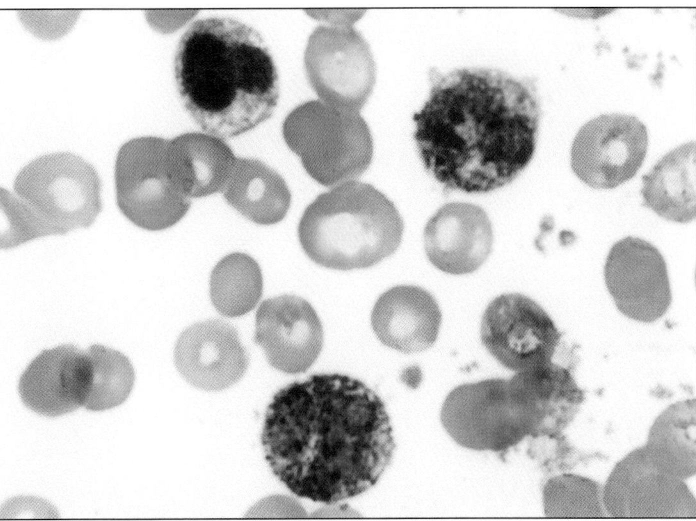

i4.19 Increased number of mature basophils associated with chronic myeloid leukemia in the accelerated phase

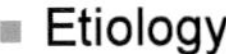

- Etiology
  - Most often reactive condition associated with allergies or parasitic infections
  - Other causes include connective tissue or immunodeficiency diseases, chronic myeloid leukemia, asthma, eosinophilic leukemia, hypereosinophilia syndrome & granulocyte macrophage-colony-stimulating factor treatment
- Peripheral blood findings i4.18
  - Eosinophils are normal & mature with a few bands possible

4.8.1.4 Basophilia

- Definition
  - Increase in circulating basophils >200/μL (>0.2×10^9/L)
- Etiology
  - Associated with immediate hypersensitivity reactions, chronic myeloid leukemia, basophilic leukemia, some endocrinopathies & infectious diseases
- Peripheral blood findings i4.19
  - Basophils are normal & mature
  - May sometimes appear immature and/or abnormal in malignancies

4.8.2 Qualitative granulocytic

- Disorders of granulocytes including Alder-Reilly, May-Hegglin, and Pelger-Huët anomalies, Chédiak-Higashi syndrome, and chronic granulomatous disease
- Pelger-Huët anomaly is benign and the most common condition in this group
- Alder-Reilly, Chédiak-Higashi, May-Hegglin & chronic granulomatous disease are rare disorders with varying degrees of clinical severity
- Etiology
  - All these conditions are inherited
- Pathophysiology
  - Alder-Reilly anomaly
    - Associated with mucopolysaccharidoses
    - Mucopolyssacharides are incompletely degraded and accumulate in cellular lysosomes
  - Chédiak-Higashi syndrome
    - Mutation in the lysosomal trafficking regulatory gene (*CHS1/LYST*) results in the abnormal fusion of primary & secondary granules
    - Granule contents are ineffectively delivered to destroy ingested bacteria
    - Patients susceptible to severe & recurrent bacterial infections
  - May-Hegglin anomaly
    - Mutation in the *MYH9* gene results in defective production of nonmuscle myosin heavy chain IIA (MHIIA)
    - MHIIA functions in maintaining cell motility and shape as well as in cellular processes like cytokinetics & phagocytosis
    - Patients may have thrombocytopenia & subsequent bleeding
  - Chronic granulomatous disease
    - Ineffective intracellular destruction of ingested organisms results from defects in the cellular respiratory or oxidative burst system
    - Patients susceptible to severe & recurrent infection from opportunistic pathogens
    - Granuloma formation occurs at sites of infection

 ISBN 978-089189-6616

Nonmalignant disorders of leukocytes>Qualitative granulocytic

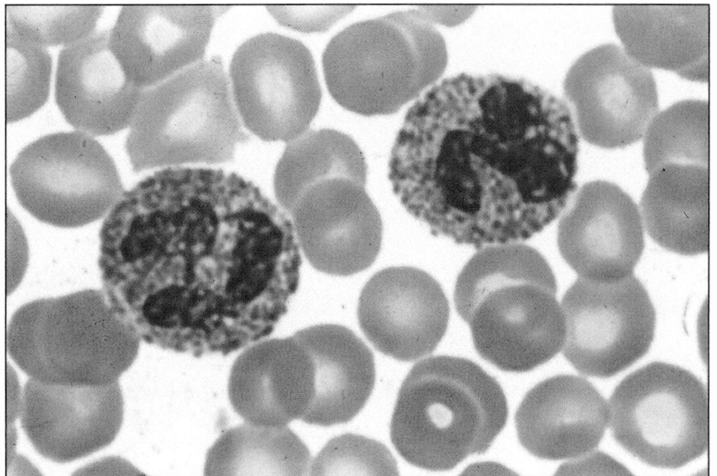

i4.20 Alder-Reilly inclusions in neutrophils

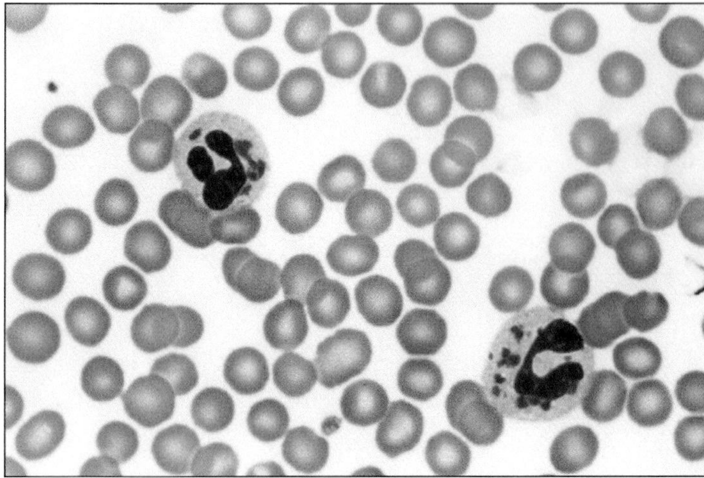

i4.21 Lysosomal granules in neutrophils

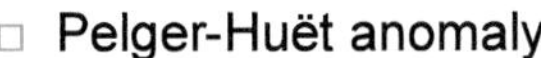

- Pelger-Huët anomaly
  - Nuclear hyposegmentation in neutrophils
  - Cells function normally
  - Acquired or pseudo−Pelger-Huët anomaly can be associated with myelodysplastic/myeloproliferative neoplasms/syndromes and in coronavirus disease 2019 (COVID-19) [Nazarullah et al, *AJCP* 2020]
- Peripheral blood findings
  - Alder-Reilly anomaly
    - Large azurophilic granules resembling toxic granulation seen in all types of leukocytes i4.20
  - Chédiak-Higashi syndrome
    - Giant cytoplasmic granules evident in granulocytes, lymphocytes & monocytes i4.21
    - Granules may appear gray-green and stain positive for myeloperoxidase & acid phosphatase
    - Neutropenia & thrombocytopenia may be seen as the condition progresses
  - May-Hegglin anomaly i4.22
    - Inclusions resembling Döhle bodies in neutrophils (and sometimes in eosinophils, basophils & monocytes)
    - Thrombocytopenia
    - Giant or large platelets
  - Chronic granulomatous disease
    - WBC count increases during infection
    - Screen using nitroblue tetrazolium (NBT) test
      - Nitroblue tetrazolium not reduced in chronic granulomatous disease
    - Flow cytometry is a newer method to measure oxidative burst (neutrophil oxidative burst assay)

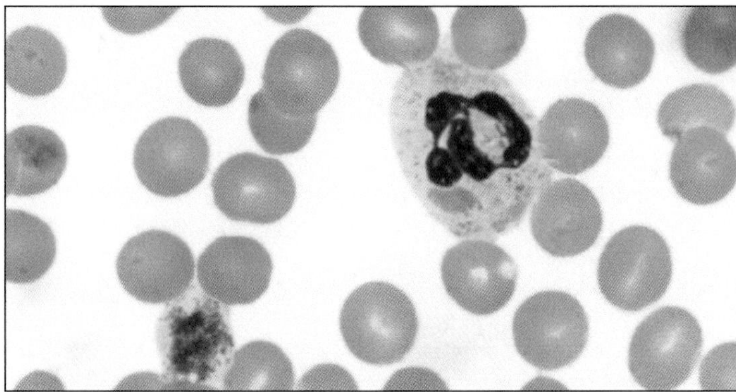

i4.22 Large Döhle body in a neutrophil, a giant platelet & thrombocytopenia

      - Dihydrorhodamine 123 (DHR 123) oxidized by neutrophils to fluorescent product measured by flow cytometry
      - Normal neutrophils display 80%-100% phagocytic activity
  - Pelger-Huët (PH) anomaly
    - Heterozygotes show primarily bilobed neutrophils with a few nonsegmented or unilobed cells
    - Bilobed cells appear with a thin strand of chromatin connecting the lobes (resembling spectacles or eye-glasses without earpieces) i4.23
    - Some bilobed nuclei look like dumbbells or peanuts
    - Homozygotes are rare and the majority of the nuclei are round and unilobed
    - Pseudo-Pelger-Huët neutrophils i4.24 may also be bilobed or unilobed but the nuclear lobes, when present, are usually not uniform in size or shape
    - Pseudo-PH cells will constitute generally >30% of the total neutrophil population in contrast to often >50% of neutrophils in inherited PH
    - Pseudo-PH neutrophils may be hypogranular

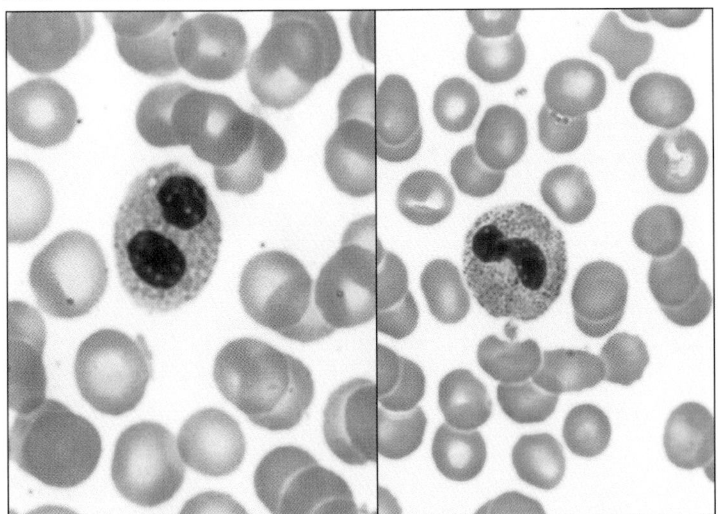

i4.23 Pelger-Huët anomaly with various forms of bilobed neutrophils

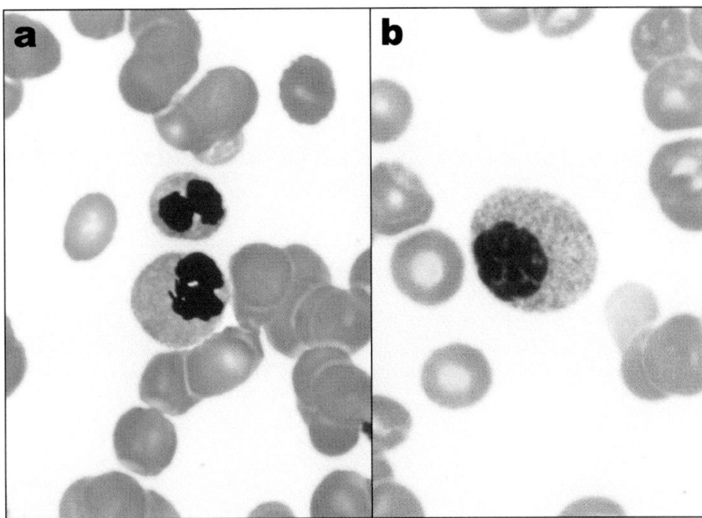

i4.24 Pseudo-Pelger-Huët anomaly: a bilobed neutrophils; b unilobed neutrophil

4.8.3 Quantitative lymphocytic

4.8.3.1 Lymphocytosis

- Definition
  - Increase in circulating lymphocytes >4000/µL (>4.0×10^9/L) in adults and approximately >8900/µL (>8.9×10^9/L) in children
- Etiology
  - Reactive process resulting from infection or inflammation
  - Lymphocytes may be morphologically mature & normal or appear reactive (atypical, variant)
  - Associated with numerous conditions to include viral infections (such as infectious mononucleosis, cytomegalovirus, human immunodeficiency virus [HIV], hepatitis, measles, mumps), toxoplasmosis, pertussis, stress, trauma & smoking
  - Lymphocytes also increased in hematologic malignancies such as acute lymphoblastic leukemia, chronic lymphocytic leukemia & the leukemic phase of non-Hodgkin lymphoma
- Peripheral blood findings
  - WBC also increased in some disorders (mono, pertussis, cytomegalovirus, leukemia)
  - Morphology of lymphocytes is variable with regard to cell size & shape, nuclear features, and cytoplasmic characteristics and dependent on underlying condition
  - Though variable in morphology, reactive lymphocytes i4.25 typically appear with distinctive features as summarized in t4.8

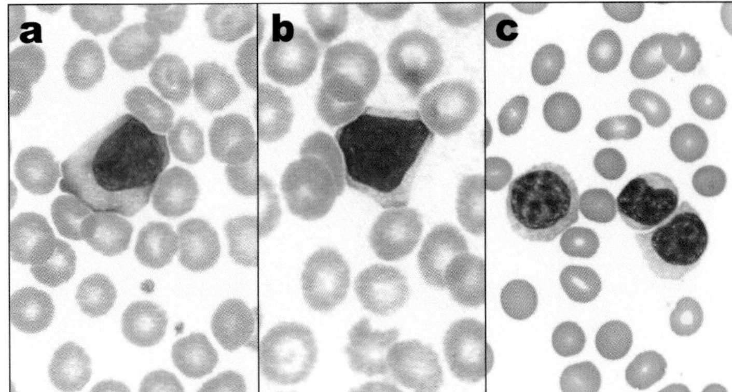

i4.25 Reactive lymphocytes: a,b atypical (reactive) lymphocytes having abundant cytoplasm with "burnt" cytoplasmic edges; c increased number of mature lymphocytes associated with whooping cough

t4.8 Features of reactive lymphocytes

Cell size	Variable, can be large (9-20 µm)
Nucleus	
Shape	Irregular (lobulated, oval, indented)
Chromatin	Coarse & moderately fine
Parachromatin	More evident & white
Nucleoli	May be prominent
Cytoplasm	Abundant, often deep, intense blue with darker or "burnt" edges at contact points with other cells, like red blood cells

4.8.3.2 Lymphocytopenia

- Definition
  - Decrease in circulating lymphocytes <2000/µL (<2.0×10^9/L) in children and <1000/µL (<1.0×10^9/L) in adults

ISBN 978-089189-6616

- Etiology
  - Associated with systemic lupus erythematosus, steroid therapy, immune deficiency disorders, HIV infection, malnutrition, renal disease, chemotherapy & radiation therapy, carcinoma, tuberculosis, Hodgkin disease & other conditions (eg, COVID-19)
- Peripheral blood findings
  - Lymphocytes are morphologically normal
  - Granulocytopenia, normocytic, normochromic anemia & thrombocytopenia may be present depending on the underlying condition

4.8.4 Monocytosis

- Definition
  - Increase in circulating monocytes >1000/µL (>1.0×10^9/L) in adults
- Etiology
  - Reactive process associated with collagen vascular diseases, chronic infections (like tuberculosis), as a compensatory response during neutropenia, after treatment with growth factors (granulocyte macrophage-colony-stimulating factor or macrophage colony-stimulating factor) & in other conditions
  - Also increased in myelodysplastic syndromes, myeloproliferative neoplasms & monocytic leukemias
- Peripheral blood findings
  - Monocytes seen in reactive conditions are morphologically normal
  - In malignancy, immature monocytes may be seen (promonocytes & monoblasts)
  - Increased WBC, anemia & thrombocytopenia may be seen in malignancies

4.9 Malignant disorders of leukocytes

4.9.1 Acute myeloid (myelogenous/ myeloblastic) leukemia (AML)

- General features
  - Typically this comprises most leukemia seen in adults & infants
  - Median age 65 years
  - Typically presents with elevated WBC count because of numerous circulating blasts
  - Blasts ≥20% of all nucleated cells (peripheral blood & bone marrow) establishes diagnosis
    - In some conditions, other cells are included in the "blast" percentage (promyelocytes in acute promyelocytic leukemia [APL] and promonocytes in acute monocytic leukemia)

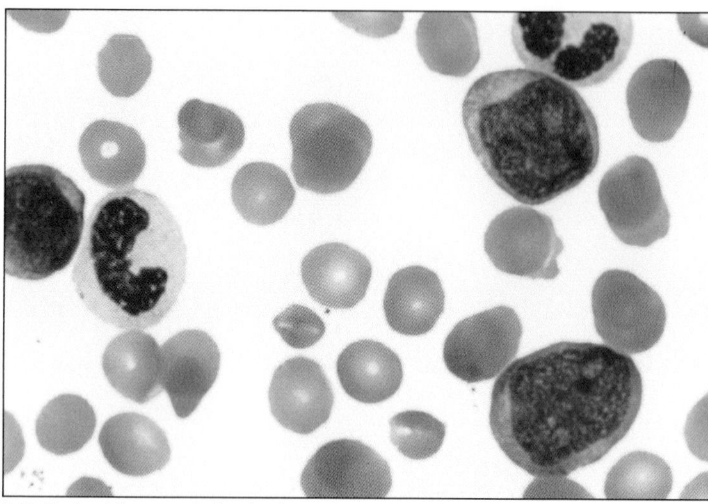

i4.26 Evolved from myelodysplastic syndrome: blasts, hypogranular neutrophil & a band

- Laboratory findings
  - WBC count variable in most acute myeloid leukemias
  - Normocytic, normochromic anemia
  - Decreased platelet count
  - Morphology of abnormal cells i4.26 includes:
    - Typically large myeloblasts with high nuclear-to-cytoplasmic ratio, prominent (and possibly multiple) nucleoli, loose & open chromatin, and moderate amount of blue cytoplasm that may have granules or Auer rods
    - Other blast types & myeloid cells may be present depending on classification
  - Cytochemical stains can be useful in the initial evaluation
    - Myeloperoxidase (MPO) and specific esterase generally positive in granulocytic cells (myeloblasts) but negative in lymphoid cells & monocytes
    - Nonspecific esterase (NSE) usually positive in monoblasts & megakaryoblasts (acetate substrate)
  - Immunophenotyping
    - Blasts in acute myeloid leukemia generally express CD34, CD13, CD33, HLA-DR & CD45, though acute promyelocytic leukemia usually negative for CD34 & HLA-DR
    - Lymphoid markers typically negative
    - Terminal deoxynucleotidyl transferase (TdT) marker for primitive lymphoid cells (generally negative in acute myeloid leukemia)
  - Molecular techniques detect specific genetic abnormalities unique to certain classifications of AML (such as *PML/RARα* in APL)

4.9.1.1 Classification t4.9

- Current World Health Organization (WHO) scheme based on morphology, cytogenetics, molecular testing, and immunophenotyping
- Earlier French-American-British (FAB) system retained in the WHO acute myeloid leukemia not otherwise specified (NOS) category
- The WHO categories of acute myeloid leukemia & related neoplasms are as follows
  - Acute myeloid leukemia (AML) with recurrent genetic abnormalities
    - AML with t(8;21)(q22;q22.1); *RUNX1-RUNX1T1**
    - AML with inv(16)(p13.1;q22) or t(16;16)(p13.1;q22); *CBFB-MYH11**
    - Acute promyelocytic leukemia with t(15;17)(q22;q12); *PML-RARα**
    - AML with t(9;11)(p21.3;q23.3); *MLLT3-KMT2A**
    - AML with t(6;9)(q23;q34.1); *DEX-NUP214**
    - AML with inv(3)(q21.3;q26.2) or t(3;3)(q21.3;q26.2); *GATA2, MECOM**
    - AML (megakaryoblastic) with t(1;22)(p13.3;q13.3); *RBM15-MKL1**
    - AML with *BCR-ABL1*
    - AML with mutated *NPM1*
    - AML with biallelic mutation of *CEBPA*
    - AML with mutated *RUNX1*

  *[*These abbreviations refer to specific genes or regions where abnormalities occur]*

  - Acute myeloid leukemia (AML) with myelodysplasia-related changes
  - Therapy-related myeloid neoplasms (includes therapy-related AML)
  - Acute myeloid leukemia, not otherwise specified (NOS)
    - M0-M7 (FAB groups):
      - AML with minimal differentiation (M0)
      - AML without maturation (M1)
      - AML with maturation (M2)
      - Acute myelomonocytic leukemia (M4)
      - Acute monoblastic/monocytic leukemia (M5a & M5b)
      - Pure erythroid leukemia (M6)
      - Acute megakaryoblastic leukemia (M7)
      - Acute basophilic leukemia
      - Acute panmyelosis with myelofibrosis
      - Myeloid sarcoma

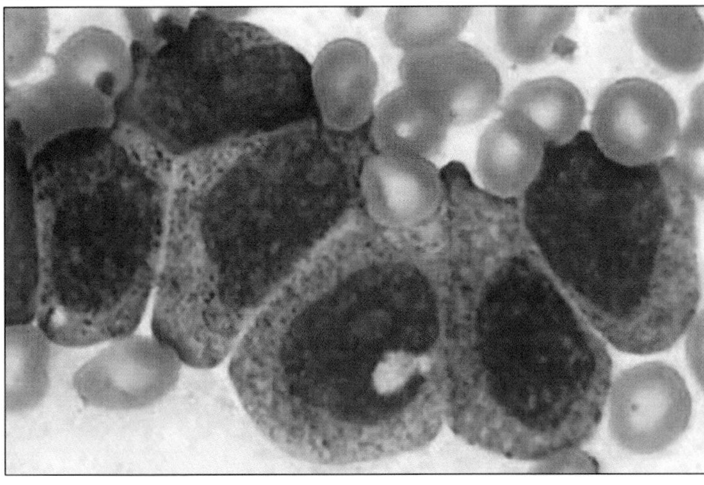

i4.27 AML with t(8;21)

    - Myeloid proliferations related to Down syndrome
      - Transient abnormal myelopoiesis (TAM)
      - Myeloid leukemia associated with Down syndrome
      - Blastic plasmacytoid dendritic cell neoplasm
    - Acute leukemia of ambiguous lineage
      - Acute undifferentiated leukemia
      - Mixed phenotypic leukemia (MPAL) with t(9;22)(q34.1;q11.2); *BCR-ABL1*
      - MPAL with t(v;11q23.3); *KMT2A* rearranged
      - MPAL, B/myeloid, NOS
      - MPAL, T/myeloid, NOS

4.9.1.2 Characteristics of selected WHO classifications of acute myeloid leukemia (AML) & related neoplasms

- AML with recurrent genetic abnormalities
  - AML with t(8;21)(q22;q22.1) i4.27
    - Represents 8%-10% of all de novo cases of AML
    - *RUNX1* gene encodes the α chain of core binding factor (CBFα)
    - Blasts are characterized by pronounced, sometimes large, azurophilic granules & Auer rods
    - Morphologic features almost always like FAB/NOS M2
    - Dysplasia in granulocytes is present in the blood & bone marrow, with pseudo-Pelger-Huët nuclei and homogeneous pink cytoplasm
    - Immunophenotypically, the blasts sometimes express CD19 & CD56, highly suggestive of t(8;21); CD13, CD34, HLA-DR also positive
    - Affects young adults and is relatively sensitive to chemotherapy

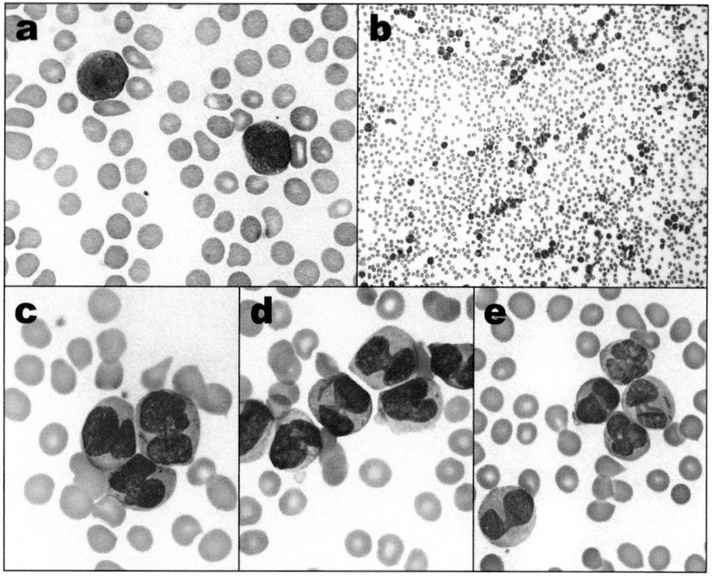

i4.28 Acute myelogenous leukemia with t(15;17)(q22;q12)
a In the classic variant, there is usually a low blast count & cytoplasmic granules are prominent
b-e In the microgranular variant, there is usually a high blast count & granules are absent; the cells are notable for indented nuclei & occasional Auer rods

- AML with inv(16)(p13.1q22) or t(16;16)(p13;q22)
    - Blasts demonstrate myelomonocytic (FAB/NOS M4) differentiation and are found in association with dysplastic eosinophils
    - Immunophenotypically, the blasts express CD13, CD33, CD34, CD14, CD64, CD11b, CD2, HLA-DR & lysozyme
    - Affects younger adults and is relatively sensitive to chemotherapy
- AML with t(15;17)(q22;q12)(acute promyelocytic leukemia [APL]) i4.28
    - Disseminated intravascular coagulation (DIC) is often the presenting condition of patients
    - Age-associated incidence beginning in the late teen years and extending to 60 years
    - Abnormal promyelocytes with kidney-shaped or bilobed nuclei, cytoplasm varying from intensely granulated to agranular (microgranular variant)
    - Typical (hypergranular) variant often presents with very few leukemic cells in the peripheral blood
    - MPO strongly positive in both variants, and is weak or negative in monoblasts
    - Neoplastic cells express CD33 and CD13 and express CD15 weakly (in contrast to normal promyelocytes that are CD15 bright)
        - Cells are negative for HLA-DR & CD34
        - CD34 & HLA-DR expression may be seen in microgranular variant, in addition to expression of CD2
    - Patients responsive to all trans retinoic acid (ATRA) therapy
- AML with t(9;11)(p21.3;q23.3); *MLLT3-KMT2A*
    - Common in children
    - Monoblastic differentiation (resembling FAB/NOS M4 or M5) with expression of CD4, CD14, CD64, CD11b & lysozyme
    - CD34 is usually negative
    - Patients may have extramedullary and/or tissue infiltration; DIC is possible
    - Poor prognosis, but better prognosis than other 11q23 aberrations
- AML with t(6;9) DEK-NUP214
    - Associated with basophilia & multilineage dysplasia
    - Blasts often morphologically like FAB/NOS M1 or M4
    - Seen in children & younger adults
    - Poor prognosis
- AML with inv(3) or t(3;3)GATA2-MECOM
    - Seen de novo or after a myelodysplastic syndrome
    - Blasts seen in association with dysplastic small, hypolobated megakaryocytes
    - Morphologic features of blasts like FAB/NOS M0, M1, or M7
    - Multilineage dysplasia
    - Poor prognosis
- AML (megakaryoblastic) with t(1;22)(p13.3;q13.3); RBM15-MKL1
    - Often in infants without trisomy 21
    - Female predominance
    - Megakaryoblastic differentiation, expressing CD41, CD61 & CD42b; CD13 & CD33 also positive

AML with myelodysplasia-related changes
- Affects mainly the elderly
- Multilineage dysplasia and ≥20% blasts in peripheral blood or bone marrow
- May arise from existing or current myelodysplastic syndrome (MDS)
- Typically CD34, CD13 & CD33 positive
- Myeloperoxidase (MPO) positive in blasts
- Poor prognosis & unresponsive to therapy

Malignant disorders of leukocytes>Acute myeloid (myelogenous/myeloblastic) leukemia (AML)

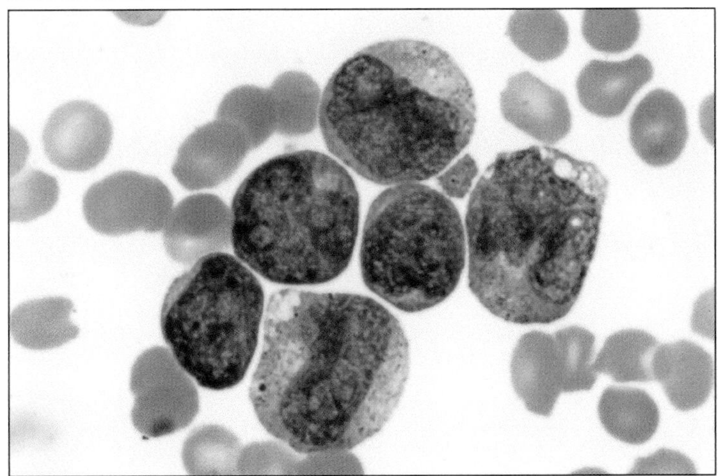

i4.29 AML-M4: 3 blasts, a myelocyte, a metamyelocyte, a monocyte & lack of platelets

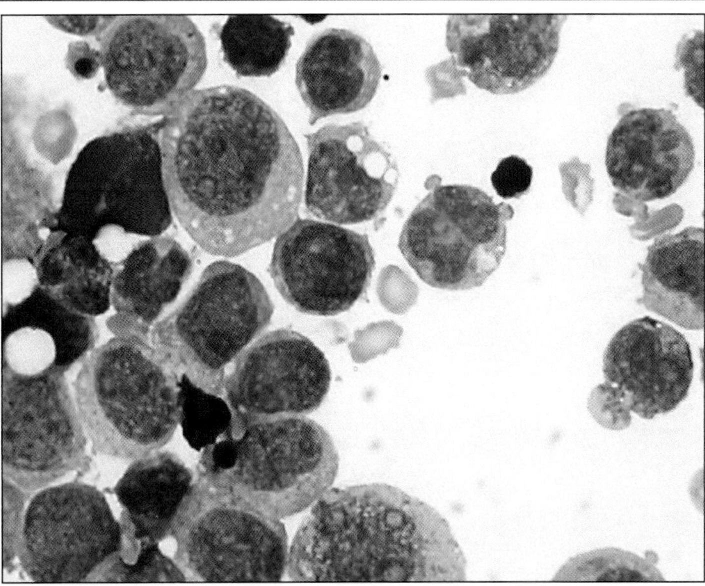

i4.30 AML, NOS, with monoblastic differentiation; the blasts have prominent nucleoli & an abundance of pale blue cytoplasm with occasional vacuoles

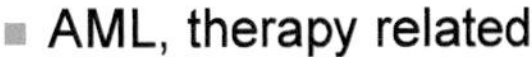

- AML, therapy related
  - Occurs in patients who have received chemotherapy and/or radiation therapy for a neoplastic or non-neoplastic disorder
  - Associated with alkylating agents, ionizing radiation & topoisomerase II inhibitors
  - Median onset varies depending on type of therapy, but can be 1-10 years after treatment
  - Any age group affected, though risk increases with age for some types of therapy (alkylating agents & radiation)
  - Associated with multilineage dysplasia and ≥1 peripheral blood cytopenias
  - Blasts express CD13, CD33, CD34 & HLA-DR
  - Poor prognosis
- AML, not otherwise specified
  - Acute myeloid leukemia, not otherwise specified, minimally differentiated (FAB M0)
    - Blasts show no evidence of myeloid differentiation using morphology or cytochemistry
    - Blasts do typically express myeloid markers such as CD13, CD33, CD117, CD34 & HLA-DR
    - Poor prognosis
  - Acute myeloid leukemia, not otherwise specified, without maturation (FAB M1)
    - >90% of blasts show no maturation (maturation in ≤10% blasts)
    - At least 3% of the blasts stain with MPO
    - Auer rods or granules may be present
    - Blasts express CD34, CD13, CD33, HLA-DR & CD117
    - Poor prognosis
  - AML, not otherwise specified, with maturation (FAB M2)
    - At least 20% blasts in peripheral blood or bone marrow
    - At least 10% of cells are maturing in the myeloid lineage
    - Auer rods & cytoplasmic granules may be present
    - Blasts may or may not express CD34, but they are usually positive for HLA-DR, CD13, CD33 & CD117
    - Often responds to treatment
  - Acute myelomonocytic leukemia (FAB M4) i4.29
    - Among all nonerythroid cells, at least 20% display monocytic maturation and at least 20% show neutrophilic maturation
    - Cells are positive for CD13, CD33, CD4, CD14, CD64, CD11b & lysozyme
    - Often responds to treatment
  - Acute monocytic/monoblastic leukemia (FAB M5a & M5b) i4.30
    - Monoblasts, promonocytes & monocytes predominate and constitute at least 80% of all nonerythroid cells
    - Cells express HLA-DR, monocytic markers (CD4, CD14, CD64, CD11b, lysozyme)
    - Myeloid markers variable (CD13, CD33, CD117)
    - t(8;16) sometimes present and is associated with hemophagocytosis
    - Patients may present with bleeding, gingival enlargement & central nervous system involvement
    - Poor prognosis

Malignant disorders of leukocytes>Acute myeloid (myelogenous/myeloblastic) leukemia (AML)

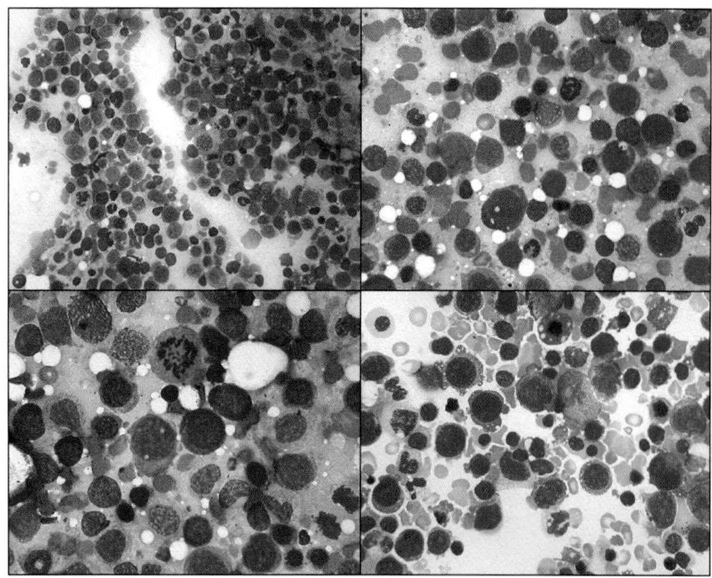

i4.31 AML, NOS, with erythroid maturation; note the predominance of erythroid precursors, many of which have dyspoietic morphology

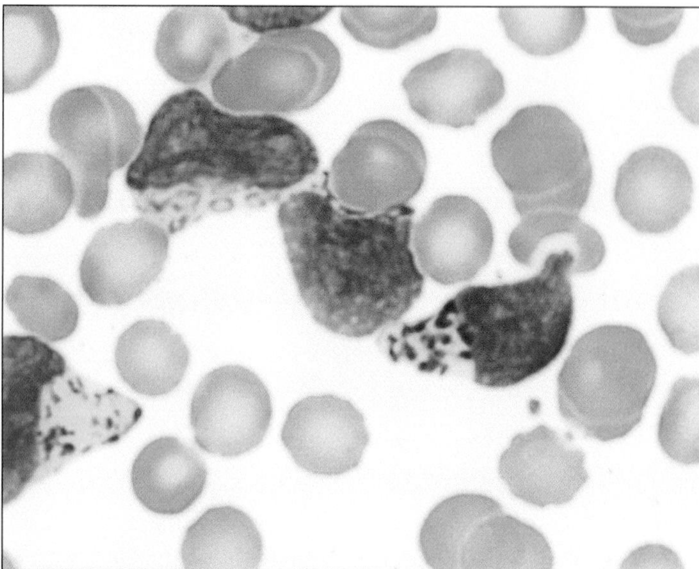

i4.32 Blasts with basophilic granules & thrombocytopenia

- Acute (pure) erythroid leukemia (FAB M6) i4.31
  - Undifferentiated/proerythroblastic (pronormoblastic) differentiation
    - >80% immature erythroid precursors with at least 30% proerythroblasts, myeloblasts <20%
  - Dysplastic morphology may be seen
  - Cells express HLA-DR, CD34, glycophorin (CD235a) & CD71 (which may be aberrantly dim)
  - Poor prognosis & poor response to therapy
- Acute megakaryoblastic leukemia (FAB M7)
  - >50% of blasts show megakaryocytic differentiation
  - Acute myeloid leukemias & transient myeloproliferative disorders (TMDs) that are associated with Down syndrome most often present as M7
  - Megakaryocytic cells express CD41 & CD61 and myeloblasts may express CD13 & CD33
  - Megakaryoblasts may display cytoplasmic blebs
  - Cytopenia with or without thrombocytopenia
  - Poor prognosis
- Acute basophilic leukemia i4.32
  - Basophil precursors in peripheral blood & bone marrow
  - Cells show metachromatic positivity with toluidine blue
  - Cells express CD13, CD33, CD34, HLA-DR but are CD117 negative
  - Symptoms associated with hyperhistaminemia
  - Rare disorder
- Acute panmyelosis with myelofibrosis
  - Panmyeloid proliferation & fibrosis of the bone marrow
  - Blasts, pancytopenia, dysplastic neutrophils & platelets in peripheral blood
  - Megakaryocytic abnormalities may be seen
  - CD13, CD33, CD117 positive; C41, CD61 variable
  - Rare disorder

t4.9 Features of selected WHO subgroups of AML

Subgroup	Morphology	Cytochemistry	Major immunophenotype	Special notes
With recurrent genetic abnormalities (abnormalities abbreviated)				
t(8;21)(q22;q22.1)	Neutrophil lineage maturation; Auer rods; neutrophilic dysplasia	MPO positive	MPO, CD34, CD13, HLA-DR positive; sometimes CD56 & CD19 positive	Resembles M2 morphology in PB
in(16)(p13.1q22) or t(16;16)(p13;q22)	Neutrophil & monocytic maturation; increased & abnormal eosinophils in BM	MPO positive, NSE positive; eosinophils positive with naphthyl esterase	CD34, CD13, CD33, CD14, CD2, CD11b, CD11c, CD64, lysozyme positive	Resembles M4 morphology in PB
t(15;17)(q22;q12)	Hypergranular variant Abnormal promyelocytes Bundles of Auer rods Microgranular variant Bilobed nuclei Granules not visible	MPO strongly positive	CD33, CD13 positive; CD15, HLA-DR both weakly positive; CD2, CD34 may be positive in microgranular variant	APL; DIC common clinical finding
t(9;11)(p21.3;q23.3)	Monoblasts & promonocytes predominate	MPO negative, NSE positive	CD33,CD64,CD4 HLA-DR,CD11b, CD14, lysozyme positive	Clinical findings can include DIC, extramedullary and/or tissue infiltration
t(6;9)(q23;q34.1)	Monocytic component may or may not be seen; basophilia & multilineage dysplasia common	MPO positive in myeloblasts, NSE positive in monocytic cells	MPO, CD13, CD33, CD38, HLA-DR consistently positive; CD117, CD34, CD15 may be positive; CD64 positive in some cases	Often resembles M1 or M4 morphology
inv(3) or t(3;3)	Multilineage dysplasia (especially with platelets & megakaryocytes) in PB & BM	Dependent on predominate cell type	CD13, CD33, HLA-DR, CD34, CD38 positive; subsets may be CD41, CD61 positive	Often resembles M1, M4 or M7 morphology
t(1;22)(p13.3;q13.3)	Megakaryoblasts & micromegakaryocytes	MPO negative	CD41, CD42b, CD61, CD13, CD33 positive	Seen in female infants without Down syndrome
With myelodysplasia-related changes	Multilineage dysplasia ≥50% of cells in at least 2 BM lineages; ≥20% blasts in PB or BM	MPO positive in myeloblasts	Variable because of heterogeneity of genetic events; CD13 & CD33, CD34 often positive	Disease of the elderly
Therapy-related myeloid neoplasms	Multilineage dysplasia ≥1 PB cytopenias	No specific cytochemistry helpful	CD13, CD33, CD34 usually positive	Associated with alkylating agents, topoisomerase II inhibitors, ionizing radiation
AML, not otherwise specified (NOS)				
With minimal differentiation (FAB M0)	No evidence myeloid differentiation or maturation	MPO negative	CD34, HLA-DR, CD13, CD33, CD117 positive	Diagnosis requires immunophenotyping
Without maturation (FAB M1)	Evidence of myeloid differentiation, but no maturation	MPO positive (at least 3%)	CD13, CD33, CD34, CD117, HLA-DR positive	Auer rods or cytoplasmic granules may be present
With maturation (FAB M2)	≥20% blasts in PB or BM; all stages of neutrophils (at least 10%)	MPO positive (at least 3%)	CD13, CD33, CD117, HLA-DR, CD15 positive; variable expression of HLA-DR, CD34	Auer rods & cytoplasmic granules may be present
Acute myelomonocytic leukemia (FAB M4)	Both neutrophil & monocyte precursors present	MPO positive, NSE positive	CD13, CD33, CD14, CD4, CD11b, CD64, lysozyme all positive	Often responds to treatment
Acute monoblastic & monocytic leukemia (FAB M5a, M5b)	Monoblasts, promonocytes, monocytes predominate	MPO negative, NSE positive	CD13,CD33,CD117 variable; CD14, CD4, CD11b, CD64, lysozyme positive	Tissue infiltrates, CNS involvement; sometimes t(8;16) & hemophagocytosis present
Acute (pure) erythroid leukemia (FAB M6) (erythroleukemia)	≥80% immature erythroid precursors with at least 30% proerythroblasts; myeloblasts <20%; dysplasia in erythroid cells	MPO positive in myeloblasts	Glycophorin A (CD235); CD34, CD71 positive	Rare subgroup with poor prognosis
Acute megakaryoblastic leukemia (FAB M7)	≥20% blasts with at least 50% megakaryoblasts; cytoplasmic blebs	MPO negative, NSE positive (acetate substrate)	CD41 and/or CD61, CD13, CD33 positive	Cytopenia with or without thrombocytopenia
Acute basophilic leukemia	Basophil precursors	Metachromatic positivity with toluidine blue	CD13, CD33, CD34, HLA-DR positive; CD117 negative	Very rare (<10% of all AMLs); symptoms relate to hyperhistaminemia
Acute panmyelosis with myelofibrosis	Blasts increased; dysplasia in neutrophils & platelets	MPO positive	CD13, CD33, CD117 positive; CD41, CD61 variable	Marked PB pancytopenia, BM panmyelosis with fibrosis; variable megakaryocytic abnormalities

AML, acute myeloid leukemia; APL, acute promyelocytic leukemia; BM, bone marrow; CD, cluster of differentiation; DIC, disseminated intravascular coagulation; FAB, French-American-British; HLA, human leukocyte antigen; MPO, myeloperoxidase; NSE, nonspecific esterase; PB, peripheral blood; WHO, World Health Organization

ISBN 978-089189-6616

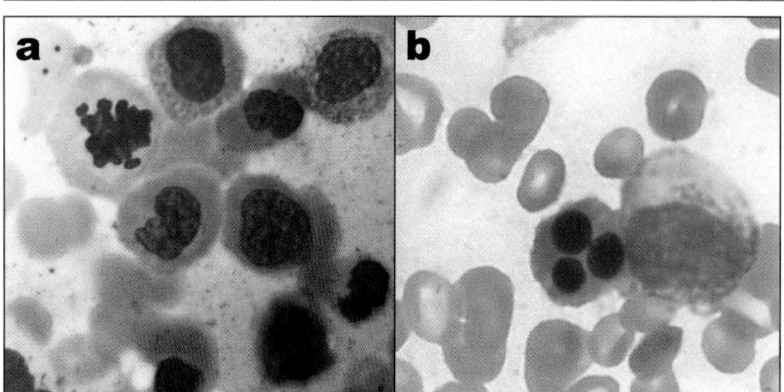

i4.33 Myelodysplastic syndrome (MDS): a multinucleate erythroid precursors; b irregular nuclear contours & karyorrhexis

i4.34 a Dysgranulopoiesis: pseudo Pelger-Huët cells (bilobed neutrophils) & a hypogranular myelocyte. b Dysmegakaryocytopoiesis: small mononuclear megakaryocyte

4.9.2 Myelodysplastic syndromes (MDSs)

- General features
  - Myeloid neoplasms characterized by ineffective hematopoiesis that displays as cytopenias, dyspoiesis in ≥1 of the major myeloid lineages, and increased risk of developing into acute myeloid leukemia
  - Usually seen in older adults
    - Associated in younger adults as a secondary condition with chemotherapy, radiation, benzene, or inherited bone marrow failure conditions (such as Fanconi anemia)
- Laboratory findings t4.10
  - High quality smears (both in preparation & staining) critical to assess dysplasia
  - Hypercellular bone marrow
  - Blasts represent <20% of cells
  - Many different dysplastic changes are possible in each lineage both in peripheral blood & bone marrow
  - Dyserythropoiesis
    - Anisocytosis & poikilocytosis
    - Multinuclearity i4.33a
    - Basophilic stippling & possible other inclusions (Pappenheimer bodies, Howell-Jolly bodies)
    - Oval macrocytes, megaloblastoid cells & nuclear fragments
    - Irregular cytoplasmic staining
    - Ringed sideroblasts
    - Karyorrhexis i4.33b
    - Dimorphism
  - Dysgranulopoiesis
    - Hypogranulation & abnormal granulation
    - Pseudo-Pelger-Huët (hyposegmentation) i4.34a
    - Hypersegmentation
    - Ring nuclei
    - Increase in granular & agranular blasts
    - Abnormal staining granules in promyelocytes
    - Absence of secondary granules
    - Possible Auer rods
  - Dysmegakaryocytopoiesis
  - Micromegakaryocytes
  - Hypogranulation or large abnormal granules
  - Giant platelets
  - Platelet functional abnormalities
  - Abnormally multinucleated megakaryocytes
  - Large or small mononuclear megakaryocytes i4.34b
- Classification t4.10
  - WHO scheme based on degree of dysplasia & cytopenia, the percentage of blasts in the peripheral blood & bone marrow, and the percentage of ringed sideroblasts in the bone marrow
  - Seven major categories
  - Prognosis variable depending on percentage of blasts, the number of cell lines showing dysplasia & cytopenia, and cytogenetics
  - MDS with 5q– has a favorable prognosis
  - Cytopenias defined as:
    - Hemoglobin of <10 g/dL (<100 g/L)
    - Platelet count of $<100\times10^3/\mu L$ ($100\times10^9/L$)
    - Absolute neutrophil count $<1800/\mu L$ ($<1.8\times10^9/L$)
    - Peripheral blood monocytes must also be $<1000/\mu L$ ($1.0\times10^9/L$)

t4.10 Myelodysplastic syndromes

Type	Peripheral blood	Bone marrow
MDS with single lineage dysplasia	Anemia or thrombocytopenia or neutropenia No blasts (<1%) or Auer rods No monocytosis (<1000/μL [<1.0 × 10^9/L])	Unilineage dysplasia <5% blasts & no Auer rods ≤15% ringed sideroblasts
MDS with single lineage dysplasia & ring sideroblasts	Anemia ± dimorphic RBCs & Pappenheimer bodies No blasts (<1%) or Auer rods No monocytosis (<1000/μL [1.0 × 10^9/L])	Dysplastic erythroids <5% blasts & no Auer rods >15% ringed sideroblasts
MDS with multilineage dysplasia	Bi- or pancytopenia <1% blasts No Auer rods	<5% blasts & no Auer rods Dysplasia in >10% of >1 cell line ≤15% ringed sideroblasts
MDS with multilineage dysplasia & ringed sideroblasts	Bi- or pancytopenia <1% blasts No Auer rods	<5% blasts & no Auer rods dysplasia in >10% of >1 cell line >15% ringed sideroblasts,
MDS with EB MDS-EB1 MDS-EB2	Bi- or pancytopenia <5% blasts, no Auer rods 5%-19% blasts or Auer rods	Dysplasia 5%-9% blasts, no Auer rods 10-19% blasts or Auer rods
MDS with isolated del(5q)	Anemia, normal to increased platelets <5% blasts No Auer rods	Hypolobated megakaryocytes <5% blasts & no Auer rods Karyotype: 5q– with 1 additional abnormality, except 7q–
MDS, unclassifiable		
with 1% blasts	<1% blasts, no Auer rods; cytopenia in 1-3 cell lines	<5% blasts, dysplasia in 1-3 cell lines
with single lineage dysplasia & pancytopenia	<1% blasts, no Auer rods; cytopenia in 1-3 cell lines	<5% blasts, dysplasia in 1 cell line
based on defining cytogenetic abnormality	<1% blasts, no Auer rods; cytopenia in 1-3 cell lines	<5%blasts; <15% ringed sideroblasts; MDS-defining abnormality, no dysplastic lineages
Refractory cytopenia of childhood	<2% blasts; cytopenia in 1-3 cell lines	<5% blasts; dysplasia in 1-3 cell lines

EB, excess blasts; MDS, myelodysplastic syndrome; RBC, red blood cells

4.9.3 Myeloproliferative neoplasms (MPNs)

- Group of closely related malignant disorders that share common clinical & hematologic features
- Result from autonomous clonal proliferation of hematopoietic stem cells
- Although characterized by abnormal proliferation of all myeloid lineages, 1 cell line typically more prominently involved
- General features
    - Condition seen in middle-aged & older adults
    - Overlap in clinical features, morphologic characteristics & laboratory findings often seen with the specific disorders

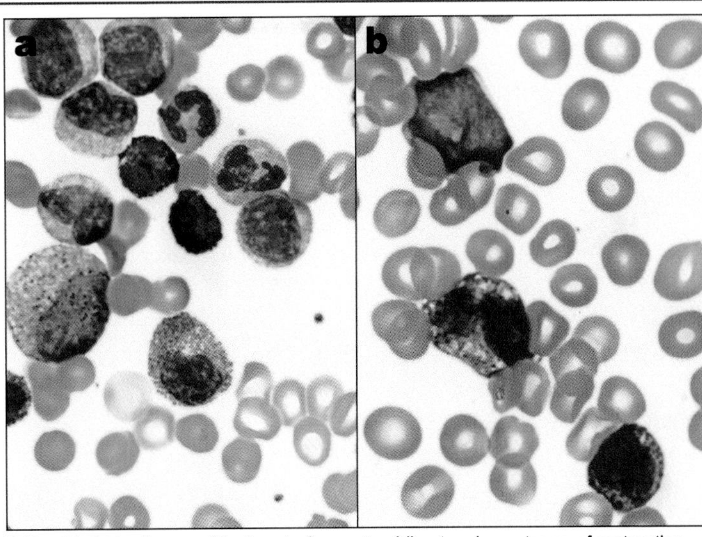

i4.35 a Variable degree of leukocytosis, neutrophils at various stages of maturation & basophils; b in accelerated phase: a blast & 2 basophils

4.9.3.1 Classification

4.9.3.1.1 WHO subgroups

- Chronic myeloid leukemia (CML), BCR-ABL1
- Chronic neutrophilic leukemia (CNL)
- Polycythemia vera (PV)
- Primary myelofibrosis (PMF)
    - PMF, prefibrotic/early stage
    - PMF, overt fibrotic stage
- Essential thrombocythemia (ET)
- Chronic eosinophilic leukemia, not otherwise specified (NOS)
- MPN, unclassifiable

4.9.3.1.2 Features of selected subgroups t4.11

4.9.3.1.2.1 CML

- Splenomegaly common at presentation
- Blasts <20% in chronic phase (and often <1%) i4.35a
- Accelerated phase characterized by progressive basophilia, thrombocytopenia, thrombocytosis, or leukocytosis i4.35b
- Elevated myeloid-to-erythroid (M:E) ratio
- >20% blasts (accellerated phase) in peripheral blood or bone marrow: 70% AML progression, 30% ALL progression
    - Tyrosine kinase inhibitors result in prolonged survival

ISBN 978-089189-6616

Malignant disorders of leukocytes>Myeloproliferative neoplasms (MPNs)

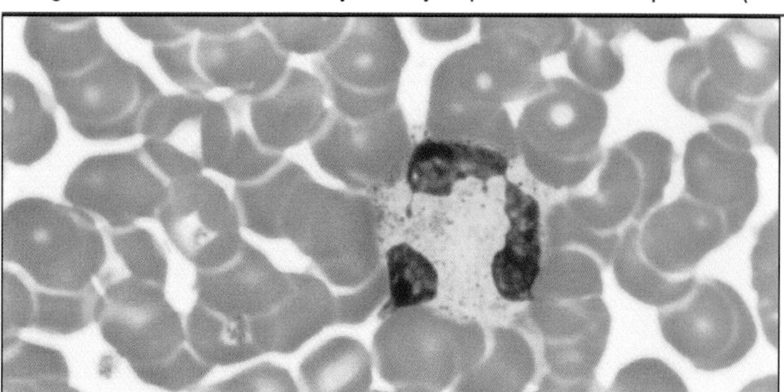

i4.36 Polycythemia vera with erythrocytosis & a neutrophil

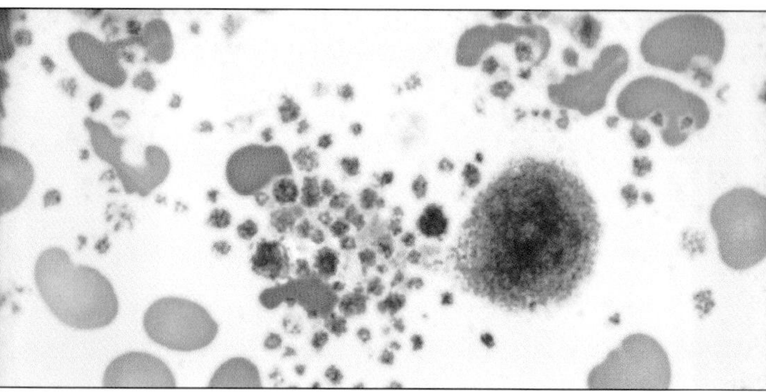

i4.38 Essential thrombocythemia showing marked thrombocytosis, a giant platelet, clumping of platelets, poikilocytosis & anisocytosis

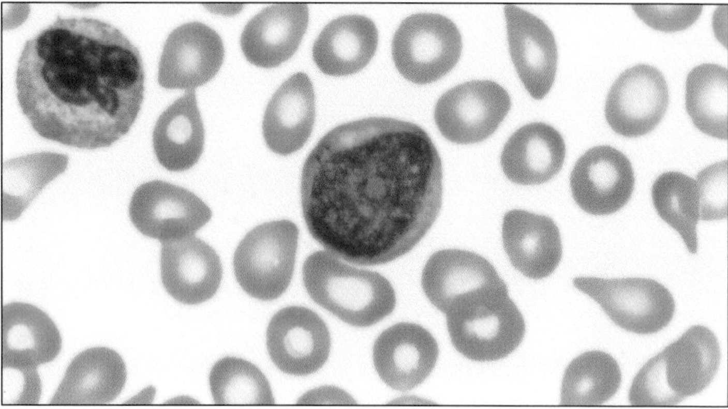

i4.37 Primary myelofibrosis with many teardrop cells, a blast cell, a dysplastic normoblast & decreased number of platelets

4.9.3.1.2.2 Polycythemia vera (PV) i4.36

- Splenomegaly common at presentation
- Other possible symptoms include hypertension, pruritis, plethora, erythromelalgia & headache
- Must be distinguished from relative & secondary causes of erythrocytosis as well as other MPNs

4.9.3.1.3 Primary myelofibrosis (PMF) i4.37

- Prefibrotic stage presents with anemia, mild leukocytosis & thrombocytosis
- Fibrotic stage characterized by leukoerythroblastosis in peripheral blood to include dacryocytes & anisocytosis
- Dry tap bone marrow aspirate

4.9.3.1.4 Essential thrombocythemia (ET) i4.38

- Bimodal age distribution to include peaks at 30 & 60 years of age with female prevalence
- Some patients present with thrombotic symptoms & mucosal hemorrhage
    - Must be distinguished from reactive thrombocytosis as may occur in iron-deficiency anemia, chronic inflammation, asplenia, and some hematologic malignancies (chronic myeloid leukemia)

t4.11 Laboratory findings in selected myeloproliferative neoplasms

	Chronic myeloid leukemia	Polycythemia vera	Primary myelofibrosis	Essential thrombocythemia
White blood cells	Markedly elevated (>50,000/µL [$>50\times10^9$/L])	Moderately elevated (<30,000/µL [$<30\times10^9$/L])	Variable	Normal or elevated (<30,000/µL [$<30\times10^9$/L])
Hemoglobin	Normal or decreased	Markedly elevated	Decreased	Variable
Platelets	Variable	Normal or elevated	Variable	Markedly elevated (>450×10^3/µL [$>450\times10^9$/L])
Peripheral blood morphologic changes				
White blood cells	Immature granulocytes	None	Immature granulocytes	Occasional immature granulocyte
	Eosinophilia, basophilia	Occasionally eosinophils ↑ & basophilia	Occasionally eosinophils ↑ & basophilia	Mild eosinophilia, basophilia possible
Red blood cells	Normocytic, normochromic	Normocytic, normochromic	Dacryocytes, nucleated red blood cells	Normocytic, normochromic
Platelets	Occasional enlarged, giant	Megakaryocytic fragments	Megakaryocytic fragments, giant	Marked variation in size & shape
Molecular tests				
Philadelphia chromosome/ *BCR-ABL* gene rearrangement	Present	Absent	Absent	Absent
JAK 2	Absent	~95%-100% of cases	~95%-100% of cases	~55% of cases
Marrow fibrosis	Progressively increases	Progressively increases	Markedly elevated	Progressively increases

4.9.4 Myelodysplastic/myeloproliferative neoplasms

- General features
  - Clonal hematopoietic neoplasms
  - Some disorders overlap myelodysplastic syndromes & myeloproliferative neoplasms in clinical presentation and laboratory findings, including morphologic features
  - Incidence & disease progression vary depending on subgroup
- Laboratory findings
  - Proliferation can be effective or ineffective
    - Hyperproliferation seen in effective cellular production
    - Cytopenias seen in ineffective cellular production
  - Dysplasia in ≥1 cell lineages
  - Blasts <20% in peripheral blood & bone marrow
  - No specific associated genetic defects
- Classification: The WHO scheme includes 5 subgroups
  - Chronic myelomonocytic leukemia (CMML) i4.39
    - Persistent peripheral blood monocytosis (>1000/µL [>1.0×10^9/L])
    - Dysplasia in ≥1 myeloid lineages
    - <20% blasts (including promonocytes)
    - If eosinophilia (>1500/µL [>1.5×10^9/L]) mutations of *PDGFRα*, *PDGFRβ*, *FGFR1* & *PCMi-JAK2* should be excluded
  - Atypical chronic myelogenous leukemia (aCML)
    - Leukocytosis (>13,000/µL [>13.0×10^9/L])
    - Spectrum of neutrophils & neutrophil precursors
    - <20% blasts
    - Dysgranulopoiesis in bone marrow
    - Philadelphia chromosome negative
  - Juvenile myelomonocytic leukemia (JMML)
    - Disorder of children
    - Monocytosis (>1000/µL [>1.0×10^9/L]) and/or granulocytosis
    - Blasts <20%
    - Anemia & thrombocytopenia may be present
    - Seen in ~10% of children with neurofibromatosis type 1
    - Hypersensitivity to granulocyte macrophage-colony-stimulating factor
    - Increased hemoglobin F levels
    - Monosomy 7 in 25% of patients
    - Recurrent mutations may be seen, such as *KRAS* & *NRAS*

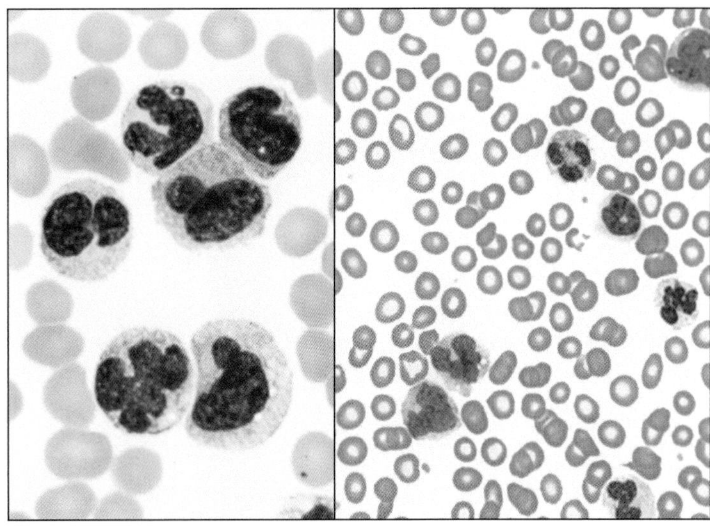

i4.39 Chronic myelomonocytic leukemia: a monocytosis; b dyspoietic neutrophils & monocytes

  - MDS/MPN, unclassifiable
    - Cases do not satisfy criteria for any other subgroup in classification
    - Clinical, laboratory & morphologic features overlap both myelodysplastic syndromes & myeloproliferative neoplasms
    - Ineffective and/or dysplastic proliferation of ≥1 myeloid lineages
    - Effective proliferation with or without dysplasia in other cell lines
    - Blasts <20%
    - Philadelphia chromosome negative
    - Anemia
    - No specific cytogenetic or molecular abnormalities identified
  - MDS/MPN with ring sideroblasts and thrombocytosis
    - Anemia associated with erythroid lineage dysplasia with or without multilineage dysplasia
      - ≥15 ring sideroblasts
      - <1% blasts in perepheral blood and bone marrow
    - Persistent thrombocytosis (≥450×10^3/µL [≥450×10^9/L])
    - Presence of *SF3B1* mutation (if absent, no recent therapy to explain MDS/MPN features)
    - No *BCR-ABL1* fusion gene or *PDGF*-related rearrangements

4.9.5 Lymphoblastic leukemia/lymphoma

- Acute lymphoblastic leukemia (ALL) and lymphoblastic lymphoma (LBL) are considered to be the same disease with different clinical presentations

ISBN 978-089189-6616

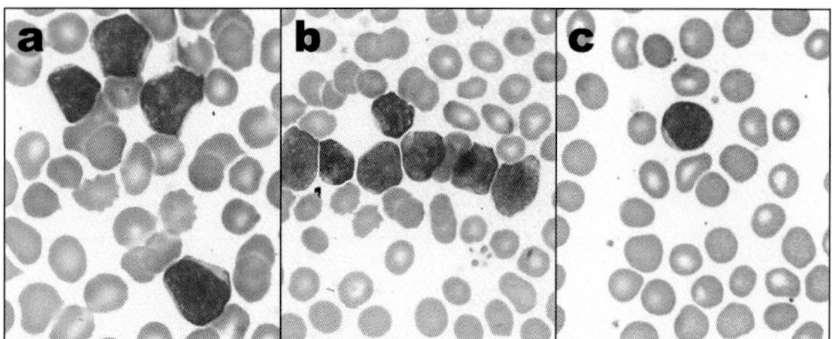

i4.40 Acute lymphoblastic leukemia
a & b Large B lymphoblasts with relatively sparse agranular cytoplasm
c T lymphoblasts which are morphologically identical to B lymphoblasts

- ALL primarily involves bone marrow and peripheral blood, though some tissue overlap is possible
- LBL primarily involves lymphoid organs, though some bone marrow & peripheral blood overlap is possible

- Neoplastic cells are precursor or immature lymphoid cells
- Many treatment protocols require at least 25% blasts in bone marrow or peripheral blood to define ALL

4.9.5.1 B-cell acute lymphoblastic leukemia (precursor)

- Malignant lymphoblasts are B cells
- General features
  - More common than T cell
  - Peak incidence at 3 years of age and again in the 6th decade
  - Some patients have central nervous system involvement
  - Good prognosis in children (complete remission in >95% of cases) and fair in adults (complete remission ~80%)
- Laboratory findings i4.40a,b
  - White blood cell count is variable, but elevated numbers common
  - Normocytic, normochromic anemia & thrombocytopenia typical
  - Proliferation of undifferentiated blasts that vary from small cells with scant cytoplasm, more condensed chromatin and indistinct nucleoli to larger cells with moderate amounts of light blue cytoplasm, dispersed nuclear chromatin & several nucleoli
  - Blasts generally myeloperoxidase negative & terminal deoxynucleotidyl transferase (TdT) positive
  - B-cell immunophenotype
- Classification t4.12
  - The WHO scheme includes precursor B-cell acute lymphoblastic leukemia/lymphoblastic lymphoma, not otherwise specified (NOS), and B-cell acute lymphoblastic leukemia with recurrent cytogenetic abnormalities

t4.12 WHO classification of B-lymphoblastic leukemia/ lymphoma

B-lymphoblastic leukemia/lymphoma, not otherwise specified
B-lymphoblastic leukemia/lymphoma with recurrent genetic abnormalities
B-lymphoblastic leukemia/lymphoma with t(9;22)(q34.1;q11.2); *BCR-ABL1*
B-lymphoblastic leukemia/lymphoma with t(v;11q23.3);KMT2A (MLL) rearranged
B-lymphoblastic leukemia/lymphoma with t(12;21)(p13.2;q22.1); *TEL-AML1 (ETV6-RUNX1)*
B-lymphoblastic leukemia/lymphoma with hyperdiploidy
B-lymphoblastic leukemia/lymphoma with hypodiploidy
B-lymphoblastic leukemia/lymphoma with t(5;14)(q31.1;q32.1) IL3-IGH
B-lymphoblastic leukemia/lymphoma with t(1;19)(q23;p13.3);TCF3-PBX1
B-lymphoblastic leukemia/lymphoma, BCR-ABL1–like
B-lymphoblastic leukemia/lymphoma with iAMP21

- Cytogenetic abnormalities are biologically distinct and grouped based on clinical features and prognostic significance
- **t4.13** highlights features of selected subgroups of B-cell acute lymphoblastic leukemia with recurrent cytogenetic abnormalities

t4.13 B ALL/LBL with recurrent genetic abnormalities

Abnormality	Genetics	Age group	Prognosis	Immunophenotype
t(9;22) (q34.1;q11.2)	*BCR/ABL1*	25% of adults 3% of children	Worst of all in this category	CD19+, CD10+, TdT+, CD34+ CD13/33+ (weak), CD25+
t(v;11)(q23.3), usually t(4;11)	*KMT2A* rearranged	80% of infants express t(4;11)	Poor	CD19+, CD10–, CD15+ overexpress FLT3
t(12;21) (p13.2;q22.1)	*ETV6-RUNX1*	25% of children	Good	CD19+, CD10+, CD9– CD13/33+ (weak)
Hyperdiploid	>50 extra copies esp of 21, 4, 14, X	25% of children	Good	CD19+, CD10+, TdT+, CD34+
Hypodiploid	<46	<5% of children & adults	Poor	CD19+, CD10+, TdT+, CD34+
t(5;14) (q31.1;q32.1)	*IL3-IGH*	<1% of children & adults	Intermediate	CD19+, CD10+, TdT+, CD34+
t(1;19) (q23;p13.3)	*TCF3-PBX1*	5% of children	Poor	CD19+, CD10+, CD34–

4.9.5.2 T-cell acute lymphoblastic leukemia (precursor)

- Malignant lymphoblasts are T cells
- Cannot be distinguished morphologically from B cells
- General features
  - Commonly presents in adolescence
  - Often involvement of thymus expressed as a mediastinal mass

- May be more aggressive disease than B-cell acute lymphoblastic leukemia
- Laboratory findings i4.40c
  - WBC count often elevated
  - Normocytic, normochromic anemia & thrombocytopenia typical
  - Proliferation of undifferentiated blasts with variable morphology as previously described
  - T-cell immunophenotype
- Classification
  - The World Health Organization scheme includes provisional entities
    - Provisional entity: Early T-cell precursor lymphoblastic leukemia
    - Provisional entity: Natural killer (NK) cell lymphoblastic leukemia/lymphoma

4.9.6 Mature lymphoproliferative (lymphoid) disorders

- Heterogeneous group of conditions that include both mature B- and T-cell malignancies as well as plasma cell disorders
- The WHO classification (2016) includes mature B-cell, mature T-cell, and natural killer cell (NK) neoplasms, Hodgkin lymphoma, and posttransplant lymphoproliferative disorders (PTLD)

4.9.6.1 Selected B-cell neoplasms

4.9.6.1.1 Chronic lymphocytic leukemia (CLL)/ small lymphocytic lymphoma (SLL) i4.41

- CLL is a malignancy of bone marrow & peripheral blood
- SLL is a malignancy that presents as tumor masses primarily in lymphoid organs
- SLL represents a different clinical manifestation of the same disease as CLL
- General features of CLL
  - Most common B-cell leukemia in the Western hemisphere
  - Strong genetic component
    - Familial clustering seen in 5% of cases
    - Five-fold increased risk in first-degree relatives of those affected
    - Incidence increases with age (median age at diagnosis 65 years)
    - Risk factors include autoimmunity & immunodeficiency
- Laboratory findings of CLL
  - Increased WBC count (typically $20\times10^3/\mu L$-$100\times10^3/\mu L$ [20-$100\times10^9/L$])

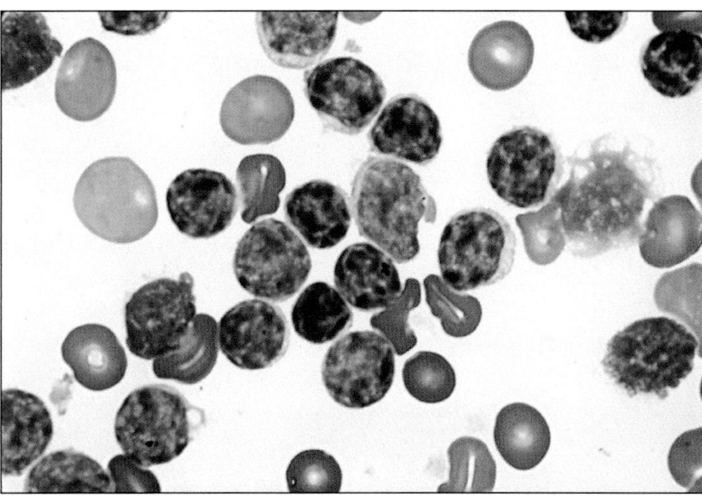

i4.41 Chronic lymphocytic leukemia (CLL)/small lymphocytic lymphoma (SLL) showing marked lymphocytosis with many mature lymphocytes & a smudge cell

  - Lymphocytosis usually $>5\times10^3/\mu L$ ($>5.0\times10^9/L$)
  - Normocytic, normochromic anemia
  - Small to medium-sized, mature-appearing lymphocytes
    - Scanty blue cytoplasm
    - Round nuclei with no or inconspicuous nucleoli & clumped chromatin (blocklike or checkerboard)
  - Many smudge cells
  - Prolymphocytes may be seen (<10%)
  - Possible thrombocytopenia
  - Cells express CD19, CD20, CD23, CD5, sIg
  - CD38 & ZAP70 expression associated with atypical cellular morphology, unmutated *IgVH* gene (immune globulin heavy chain variable region), and an unfavorable prognosis
  - Several cytogenetic abnormalities possible [trisomy 12, del(13q14), del(11q), del(14q), del(17p)], but none specific

4.9.6.1.2 Prolymphocytic leukemia

- General features
  - 80% of cases B cell
  - Often acute onset
  - Patients typically have prominent splenomegaly
  - Rare but aggressive disease
  - Poor prognosis
- Laboratory findings
  - Markedly elevated WBC count (often $>100\times10^3/\mu L$ [$>100\times10^9/L$])
  - Anemia & thrombocytopenia present at diagnosis
  - Prolymphocytes represent >55% of lymphoid cells

ISBN 978-089189-6616

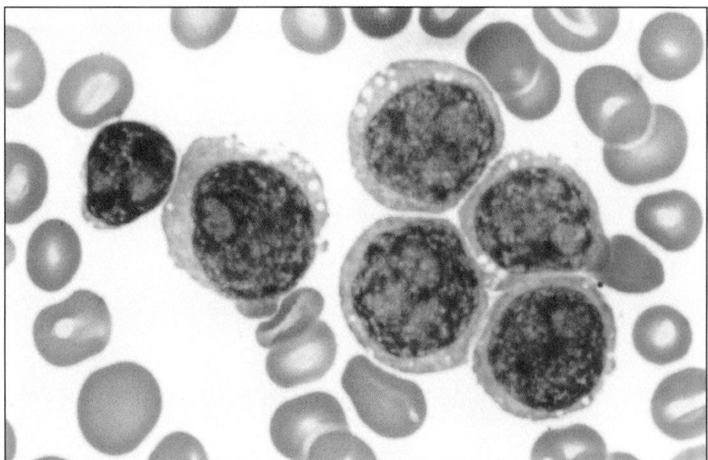

i4.42 Prolymphocytic leukemia: 5 prolymphocytes

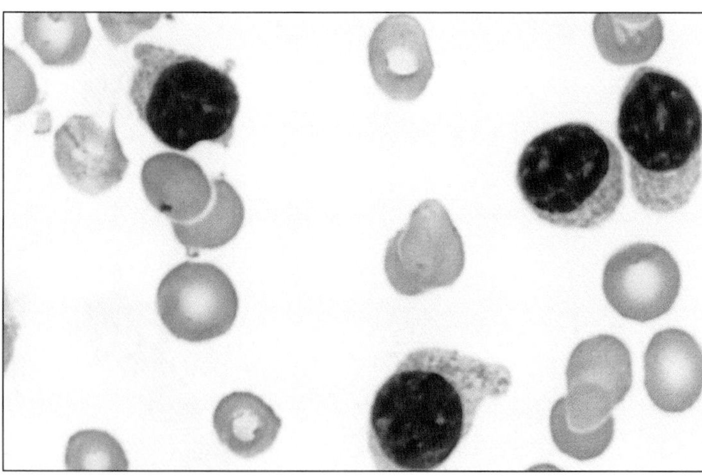

i4.44 Large granular lymphocytosis: several granular lymphocytes

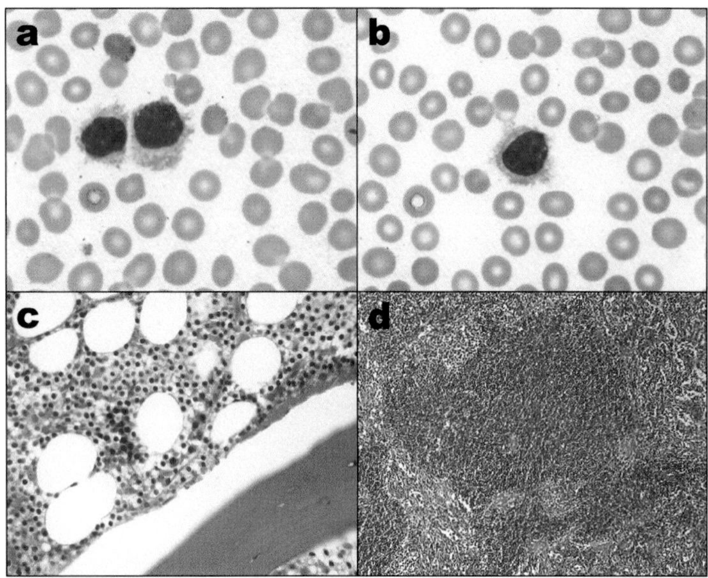

i4.43 Hairy cell leukemia (HCL)
a & b Peripheral blood involvement by cells with large nuclei, approximately twice the size of a red cell, no nucleoli & an abundance of cytoplasm with frayed edges (hairy projections)
c Marrow involvement by cells with abundant clear cytoplasm ("fried eggs")
d Blood lake in the spleen

- Characteristic morphology i4.42
  - Large cells with moderate amount of blue cytoplasm
  - Nuclear chromatin moderately condensed
  - Usually single, prominent nucleolus
- Cells express CD19, CD20, CD22, FMC7, CD79a & sIg

4.9.6.1.3 Hairy cell leukemia

- General features
  - Rare condition affecting primarily middle-aged men
  - Patients typically present with massive splenomegaly
- Laboratory findings i4.43
  - Pancytopenia often present
  - Hairy cells visible in peripheral blood
    - Medium-sized cells
    - Nuclei are round, oval, or reniform with generally fine chromatin; nucleoli are absent or indistinct
    - Pale blue cytoplasm with projections ("hairs") that are circumferential, sometimes indistinct, and may appear frayed
  - Bone marrow may be hypocellular and fibrosis is common
    - May result in dry tap bone marrow aspirate
  - Cells express CD19, CD20, CD22, CD25, CD11c, CD103, TRAP (tartrate resistant acid phosphatase) & sIg
  - Almost all cases associated with *BRAFV600E* mutation

4.9.6.2 Selected T-cell neoplasms

4.9.6.2.1 Large granular lymphocytic leukemia (LGLL)

- General features
  - Sustained (>6 months) increase in large granular lymphocytes (LGLs) not associated with any cause
  - Splenomegaly common symptom
  - Indolent disease progression
- Laboratory findings i4.44
  - Absolute increase in LGLs (≥2000/µL [$\geq 2.0 \times 10^9$/L])
    - Large cells with abundant, pale blue cytoplasm
    - Azurophilic granules present in cytoplasm
    - Round or oval nuclei with clumped chromatin and no visible nucleoli

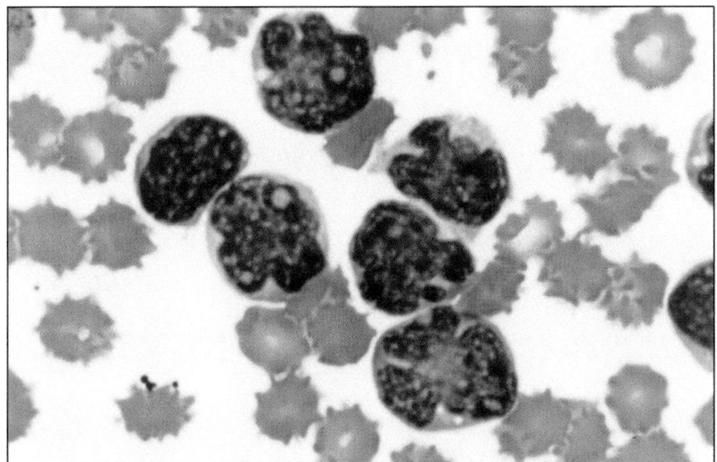

i4.45 Adult T-cell leukemia/lymphoma: lymphoma cells with multilobated nuclei

- Absolute lymphocytosis (2000-20,000/µL [2-20×10^9/L])
- Clonality demonstrated by T-cell receptor (TCR) gene rearrangement
- Cells express CD2, CD3, CD8, CD16 & CD57

4.9.6.2.2 Adult T-cell leukemia/lymphoma (ATLL)

- General features
  - Associated in adults with human T-cell lymphotropic virus type 1 (HTLV-1)
  - Endemic in southern Japan, some locations in the South Pacific & sections of the Caribbean
  - Widespread lymphadenopathy & hepatosplenomegaly seen in patients
- Laboratory findings i4.45
  - Peripheral blood involvement (as well as tissue) often present
  - Leukemic cells have lobulated nuclei that appear like flowers or cloverleaves
  - Cells express CD2, CD3, CD4, CD5 & CD25

4.9.6.2.3 Sézary sydrome

- General features
  - Malignancy of mature T cells
  - Related to mycosis fungoides, a T-cell malignancy of the skin, which may or may not have peripheral blood involvement
    - Cutaneous lesions appear as patches or plaques on the skin
  - Abnormal T cells in Sézary syndrome may be seen in skin, lymph nodes & peripheral blood
    - Patients demonstrate erythroderma & generalized lymphadenopathy

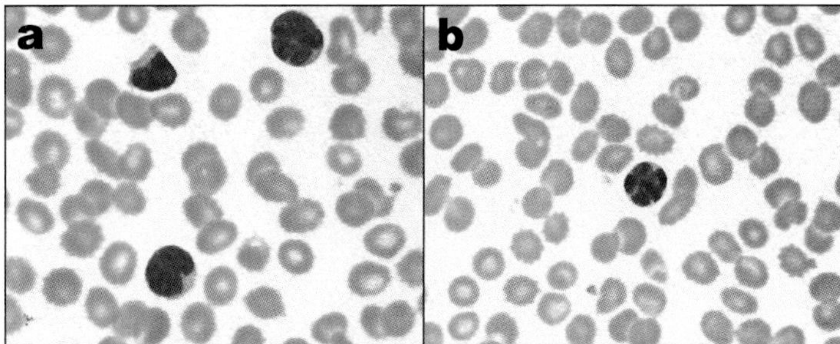

i4.46 a-b Peripheral blood involvement by mycosis fungoides (Sézary syndrome) consisting of cells with markedly irregular (cerebriform) nuclear contours

- Laboratory findings i4.46
  - Sézary cells seen in peripheral blood
    - Small to large cells with cerebriform or convoluted nuclei
    - Nucleoli are usually not visible and chromatin is fine
  - Cells are CD4-positive lymphocytes but also express CD2, CD3 & CD5
  - Loss of at least 1 T-cell antigen (usually CD7) characteristic

Plasma cell neoplasms

- Group of disorders characterized by abnormal clone of plasma cells that produce increased amounts of immunoglobulin (monoclonal)

4.9.6.2.4 Multiple myeloma

- General features
  - Affects older adults with median age at onset 70 years
  - More common in African Americans
  - Familial clustering seen with increased risk in first-degree relatives (3-4 time increased risk)
  - Mean survival 3-5 years
  - Many clinical manifestations that may include:
    - Renal insufficiency
    - Hypercalcemia
    - Lytic bone lesions
    - Hyperviscosity syndrome
- Laboratory findings
  - Bone marrow plasmacytosis (>10%)
    - Cells may appear in clusters or sheets
    - Immature & abnormal cells may be seen
    - Nuclear & cytoplasmic inclusions are possible, but not diagnostic
  - Monoclonal protein (M spike) in serum and/or urine
    - M protein usually represents complete immunoglobulin molecule with a heavy chain, but only 1 of 2 possible light chains (κ or λ)

ISBN 978-089189-6616

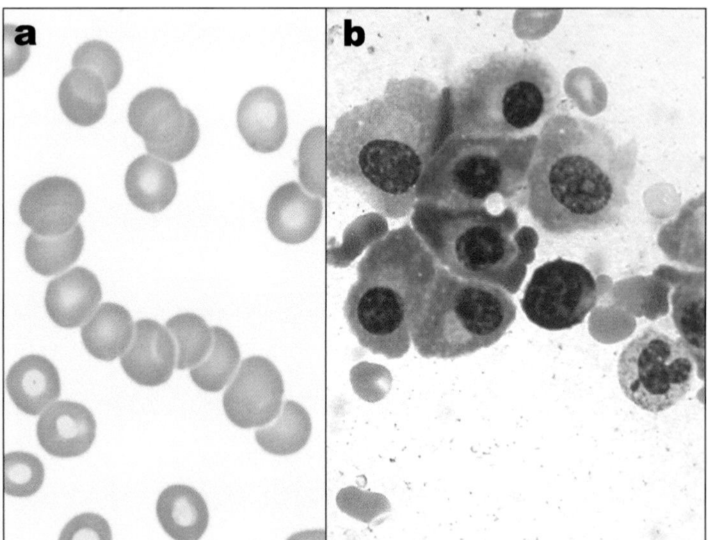

i4.47 Multiple myeloma: a red cell rouleaux; b prominent paranuclear hofs are evident

    - Most cases are IgG followed by IgA, light chains only, and rarely IgD and IgE
    - Bence Jones protein (free light chains) seen in urine of about 2/3 of cases
  - Normocytic, normochromic anemia
  - Rouleaux i4.47a & elevated ESR
  - Paranuclear hof represents the golgi apparatus i4.47b
  - Thrombocytopenia
  - Neutropenia as disease progresses
  - Plasma cells seen in peripheral blood in advanced stages
  - Cells express cytoplasmic κ or λ, CD38 CD138, CD56 (and characteristically do not express B-cell antigens)
  - Common cytogenetic findings include 14q32 (*IgH* gene), t(11;14)(q13;q32), CCND1/IgH, but none are specific

4.9.6.2.5 Waldenström macroglobulinemia

- General features
  - Represents a lymphoplasmacytic lymphoma (LPL) with an IgM monoclonal gammopathy & bone marrow involvement
  - Hyperviscosity syndrome results in poor circulation, visual difficulties, headache & other symptoms
  - Lymphadenopathy, hepatosplenomegaly seen in patients
  - Some cases associated with cryoglobulinemia
  - In contrast to multiple myeloma, patients do not have lytic bone lesions
- Laboratory findings
  - Elevated IgM (with M spike on protein electrophoresis)
  - Small lymphocytes, plasmacytoid lymphocytes, and plasma cells predominate in bone marrow (≥10% lymphoplasmacytic infiltration)
  - Normocytic, normochromic anemia possible
  - Cells express CD19, CD20, CD38, sIg & cIg (plasma cells)
  - Associated mutations include *MYD88* L265P (>90% of LPL cases) & CXCR4

4.9.6.2.6 Plasma cell leukemia

- General features
  - May arise de novo or as a terminal phase of multiple myeloma
  - Aggressive disease
  - Poor response to treatment & poor prognosis
- Laboratory findings
  - Defined by $>2\times10^3/\mu L$ ($>2.0\times10^9/L$; or 20% of WBCs) plasma cells in the peripheral blood
  - Most plasma cells are immature
  - Features seen in bone marrow & peripheral blood similar to multiple myeloma
  - Cells express CD20 but no CD56

4.9.6.2.7 Monoclonal gammopathy of undetermined significance (MGUS)

- General features
  - Patients present with monoclonal gammopathy, but essentially lack a B-cell malignancy that results in an M spike
  - No evidence to support known plasma cell dyscrasias
    - No organ damage
- Laboratory findings
  - Serum monoclonal protein <3.0 g/dL
  - <10% plasma cells in bone marrow
  - No specific peripheral blood changes

4.9.7 Lymphomas

- Represent diverse group of lymphoid neoplasms
- Broadly divided into 2 major classifications: Hodgkin lymphoma (HL) & non-Hodgkin lymphoma (NHL)
- Most are B cell in origin
- May or may not have bone marrow and/or peripheral blood involvement
- Some previously summarized (chronic lymphocytic leukemia/small lymphocytic lymphoma, adult T-cell leukemia/lymphoma, Sézary syndrome, mycosis fungoides, lymphoplasmacytic lymphoma)

4.9.7.1 Hodgkin lymphoma

- General features
  - Two main histologic subtypes with unique clinical & biologic profiles
  - Classic Hodgkin lymphoma (HL) represents 95% of cases
    - Classic HL is further subdivided by histologic characteristics into 4 additional groups
  - Lymphocyte predominant HL (LPHL) accounts for the remaining 5%
  - No bone marrow or peripheral blood involvement
  - Characteristic bimodal age distribution (classic HL) in patients
    - Peak in patients aged 15-35 years
    - Second peak in patients >50 years
  - Commonly presents as painless swelling of lymph nodes
  - Lymphadenopathy spreads in contiguous manner
  - Lymphocyte predominant HL affects younger adults and lymph node involvement not contiguous
- Laboratory findings
  - Classic HL
    - Reed-Sternberg (RS) cells or RS variants seen in tissue
    - RS cells express CD15 & CD30, but not common B-cell markers
  - LPHL
    - Malignant histiocytes described as "popcorn" cells because of folded nuclei
    - Do not express CD15 & CD30

4.9.7.2 Non-Hodgkin

- General features
  - Most seen in adults >60 years old
  - Variable presenting symptoms, but often associated with painless swelling of ≥1 lymph nodes
  - Spread of disease is noncontiguous
  - Most types originate in lymph nodes, but disease can begin in extranodal sites
  - Bone marrow and/or peripheral blood involvement may be seen
  - Many types
- Laboratory findings & selected subtypes
  - **t4.14** summarizes important features of selected B-cell non-Hodgkin lymphomas (NHLs) that have bone marrow and/or peripheral blood involvement

t4.14 Important features of selected B-cell non-Hodgkin lymphomas

Lymphoma type	BM/PB morphology	Immunophenotype	Cytogenetics	Notes
Burkitt lymphoma/leukemia	Intermediate-sized lymphs with round nuclei, fine chromatin, multiple nucleoli, scanty, deeply basophilic & vacuolated cytoplasm	Express CD19, CD20, CD22, CD10, sIg, Myc, Ki67	*MYC* gene rearrangement from t(8:14)	2 subtypes associated with either EBV or HIV; extranodal sites often involved (jaw)
Diffuse large cell	Large cells, moderate amount of blue cytoplasm, multiple nuclei with open chromatin	Express CD19, CD20, CD22, CD45	*BCL2*, t(14;18), *BCL6*, t(3;x) rearrangements	Most often presents as GI mass; 2 phenotypes
Follicular	Small cells with condensed nuclear chromatin, scanty blue cytoplasm; distinct nuclear clefting; large cells with pleomorphic features may also be seen	Express CD19, CD20, FMC7, CD22, CD10, sIg, bcl2, bcl6	t(14;18) results in *BCL2* rearrangement	Duodenal & testicular sites possible
Mantle cell	Variable with small cells & clumped nuclear chromatin, scanty, blue cytoplasm; or larger, blastlike cells	Express CD19, CD20, CD22, FMC7, CD5, sIg, CD43, bcl1 (cyclin D1), SOX11 (need when cyclin D1 negative)	t(11;14) results in translocation of *IgH* gene to CCND1 [11q13]	Men often affected; detect cyclin D1 by FISH
Marginal zone, splenic	Small to medium cells with clumped nuclear chromatin, inconspicuous nucleoli, scant to moderate blue cytoplasm & irregular cytoplasmic margins with polar villous projections	Express CD19, CD20, CD79a, FMC7, bcl2, sIg	7q31-32, trisomy 3	White pulp spleen; 2 other subtypes possible

BM, bone marrow; EBV, Epstein-Barr virus; GI, gastrointestinal; HIV, human immunodeficiency virus; PB, peripheral blood

ISBN 978-089189-6616

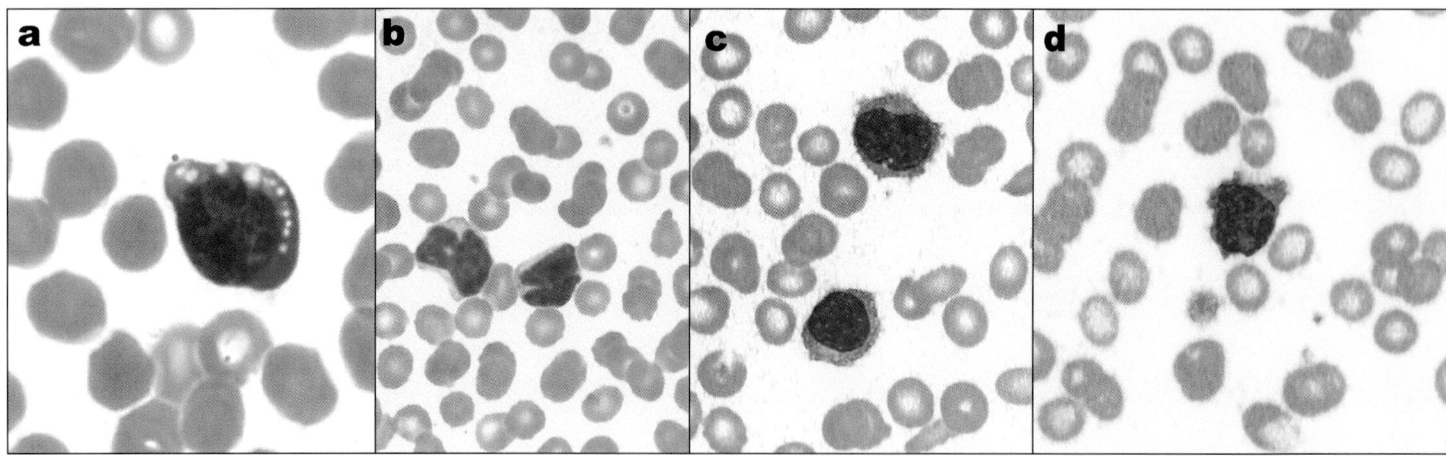

i4.48 Selected B cell lymphomas: a Burkitt lymphoma in peripheral blood (& in touch imprints) has deep blue vacuolated cytoplasm; b Follicular lymphoma (FL) involving the peripheral blood; c-d splenic marginal zone lymphoma with villous lymphocytes, in which lymphocytes with distinct nucleoli are associated with voluminous cytoplasm that is bipolar & has polar villi

- Morphologic features of selected B cell lymphomas
  - Burkitt lymphoma/leukemia i4.48a
  - Follicular lymphoma i4.48b
  - Splenic marginal zone lymphoma i4.48c-d

4.10 Laboratory procedures

4.10.1 Cell counts for WBCs & platelets

4.10.1.1 Manual method (hemacytometer—Levy chamber with improved Neubauer ruling)

- Principle
  - Whole blood is added to diluent (1% buffered ammonium oxalate, 3% acetic acid, or 1% hydrochloric acid) which lyses RBCs
  - White blood cells & platelets preserved
  - Diluted sample added to a hemacytometer (chamber)
  - Microscope used to count the number of cells in all 9 large squares of the chamber
- Reporting results
  - Number of cells per microliter (µL) of whole blood calculated using number of cells counted (average both sides of chamber), dilution factor, volume used
  - General formula

$$\text{total count} = \frac{\text{\# cells counted} \times \text{dilution factor}}{\text{area (mm}^2\text{)} \times \text{depth}}$$

  - Typically 1:100 dilution of sample used (1.98 mL diluent & 20 µL blood)
  - Area of chamber = 1 mm×1 mm × 9 = 0.9 mm^2
  - Depth of chamber = 0.1 mm
  - Final result

$$\text{total count} = \frac{\text{\# cells counted} \times 100}{0.9\ \text{mm}^2 \times 0.1\ \text{mm}}$$

  - Note that for manual platelet counts, 1% ammonium oxalate is the diluent, the dilution is 1:100, and platelets are counted in 25 small squares in the large center square of the hemacytometer (1 mm^2)
  - See chapter 3, Body Fluids, for manual cell counts on cerebrospinal fluid (3.3.6), serous fluids (3.4.5) & synovial fluid (3.5.6)
- Sources of error
  - Improper dilution
  - Dirty hemacytometer
  - Improper charging of chamber
  - Failure to allow cells to settle before counting
  - Improper counting or counting debris
  - Presence of nucleated RBCs (for WBC counts)
    - The WBC count can be corrected for nucleated RBCs (NRBCs) using the following formula

$$\frac{\text{uncorrected WBC count} \times 100}{\text{number of NRBCs per 100 WBCs} + 100}$$

  - Inaccurate calculation of results

4.10.1.2 Automated methods

- Principles
  - 2 basic methods used in automated cell counting instruments
  - Electrical impedance

- When cells suspended in a conductive diluent traverse a small aperture, they cause an increase in electrical resistance to the flow of current between 2 electrodes
- These voltage changes (pulses) can be detected & measured
- The number of pulses detected is proportional to the number of cells passing through the aperture
- The height of each voltage pulse is directly proportional to the volume (size) of each cell
- Sometimes radio frequency supplements impedance counting instruments
  - Radio frequency measures conductivity and allows further discrimination of each cell's internal characteristics and separation of leukocyte subtypes

- Optical (light scatter)
  - Cells suspended in a diluent pass through a sensing zone and interrupt light generated by a laser
  - The interruption allows cells to be counted
  - Light is also scattered
  - Photodetectors capture scattered light
  - The degree of forward light scatter determines cell size and side scatter data measures cell granularity, which allows separation of cell types & leukocyte subgroups
  - Note that many automated hematology analyzers have a dedicated body fluid channel or mode for performing cell counts on selected fluids

- Interferences
  - Several conditions can interfere with automated cell counting and cause spurious or erroneous results
  - Cold agglutinins can decrease RBC counts as erythrocytes clump
  - Hemolysis can cause decreased RBC counts as erythrocytes are lysed and not counted
  - RBCs in some abnormal hemoglobins are lysis-resistant and these erythrocytes are counted as WBCs (increase WBC counts)
  - Microcytes & schistocytes may be counted as platelets (increase platelet counts) and decrease RBC count
  - Older instruments cannot discriminate among nucleated RBCs, megakaryocyte fragments, or very large platelets, and cause increased WBC counts
  - Platelet clumps cause platelets to be counted as WBCs and increase WBC counts and decrease platelet counts

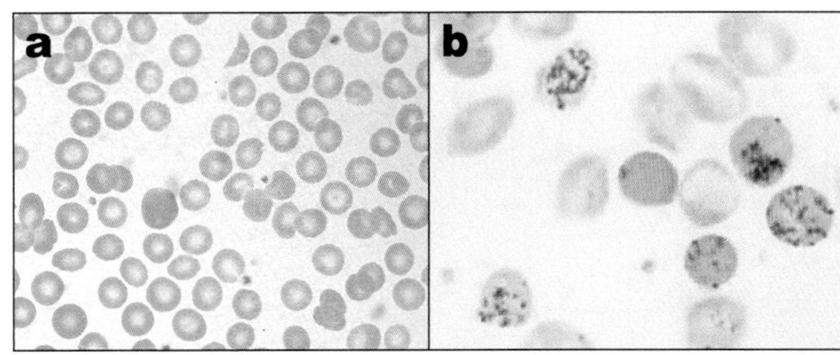

i4.49 Reticulocytes on a Wright stained smear & b supravital stain

  - Extremely elevated WBC counts with associated turbidity can interfere with spectrophotometric determination of hemoglobin (increase); RBC count can be increased when WBCs are counted with RBCs
  - Fragile WBCs (seen in leukemia) may decrease WBC counts

- Leukocyte differential counts
  - In addition to total WBC counts, automated hematology analyzers can provide leukocyte differentials to include relative and absolute values for all WBC subtypes
  - Some of these instruments can also measure the populations of immature granulocytes (promyelocytes, myelocytes, metamyelocytes)

4.10.2 Cell counts for reticulocytes

4.10.2.1 Manual method

- Principle
  - Reticulocytes are young, non-nucleated RBCs
  - On Wright-stained peripheral blood smears, reticulocytes are identified as polychromatophilic cells i4.49a
  - The blue tint of polychromatophilic RBCs results from ribosomal RNA retained in the cytoplasm
  - To enumerate reticulocytes, RBCs are stained with a supravital stain, typically new methylene blue i4.49b
  - The stain causes the ribosomal RNA to precipitate as blue granular filaments or "reticulum"
  - The younger the RBC, the more reticulum or network will be seen
  - Reticulocytes are counted per 1000 RBCs (note that each reticulocyte is counted twice, once as a reticulocyte and once as an erythrocyte)
  - Note that a Miller disc can be used to facilitate easier counting of the large number of RBCs
- Reporting results
  - Reticulocytes are reported as a percentage

$$\text{reticulocyte \%} = \frac{\text{\# reticulocytes} \times 100}{\text{1000 RBCs}}$$

ISBN 978-089189-6616

- General normal is 0.5%-1.5%
- In an anemic patient, a correction is needed; the percentage of reticulocytes may be falsely increased because of a fewer number of RBCs that are present

$$\text{corrected reticulocyte (\%)} = \frac{\text{reticulocyte \%} \times \text{patient hematocrit (\%)}}{\text{45 (average normal hematocrit)}}$$

- When "shift" reticulocytes are seen on a Wright-stained peripheral blood smear (polychromatophilic cells), an adjustment is needed to account for RBCs that are maturing longer than the usual 1 day in the circulation
- This adjustment is the reticulocyte production index (RPI)

$$\text{RPI} = \frac{\text{corrected reticulocyte count (\%)}}{\text{maturation time}}$$

- The maturation time varies by patient hematocrit as shown in **t4.15**

t4.15 Maturation time by hematocrit

Patient hematocrit	Maturation time (days)
36-45	1.0
26-35	1.5
16-25	2.0
≤15	2.5

- The absolute reticulocyte count can also be determined

$$\text{absolute reticulocyte count } (\times 10^6/\mu L \text{ or } \times 10^{12}/L) = \text{\% reticulocytes} \times \text{RBC count } (\times 10^6/\mu L \text{ or } \times 10^{12}/L)$$

- Sources of error
  - More or less blood to be added to stain for anemic or polycythemic patients, respectively
  - Failure to mix blood before adding to stain or to mix blood/stain mixture prior to making smears for counting
  - Artifacts like refractile areas caused by slow drying, which can be confused with reticulocytes
  - Improper counting of reticulocytes
  - Counting other RBC inclusions as reticulocytes (Heinz bodies, Howell-Jolly bodies, Pappenheimer bodies)

4.10.2.2 Automated method

- Principle
  - RBCs treated with fluorescent dyes or nucleic acid stains to highlight residual RNA in reticulocytes and then analyzed based on light (optical) scatter or fluorescence
- Reporting results
  - Relative & absolute reticulocyte values determined and reported as percentage or $\times 10^6/\mu L$ ($\times 10^{12}/L$) respectively
  - Additional parameters available on some instruments
    - Imature reticulocyte fraction (IRF) as an early indicator of erythropoiesis
    - Reticulocyte hemoglobin content (CHr or Ret-He) reflects the availability of bone marrow iron
    - Mean reticulocyte volume (similar to mean cell volume as a measure of reticulocyte size)
    - Reticulocyte distribution width (similar to red cell distribution width as an indicator of variation in reticulocyte size)

4.10.3 Making & staining peripheral blood smears

4.10.3.1 Making a good smear (wedge)

- Steps
  - Select a glass slide free of dust & debris and place a well-mixed drop of blood (about 2-3 mm) at approximately 1 cm from one end of the slide
  - Using another glass slide (spreader slide) held at about a 30°-45° angle, place the spreader slide on the first slide in front of the blood drop or on the slide toward the long end of the first slide
  - Pull the spreader slide into the drop of blood, allowing the blood to spread evenly across the width of the spreader slide
  - Maintaining the spreader slide at a constant angle, push the spreader slide quickly & smoothly forward in a rapid motion
  - Label the slide and allow it to air dry
- Characteristics of a good smear
  - Smooth, no vacuoles, jerks, streaks, ridges, or other irregularities
  - 2/3 to 3/4 the length of the slide
  - Straight or only slightly rounded feathered edge
  - Visible lateral edges
  - Absence of visible clotting
  - Not too thick, with transition from thick to thin
  - No clumping of cells near feathered edge, especially platelets
  - Even distribution of cells; RBCs barely touching or overlapping

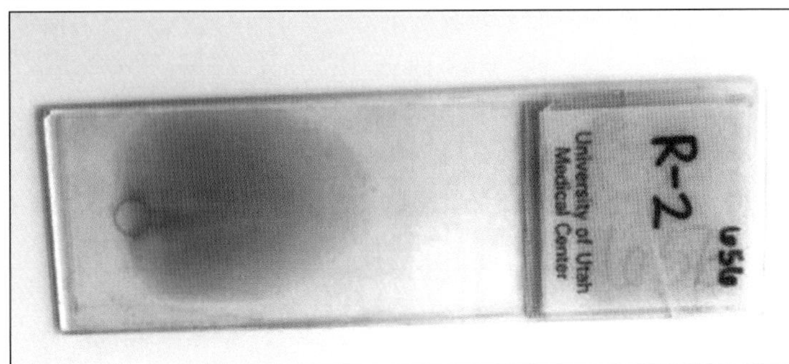

i4.50 Macroscopic view of a properly made & well-stained peripheral blood smear

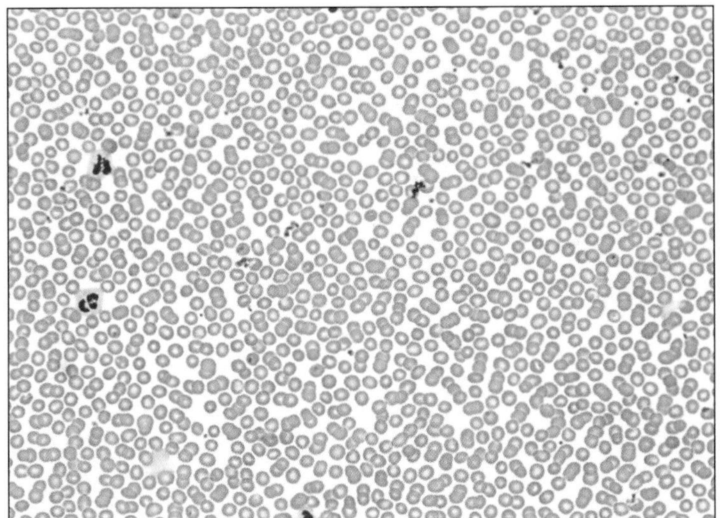

i4.51 Microscopic view of a properly prepared & well-stained peripheral blood smear (low magnification)

4.10.3.2 Staining smears

- Components & function of the Wright stain
  - Wright stain makes cells more visible and enhances cellular detail and morphologic features for better evaluation
  - Wright stain is a polychrome stain because dyes present produce multiple colors when applied to cells
  - Mixture of methylene blue & eosin
  - Methylene blue is basic (and positively charged) and stains acidic components of the cell various shades of blue to purple
  - Eosin is acidic (and negatively charged) and stains basic components of cells varying shades of orange to pink
  - Staining reactions are pH dependent and pH of buffer is important
  - Neutral cellular structures are stained by both dyes
  - Methanol needed as a fixative so that cells adhere to the glass slide
- Characteristics of a well-stained smear
  - Macroscopic i4.50
    - Smear is a purple-pinkish color
  - Microscopic i4.51
    - No precipitated stain or artifacts between cells (bubbles or water droplets)
    - Pink or orange-red RBCs
    - Pale central area evident with erythrocytes
    - Nuclei in WBCs are purple & chromatin/parachromatin evident
    - Light pink cytoplasm with lilac granules in neutrophils
    - Large, bright, orange-red individual granules in eosinophils
    - Large, dark blue, or purple (may look black) individual granules in basophils
    - Varying shades of blue cytoplasm in lymphocytes
    - Gray-blue cytoplasm in monocytes
    - Purple or bluish platelets
- Automation
  - Some automated hematology instruments have capabilities of making and staining peripheral blood smears

4.10.4 Examining a peripheral blood smear

- One of the most important procedures in the hematology laboratory
  - Provides information for diagnosis
  - Is the basis for selection of additional laboratory analyses to help establish a diagnosis
  - Guides clinicians to choose & monitor treatment
  - Indicates possible harmful effects of therapy

4.10.4.1 The differential WBC count

- Procedure
  - First examine the smear using low power (10×) to evaluate quality of the smear & distribution of cells
  - Select good area of the smear to begin the differential cell count using the high dry (40×) or 50× oil immersion lens
    - Good area (~200 cells in field) near feathered edge, with RBCs slightly overlapping and areas of central pallor visible
    - The high dry objective can also be used to perform a WBC estimate by averaging the number of WBCs seen in 10 fields and multiplying by 2000

ISBN 978-089189-6616

Laboratory procedures>Examining a peripheral blood smear

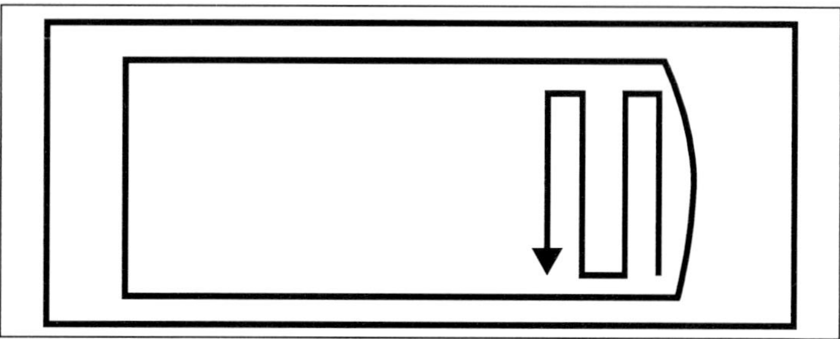

f4.5 Battlement pattern for counting WBCs in a manual differential cell count

- Use an oil immersion objective (50× or 100×) for the differential count
- Count 100 WBCs using a battlement pattern or by tracking top to bottom on the slide f4.5
- Classify each WBC seen and record on a counter until 100 cells have been identified
- Note & record any WBC abnormalities while counting
- Examine & note any changes in RBC morphology
- Examine platelets for number & morphology
- Results are reported as percentage for each type of WBC seen
- Manual differential cell counts can also be performed on body fluids; see chapter 3 Body Fluids
- Note that body fluid WBC differential cell counts may be performed with hematology instruments that have a dedicated body fluid mode
- The body fluid differential is usually limited to only multilobed cells & mononuclear cells

- Distinguishing WBCs
  - Major types of WBCs are granulocytes, lymphocytes & monocytes
  - There are 3 types of granulocytes: neutrophils, eosinophils & basophils
  - t4.16 summarizes the granulocytic maturation sequence and selected characteristics associated with each stage of development

t4.16 Summary of characteristics of the granulocytic maturation sequence

Cell	Morphology	Size	N:C	Nucleus	Cytoplasm
Myeloblast		Large	High	Large Round or oval with 2 or more nucleoli Fine chromatin pattern Reddish purple	Deeply basophilic Scanty Usually lacks granules
Promyelocyte		Large; may be slightly larger than myeloblast	High	Still large Round or oval with 2 or more nucleoli visible Fine chromatin pattern Reddish purple	Basophilic cytoplasm Few to many prominent dark red or purple primary granules
Myelocyte		Decreased from blast	Slightly high	Becoming more clumped & coarse No nucleoli visible Often eccentrically located; may be oval Reddish purple;	Few primary granules but specific (secondary) granules begin to appear: neutrophilic, eosinophilic or basophilic Bluish pink cytoplasm
Metamyelocyte		Decreased from blast	Equal	Chromatin condensed & clumped; darker purple; indented or kidney bean shaped; no nucleoli	Many neutrophilic, eosinophilic or basophilic granules Pink cytoplasm
Band		Slightly smaller than meta; cell will not decrease in size any more	Low	U or C shape of uniform thickness Clumped & condensed chromatin No nucleoli Deep purple	Many neutrophilic, eosinophilic or basophilic granules Pink cytoplasm
Polymorphonuclear neutrophil (PMN, seg)		About same as band; segs are 2× the size of normal RBCs	Low	Distinct lobes visible connected by chromatin strand; 2-5 lobes possible Clumped chromatin Deep purple	Many tan, pink or violet pink granules Faint pink cytoplasm
Eosinophil		About same as seg	Low	Only 2 lobes usually present Clumped chromatin Deep purple but almost obscured by specific granules in cytoplasm	Many large, coarse, orange granules Faint pink cytoplasm when visible
Basophil		About same as seg	Low	Only 2 lobes usually present Clumped chromatin Deep purple but almost obscured by specific granules in cytoplasm	Many large, coarse, bluish-black granules Faint pink cytoplasm when visible

N:C, nuclear to cytoplasmic ratio

- t4.17 summarizes characteristics of lymphocytes & monocytes, including reactive lymphocytes

t4.17 Lymphocyte & monocyte characteristics

	Small lymph	Reactive lymph	Monocyte
Cell size	8-12 µm	Variable, can be large (9-30 µm)	Large (15-18 µm)
Nuclear shape	Round	Irregular (lobulated, oval, notched)	Horseshoe, round, folded
Nuclear chromatin	Clumped; parachromatin not evident & more lavender	More fine (but not like blasts) Parachromatin more evident & white	Lacy, loose strands, brainlike
Nucleoli	Usually not present	May be prominent	Absent
Cytoplasm amount	Scant	Abundant	Abundant
Cytoplasm color	Blue	Often deep, intense blue with darker edges at contact points with other cells	Light bluish-gray

- Quantitative & morphologic WBC changes associated with nonmalignant disorders
  - Seen when neutrophils are activated by cytokines, such as granulocyte-colony-stimulating factor (G-CSF) or an infection
  - Quantitative change usually is neutrophilia accompanied by a neutrophilic left shift
  - Morphologic changes include Döhle bodies, toxic granulation & toxic vacuolation
  - Morphologic changes in WBCs (including reactive lymphocytes) need to be reported according to individual laboratory protocol and may use specific terminology (slight, moderate, marked) or graded on a scale (1+, 2+, 3+)
  - Döhle bodies
    - Light blue, usually single inclusions of varying size & shape in the cytoplasm of neutrophils & bands
    - Remnants of rough endoplasmic reticulum or aggregates of denatured free ribosomes
    - Often seen in combination with toxic granulation & toxic vacuolation
    - Toxic granulation
      - Large, purplish or blue-violet granules in the cytoplasm of neutrophils & bands
      - Primary granules that have retained their basophilia
    - Toxic vacuolation
      - Round or oval unstained areas of varying sizes in the cytoplasm of neutrophils & bands
      - End stage of phagocytosis

4.10.4.2 Evaluating RBC morphology

- RBCs are evaluated for size, shape, hemoglobin content (chromicity), distribution & inclusions
- Morphologic changes are reported according to individual laboratory protocol and may include specific terminology (slight, moderate, marked) or a grading scale (1+, 2+, 3+)
- Size
  - Normal RBCs are generally uniform in size and have no nucleus
  - They are about the same size as the nucleus of a normal small lymphocyte
  - Macrocytosis occurs when many larger-than-normal RBCs are present
  - Microcytosis occurs when many smaller-than-normal RBCs are present
  - Mean corpuscular volume (MCV) useful in evaluating
- Shape
  - Many variations in RBC shape are possible because of the erythrocyte's flexibility, changes that may occur in the vessels, and alterations that occur with the cellular environment, metabolic state & age
  - t4.18 lists common changes and associated disease states & conditions
- Hemoglobin content (chromicity)
  - Direct relationship between amount of hemoglobin produced by RBC and the appearance of the RBC when properly stained
  - RBCs with normal hemoglobin content have a clear central pallor that occupies about 1/3 of the cell diameter
  - Mean corpuscular hemoglobin (MCH)/mean corpuscular hemoglobin concentration (MCHC) useful in evaluating
  - Hypochromia usually associated with microcytosis
  - "Hyperchromia" seen in spherocytes because of their decreased surface to volume ratio
- Distribution (rouleaux & agglutination)
  - Two types of abnormal distribution patterns may be seen in RBCs
  - Common changes & associated disease conditions
  - Rouleaux: RBCs not separated from one another but appear in linear stacks that resemble coins; characteristic in monoclonal gammopathies like multiple myeloma & hyperproteinemia
  - Agglutination: Random clusters, clumps, or masses of RBCs; Characteristic of cold agglutinin syndrome & other immune-associated conditions
    - Unlike rouleaux, do not easily disperse when diluted and may affect several automated complete blood cell count (CBC) parameters

ISBN 978-089189-6616

t4.18 Common RBC shape changes & associated conditions

Finding	Definition	Associated conditions
Acanthocytes (spur cells)	RBCs that have unevenly distributed, blunt & spiny projections with bulbous tips i4.52	Liver disease Abetalipoproteinemia McLeod (Kell-null) phenotype
Basophilic stippling	Small blue dots in RBCs, caused by clusters of ribosomes (RNA) Do not stain for iron i4.53	Hemolytic anemias Lead poisoning Arsenic poisoning Thalassemia Megaloblastic anemia Alcoholism Pyrimidine 5' nucleotidase deficiency
Dacryocytes (teardrop cells)	Teardrop- or pear-shaped erythrocytes i4.54	Can be seen in relatively benign conditions (thalassemia, megaloblastic anemia) Often seen in myelophthisis
Echinocytes (burr cells)	RBCs that have circumferential undulations or spiny projections with pointed tips	Uremia Gastric cancer Pyruvate kinase deficiency Postsplenectomy Often artifact
Elliptocytes	RBCs twice as long as they are wide	Iron deficiency B_{12} & folate deficiency Myelodysplasia Hereditary elliptocytosis
Heinz bodies; Bite cells	Heinz bodies: gray-black round inclusions, seen only with supravital stains (crystal violet) Bite cells: sharp bitelike defects in RBCs where a Heinz body has been removed in the spleen Both are due to denatured hemoglobin	Oxidative injury: G6PD deficiency or unstable hemoglobins
HbC crystals	Densely red, hexagonal or rod-shaped crystals	HbC disease
Howell-Jolly bodies	Dotlike dark purple inclusion Represent nuclear fragment i4.55	Asplenia Myelodysplasia, megaloblastic anemia Hemoglobinopathies
Cabot rings	Ring shaped dark purple inclusion Represent a residual nuclear fragment	Severe megaloblastic anemia & congenital dyserythropoietic anemia
Macrocytosis	Enlarged RBCs (confirm with MCV, with age appropriate reference range)	Reticulocytosis Oval macrocytes: megaloblastic (folate or B_{12} deficiency) Round macrocytes: chronic liver failure, hypothyroidism, myelodysplasia
Malaria parasites	*Plasmodium* species	Commonly small blue ring with red nucleus; any stage of developing gametocyte may be seen

t4.18 Common RBC shape changes & associated conditions

Finding	Definition	Associated conditions
Microcytosis	Small RBCs (confirm with MCV)	Iron deficiency Thalassemia Anemia of chronic disease (usually normocytic) Immune hemolysis Lead poisoning Sideroblastic anemia
Pappenheimer bodies (siderocytes with Prussian blue)	Larger, more irregular & grayer than basophilic stippling, caused by iron containing mitochondria i4.56	Asplenia Sideroblastic anemia
Rouleaux	Adherent RBCs lying side by side, usually caused by abnormal plasma proteins (immunoglobulin or fibrinogen) Unlike RBC aggregates caused by immune phenomena, rouleaux are reversible with dilution & do not affect automated CBC parameters i4.57	Monoclonal immunoglobulin Marked hyperfibrinogenemia
Agglutination	Random clusters of RBCs	Immune-associated anemias
Schistocytes	Fragmented RBCs, taking shapes such as helmet shaped cells, due to mechanical RBC fragmentation i4.58	Microangiopathic hemolytic anemias (MHA): DIC, TTP, HUS, HELLP Mechanical heart valves 58% of normal adults have schistocytes, with mean of 0.05% of RBCs, Range 0.00-0.27%
Spherocytes	RBCs without central pallor, due to decreased RBC membrane, often with high MCHC	Immune hemolytic anemia Hereditary spherocytosis
Sickle cells (drepanocytes)	RBCs shaped like holly leaves, boats, envelopes, crescents with 2 elongated & pointed ends	Sickle cell anemia, sickle-thalassemia, hemoglobin SC disease & other sickle cell diseases
Target cells (codocytes)	RBCs with a dark circle within the central area of pallor, reflecting redundant membrane i4.59	Thalassemia Hemoglobin C Liver disease

DIC, disseminated intravascular coagulation; G6PD, glucose-6-phosphate dehydrogenase; HELLP, hemolysis, elevated liver enzymes, low platelet count; HUS, hemolytic uremic syndrome; MCHC, mean corpuscular hemoglobin concentration; MCV, mean corpuscular volume; RBC, red blood cell; TTP, thrombotic thrombocytopenic purpura

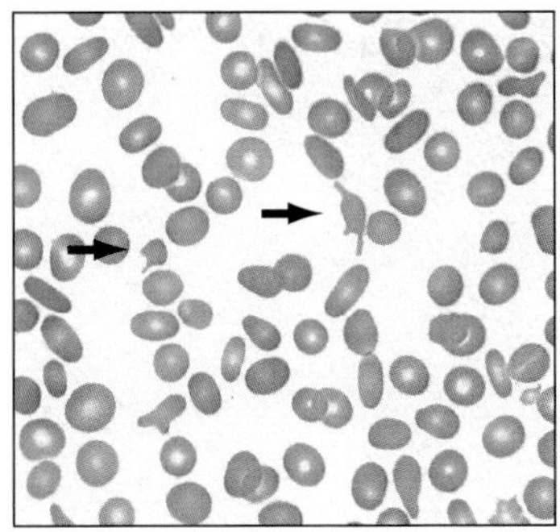

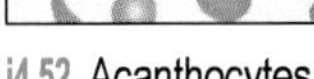

i4.52 Acanthocytes

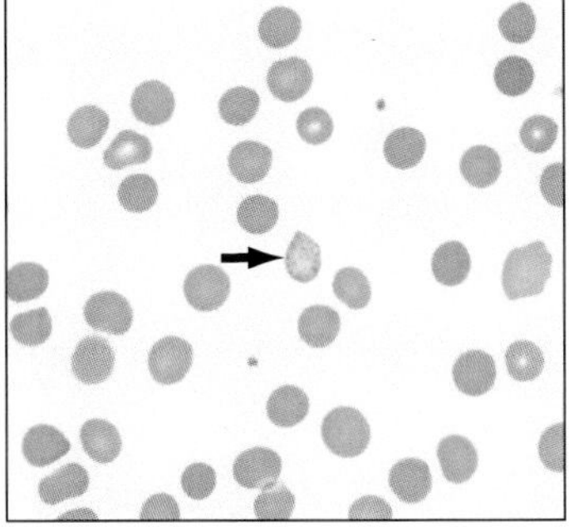

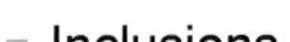

i4.53 Basophilic stippling

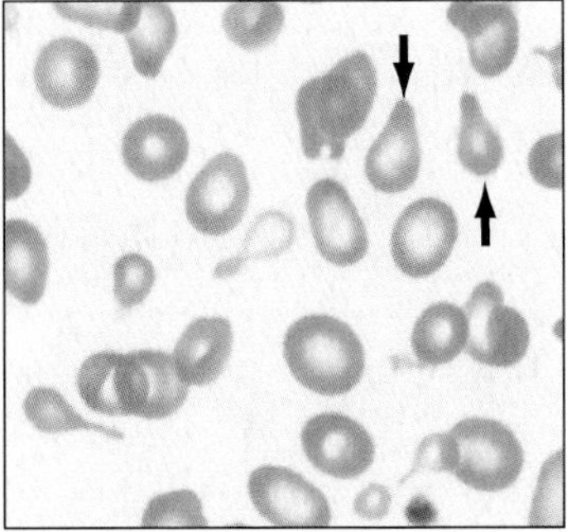

i4.54 Teardrop cells (dacryocytes)

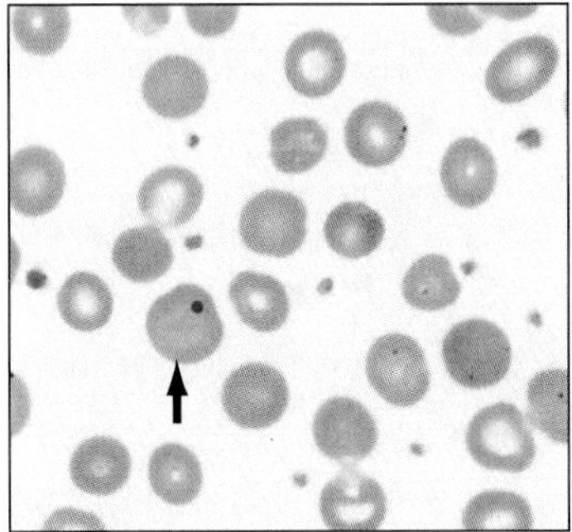

i4.55 Howell-Jolly body

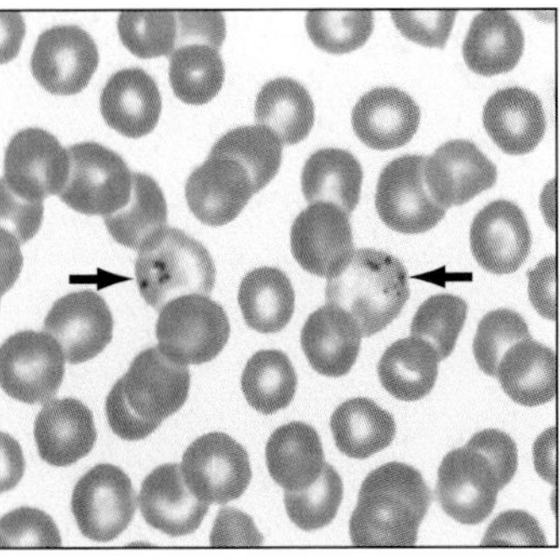

i4.56 Pappenheimer bodies

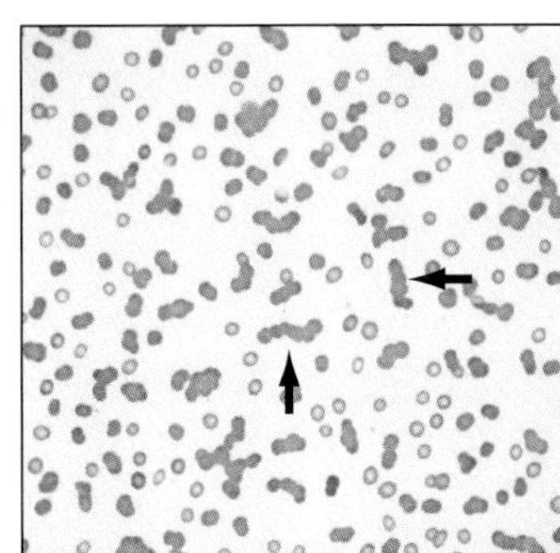

i4.57 Rouleaux

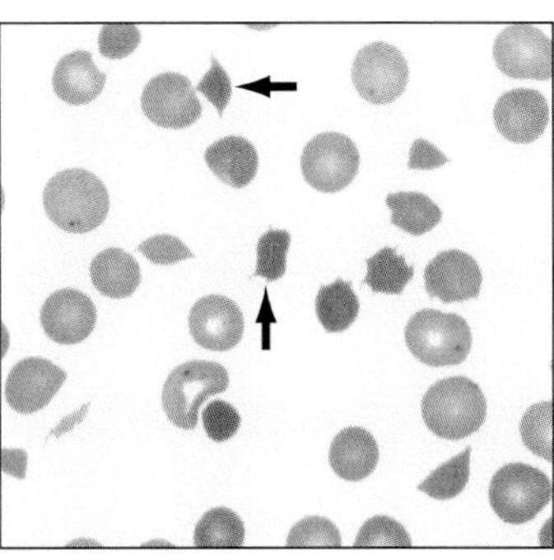

i4.58 Schistocytes

i4.59 Target cells

- Inclusions
  - RBCs normally have no inclusions
- Definition & composition
  - Basophilic stippling
    - Small, deep blue or blue-gray granules of ribosomes (RNA) evenly distributed in cells
  - Heinz bodies (only seen with supravital stains)
    - Purple or blue-gray, usually round or oval, particles of denatured hemoglobin
  - Cabot rings
    - Purple or reddish-purple rings or loops consisting of remnants of the mitotic spindle
  - Howell-Jolly bodies
    - Smooth, round, small dense purple inclusions representing a nuclear fragment
  - Pappenheimer bodies (siderocytes with Prussian blue)
    - Irregularly shaped, blue-gray clusters consisting of iron containing mitochondria
  - Hemoglobin C crystals
    - Densely red, hexagonal or rod-shaped crystals
  - Malaria parasites
    - Commonly small blue rings with red nucleus; any stage of developing gametocyte may be seen
- Associated disease states & conditions
  - **t4.17** summarizes various RBC inclusions and associated disease conditions as well as RBC morphologic findings and associated disease states as related to RBC size, shape & distribution
- Automation & RBC morphology
  - Some automated hematology instruments are capable of measuring RBC subpopulations
  - These new parameters assess the percentage of hypochromia, hyperchromia, microcytic & macrocytic RBCs

4.10.4.3 Evaluating platelet numbers & morphology

- Performed as part of differential cell count
- Platelet estimate
  - Obtained by averaging the number of platelets in approximately 10 oil immersion fields and multiplying by 20,000
  - This estimate should correlate with the automated platelet count
- Size & shape
  - Variable (smaller than RBCs), generally round or ovoid, bluish-gray, often with a central granular core & a surrounding clear zone
  - A platelet that is larger than normal may be referred to as enlarged or large
  - A platelet the size of a normal RBC or larger is called "giant"
  - Automated analyzers determine total platelet counts as well as the mean platelet volume (MPV); some instruments also provide an immature platelet fraction (IPF) or reticulated platelets, which reflect platelet size & age, respectively

 ISBN 978-089189-6616

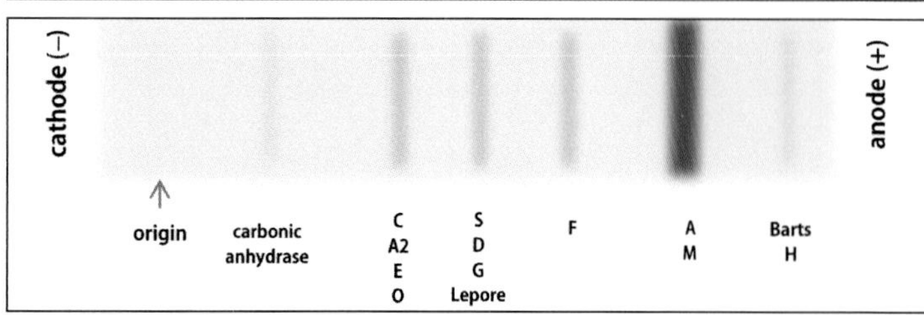

i4.60 Hemoglobin electrophoresis at pH 8.6 (alkaline electrophoresis), showing the positions of the various hemoglobin variants

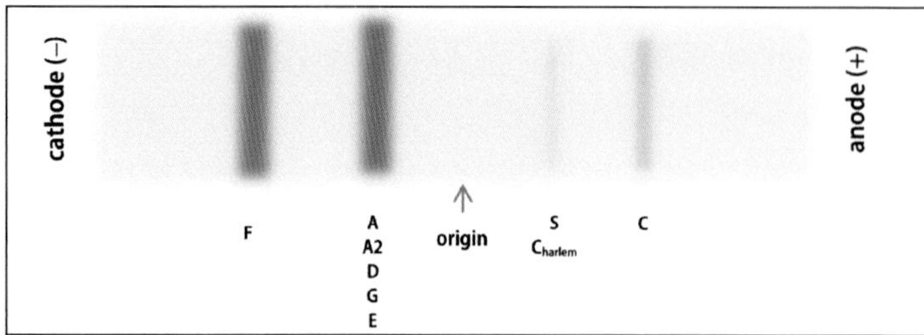

i4.61 Hemoglobin electrophoresis at pH 6.8 (acid electrophoresis), showing the positions of the various hemoglobins

4.10.5 Examining bone marrow

4.10.5.1 Collection techniques

- Aspiration
  - Marrow is aspirated into a syringe
  - Smears are made directly from the aspirate or the aspirate is added to EDTA and then smears are made
- Core biopsy
  - The inner medullary cavity of the bone is penetrated
  - A core cylinder of marrow is removed
  - Imprints (touch preps) are made on glass slides
  - Core is placed in fixative for histologic processing

4.10.5.2 Staining smears

- Wright stain
  - Aspirate & core biopsy slides are stained using the same procedure as is used for peripheral blood slides
- Prussian blue
  - Detects marrow storage iron to assess iron metabolism disorders

4.10.6 Hemoglobin determinations

4.10.6.1 Quantitative methods

- Manual
  - Cyanmethemoglobin method
    - Whole blood added to reagent (Drabkin solution)
    - Potassium ferricyanide converts hemoglobin from ferrous to ferric state and forms methemoglobin
    - Methemoglobin combines with potassium cyanide to form the stable pigment cyanmethemoglobin
    - Color intensity (absorbance) is directly proportional to hemoglobin concentration

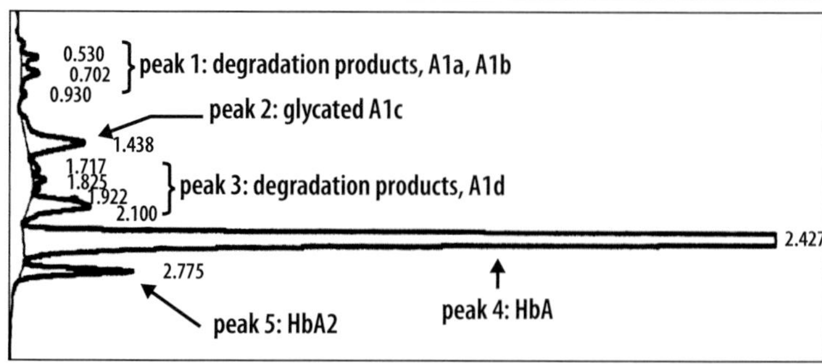

f4.6 High pressure liquid chromatography in a patient with normal hemoglobin genotype; 5 major peak regions are present, including some caused by degradation products (peaks 1 & 3), the HbA1c peak (peak 2), the HbA peak (peak 4), and the HbA2 peak (peak 5)

- Automated
  - Hematology analyzers use a modified cyanmethemoglobin method or the lauryl sulfate method

4.10.6.2 Detecting normal & variant hemoglobins

- Electrophoretic methods
  - Separate, identify & quantitate normal and abnormal hemoglobins based on relative rates of migration through various mediums while an electric current is applied
    - Migration rates primarily depend on net charge of the hemoglobin molecules
  - Routine hemoglobin electrophoresis at pH 8.6 (alkaline)
  - Normal adult has >97% HbA, <3% HbA_2 (migrates with HbC)
  - When results are ambiguous, electrophoresis on citrate agar at pH 6.2 (acid) produces different electrophoretic mobility patterns and allows separation of abnormal hemoglobins
  - Fast hemoglobins (HbH & HbBart) migrate beyond HbA on alkaline electrophoresis
  - Any band in the S region on alkaline electrophoresis can be confirmed by a sickle screening test or hemoglobin solubility test
  - Disadvantages of electrophoresis include inability to quantitate HbA_2 & HbF; on alkaline electrophoresis, HbS, HbD & HbG migrate together; HbA_2, HbC, HbO & HbE also all migrate to same position and cannot be separated
    - HbA, HbA_2, HbD, HbG & HbE migrate together on acid electrophoresis i4.60 & i4.61
- High-pressure liquid chromatography (HPLC) **f4.6**
  - Separates normal & abnormal hemoglobins in a cation exchange column under high pressure
  - Individual molecules elute at different and characteristic rates, allowing separation and identification of hemoglobin variants
  - HbA_2 & HbF can be quantitated

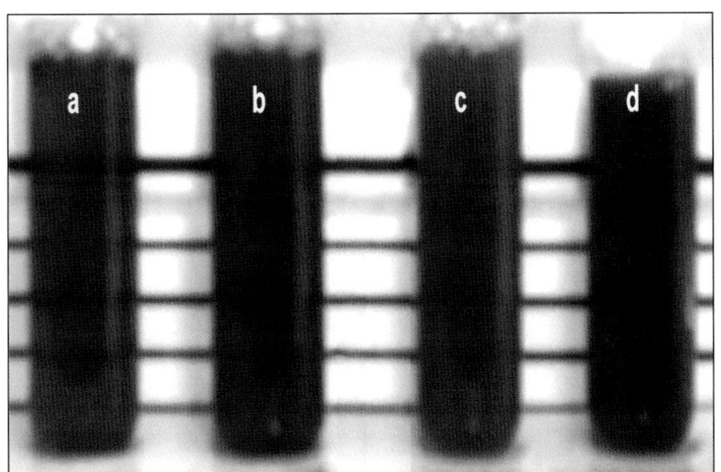

i4.62 Sickle cell screen; tubes a & b are negative (background lines can be seen throughout); tubes c (sickle trait) & d (sickle cell disease) are positive (lines obscured)

- Sickle solubility i4.62
  - Abnormal & insoluble HbS is precipitated causing a turbid solution
  - Turbidity is a positive result
  - Sickling & nonsickling hemoglobins can be detected, but not specific type of hemoglobin or if patient is homozygous or heterozygous for the abnormal hemoglobin
    - May be positive with HbSS, HbAS, HbSC, HBSD & HbC_{Harlem}

4.10.7 Hematocrit

- Also called packed cell volume (PCV)
- Represents the proportion of whole blood that consists of RBCs
- Values closely parallel hemoglobin levels

4.10.7.1 Manual

- Capillary tubes are filled with whole blood and centrifuged to achieve maximum RBC packing
- Space occupied by RBCs is measured & reported as a percentage of the total volume of blood in the tube
- Errors result when sample is improperly mixed, centrifugation time is inadequate, blood is over-anticoagulated, tubes are incompletely sealed, hematocrit tubes are inaccurately read

4.10.7.2 Automated

- Most hematology analyzers calculate the hematocrit using directly measured RBC counts and mean corpuscular volume (MCV) data

4.10.8 Red blood cell indices

4.10.8.1 Calculations

- Mean cell (corpuscular) volume (MCV)
  - Indicates average size of RBCs, though it is expressed as a volume (femtoliters [fL])
  - Determined by the formula

$$\frac{\text{hematocrit (\%)} \times 10}{\text{RBC count (in millions/}\mu\text{L)}}$$

- Mean cell hemoglobin (MCH)
  - Indicates average weight of hemoglobin in individual cells or the average mass of hemoglobin per RBC
  - Expressed in picograms (pg)
  - Determined using the following formula

$$\frac{\text{hemoglobin (g/dL)} \times 10}{\text{RBC count (in millions/}\mu\text{L)}}$$

- Mean cell (corpuscular) hemoglobin concentration (MCHC)
  - Represents average concentration of hemoglobin per 100 mL of packed RBCs or the percentage of RBCs filled with hemoglobin
  - Expressed as a percentage
  - Determined by the formula

$$\frac{\text{hemoglobin (g/dL)} \times 100}{\text{hematocrit (\%)}}$$

- Red cell distribution width (RDW)
  - Parameter available on automated hematology analyzers
  - Represents degree of variation in RBC size or is a measure of anisocytosis
  - Determined from the standard deviation of RBC volume

4.10.8.2 Significance

- Useful in diagnosis & classification of anemias
- Results from automated hematology analyzers can be used for internal quality control
- Mean corpuscular volume (MCV) indicates if the average RBC is normocytic, microcytic, or macrocytic
- Mean corpuscular hemoglobin (MCH) indicates whether the RBCs appear normochromic, hypochromic, or "hyperchromic"
  - Note that use of the term "hyperchromic" is usually reserved for cases in which the MCHC is increased or when spherocytes are present
  - Along with MCHC reflects amount of central pallor & staining of RBCs

ISBN 978-089189-6616

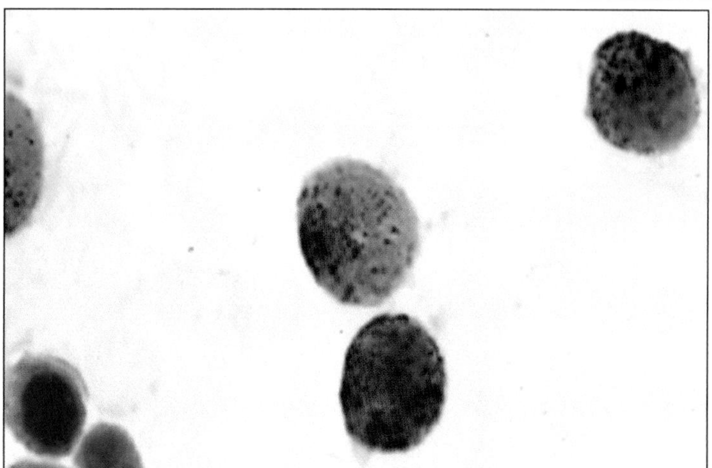

i4.63 Positive MPO in a patient with AML

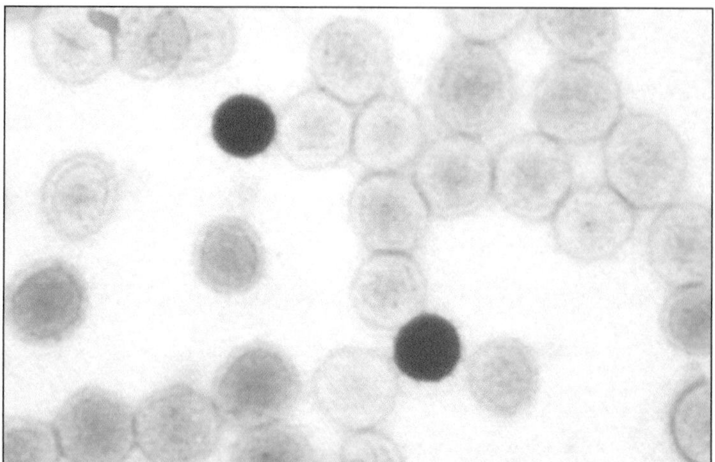

i4.64 Kleihauer-Betke preparation; the pale cells have no fetal hemoglobin, while the bright red cells have fetal hemoglobin

- MCHC indicates if RBCs appear normochromic, hypochromic, or "hyperchromic" (spherocytes)
- RDW indicator of variation in RBC size (anisocytosis)

4.10.9 Indicators of hemolytic anemia

- See also chapter 1 Chemistry for more details related to testing methods
- Bilirubin
  - Breakdown product of heme
  - Increased in extravascular & intravascular hemolysis
- Haptoglobin
  - Serum α_2-globulin glycoprotein
  - Binds free hemoglobin for transport to the liver
  - Decreased in intravascular hemolysis & severe extravascular hemolysis
- Lactate dehydrogenase (LD)
  - Enzyme
  - Activity increases in intravascular hemolysis

4.10.10 Special stains

4.10.10.1 Acute leukemias

- Several cytochemical stains can provide an easy & inexpensive method to distinguish various blast cells (especially differentiate blasts of AML from those in ALL)
  - Esterases
    - Generally used to differentiate myeloblasts & monoblasts
      - Myeloblasts positive for specific esterase (chloracetate esterase)
      - Monoblasts positive for nonspecific esterase (α-naphthyl acetate esterase or α-naphthyl butyrate esterase)
      - Note that megakaryoblasts are also positive with α-naphthyl acetate esterase (not butyrate esterase)
  - Myeloperoxidase (MPO) i4.63
    - Enzyme associated with primary granules in granulocytic cells (including myeloblasts)
    - Granulocytic cells stain positive, lymphoid cells (including lymphoblasts) do not stain

4.10.10.2 Chronic leukemias

- Leukocyte alkaline phosphatase (LAP)
  - Useful in distinguishing chronic myeloid leukemia (CML) from leukemoid reaction
  - Reported as a score derived by visually examining & grading 100 cells according to staining intensity
  - Score high in leukemoid reaction and low in CML

4.10.10.3 Detecting hemoglobin F

- Kleihauer-Betke stain i4.64
  - Acid elution technique that detects RBCs containing fetal hemoglobin
  - Smears examined microscopically for cells with persistent staining after acid elution
  - Heterocellular pattern seen in fetomaternal hemorrhage (& thalassemia)
  - Pancellular pattern associated with hereditary persistence of fetal hemoglobin (HPFH)

4.10.10.4 Detecting Heinz bodies

- Heinz bodies represent denatured hemoglobin
- Associated primarily with glucose-6-phosphate dehydrogenase (G6PD) deficiency & unstable hemoglobins
- Not visible with Wright stain
- Appear as blue or purplish (color dependent on supravital stain) single, multiple, round, oval, or irregular inclusions in RBCs i4.65

4.10.11 Evaluation of erythrocytes

4.10.11.1 Erythrocyte sedimentation rate

- Nonspecific test to primarily detect & monitor increased plasma proteins associated with inflammation
- Manual
    - Measures the settling of RBCs in diluted plasma over a specified period of time
    - Affected by numerous technical factors
        - Type & concentration of anticoagulant
        - Temperature of testing room
        - Specimen handling to include clotted sample or delay in testing
        - Increased WBC
        - Changes in erythrocytes (size, shape, inclusions)
        - Vibration & tilting of tubes
- Automated
    - Several systems available
        - Provide sample identification capability
        - Require smaller sample volume
        - Incorporate quality control
        - Can interface with laboratory information system
        - Provide rapid turnaround time
    - Some systems use an infrared reader or quantimetric photometry
- Significance
    - Although nonspecific, useful to diagnose or monitor several conditions to include:
        - Rheumatoid arthritis, malignancy, multiple myeloma, other collagen vascular diseases, bacterial infection, temporal arteritis, and inflammatory diseases

4.10.11.2 Glucose-6-phosphate dehydrogenase (G6PD)

- Quantitative assay determines enzyme activity and confirms diagnosis of deficiency
- Hemolysate incubated with a G6PD/NADP (nicotinamide adenine dinucleotide phosphate) reagent
- NADPH (reduced NADP) measured spectrophotometrically and is proportional to G6PD levels

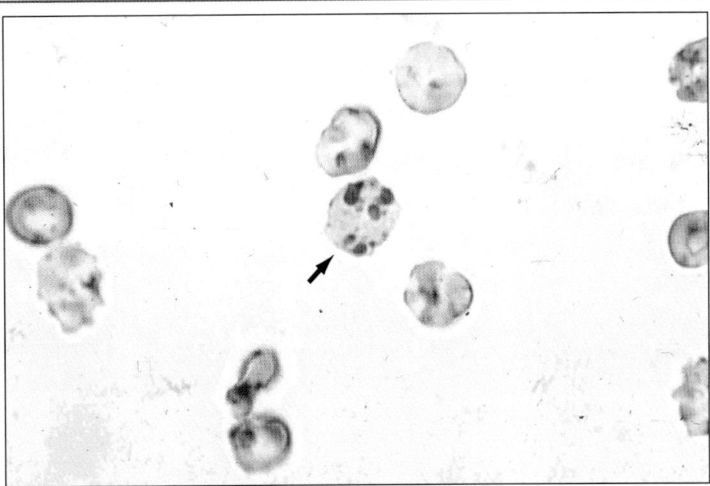

i4.65 Heinz bodies (arrow) stained with brilliant cresyl blue

4.10.12 Immunophenotyping (flow cytometry)

- See also Immunology 8.5.15
- Valuable tool in diagnosing hematology malignancy
- Use monoclonal antibodies to help subclassify leukemia and define other abnormalities
- Acute myeloid leukemia (AML)
    - See **t4.9** (page 195)
- Acute lymphoid (lymphoblastic) leukemia (ALL)
    - B cell (immunologic subgroups defined by immunophenotype)
        - Early precursor (pro-B cell) B-cell ALL expresses CD34, CD19, TdT, HLA-DR
        - Intermediate pre-B cells are positive for CD10, CD19, HLA-DR, TdT, and sometimes CD34
        - Pre-B cell sometimes expresses CD10, but also CD19, clg, HLA-DR, TdT, CD22
    - T cell
        - Express CD2, CD3, CD4, CD5, CD7, CD8, TdT
    - Selected lymphomas
        - **t4.19** summarizes immunophenotypes for selected lymphomas of mature B cells

t4.19 Immunophenotype of selected mature B-cell neoplasms

	CD19	CD20	CD79a	CD5	CD23	FMC7	CD11c	CD25	CD10	slg
CLL/SLL	+++	+	–/+	+	+	–	±	–	–	±
MCL	+++	+++	+	+	–	+	–	–	–	++
FL	++/±	+++	+	–	+	+	–	–	+	+++
MZL/SLVL	+++	+++	+	–	–	+	+	–/+	–	+++

CLL, chronic lymphocytic leukemia; FL, follicular lymphoma; MCL, mantle cell lymphoma; MZL/SLVL, marginal zone lymphoma/splenic lymphoma with villous lymphocytes

ISBN 978-089189-6616

4.10.13 Cytogenetic & molecular testing

- WHO classifications of acute myeloid leukemia (AML) & acute lymphoblastic leukemia (ALL) include subgroups with recurrent genetic abnormalities
- Subtypes also indicate molecular mutations associated with each cytogenetic abnormality
- Genetic abnormalities identified through chromosome analysis by conventional karyotyping or chromosomal microarrays
- Most molecular techniques isolate and amplify DNA or RNA sequences
- Methods include polymerase chain reaction (PCR) and fluorescence in situ hybridization (FISH), among others (see chapter 9 Molecular Biology)
- Myeloid malignancies
  - AML with recurrent genetic abnormalities previously summarized in **t4.9** (page 195)
  - Myeloproliferative neoplasms (MPNs) also associated with important cytogenetic & molecular abnormalities
    - CML defined by presence of the Philadelphia chromosome [t(9;22)(q34;q11)] that produces the *BCR/ABL-1* fusion gene
    - Other MPNs present with *JAK2* (Janus kinase 2) mutations (>90% in polycythemia vera, 50% in essential thrombocythemia, and 50% in primary myelofibrosis)
    - The common *JAK2* mutation results in a valine to phenylalanine substitution at codon 617 (*JAK2* V617F)
- Lymphoid malignancies
  - B-ALL with recurrent genetic abnormalities previously summarized in **t4.13** (page 200)
  - Some mature lymphoid malignancies associated with specific genetic & molecular findings
  - **t4.20** summarizes cytogenetic & molecular abnormalities in selected mature lymphoid neoplasms

t4.20 Selected molecular genetic associations

Disease	Rearrangement	Notes
Burkitt lymphoma	t(8;14), t(8;22), t(2;8)	cMyc/IgH; cMyc/Igλ; cMyc/Igκ
Chronic lymphocytic leukemia/small lymphocytic lymphoma (CLL/SLL)	del(13q), del(11q), +12, del(17p), del(14q)	20% have normal chromosomes 30% of cases have complex abnormalities
Follicular lymphoma (FL)	t(14;18)(q32;q21)	BCL2/IgH
Mantle cell lymphoma (MCL)	t(11;14)(q13;q32)	BCL1/IgH
MALT lymphoma	t(11;18)(q21;q21) & others	MLT/API2
Lymphoplasmacytic lymphoma (LPL)	t(9;14)(p13;q32)	PAX5/IgH
Diffuse large B-cell lymphoma	BCL2, t(14;18) & BCL6, t(3;x)	Rearrangements vary per 1 of 2 possible phenotypes
Hairy cell	*BRAF* V660E	

4.11 Selected readings

4.11.1 Books

Gulati G, Caro J. *Blood Cells: Morphology & Clinical Significance*. 3rd ed. ASCP Press. 2021. ISBN 978-0891896791

Gulati G, Krause J. *Bone Marrow and Blood Cells: Morphology, Histology & Clinical Relevance*. ASCP Press. 2021. ISBN 978-0891896784

Keohane EM, Otto CN, Walenga JM. *Rodak's Hematology Clinical Principles and Applications*. 6th ed. Elsevier. 2019. ISBN 978-0323520453

Kjeldsberg C, Perkins S. *Practical Diagnosis of Hematologic Disorders*. 5th ed. ASCP Press. 2010. ISBN 978-0891895718

McKenzie SB, Landis PK, Williams JL. *Clinical Laboratory Hematology*. 4th ed. Pearson. 2019. ISBN 978-0134709390

4.11.2 Journals & online

Arber DA, Orazi A, Hasserjian R, et al. The 2016 revision to the World Health Organization (WHO) classification of myeloid neoplasms and acute leukemia. *Blood* 2016; 127:2391-2405. doi: 10.1182/blood-2016-06-721662

Nazarullah A, Liang C, Villareal A, et al. *Peripheral blood findings in SARS-CoV-2* infection. *AJCP* 2020 Aug 5;154(3):319-329. doi: 10.1093/ajcp/aqaa108

Swerdlow SH, Campo E, Pileri SA, et al. The 2016 revision of the World Health Organization classification of lymphoid neoplasms. *Blood* 2016;127(20):2375-2390. doi: 10.1182/blood-2016-01-643569

Wagner J, DuPont A, Larson S, et al. Absolute lymphocyte count is a prognostic marker in Covid-19: A retrospective cohort review. *International Journal of Laboratory Hematology*, 2020 Jul 10. doi: 10.1111/ijlh.13288

Chapter 5

Hemostasis

ISBN 978-089189-6616

5.1 Overview of hemostasis

- This is a system of checks and balances in which the blood vascular system, platelets, and coagulation proteins, in a series of enzymatic reactions, work together to ensure the fluidity of the blood
- It consists of primary hemostasis, secondary hemostasis & fibrinolysis
- Vascular system
  - Comprised of arteries, veins & capillaries
  - Various clinical abnormalities are due to a structural abnormality or rupture of the endothelial lining or the subendothelial structures
- Primary hemostasis: Platelets
  - Platelets interact with damaged endothelium using specialized glycoproteins
  - Primary hemostatic plug forms to arrest bleeding (primary platelet plug)
  - The primary platelet plug is fragile and easily dislodges
- Secondary hemostasis: Coagulation factors
  - Formation of insoluble fibrin strands leads to a more stable clot
  - Secondary hemostatic plug (secondary platelet plug) is formed
  - Allows healing of the damaged tissue
  - Involves the coagulation cascade proteins that interact with each other and the platelet plug, resulting in fibrin formation
- Fibrinolysis
  - The final stage of coagulation in which the clot must be lysed to prevent occlusion of the vessel, and when wound healing occurs

5.2 Vasoconstriction

5.2.1 Vascular structure & function

- Endothelial cells play a key role in hemostasis
  - Procoagulant role: To induce activation of coagulation cascade, platelet adhesion at site of injury
  - Anticoagulant role: To prevent platelet activation in areas where the endothelium is intact
  - Capillaries are the smallest and most numerous of the vessels. Every cell in the body is within 0.13 mm of a capillary
- Involved in metabolic exchange between blood and tissues. Lumen of the capillary is surrounded by a single endothelial cell, just large enough for a single red blood cell (RBC) or white blood cell to pass through
- When the endothelial lining is disrupted, the vascular system acts to prevent bleeding and promotes the rapid vasoconstriction of the injured vessel and adjacent vessels. This diverts blood flow around the damaged vessels and enhances contact activation of platelets with coagulation factors
- Thromboxane A2 promotes vasoconstriction and platelet aggregation; serotonin released from platelets is a vasoconstrictor that binds endothelial cells and platelet membranes

5.2.2 Disorders of vasoconstriction

5.2.2.1 Hereditary or congenital defects

- Vascular malformations
  - Cavernous hemangioma (Kassabach-Merritt syndrome)
  - Hereditary hemorrhagic telangiectasia (Rendu-Osler-Weber): Blood vessels lack capillaries between artery and vein, and are fragile and rupture easily
- Connective tissue disorders
  - Ehlers-Danlos syndrome: Characterized by joint hypermobility, cutaneous fragility associated with arterial rupture, and visceral perforation
  - Marfan syndrome characterized by connective tissue abnormalities and skeletal defects, resulting in long limbs and a predisposition to cardiovascular disease

5.2.2.2 Acquired defects

- Disorders caused by an underlying disease or condition
- The supportive connective tissue in the blood vessel wall is decreased
  - Senile purpura: More commonly seen in the elderly
  - Cushing syndrome and corticosteroid therapy
  - Scurvy: Insufficient dietary intake of vitamin C
  - Henoch-Schönlein purpura: Primarily a disease of children
  - Drugs: Often involve immune reactions leading to changes in the vessel wall
  - Amyloidosis

5.3 Primary hemostasis

5.3.1 Platelets: Background, structure & function

- Background information
  - Anucleated cytoplasmic fragment
  - Measure 2-4 µm in diameter
  - Originate from megakaryocyte in bone marrow

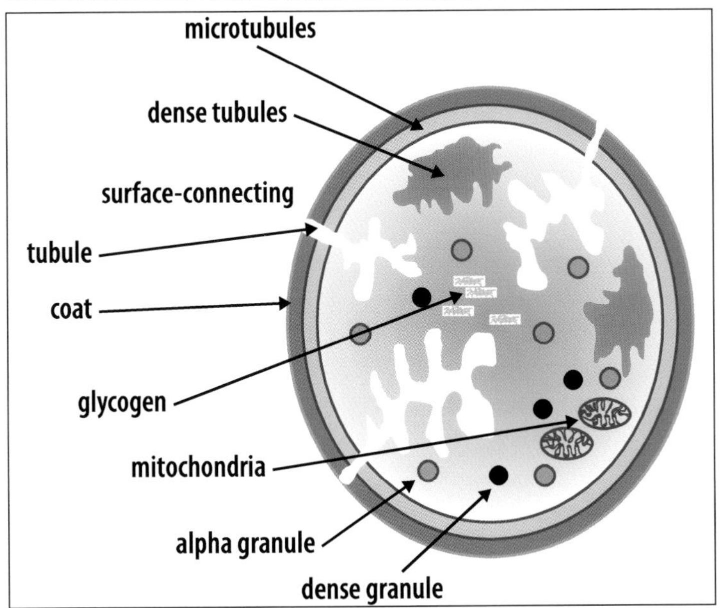

f5.1 Platelet structure
Peripheral zone: Glycocalyx: outermost membrane. Contains platelet phospholipids which binds clotting factors onto the platelet surface. Glycoprotein receptor sites
Sol gel zone: Platelet retraction/contraction function & platelet shape; microtubules/ microfilaments
Membrane zone: Open canalicular system, dense tubular system
Organelle zone: Storage & platelet release function; contains granules; dense bodies, α granules, lysosomal granules

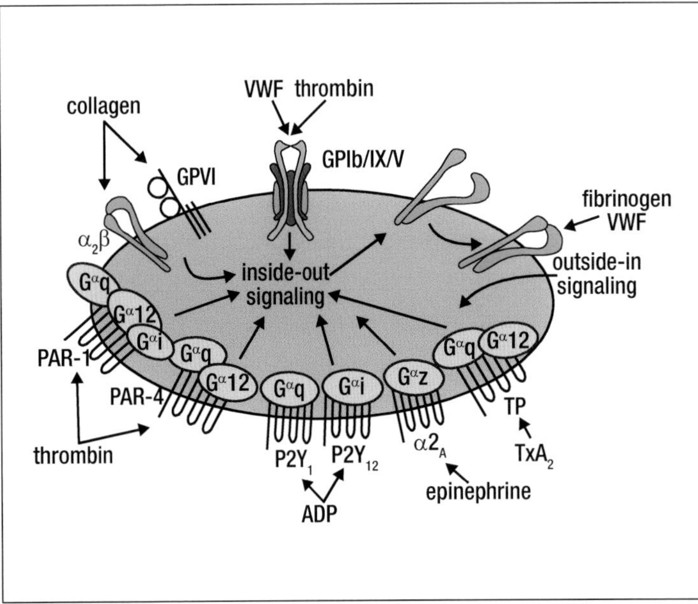

f5.2 Adhesion of platelets to the exposed subendothelium is mediated by glycoprotein (GP) Ib/IX/V complex & collagen receptors, GP VI & $\alpha_2\beta_1$ integrin, in the platelet surface, and by von Willebrand factor (vWF) & fibrillar collagen in the vascular site. Interactions between these are the result of signaling events that reinforce adhesion & promote platelet activation. The agonists of adenosine diphosphate (ADP), thrombin, and thromboxane that are produced & released at the site of vascular injury amplify platelet activation & recruit other circulating platelets to aid in the formation of a clot

- On stained blood smear, platelets appear as pale blue cells with azurophilic granules
- 70%-80% circulate in the blood, with a lifespan of 7-10 days
- 20%-30% of released platelets pool in the spleen
- Thrombopoietin is generated by the kidneys in response to a demand for platelets
- Megakaryocytopoiesis: Takes ~1 week for a megakaryoblast to create platelets

- Structure f5.1

5.3.2 Primary hemostasis in the injured vessel

- The vessel is cut or injured, exposing subendothelial collagen microfibrils
- The vessel constricts, slows down the blood flow, and diverts the flow away from the injured vessel; platelets undergo a shape change—from a disc to a spiny sphere
- Platelet activation is stimulated by von Willebrand factor (vWF), collagen, epinephrine, adenosine diphosphate (ADP), thrombin, thromboxane A2 (TXA2)

5.3.3 Three phases of platelet activation

- Adhesion: Platelets adhere to exposed collagen (receptor glycoprotein [GP] VI) within the endothelium of the vessel wall. GPIb-IX-V complex, which is the receptor for von Willebrand factor (vWF), is activated by shear stress and ristocetin. This is the initial reaction in clot formation, however, the clot is unstable and reversible f5.2, t5.1
- Secretion: Release from α granules and dense bodies, as well as the synthesis and release of TXA2, results in the recruitment of more platelets to the vessel wall. Occurring during aggregation, this step is irreversible and leads to the formation of the primary platelet plug
- Aggregation: Adherence of platelets to each other and mediated by the GPIIb/IIIa receptor on the platelet, which binds to fibrinogen in the presence of ionized calcium

t5.1 Platelet cell surface receptors

Antigen	Notes
GPIb/IX/V complex	Receptor for vWF; adherence to collagen
GPIIb/IIIa	Fibrinogen receptor; platelet plug stabilization
GPVI; $\alpha_2\beta_1$ (GPIa/IIa)	Collagen receptors
GPIc/IIa complex	Fibronectin receptor
GPIa/IIa	Adherence of platelets to negatively charged phospholipids

GP, glycoprotein; vWF, von Willebrand factor

ISBN 978-089189-6616

5.4 Secondary hemostasis

5.4.1 Coagulation factors t5.2

- These consist of plasma proteins produced in the liver (except for factor VIII (FVIII) which is partially made in the liver) The reticuloendothelial system of the liver helps to regulate coagulation and fibrinolysis by clearing these coagulation factors from circulation
- Coagulation factors circulate in plasma in an inactive form
- FVIII is unstable in plasma and so it circulates in a complex with von Willebrand factor (vWF)
- After activation, they are kept in check (or inactivated) by specific factor inhibitors
- Sequential activation of coagulation factors with the final step being the conversion of fibrinogen to fibrin

5.4.2 Coagulation pathways f5.3

- Extrinsic: Initiated by tissue factor (TF): TF:VIIa complex converts FX to FXa
  - TF:VIIa + Ca^{2+} + PF3 complex known as the "extrinsic tenase" complex
- Intrinsic: Initiated by negatively charges phospholipids:
  - FIXa + FVIIIa + Ca^{2+} + PF3 complex → "intrinsic tenase" complex converts FX to FXa

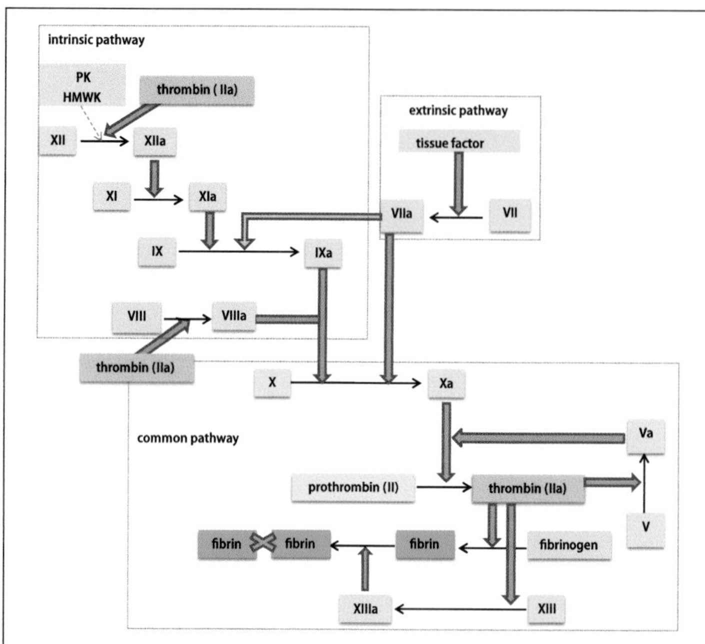

f5.3 The clotting cascades. The intrinsic cascade (left) is thought to have a minor in vivo significance. The extrinsic pathway (right) is initiated upon vascular injury, which leads to exposure of tissue factor (TF, factor III). There is thought to be a biologically significant interrelation of the extrinsic & intrinsic pathways, mediated by (1) factor VIIa crossing over & activating factor IX and (2) factor VIIa activating thrombin, which in fact drives the intrinsic pathway. PK & HMWK were once thought to activate the intrinsic pathway, but their biologic significance is now unclear

t5.2 Coagulation factors

Factor	Other names	Function	Half-life (h)	% activity required for normal coagulation	Pathway	Coagulation protein group
I	Fibrinogen	Thrombin substrate	100-150	30	Common	Fibrinogen[*]
II	Prothrombin	Activated on surface of platelets by the prothrombinase complex	50-80	30	Common	Zymogens[†] Prothrombin[‡]
V	Labile factor	Activated by thrombin, factor Va is a cofactor in the activation of prothrombin by factor Xa	24	20	Common	Cofactor Fibrinogen[*]
VII	Stable factor	Activated by thrombin in the presence of Ca^{2+}	6	20	Extrinsic	Zymogens[†] Prothrombin[‡]
VIII	Antihemophilic factor	Activated by thrombin, factor VIIIa is a cofactor in the activation of factor X by factor IXa; labile factor	12	30	Intrinsic	Cofactor Fibrinogen[*]
IX	Christmas factor	Activated by factor XIa in the presence of Ca^{2+}	24	30	Intrinsic	Zymogens[†] Prothrombin[‡]
X	Stuart-Prower factor	Activated on the surface of activated platelets by tenase complex & by factor VIIa in the presence of TF & Ca^{2+}	25-60	20	Common	Zymogens[†] Prothrombin[‡]
XI	Partial thromboplastin anticedent	Activated by factor XIIa	40-80	20	Intrinsic	Zymogens[†] Contact[§]
XII	Hagemann factor	Binds to exposed collagen at site of vessel injury; activated by HMWK & kallikrein	50-70	<5	Intrinsic	Zymogens[†] Contact[§]
XIII	Fibrin stabilizing factor		150	<5	Common	Fibrinogen[*]
Prekallikrein	Fletcher factor	Activates factor XII to XIIa	35	<5	Contact	Kinin[¶]; Contact[§]
HMWK	Fitzgerald factor	Cofactor; binds to factor XIIa & prekallikrein	150	<5	Contact	Kinin[¶]; Contact[§]

HMWK, high-molecular-weight kininogen; TF, tissue factor
[*]Most labile, consumed in coagulation, found on platelets
[†]When activated, become serine proteases (designated by "a")
[‡]Vitamin K dependent, may be affected by warfarin, diet, antibiotics
[§]Initiate intrinsic pathway and fibrinolysis
[¶]Roles include coagulation activation & fibrinolytic activation

- They result in a common, final pathway
  - Initiated by activation of factor X to Xa
  - FXa + FVa + PF3 + Ca^{2+} – "prothrombinase" complex converts prothrombin (II) to thrombin (IIa)
- Thrombin converts fibrinogen to fibrin monomers (Ia); fibrin monomers then polymerize end to end and associate noncovalently, ultimately cross-linked covalently by factor XIII
- FXIIIa cross-links the fibrin monomers into an insoluble fibrin polymer (clot)

5.4.3 Cell-based model of coagulation

- This is proposed to replace the traditional cascade; it more accurately explains coagulation in vivo **t5.3**
- It occurs in 3 overlapping stages
  - Initiation, which occurs on a TF-bearing cell
  - Amplification, in which platelets and cofactors are activated to set the stage for large-scale thrombin generation
  - Propagation, in which large amounts of thrombin are generated on the platelet surface
- Platelets and thrombin are central to the process
- This cell-based model explains some aspects of hemostasis that a protein-centric model does not

t5.3 Cell-based model of coagulation

Initiation	Amplification	Propagation
Vascular endothelium & circulating blood cells are disrupted; interaction of FVII with TF	Platelets, FV, FVIII & FXI are activated by thrombin on the platelet's surface	Results in production of an adequate amount of thrombin activity, production of temporary plug at the site of injury & stops the interruption of the blood supply

- Extrinsic pathway operates on the TF-bearing cell to initiate and amplify coagulation
- Intrinsic pathway operates on the activated platelet surface to produce the burst of thrombin that stabilizes the clot
- Cellular components play a large role in blood clotting
- Platelets function throughout the process
- Thrombin is generated in bursts and its feedback mechanisms are important in final clot formation

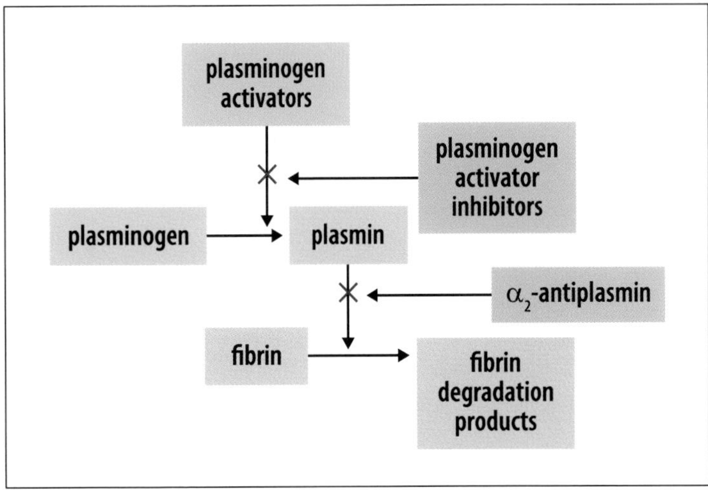

f5.4 Schematic of the fibinolytic system

5.4.4 Regulatory mechanisms of the coagulation pathway

- Fibrinolysis **f5.4**
  - Plasminogen
    - Becomes bound to fibrin at the time of fibrin polymerization
    - Bound plasminogen is converted to active plasmin molecule
  - Plasmin
    - Serine protease that systematically digests fibrin
    - Also digests FV, FVIII, fibrinogen
    - Binding to fibrin clot via lysine bonds prevents systemic activity
    - Plasmin is the main enzyme in fibrinolytic system

5.5 Disorders of primary hemostasis

- These include abnormalities that result in bleeding because of defects in formation of the primary hemostatic (platelet) plug
- Defects in primary hemostasis are classified as:
  - Qualitative defects, involving platelet function
  - Quantitative defects, involving the number of circulating platelets
- Defects in primary hemostasis are also classified as acquired or congenital
  - Acquired defects are those in which bleeding usually presents in adulthood
  - Congenital defects are those in which bleeding episodes present during early childhood
- Types of bleeding
  - Purpura—refers to petechiae and ecchymoses

ISBN 978-089189-6616

- Easy bruisability—excessive petechiae and ecchymoses following less than "usual" trauma
- Excess bleeding—involves both platelets and coagulation abnormalities

- Morphologic examination of platelets
  - Unexpectedly low platelet counts should be confirmed by examining a peripheral smear
  - Platelet aggregation (platelet-platelet binding) and/or satellitosis (platelet-neutrophil binding) are common causes of pseudothrombocytopenia (usually caused by the anticoagulant EDTA). Recollecting the patient's sample using sodium citrate as the anticoagulant should normalize the EDTA-induced artifacts
  - Note platelet size:
    - The mean platelet volume (MPV) is the automated measurement of platelet size
  - In general, consumptive platelet conditions (hyperproliferative thrombocytopenias) are associated with higher MPV and hypoproliferative thrombocytopenias generally are not

5.5.1 Quantitative disorders of primary hemostasis

- These are caused by:
  - Deficient platelet production
  - Increased destruction
  - Abnormal platelet distribution (splenic sequestration)
  - Secondary to an underlying disease
- Clinical symptoms typically are not seen until $<100 \times 10^3/\mu L$ ($<100 \times 10^9/L$)
- More often $<50 \times 10^3/\mu L$ ($<50 \times 10^9/L$)
- Spontaneous bleeding occurs at $<20 \times 10^3/\mu L$ ($<20 \times 10^9/L$)
- Life-threatening at $<10 \times 10^3/\mu L$ ($<10 \times 10^9/L$)
- Clinical manifestation
  - Petechiae, menorrhagia, spontaneous bruising, central nervous system (CNS) bleeding, gastrointestinal (GI) and genitourinary bleeding, and nosebleeds

5.5.1.1 Deficient platelet production

- Ineffective thrombopoiesis
  - Conditions associated with normal to increased marrow cellularity but peripheral blood cytopenias persist, such as in megaloblastic anemia, myelodysplastic syndromes, and alcohol use
  - Congenital megakaryocytic hypoplasia: Decrease in bone marrow megakaryocytes seen in thrombocytopenia with absent radii (TAR), Wiskott-Aldrich syndrome, May-Hegglin anomaly, and Fanconi anemia
  - Bernard-Soulier initially presents with thrombocytopenia caused by a deficiency of the GpIa/IX,V receptor
  - Congenital amegakaryocytic thrombocytopenia reflects bone marrow failure
  - Neonatal thrombocytopenia occurs in 1%-5% of infants as a result of certain infections
  - Certain viruses and chemotherapeutic drugs may suppress bone marrow megakaryocyte production

5.5.1.2 Increased platelet destruction

- Immune-mediated mechanism causes increased destruction of platelets
  - Primary (idiopathic): Defects that are intrinsic to the platelet
  - Secondary: Defect that is extrinsic to the platelet and is caused by underlying disease

5.5.1.2.1 Autoimmune thrombocytopenia (immune thrombocytopenic purpura [ITP])

- This is an autoimmune disorder characterized by:
  - Immune-mediated destruction of platelets
  - Impaired platelet production
- Autoantibodies—mostly immunoglobulin (Ig) G—directed against GPIIb/IIIa, GPIb/IX, GPV
- Two types: Chronic and acute t5.4

t5.4 Acute vs chronic ITP

Feature	Acute ITP	Chronic ITP
Peak age	Children: 2-4 years	Adults: 20-40 years
Platelet count (initial)	$<20 \times 10^3/\mu L$ ($<20 \times 10^9/L$)	$<30\text{-}80 \times 10^3/\mu L$ ($30\text{-}80 \times 10^9/L$)
Onset	Abrupt	Insidious
Antecedent infection	Common: 1-3 weeks	Unusual
Spontaneous remission	~93% of cases	Rare Course of disease fluctuates
Therapy	Corticosteroids Anti-D IVIg	Corticosteroids Splenectomy

ITP, immune thrombocytopenic purpura; IVIg, intravenous immunoglobulin

- One of the most common disorders causing severe isolated thrombocytopenia
- Most cases asymptomatic
- Low platelet counts can lead to a bleeding diathesis and purpura
- There is no specific test that readily confirms the diagnosis of ITP; therefore, it is a diagnosis of exclusion: antiplatelet antibodies + bone marrow examination + clinical presentation

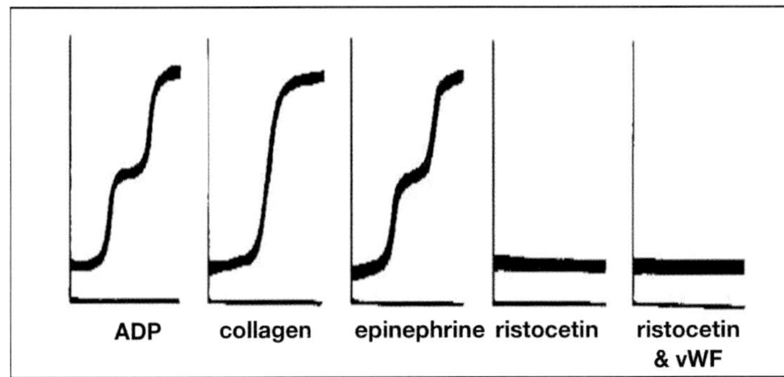

f5.5 Platelet aggregation study in hemolytic uremic syndrome with absent aggregation with ristocetin; normal aggregation with all other agonists

- Clinical features
  - Bruising, petechiae, epistaxis, gingival bleeding
  - Thrombocytopenia (platelet count <30 × 10^3/µL [<30 × 10^9/L])

5.5.1.2.2 Other causes of thrombocytopenia

- Neonatal alloimmune thrombocytopenia (NAITP): Fetal maternal incompatibility of platelet antigens. Antibody is anti-HPA, an IgG alloantibody
- ITP in pregnancy: Gestational thrombocytopenia, antibodies against platelet antigen PLA-1A (HPA-1a)
- Posttransfusion purpura: Severe thrombocytopenia 3-12 days after a blood transfusion, caused by antibody-related platelet destruction against platelet antigen PLA-1a (HPA-1a)
- Thrombotic microangiopathies (TMA)
  - Presents with a microangiopathic hemolytic anemia, thrombocytopenia, and microvascular thrombosis
  - Includes thrombotic thrombocytopenic purpura (TTP) and hemolytic uremic syndrome (HUS)
- Congenital TTP—Upshaw-Schulman syndrome—a deficiency of ADAMTS-13 (a disintegrin-like and metalloprotease with thrombospondin type 1 motif) that occurs during childhood
  - Presence of large von Willebrand factor (vWF) multimers found in the plasma of patients with TTP, because of the lack of a cleaving protease
  - vWF-cleaving protease cleaves the ultra-large vWF into inactive monomers to prevent interaction with platelets
- Hemolytic uremic syndrome (HUS) **f5.5, t5.5**
  - Generally encompasses several diverse disorders
  - Associated with diarrhea caused by verotoxin-producing *Escherichia coli* (O157:H7), with 95% of all cases occurring in children
  - Associated with deficiencies in proteins that regulate the alternative pathway of complement activation
  - Adult-onset HUS can be associated with bacterial infections, connective tissue disease, and some types of cancer

5.5.2 Qualitative disorders of primary hemostasis

5.5.2.1 Inherited platelet disorders t5.6

t5.5 Distinguishing features between TTP & HUS

TTP	HUS
Adults: 20-50 years old	Children: <5 years old
Pentad	Tetrad
Hemolytic anemia with RBC fragmentation	Hemolytic anemia with RBC fragmentation
Renal dysfunction	Acute renal failure
Thrombocytopenia (35 × 10^3/µL [35 × 10^9/L])	Thrombocytopenia (95 × 10^3/µL [95 × 10^9/L])
Severe CNS symptoms	Mild CNS symptoms
Fever	

CNS, central nervous system; HUS, hemolytic uremic syndrome; RBC, red blood cells; TTP, thrombotic thrombocytopenic purpura

t5.6 Types of platelet disorders

Defect	Disorder type	Disease	Cause
Platelet-vessel wall interaction	Adhesion	Congenital	
		von Willebrand disease	Deficiency or defect in plasma vWF
		Bernard-Soulier syndrome	Defect in GPIb/IX/V
		Acquired	
		Paraproteinemia	
Platelet-platelet interaction	Aggregation	Congenital	
		Afibrinogenemia	Deficiency of plasma fibrinogen
		Glanzmann thrombasthenia	Deficiency or defect in GPIIb/IIIa
		Acquired	
		Dysfibrinogenemia	
Platelet secretion & signal transduction	Impaired secretion of granule contents	Storage pool disorders	Abnormal aggregation during platelet activation
		α-SPD (gray platelet syndrome)	Abnormalities of platelet granules
		δ-SPD	
		αδ-SPD	
		Chédiak-Higashi syndrome	
		Hermansky-Pudlak syndrome	
		Acquired	
		Aspirin, NSAIDS	

GP, glycoprotein; NSAIDs, nonsteroidal anti-inflammatory drugs; SPD, storage pool disorder; vWF, von Willebrand factor

ISBN 978-089189-6616

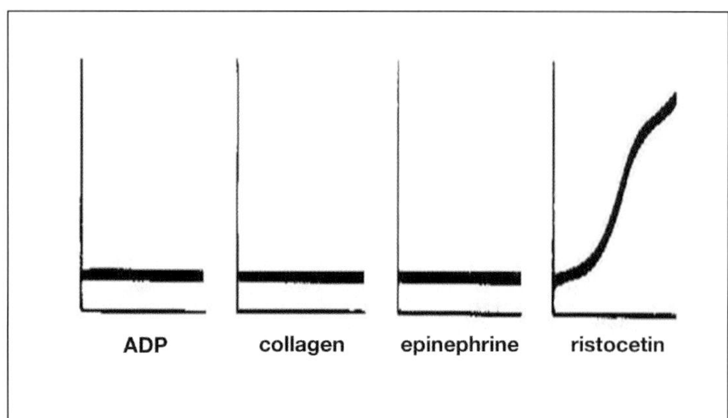

f5.6 Platelet aggregation study in Glanzmann thombasthenia showing normal aggregation with ristocetin; absent aggregation with all other agonists

- Bernard-Soulier syndrome
  - Abnormal recessive: GPIb deficiency or defect
  - Mild to moderate thrombocytopenia, commonly 30-200 × 10^3/μL (30-200 × 10^9/L)
  - Giant platelets on peripheral blood smear
- Glanzmann thrombasthenia **f5.6**
  - Abnormal recessive: Deficiency of GPIIb/IIIa
  - Normal platelet count
  - Prolonged PFA
  - Abnormal platelet aggregation response to adenosine diphosphate (ADP), arachidonic acid, collagen, epinephrine
  - Normal platelet aggregation response to ristocetin
  - Flow cytometry provides confirmatory diagnosis by demonstrating decreased expression of:
    - GPIIb (CD41) or
    - GPIIIa (CD61)
  - In Glanzmann thrombasthenia, aggregation by ADP, collagen & thrombin are abnormal, due to the absence of GpIIb/IIIa, but aggregation by ristocetin is normal because GpIb/IX/V receptors are available
- Storage pool diseases
  - Affect the secretion phase of platelet function
  - Autosomal dominant or autosomal recessive mode of inheritance
  - Dense granule deficiency
    - Decrease or absence of dense granules on electron microscopy
    - Morphologically normal-appearing platelets on peripheral blood smear
    - Prolonged PFA
    - Abnormal aggregation because of lack of ADP in dense granules
    - Abnormal aggregation with ADP, epinephrine → normal primary wave BUT blunted secondary wave
    - Low doses of collagen result in decreased or absent response because of lack of required endogenous ADP
  - α-granule deficiency
    - Absence of the α-granules causes the platelets to appear agranular on peripheral blood smear
    - Synthesis of the α-granules is normal BUT there are defects involving targeting endogenously synthesized proteins to developing α-granules
    - Platelet aggregation studies are normal/decreased in α-granule deficiency
    - AKA gray platelet syndrome
  - Dense granule deficiency
    - Albinism
    - Thrombocytopenia
    - Chédiak-Higashi syndrome: Frequent pyogenic infections, giant lysosomal granules in cells
    - Hermansky-Pudlak syndrome: Inclusions in the cells of the reticuloendothelial system, common in Puerto Rico
- Laboratory findings
  - Normal prothrombin time (PT)/partial thromboplastin time (PTT)
  - Platelet aggregation shows blunted response in biphasic curves
  - Diagnosis made with electron microscopy → absence of dense granules

5.5.2.2 Acquired qualitative platelet disorders

- Chronic renal failure: Uremia
  - Platelet dysfunction associated with uremic plasma because of guanidinosuccinic acid
    - Dialysis corrects abnormal test results
    - Clinical effects are hemorrhage, often in the gastrointestinal and genitourinary tracts
- Cardiopulmonary bypass surgery
  - Thrombocytopenia
  - Abnormal platelet function, which correlates with duration of the bypass procedure
  - Platelet defect likely because of the effects of platelet activation and fragmentation in extracorporeal circulation
- Liver disease
  - Thrombocytopenia caused by splenomegaly from portal hypertension & alcohol toxicity

- Paraproteinemias
  - Clinical bleeding and platelet dysfunction are particularly common in IgA and IgM paraproteinemia but may be seen with any class
  - Platelet dysfunction results from coating of platelets by paraproteins
- Platelet defects in myeloproliferative & myelodysplastic disorders
  - Thrombosis and less commonly hemorrhage are common in these disorders
  - Hepatic vein thrombosis (Budd-Chiari syndrome) is common in polycythemia vera and essential thrombocythemia
  - Abnormal aggregometry; most common finding is decreased aggregation and secretion in response to epinephrine, ADP, and/or collagen
- HELLP syndrome
  - Presents with hemolysis, elevated liver enzymes & decreased platelet count
  - Occurs in 4%-12% of pregnancies with severe pre-eclampsia
- Aspirin & nonsteroidal anti-inflammatory drugs (NSAIDs)
  - Inhibit cyclooxygenase type 1 (COX-1), which is involved in the production of TXA2; TXA2 stimulates dense granule release and the secondary wave of aggregation
  - The inhibitory effect of aspirin persists for the lifetime of the platelet; the effect of other NSAIDs is reversible
  - The aspirin effect is detectable in aggregometry responses to epinephrine, ADP, arachidonate, low-dose collagen, and low-dose thrombin; these are considered "weak" agonists because, by themselves, they are capable of producing only the first wave of aggregation; they depend on TXA2 to generate the secondary wave

5.5.2.3 von Willebrand disease (vWD)

- Most common of the congenital bleeding disorders, affecting 1%-2% of the general population
- Symptomatic in 1:10,000
- Mucocutaneous bleeding of varying severity in males and females
- Includes ecchymoses, epistaxis, GI bleeding, menorrhagia
- Defect of platelet adhesion with reduced FVIII levels
- von Willebrand factor (vWF) synthesized in endothelial cells & megakaryocytes
- Stored in Weibel-Palade bodies of endothelial cells
- Stored in α-granules of platelets
- Secreted into circulation as ultra-large multimers
- Multimers are immediately broken down by a cleaving protease and circulate as variably sized multimers
- vWD is an extremely heterogeneous, complex disorder with >20 distinct subtypes
- vWF serves 2 important biologic functions
  - Serves as a carrier protein for plasma FVIII: vWF protects FVIII in circulation and colocalizes FVIII at sites of vascular injury
  - Serves as a ligand that binds to the GPIb receptor on platelets to initiate platelet adhesion to the damaged endothelium: vWF binds to extravascular collagen; platelets adhere to the bound vWF; adherent platelets become activated

5.5.2.3.1 Types of vWD t5.7

5.5.2.3.1.1 Quantitative defects

- Type 1
  - Most common, 70%-80% of cases
  - Overall a mild quantitative defect in vWF
  - Normal prothrombin time (PT) and platelet count, normal to prolonged activated partial thromboplastin time (aPTT) and PFA

t5.7 Types of vWD

Type	Ristocetin cofactor (vWF:Rco)	vWF antigen (vWF:Ag)	Ratio vWF Rco:Ag	Factor VIII activity	RIPA	Platelet count	Multimer pattern
1	↓	↓	Nl	↓Nl	↓Nl	Nl	Normal distribution, all diminished
2A	↓	↓	↓	↓Nl	Nl↓	Nl	↓ HMW multimers
2B	↓	↓	Nl↓	↓Nl	↑with low dose	↓	↓ HMW multimers
Platelet type	↓	↓	Nl	Nl	↑ with low dose	↓	↓ HMW multimers
2N	↓Nl	↓Nl	Nl	↓	Nl	Nl	Normal
2M	↓	↓	↓	↓Nl	Nl↓	Nl	Normal
3	↓↓	↓↓	Nl	↓↓	↓	Nl	Absent multimers

Ag, antigen; HMW, high molecular weight; Nl, normal; Rco, ristocetin cofactor; vWD, von Willebrand disease; vWF, von Willebrand factor

ISBN 978-089189-6616

- Decreased FVIII, vWF antigen, and vWF activity
- The decreases in these 3 analytes are "concordant," and the ratio of vWF activity to vWF antigen approaches 1:1
- Normal multimer pattern

- Type III
  - Severe bleeding disorder
  - Both vWF and FVIII are markedly decreased

5.5.2.3.1.2 Qualitative defects

- Type 2A
  - Second most common, 10%-15% of cases
  - Moderately severe bleeding disorder
  - Normal prothrombin time (PT), while the activated partial thromboplastin time (aPTT) may be slightly prolonged
  - Normal to decreased FVIII and von Willebrand factor (vWF) antigen, with decreased vWF activity
  - There is "discordance," with markedly decreased vWF activity (ristocetin cofactor activity) and normal to only mildly decreased FVIII and vWF antigen; the ratio of vWF antigen to vWF activity is usually <0.7
  - Absence of high- and intermediate-molecular-weight multimers
- Type 2B
  - Like type 2A, has decreased high molecular weight multimers
  - Enhanced ristocetin-induced platelet aggregation
  - Desmopressin may cause severe thrombocytopenia & thrombosis
- Type 2M
  - Mutation in the *VWF* gene affecting the GP1b binding domain
  - Multimer analysis appears normal
- Type 2N (Normandy)
  - Mutations in the *VWF* gene affecting the domain that binds FVIII
  - This results in low levels of circulating FVIII, mimicking hemophilia A
  - Clinical picture resembles mild hemophilia A with the exception of autosomal pattern of inheritance

5.5.2.3.1.3 Pseudo-vWD

- No genetic defect of the vWF molecule—vWF molecule is normal
- Gain-of-function mutation in the platelet GPIb receptor
- Increased affinity of platelets for vWF

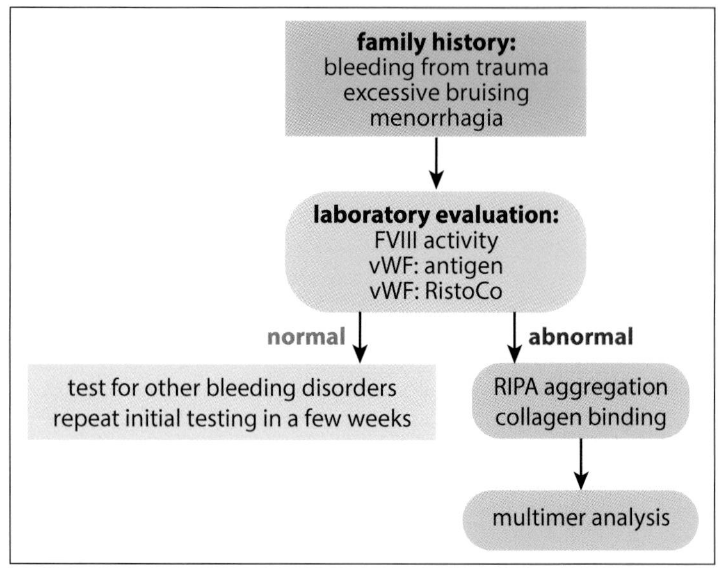

f5.7 Algorithm for laboratory evaluation of von Willebrand disease (vWD)

- Enhanced clearance of vWF and platelets from circulation
- Laboratory findings
  - Loss of high-molecular-weight multimers
  - Platelet count is low
  - Enhanced platelet aggregation with low-dose ristocetin (RIPA)

5.5.2.3.1.4 Acquired vWD

- Qualitative, structural, or functional disorder of vWF, which is not inherited and is associated with an increased risk of bleeding
- Associated with
  - Autoimmune clearance: Lymphoproliferative, monoclonal gammopathy of undetermined significance, systemic lupus erythematosus (SLE), hypothyroidism
  - Autoantibodies → increased clearance of vWF from plasma
  - Fluid shear stress-induced proteolysis: Aortic stenosis, left ventricular assist device
  - Essential thrombocythemia and aortic stenosis

5.5.2.3.2 Laboratory diagnosis of vWD f5.7

- A panel of tests is needed for laboratory diagnosis of vWD
- Quantitative assays: Normal range, 50%-150%
  - vWF activity: Functional ability of vWF to bind and agglutinate platelets
  - Ristocetin cofactor activity (manual or automated aggregation method)
  - Latex immunoturbidimetric assay, which measures GPIB binding

t5.8 Congenital disorders of secondary hemostasis

Factor	Deficiency	Half-life (h)	Laboratory finding	Clinical finding
I	Afibrinogenemia		No clot, prolonged PT, aPTT, TT, no fibrinogen	Umbilical stump bleeding, easy bruising, ecchymoses, oozing, poor wound healing, hematuria
	Hypofibrinogenemia		Prolonged PT, aPTT, TT, low fibrinogen	Mild bleeding
	Dysfibrinogenemia		Normal Fib antigen with low activity (clot)	Possible hemorrhage/thrombosis Possibly asymptomatic
II	Hypoprothrombinemia	100	Prolonged PT & aPTT	Postoperative bleeding, epistaxis, menorrhagia, easy bruising
V	Parahemophilia	25	Prolonged PT, aPTT, BT	Epistaxis, menorrhagia, easy bruising
VII	Hypoproconvertinemia	5	Prolonged PT, normal aPTT	Epistaxis, menorrhagia, cerebral hemorrhage
VIII	Hemophilia A	8-12	Normal PT, prolonged aPTT, normal BT, normal platelet function	Mild, moderate, severe
	vWF	16-24	Normal PT, variable aPTT & BT	Mild, moderate, severe
IX	Hemophilia B (Christmas disease)	20	Normal PT, prolonged aPTT	Mild, moderate, severe
X	Stuart-Prower deficiency	65	Prolonged PT & aPTT	Menorrhagia, bruising, epistaxis, CNS bleeding
XI	Hemophilia C	65	Normal PT, prolonged aPTT	Mild bleeding, bruising, epistaxis
XII	Hageman trait	60	Normal PT, prolonged aPTT	Thrombotic tendency, no bleeding
XIII	Factor XIII deficiency	150	Normal PT & aPTT, abnormal 5M urea solubility assay	Umbilical stump bleeding, poor wound healing, excessive fibrinolysis, male sterility, difficulty conceiving, intracranial hemorrhage
PK	Prekallikrein (Fletcher factor)	35	Normal PT, prolonged aPTT	Thrombotic tendency, no bleeding
HMWK	Fitzgerald factor	156	Normal PT, prolonged aPTT	Thrombotic tendency, no bleeding

BT, bleeding time; PT, prothrombin time; aPTT, partial thromboplastin time; TT, thrombin time, vWF, von Willebrand factor

- vWF antigen: Amount of vWF protein present (line immunoassay-based testing)
- Functional assay of FVIII (clot-based testing)
- "Discriminating" studies for vWD subtype
  - Multimer analysis ("size" of vWF molecules measured by quantitative electrophoresis)
  - Ristocetin-induced platelet aggregation
  - Special binding assays
    - Platelet, FVIII, and collagen-binding assays
  - Genetic analysis
- Low vWF antigen and vWF activity (ristocetin cofactor activity) help in diagnosing the most common forms of vWD
- Interpretations
  - If vWF antigen, vWF activity, and FVIII are normal, then vWD is unlikely, though in some instances repeat testing after an appropriate interval should be considered
  - If all 3 tests are reduced mildly and proportionately, most likely type 1 vWD
    - Treatment is desmopressin as needed, eg, for surgical interventions
  - If all 3 tests are reduced profoundly, most likely type 3 vWD
    - Treatment with the administration of vWF, often in the form of fresh frozen plasma (FFP) or commercially available concentrates, with or without aminocaproic acid
  - When vWD activity is reduced out of proportion to vWF antigen and FVIII, it is most consistent with type 2; multimer analysis and low-dose ristocetin aggregation are necessary to further elucidate
  - Treatment for type 2A or 2B is similar to type 3; desmopressin is contraindicated in type 2B

5.5.2.3.3 Factors that affect vWD diagnosis

- Physiologic stimuli elevate vWF level
  - Stress, trauma, exercise & estrogen therapy
- Inflammation
- Thyroid status (hyperthyroid have higher levels)
- Phase of menstrual cycle (lowest in early follicular phase)
- Levels rise during pregnancy
  - Newborns have higher vWF activity; vWD may not be detectable until 1 year of age
- VWF levels fluctuate day to day and increase with age
- Acute-phase reactions cause FVIII and vWF to become elevated and may mask vWD
  - Helpful to run another acute-phase reactant such as fibrinogen to aid in the diagnosis of vWD
- Blood group (ABO, Lewis)
  - Blood group O individuals have vWF levels that are ~25%-35% lower than people with A, B, or AB

5.6 Disorders of secondary hemostasis

- Disorders of secondary hemostasis can be acquired or hereditary **t5.8**, **f5.8**

ISBN 978-089189-6616

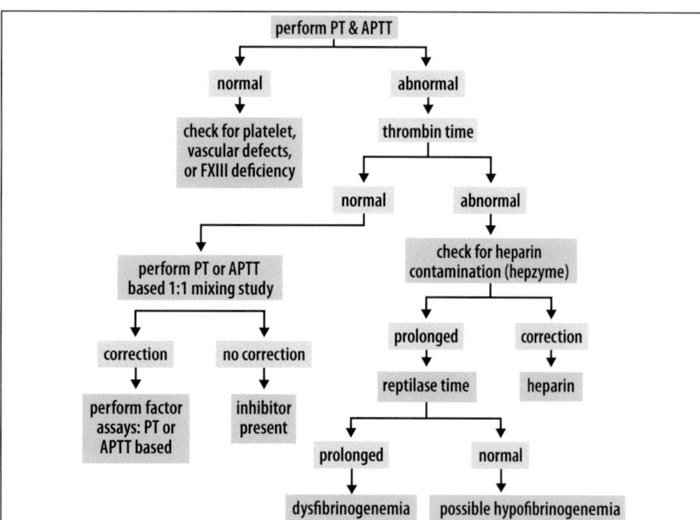

f5.8 Evaluation of secondary bleeding disorders

- Hereditary disorders usually present in childhood, as opposed to acquired disorders which develop in adulthood because of an underlying disease process
- Screening assays will be abnormal in these patients, with the exception of those who are deficient in FXIII, because FXIII is not measured by the coagulation cascade screening tests

5.6.1 Hereditary disorders of secondary hemostasis t5.14

- Prevalence
  - FI, FV, FX, FXII, FXIII: 1/million
  - FVII: 1/500,000
  - FVIII: 1/10,000
  - FIX: 1/30,000
  - FII: 1 in 2 million
  - FXI: 1 in a million, higher in Ashkenazi Jews
- Family history
  - A family history is important when evaluating a disorder of hemostasis
  - Type, location, frequency and severity of bleeding are all considered
  - Patients may be evaluated with a scoring system to assess bleeding risks
- Types of bleeding
  - In secondary hemostasis bleeding can occur spontaneously within minutes to several hours after minor trauma, surgery, or tooth extraction. Types of bleeding include:
    - Large ecchymoses (hematomas)
    - Hemorrhage into body cavities (hemoperitoneum)
    - Bleeding into joints (hemarthrosis)
- Physical examination
  - Petechiae, ecchymoses, hematomas, joint deformities
- Laboratory examination
  - Complete blood cell count including platelet count, prothrombin time (PT), activated partial thromboplastin time (aPTT), fibrinogen, thrombin time (TT)

5.6.1.1 Hemophilia

5.6.1.1.1 Hemophilia A t5.8

- Factor assays demonstrate isolated deficiency of FVIII
- Primarily affects males
- Female carriers (produced by hemophiliac male and normal female)
  - Have about 50% FVIII activity
  - Normal aPTT and no history of abnormal bleeding
- Genetics
  - The *F8* gene is found at Xq28
  - A single inversion mutation of intron 22, the "common partial inversion," causes 40%-45% of cases

5.6.1.1.2 Hemophilia B t5.9

- Factor assays show an isolated deficiency of FIX and is inherited as a recessive X-linked disorder affecting males, with females being carriers

t5.9 Hemophilia A vs hemophilia B

Factor deficiency	Hemophilia A Factor VIII	Hemophilia B (Christmas disease) Factor IX
Inheritance	X-linked recessive	X-linked recessive
Gene	*FVIII* gene on X chromosome—cloned 1984 Large gene—187 kb, 26 exons 98% of patients have mutation on *locus Xq28*, 48% of individuals with severe have inversion of intron 22	*FIX* gene on X chromosome—cloned 1982 34 kb, 8 exons 99% of mutations on Xq27.1-q27.2
Incidence	1/10,000 males	1/30,000 males
Severity	Related to factor level for both hemophilia A & B	
Severe	≤1% activity	Bleeding after major trauma, major surgery, dental extraction; no spontaneous bleeding seen, often seen in early infancy (<1 year of age)
Moderately severe	1%-5% activity	Muscle & joint bleeding after minor trauma; excessive bleeding after minor surgery & dental extractions; occasional spontaneous bleeding occurs, often seen <5-6 years of age
Mild	6%-30% activity	Bleeding after major trauma, major surgery, dental extraction; no spontaneous bleeding seen, often seen only in adulthood
Complications	Soft-tissue bleed, intramuscular bleed, hemarthrosis, urinary tract bleeding, central nervous system (major life-threatening bleed)	

5.6.1.1.3 Hemophilia C—factor XI deficiency (plasma thromboplastin antecedent)

- Also called Rosenthal syndrome (described in 1953)
- Autosomal dominant or recessive → occurs in males and females
- 2 common mutations (1 nonsense, 1 missense)
- 50% of patients with FXI deficiency bleed & 50% do not bleed
- Different from hemophilias A and B which are sex-linked
- Rare in the general population 1 in million
- More common in the Ashkenazi Jewish population—1 in 450

5.6.1.1.4 Hemophilia treatment

- Fresh frozen plasma (FFP) & antifibrinolytic agents for A, B, C
- Replacement therapy plasma (FVII, FIX, FXI) (for A, B, C)
- Cryoprecipitate: Contains high levels of FVIII, fibrinogen, von Willebrand factor (vWF) & FXIII; 1 unit of FFP prepared by cryoprecipitate contains 50-120 U of VIII
- Hemophilia A: Recombinant FVIII, extended half-life FVIII
- Hemophilia B: Recombinant FIX, extended half-life FIX
- Hemophilia C: FXI concentrates

5.6.1.2 Inherited deficiency of factors II, V, VII, X

- All display autosomal recessive inheritance
- FVII deficiency
  - Most common autosomal recessive coagulation factor deficiency
  - Poor association between FVII levels & bleeding severity
  - Prolonged prothrombin time (PT); normal activated partial thromboplastin time (aPTT) & TT
- FV deficiency
  - Prolonged PT & aPTT, TT is normal
- FX deficiency
  - Prolonged PT, aPTT & dilute Russell viper venom test (DRVVT); normal TT
- FXIII deficiency
  - FXIII is a tetrameric zymogen that is converted into an active transglutaminase by thrombin and Ca^{2+} in the terminal phase of the clotting cascade
  - Autosomal recessive; rare
  - Heterozygotes can have mild bleeding symptoms; particularly delayed bleeding, umbilical stump bleeding, frequent miscarriages, delayed wound healing
  - Homozygous FXIII deficiency is associated with essentially normal PT, aPTT, and TT, and a severe bleeding diathesis
  - Delayed bleeding can occur
  - Diagnosis
    - Urea solubility test
    - Quantitative measurement of FXIII activity
  - FXIII concentrates available (long half-life)
- FXII deficiency
  - Markedly prolonged aPTT
  - Patients do NOT exhibit a bleeding tendency
  - Patients have thrombotic tendency
- Contact factors
  - Prekallikrein deficiency (Fletcher trait)
    - Prolonged aPTT
    - Patients do NOT exhibit a bleeding tendency
    - Patients have a thrombotic tendency
    - Prolonged aPTT will normalize by increasing the incubation time
  - High-molecular-weight kininogen (Fitzgerald factor)
    - Markedly prolonged aPTT
    - Patients do NOT exhibit a bleeding tendency
    - Patients have thrombotic tendency

5.6.1.3 Fibrinogen defects

- FI: common pathway; synthesized in the liver
- Soluble plasma protein, which is converted into fibrin, a stable insoluble polymer
- Acute-phase reactant, which becomes elevated during stress, infections, inflammation & pregnancy
- Moderate to severe bleeding (typically less than in severe hemophilia)
  - Death from intracranial bleeding in childhood may occur
  - GI and other mucosal hemorrhage
  - Menorrhagia
  - Placental abruption
  - Presents with umbilical cord bleeding
- Diagnosis
  - Prolonged PT, aPTT, thrombin & reptilase times
- Afibrinogenemia, hypofibrinogenemia, dysfibrinogenemia
  - Prevalence approximately 1:1,000,000
  - Recessive inheritance
  - Most reported cases from consanguineous parents
  - Type I: Quantitative abnormalities (afibrinogenemia and hypofibrinogenemia)
  - Type II: Qualitative abnormalities (dysfibrinogenemia and hypodysfibrinogenemia)

- Functional abnormalities of fibrinogen who carry 1 abnormal allele that may result in either bleeding or thrombosis
- Prolonged thrombin & reptilase times
- PT & aPTT may be prolonged
- Disparity (>30%) between fibrinogen activity & antigen

5.6.2 Acquired disorders of secondary hemostasis t5.10

5.6.2.1 Acquired hemophilia

- Rare, potentially life-threatening bleeding disorder
- Development of autoantibodies directed against FVIII—spontaneous autoimmune disorder—FIX autoantibodies are less common
- Alloantibodies in congenital hemophilia
- Autoantibodies in acquired hemophilia
- Type II kinetics are complex
  - Initial rapid inactivation followed by a slower inactivation curve and resulting in some level of residual FVIII
- Associated with
  - Idiopathic origins, pregnancy, autoimmune disorders, spontaneous occurrence in the elderly

t5.10 Acquired factor deficiencies

VIII	Factor VIII inhibitors (autoantibodies) in nonhemophilia patients
X	Acquired factor X deficiency associated with light chain amyloidosis (adsorption to amyloid)
Multiple	Disseminated intravascular coagulation Extracorporeal membrane oxygenation Fibrinolytic drugs Liver disease Warfarin Neonatal or dietary vitamin K deficiency Nephrotic syndrome (usually most pronounced loss of antithrombin, therefore prothrombotic)

5.6.2.2 Hepatic disease

- The liver is the principal site of synthesis of procoagulant, fibrinolytic, and coagulation inhibitory proteins
- Liver disorders present 3 challenges:
  - Decreased synthesis of coagulation, fibrinolytic & inhibitory proteins; FII, FV, FVII, FIX & FX
  - Increased FVII (partially produced in liver)
  - Impaired clearance of activated hemostatic components
- Increased PT, aPTT, TT
- Increased fibrin split products, decreased platelets (hypersplenism)
- Increased FVIII

5.6.2.3 Disseminated intravascular coagulation (DIC)

- Generalized activation of hemostasis secondary to a systemic disease
- Results from a major tissue injury
- Simultaneous formation of thrombin & plasmin
- Role of thrombin: Cleaves FI, activates FV, FVIII & FXIII, activates platelets to aggregate, causing thrombocytopenia
- Role of plasmin: Activates fibrinolytic system & adhesiveness of platelets

5.6.2.3.1 Acute DIC

- Compensatory hemostatic mechanisms overwhelmed → severe consumptive coagulopathy → hemorrhage
- Elevated PT, aPTT, fibrin/fibrinogen degradation products (FDP), and D-dimer; presence of schistocytes, no single diagnostic test
- Decreased fibrinogen, platelet count, antithrombin, and coagulation factors

5.6.2.3.2 Chronic DIC

- Compensated state
- Liver and bone marrow compensate with coagulation factors and platelets
- Little obvious clinical or laboratory indication of DIC
- PT & aPTT are normal to increased
- May be normal because of a compensatory mechanism
- Elevated FDP & D-dimer

5.6.2.3.3 Treatment

- No specific treatments—supportive therapy
  - Plasma & platelet substitution therapy
  - Anticoagulants
  - Physiologic coagulation inhibitors
  - FFP provides clotting factors, fibrinogen, inhibitors & platelets in balanced amounts
  - Platelets add fuel to the fire
  - Heparin turns off coagulation, but in a patient who is already bleeding—may be contraindicated—also requires adequate levels of antithrombin to be effective
- Inhibitor therapy
  - Antithrombin: Major inhibitor of the coagulation cascade
  - Protein C (PC) concentrate: Inhibits Va and VIIIa—decreases morbidity due to sepsis
  - TF pathway inhibitor: Inhibits thrombin generation via extrinsic pathway
- Stop the triggering process

5.6.2.4 Vitamin K deficiency

- Vitamin K deficiency seen in
  - Absence of bile salts in GI tract: Vitamin K is fat soluble → bile salts are required for adsorption
  - Malabsorption syndromes: Vitamin K is absorbed primarily through the GI tract
  - Dietary lack of phylloquinone: Because of the lack of green leafy vegetables in the diet
  - Antibiotic therapy: Kills the normal flora of the GI tract
  - Bowel surgery
  - Newborn infants: Deficient in vitamin K at birth
- Diagnosis
  - Prolonged prothrombin time (PT), activated partial thromboplastin time (aPTT) & thrombin time (TT)
  - In mild vitamin K deficiency, aPTT will be normal because only FVII will be decreased (FVII has shortest half-life)
  - Decrease in vitamin K-dependent factors: Factor assays for FII, FVII, FIX, and FX, protein C and protein S
    - FV is used to differentiate between lactate dehydrogenase & vitamin K deficiency & liver disease
    - FV is not VK-dependent, but is synthesized in the liver
    - TT is normal to prolonged in lactate dehydrogenase, whereas TT is normal in vitamin K deficiency
- Treatment
  - Vitamin K parenteral injection
  - In life-threatening situation, FFP to supply the missing vitamin K-dependent factors

5.6.2.5 Other: Renal disease, hemorrhagic disease of the newborn, trauma

- Renal disease
  - In acute and chronic renal diseases, often a bleeding tendency is associated with several hemostatic abnormalities
  - Thrombocytopenia frequently develops in uremia
  - Vitamin K deficiency caused by malnutrition, associated liver disease with FV deficiency
- Underlying pathophysiology
  - Impaired platelet function → 1 of the main determinants of uremic bleeding
  - Platelet dysfunction is the most important
  - Decreased platelet aggregation & impaired adhesiveness
  - Uremic toxins

5.7 Thrombophilia

- Definition: Abnormal tendency toward excessive thrombosis **t5.11**
- Occurs when the clotting system is activated
  - Excessive generation of prothrombotic factors
  - Failure of the regulatory mechanisms to downregulate the coagulation cascade
  - Inhibition of the fibrinolytic system

t5.11 Thrombophilia: differential diagnosis by type of thrombosis

Arterial thrombosis, eg, myocardial infarction		**Venous thrombosis, eg, deep vein thrombosis**	
Common	Antiphospholipid syndrome (aCL) Prothrombin mutation (20210) HIT syndrome	Common	Factor V Leiden Prothrombin mutation (20210) Antiphospholipid syndrome (aCL & LAC) Protein C deficiency Protein S deficiency AT deficiency
Uncommon	Elevated PAI1 activity Hyperhomocysteinemia	Uncommon	Hyperhomocysteinemia heparin cofactor II
Also consider	Anomalous coronary arteries Vasculitis	Also consider	Immobilization Trauma Pregnancy

aCL, anticardiolipin antibodies; AT, antithrombin; HIT, heparin-induced thrombocytopenia; LAC, lupus anticoagulant; PAI, plasminogen activator inhibitor

5.7.1 Indications of thrombophilia

5.7.1.1 Venous thromboembolism (VTE)

- Before age 35-40 years
- Unprovoked VTE
- VTE at unusual sites
- Recurrent fetal loss syndrome
- Recurrent first-trimester spontaneous abortions
- Investigating patients with SLE
- Recurrent thromboses
- Family history of thrombosis

5.7.1.2 Venous & arterial events

- Venous thrombosis
  - TF generates thrombin before platelet activation
  - Involves RBC clots: results in DVT & pulmonary embolism (PE), which are major manifestations
  - Anticoagulation agents are necessary for treatment

ISBN 978-089189-6616

t5.12 Prevalence of thrombophilia

Risk factor	Subjects with thrombosis, %	General population, %	Relative risk of thrombosis
Antithrombin	1	0.2	25-50
Protein C	3	0.3	10-15
Protein S	2-3	0.2	11
Factor V Leiden (heterozygous)	20-50	3-15	3-8/80 (homozygous)
Prothrombin mutation (heterozygous)	6	2	3

5.7.1.3 Arterial thrombosis

- Clots are rich in platelets & involve disrupted atherosclerotic plaque
- White cell clots
- Myocardial infarction & stroke are major manifestations
- Treated with antiplatelet agents
- Antifibrinolytic and antithrombotic agents

5.7.2 Specific causes of thrombophilia

5.7.2.1 Antithrombin deficiency

- Antithrombin is a major regulator of coagulation which functions as a naturally occurring inhibitor of the activated serine proteases
- Antithrombin inhibits factors IIa, IXa, Xa, XIa, and XIIa, and to a limited extent VIIa
- Serves as a cofactor for heparin and other heparinoids
- Autosomal dominant trait and the most severe of the inherited conditions
- Relatively uncommon **t5.12**
- Recurrent venous thrombosis
- Deficiency diminishes therapeutic response to heparin therapy because antithrombin is the binding site for heparin
- Congenital antithrombin deficiency
  - Type I: Quantitative deficiency (reduced activity and antigen levels)
  - Type II: Qualitative deficiency (reduced activity but normal antigen level)
- Acquired antithrombin deficiency
  - Liver failure (such as liver cirrhosis)
  - Nephrotic syndrome (a kidney disorder)
  - Widespread (metastatic) tumors
  - DIC
  - Pregnancy
  - Acute blood clots
  - Severe trauma
  - Severe burns

5.7.2.2 Protein C (PC) deficiency

- Synthesized in liver, vitamin K-dependent factor
- Activated by thrombin-thrombomodulin on endothelial cell surface
- Requires protein S, which acts as a cofactor to stabilize activated PC (aPC)
- Degrades FVa & FVIIIa
- Functions as a naturally occurring inhibitor of the coagulation cascade
- 50% of heterozygotes will experience VTE by 40 years of age
- Common manifestations
  - DVT
  - PE
  - Superficial thrombophlebitis
  - Cerebrovascular events
  - Myocardial events
- Qualitative & quantitative
- Heterozygous
  - Recurrent thrombosis 8-10 fold
  - Associated with warfarin-induced skin necrosis
- Homozygous
  - Neonatal purpura fulminans (<1% PC)
  - DVT/PE in adolescence in mild cases
  - 5%-25% PC
- Treatment
  - Heparin
  - Long-term warfarin therapy
  - Heparin must be administered before initiation of warfarin to reduce warfarin-induced skin necrosis
  - PC concentrates
- Acquired PC deficiency
  - DIC
  - Liver disease
  - Sepsis
  - Oral anticoagulant therapy
  - Postoperatively
  - Estrogen therapy
  - Pregnancy

5.7.2.3 Protein S deficiency

- Cofactor for PC-mediated inhibition of activated FV and FVIII
- Reversible complex with C4bBP
- Is a vitamin K dependent factor → decreased under oral anticoagulation
- Hereditary protein S deficiency:
  - Type I (quantitative): Decreased activity, free & total antigen
  - Type II (functional): Dysfunctional molecule, decreased activity, but normal free & total antigen
  - Type III (distribution): Dysfunctional molecule, decreased activity & free antigen, but normal total antigen
  - Deficiency: Hereditary or acquired
- Acquired protein S deficiency: pregnancy

5.7.2.4 aPC resistance (factor V Leiden mutation)

- Activated protein C (aPC)
  - PC—when activated becomes aPC
  - Protein S serves as a cofactor to PC
  - aPC inhibits Va and VIIIa
  - Functions as a natural anticoagulant
- aPC resistance
  - Poor anticoagulant response of aPC to degrade FVa and FVIIIa
  - Approximately 90% of aPC resistance is caused by a defect in the FV molecule, known as the FV Leiden gene mutation
  - FV Leiden is a single-point mutation which makes FV more resistant to inactivation by aPC
  - Consists of a single nucleotide substitution of adenine for guanine of the FV gene
  - Higher risk for thrombosis
- Recurrent venous thrombosis and pregnancy loss
- Found in up to 50% of patients with thrombophilia
- Particularly common in northern European populations and found in up to 5% of the white population
- Heterozygotes have a 5- to 10-fold increased risk of thrombosis

5.7.2.5 Prothrombin variant (prothrombin G20210A mutation)

- Mutation at position 20210 of the prothrombin gene
- Associated with elevated prothrombin levels (>115%)
- High prevalence
  - 1%-3% of the general population of whites
  - 5%-10% of patients with thrombosis
  - 3-fold increased risk of venous thrombosis in heterozygous individuals
  - May confer an increased risk of arterial thrombosis at a young age in patients with multiple risk factors
- Recurrent venous thrombosis, particularly cerebral vein thrombosis
- Pregnancy loss

5.7.2.6 *MTHFR* gene mutation & hyperhomocysteinemia

- Hyperhomocysteinemia & homocystinuria
  - Homocystinuria is a manifestation of severe hyperhomocysteinemia
  - Severe hyperhomocysteinemia is caused by homozygous cystathionine-β-synthase deficiency or homozygous methylenetetrahydrofolate reductase (MTHFR) deficiency
- Inherited causes: Most common cause is heterozygous *MTHFR* gene mutation
- Acquired causes: Smoking, renal failure, deficiency of folate, and deficiencies of vitamins B_6 & B_{12}

5.7.3 Antiphospholipid syndrome

- Includes both the lupus anticoagulant (LA) and anticardiolipin antibody (ACA) and anti-β_2-GPI antibody
- Disorder of recurrent venous & arterial thrombosis, pregnancy loss, and thrombocytopenia

5.7.3.1 Anticardiolipin antibody

- Autoantibodies are usually IgG & IgM
- Directed against cardiolipin & other negatively charged phospholipids

5.7.3.2 Lupus anticoagulant (LA)

- Polyclonal IgG, IgM & IgA types
- LA is an antiphospholipid antibody and, as such, interferes with coagulation testing by binding to phospholipid-protein complexes, thereby prolonging clotting times
- Antibodies are commonly found in:
  - Asymptomatic elderly individuals
  - Patients with autoimmune disorders
- Associated with 2 broad categories of phospholipid antibodies
  - Anticardiolipin antibodies
  - β_2-GPI antibodies
- More specific for thrombosis and other clinical complications of the antiphospholipid syndrome
- Prevalence in venous & arterial thrombosis

ISBN 978-089189-6616

- LA is one of the most common acquired predisposing causes of thrombosis
- Patients do not bleed, but other problems can occur concurrently that can cause bleeding
  - Thrombocytopenia
  - Isolated deficiency of prothrombin
  - Qualitative platelet defects
  - Recurrent spontaneous abortions
- Results in prolongation of phospholipid-dependent assays
- LA is often identified during routine screening with the standard aPTT (based on the sensitivity of the reagent)
  - In vitro → results in a prolonged activated partial thromboplastin time (aPTT)
  - In vivo → usually results in thrombosis rather than clinical bleeding & usually does not result in clinical bleeding
- Antibody may be persistent or transient
- Diagnosis of LA requires the following steps:
  - Prolongation of at least 1 phospholipid-dependent clotting test (usually in an assay with a reagent of low phospholipid content)
  - Evidence of inhibitory activity shown by the effect of patient plasma on pooled normal plasma (mixing studies)
  - Evidence that the inhibitory activity depends on phospholipid. This may be achieved by the addition or alteration of phospholipid, hexagonal phase phospholipid, platelets, or platelet vesicles to the test system
  - LAs must be carefully distinguished from other coagulopathies that may give similar laboratory results or may occur concurrently with LAs. Specific factor assays and the clinical history may be helpful in differentiating LAs from specific factor inhibitors
  - To exclude the presence of LA, at least 2 different screening assays need to be negative
  - The presence of LA must be confirmed after at least 12 weeks, or preferably after 1 year
- Laboratory diagnosis

5.7.4 Heparin-induced thrombocytopenia (HIT)

- Types of HIT
  - Type 1 occurs early during heparinization, and the platelet count diminishes only mildly. Platelets decrease within 1-2 days of heparinization. This type of HIT is not a danger to the patient, is not immune mediated, there is no formation of IgG antibodies, and it is not a contraindication to future heparin use
  - Type 2 is usually noted after 5-7 days of heparinization (unless there has been previous exposure to heparin), and the platelet count falls by greater than 50% of baseline. Type 2 HIT is immune mediated (formation of IgG antibodies), and there is a high risk of thrombosis, both arterial and venous
- Risk factors for HIT
  - Surgery (3- to 5-fold greater risk compared to medical patients)
  - Female sex (2-fold greater risk)
- Type of heparin: Unfractionated heparin imparts the greatest risk, but any heparin exposure, even the small amount used in intravenous catheters, may lead to HIT
- Assessing pretest probability for HIT (4Ts)
  - The diagnosis of HIT is also dependent on clinical findings. Testing is performed after implementing the 4T scoring system in which a score of 6-8 indicates a high probability of HIT and a score of <4 indicates a low probability. Each of the Ts is scored from 0-2
- The 4Ts consist of:
  - *T*iming of platelet count decline
    - Typically 5-14 days following the start of heparinization
    - Rapid-onset HIT may be seen in those recently exposed to heparin
    - Delayed-onset HIT may occur after cessation of heparin therapy, for up to 3 weeks
  - *T*hrombocytopenia
    - Typical platelet count nadir is ≤50% of baseline but is rarely severe
    - Rarely $<20 \times 10^3/\mu L$ ($<20 \times 10^9/L$)
  - *T*hrombosis
    - Thrombosis is present in about half of patients at the time of onset
    - Venous or arterial, most commonly presenting with DVT
  - O*t*her causes of thrombocytopenia
    - A score of 0 indicates that another cause may be present whereas a score of 2 indicates no other cause exists
- Pathophysiology of type 2 HIT
  - Antibodies against the platelet factor 4–heparin complex lead to platelet activation
- Laboratory diagnosis
  - The most commonly used test is an immunoassay (ELISA) that detects anti-PF4/heparin antibodies
  - The gold standard test is the serotonin release assay

5.7.5 Therapeutic agents & monitoring

- Used to prevent clotting by several different mechanisms
- Warfarin sodium (proprietary name, Coumadin) renders the vitamin K factors nonfunctional (FII, FVII, FIX, and FX)
- Heparins inhibit actions of FIIa and FXa
- Direct FXa inhibitors inhibit only FXa
- Direct FIIa inhibitors inhibit thrombin
- PT, aPTT, TT, and anti-FXa not optimum for monitoring direct FXa and FIIa inhibitors

5.7.5.1 Anticoagulants

5.7.5.1.1 Warfarin

- Warfarin is an analogue of vitamin K
- Inhibits posttranslational modification of vitamin K-dependent proteins, including
  - Coagulation factors II, VII, IX, and X
  - Naturally occurring anticoagulants PC & protein S
- The half-life of PC and protein S are shorter than that of the coagulation factors, therefore:
  - Initiation of warfarin therapy is associated with a brief thrombophilic state
  - It may manifest as warfarin skin necrosis
  - It is more pronounced in patients who are deficient in PC or protein S
- The effect of warfarin depends on a variety of factors
  - Age, race, comorbidity, diet, concomitant medications
- Genotypic effects
  - The genes with greatest impact on warfarin are *VKORC1* & *CYP2C9*
- Warfarin therapy
  - Monitor with the international normalized ratio (INR), which must fall within a narrow therapeutic range, typically 2-3, and requires frequent blood draws
  - Levels above the therapeutic range lead to an increased risk of life-threatening bleeding; below the therapeutic range, a risk of thrombosis
  - Multiple dietary & pharmacologic interactions
  - When warfarin therapy is started, its anticoagulant effects may not be apparent for several days
  - The duration of action of a single dose is 2-5 days
  - Vitamin K administration is the antidote for high levels of warfarin
  - Reversal may be indicated with supratherapeutic INR and bleeding
  - Administration of oral vitamin K, intravenous vitamin K, or prothrombin complex, depending on the situation

5.7.5.1.2 Other oral anticoagulants

- The goal of novel oral anticoagulants is, in part, to offer more specific targeting and to afford more predictable responses than current anticoagulant therapies, such as warfarin, can offer
- Oral direct FXa inhibitors
  - Apixaban, rivaroxaban, edoxaban & betrixaban are direct FXa inhibitors which can be taken orally
  - FXa inhibitors target FXa, preventing the conversion of prothrombin to thrombin
  - Cleared by the liver
  - The PT and aPTT are usually prolonged when there is a therapeutic effect, but the response is nonlinear. They are not sensitive for monitoring
  - Reversal agent for these direct FXa inhibitors is andexanet alfa
- Oral direct thrombin inhibitors
  - Dabigatran is a reversible competitive thrombin inhibitor
  - Direct thrombin inhibitors target thrombin (FIIa), blocking the conversion of fibrinogen to fibrin
  - Dabigatran blocks the last stages of the coagulation cascade: cleavage of fibrinogen into fibrin, activation of platelets & stabilization of clots
  - Dabigatran blocks both fibrin- and clot-bound thrombin, unlike heparin, which inhibits only free thrombin
  - Cleared by the kidneys; half-life of 12-17 hours
  - aPTT and TT elevation give a qualitative measure of effect
  - TT is highly sensitive to the presence of dabigatran and will be markedly prolonged
  - Effect can be reversed with idarucizumab

5.7.5.1.2.1 Parenteral anticoagulants

- These agents are administered intravenously
  - Argatroban
    - Small direct thrombin inhibitor
    - Metabolized by the liver, half-life of 50 minutes
    - Used to treat heparin induced thrombocytopenia (HIT) and percutaneous coronary intervention (PCI)
  - Bivalirudin
    - Short synthetic peptide, specific thrombin inhibitor
    - Metabolized by kidneys; half-life of 25 min
    - Used to treat HIT, PCI
  - Hirudin
    - Powerful thrombin inhibitor from leeches
    - Lepirudin
      - Recombinant hirudin from yeast cells
      - Irreversible
      - Metabolized by kidney, used to treat HIT

ISBN 978-089189-6616

- Monitoring
  - DTI will prolong thrombin time; aPTT usually prolonged; however, response is reagent dependent, and may not be linear
  - Ecarin clotting time uses an ecarin solution that measures the proteolytic activity of non-inhibited meizothrombin by the conversion of fibrinogen to fibrin
    - Measured against a standard curve constructed with the anticoagulant
  - No reversal agent; may be removed by dialysis

5.7.5.1.3 Unfractionated heparin (UH)

- It binds to antithrombin, enhancing its capacity to inactivate thrombin, FXa, FIXa, FXIa & FXIIa. Also exists physiologically as a naturally occurring anticoagulant produced by basophils & mast cells
- Treats & prevents venous thromboembolism
- 20% is excreted by the kidney
- 80% is removed from the circulation by the liver & reticuloendothelial system
- Half-life of 90 minutes
- Bolus dose of 5,000-10,000 units
- Test 4-6 hours after administration to assess therapeutic affect
- Monitor with the aPTT and anti-Xa assay. The presence of heparin may be detected using TT
- Heparin resistance
  - Most common cause is antithrombin deficiency
- Reversal
  - Withhold heparin with or without intravenous protamine sulfate

5.7.5.1.4 Low-molecular-weight heparin (LMWH)

- Binds to antithrombin via a unique pentasaccharide sequence
- LMWH-antithrombin complex binds to the active site of FXa and inhibits its activity
- Exerts its anticoagulant activity via antithrombin
- Mean molecular weight 5,000 Da with <18 saccharide units
- Therapeutic range: 0.6-1.2 U/mL
- Advantages
  - Bioavailability approaches 100%
  - Peak anti-FXa activity occurs between 3 and 5 hours after administration
  - Its association with heparin-induced thrombocytopenia (HIT) is less than that of unfractionated heparin
  - Does not cause osteoporosis
  - Monitoring is only required in certain circumstances
- Agents include enoxaparin, dalteparin, nadroparin, tinzaparin & danaparoid
  - Danaparoid is considered a "heparinoid" because it is a mixture of glycosaminoglycans, including heparan sulfate, dermatan sulfate, and chondroitin sulfate, with no heparin; however, it is similar to the other LMWH in its mechanism of action and clinical utility
  - Mechanism of action is the same as UH
  - Monitoring is usually not required
  - Monitoring may be required in patients with severe obesity or renal failure & in pediatric patients
  - LMWH assay (FXa inhibitory method)
  - Reversal with protamine sulfate does not neutralize LMWH as effectively as UH

5.7.5.1.5 Fondaparinux (Arixtra)

- Synthetic heparin analogue and irreversible FXa inhibitor
- Monitored using an anti-FXa assay
- Synthetic pentasaccharide
- Mechanism
  - Contains a unique pentasaccharide sequence
  - Binds to antithrombin → inhibits FXa
  - Indirect inhibitor of IIa

5.7.5.2 Antiplatelet agents t5.13

- Proven efficacy in the treatment of acute thrombosis & prevention of arterial thrombosis
- However, increases the risk of bleeding

t5.13 Antiplatelet drugs

Target	Drug
Cyclooxygenase inhibitors Aspirin irreversibly inhibits the enzyme COX, resulting in reduced platelet production of TXA2 (powerful vasoconstrictor that lowers cyclic AMP & initiates the platelet release reaction)	Aspirin NSAIDS Ibuprofen (Motrin) Indomethacin (Indocin) Naproxen (Aleve)
ADP receptor antagonists affects the ADP-dependent activation of IIb/IIIa complex	Thienopyridines Ticlopidine Clopidogrel
GPIIb/IIIa antagonists block a receptor on the platelet for fibrinogen & von Willebrand factor	Abciximab Tirofiban Eptifibatide
Phosphodiesterase inhibitors	Dipyridamole

ADP, adenosine diphosphate; AMP, adenosine monophosphate; COX, cyclooxygenase; GP, glycoprotein; NSAIDs, nonsteroidal anti-inflammatory drugs; TXA, thromboxane

5.7.5.2.1 Aspirin

- Aspirin (acetylsalicylic acid) is effective in the prevention of cardiovascular events
- Mechanism of action
  - Irreversibly inhibits COX-1 in platelets & megakaryocytes
  - Blocks the formation of TXA_2
  - Immediate antiplatelet effect which lasts 7-10 days
    - Inhibition of COX-1 is achieved with low doses of aspirin
    - Inhibition of COX-2 requires larger doses of aspirin
- Aspirin resistance occurs in 25% of adults
- Monitoring
  - Used primarily to establish aspirin resistance, to verify compliance, or to document reversal before surgery
  - Platelet aggregometry: Decreased response to arachidonic acid
  - PFA100: Prolonged closure time with collagen/EPI cartridge and normal closure time with collagen/adenosine diphosphate (ADP) cartridge
  - VerifyNow aspirin assay

5.7.5.2.2 Thienopyridines

- ADP receptor antagonists which block the P2Y12 receptor that mediates ADP-induced platelet activation
- Agents include ticlopidine (Ticlid), clopidogrel (Plavix) & prasugrel
  - Clopidogrel
    - Irreversibly blocks the ADP P2Y12 receptor → inhibition of GpIIb/IIIa receptor
    - Inhibits platelet aggregation
  - Ticlopidine
    - Blocks the ADP P2Y12 receptor → inhibition of GpIIb/IIIa receptor
    - Inhibits platelet aggregation and release
- Agents are prodrugs that are metabolized by hepatic CYP2C19 into active metabolites
- Monitoring
  - Monitoring is necessary to diagnose drug resistance and to document reversal prior to surgery
  - Platelet aggregometry: Decreased response to ADP
  - VerifyNow P2Y12 assay

5.7.5.2.3 Dipyridamole

- Inhibits phosphodiesterase and reduces intracellular calcium concentration
- In combination with low-dose aspirin, it is marketed as Aggrenox

5.7.5.2.4 GPIIb/IIIa receptor antagonists

- GPIIb/IIIa antagonists
  - Block the GPIIb/IIIa fibrinogen binding receptor
  - Abciximab (ReoPro)
  - Eptifibatide (Integrelin)
  - Tirofiban (Aggrastat)
- May cause thrombocytopenia
- Monitoring
  - Platelet aggregometry: Decreased response to collagen & ADP
  - VerifyNow GPIIb/IIIa platelet-induced aggregation assay
- No reversal agent

5.7.5.3 Thrombolytic therapy

- Mechanism of action
  - Plasmin lyses clots by digesting fibrin contained in clots
- Streptokinase
  - Derived from *Streptococcus*
- Urokinase
  - Direct activator of plasminogen
- Tissue plasminogen activator (tPA)
  - Converts plasminogen to plasmin

5.8 Laboratory evaluation of hemostasis

5.8.1 Laboratory evaluation of primary hemostasis

5.8.1.1 Platelet function screen (PFA-100/200)

- Test cartridges that contain:
  - Collagen/epinephrine
  - Collagen/ADP
- Measures high-shear platelet adhesion & aggregation
- Whole blood is aspirated through an aperture that is covered by a thin membrane
- Platelets adhere to the membrane and aggregate, causing occlusion of the aperture
- The time it takes for the clot to occlude the aperture is called the closure time (CT), which is reported in seconds
- CT is prolonged when platelets are defective
- Testing with the Col/Epi cartridge is most sensitive to drug-induced platelet defects (aspirin and aspirinlike agents), whereas intrinsic platelet defects tend to prolong closure with both types of membranes
- CT is dependent not only on platelet function but also on platelet number & hematocrit

 ISBN 978-089189-6616

5.8.1.2 Specific platelet antagonist testing (VerifyNow)

- A whole-blood, semiautomated, cartridge-based platelet function test used to determine the response of platelets to specific antiplatelet agents
- The assay is based on the ability of activated platelets to bind fibrinogen
- It measures the aggregation of fibrinogen -coated beads that have been stimulated by an agonist in citrated whole blood
- VerifyNow aspirin cartridge
  - Qualitative test to aid in the detection of platelet dysfunction in the presence of aspirin. The test is reported in aspirin reaction units (ARU)
- VerifyNow P2Y12 cartridge
  - Measures the extent of platelet aggregation in the presence of a P2Y12 inhibitor such as clopidogrel. Lower P2Y12 reaction units (PRU) levels are associated with expected antiplatelet effect
- VerifyNow GPIIb/IIIa cartridge
  - Measures the level of platelet inhibition in patients receiving abciximab

5.8.1.3 Platelet aggregometry

5.8.1.3.1 Light transmittance (optical) aggregation

- Performed on platelet-rich plasma (PRP)
- The sample is exposed to various agonists, including ADP, epinephrine, arachidonate, collagen, and ristocetin
- Platelet aggregation is detected by measuring the increase in light transmittance when agonists are added to a stirred sample of PRP in a cuvette
- When using an optimal dose of agonist, a biphasic curve is seen consisting of a primary and secondary wave of aggregation
- A suboptimal dose of agonist will produce only a primary wave followed by disaggregation because of a lack of granule secretion
- Primary wave
  - Reversible
  - Measures the ability of platelets to respond to an external agonist and to start to aggregate
  - Without enough stimulus or without an intact prostaglandin pathway → TXA_2 — platelets disaggregate
- Secondary wave
  - Irreversible
  - Results in complete release of dense granule contents, most importantly ADP
- Collagen
  - Membrane defects
  - General ability of platelets to aggregate
  - Storage pool disorder, RD, NSAID
- Epinephrine
  - Membrane defects
  - Cyclooxygenase (COX)
  - NSAID
- Arachidonic acid
  - Most useful in detecting aspirinlike deficiencies
  - Aspirin, NSAID
- Adenosine diphosphate (ADP)
  - Membrane defects
  - COX, SPD
  - NSAID
- Ristocetin
  - Membrane defects
  - Measures agglutination (not aggregation)
  - Differentiate between BS vs von Willebrand disease (vWD), vWD type 2B vs platelet-type vWD
- Aspirin and aspirinlike agents cause decreased aggregation with collagen & arachidonate
- Poor response to all agents (ADP, epinephrine, arachidonate, collagen) except ristocetin is typical of Glanzmann thombasthenia
- An absent secondary phase (with epinephrine & ADP) is seen with SPDs
- A poor primary aggregation response to epinephrine is seen in myeloproliferative disorders
- Normal response to all agonists except high-dose ristocetin is the hallmark of vWD; this pattern is also seen in Bernard-Soulier syndrome
- A hyperresponse to low-dose ristocetin is the hallmark of type 2B and platelet-type vWD

5.8.1.3.2 Whole blood aggregometry (WBA)

- WBA measures aggregation as the change in electrical impedance between 2 electrodes as platelets adhere and aggregate in response to agonists
- This method allows for platelets to be studied in a physiologic whole blood environment, which includes erythrocytes & leukocytes
- Sample preparation is reduced, preserving labile modulators such as prostacyclin & thromboxane A_2, and reducing the chance of platelet activation during processing

5.8.1.3.3 Lumi aggregation

- The release of adenosine triphosphate (ATP) from the platelet dense granules, reflected in the secondary wave, can be monitored during aggregation

- This method detects light emitted from ATP reacting with a bioluminescent reagent (luciferin/luciferase)

5.8.1.4 Thromboelastography (TEG)

- TEG is a viscoelastic hemostatic assay that measures the global viscoelastic properties of whole blood clot formation under low shear stress
- It measures the interaction of platelets with the coagulation cascade (aggregation, clot strengthening, fibrin cross-linking & fibrinolysis) and provides a rapid assessment of hemostasis f5.9
- Specific parameters represent the 3 phases of the cell-based model of hemostasis: initiation, amplification, and propagation

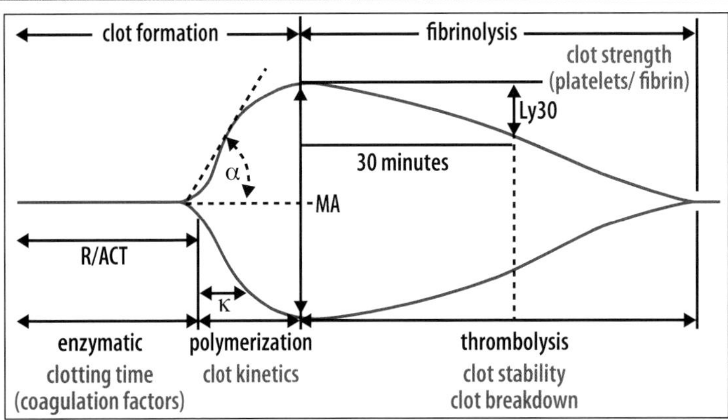

f5.9 Thromboelastography

5.8.2 Laboratory evaluation of secondary hemostasis

5.8.2.1 Coagulation analyzers

5.8.2.1.1 Optical density

- Fibrin formation is detected by a decrease in turbidity, resulting in a change in optical density
- Results are recorded as the time required for clot formation
- A curve depicting clot formation is provided on some coagulation analyzers

5.8.2.1.2 Mechanical

- Two methods are available for clot detection
  - One is based on the movement of a metal ball between 2 magnets
    - As fibrin forms, the viscosity of the sample stops the motion of the ball at the point of clot formation
  - The second method uses 2 probes, one stationary and one moving probe immersed in the patient's plasma
    - As fibrin forms, it acts as a conductor between the 2 probes and stops the timer at the clotting endpoint. This is recorded as the clotting time

5.8.2.2 Prothrombin time (PT)

- A source of tissue factor (TF)—tissue extract or recombinant TF—phospholipid, and calcium are added to citrated plasma The time to clot formation is the PT
- TF combines with FVII to form the "extrinsic" tenase complex
- Measures
  - FVII of the extrinsic pathway
  - FX, FV, FII, FI of the common pathway
  - Measures 3 of the vitamin K-dependent factors
    - FII, FVII & FX, but does not measure FIX
  - Most sensitive to deficiencies of FVII
- PT is prolonged in
  - Deficiencies of FI, FII, FV, FVII, FX
  - Liver disease
  - Warfarin (Coumadin) therapy—oral anticoagulants
  - High-dose heparin therapy and direct thrombin inhibitors
- PT is shortened after treatment with recombinant VIIa (rVIIa)
- Most common use of PT → monitoring oral anticoagulants
- Coumadin or warfarin results in the inability of the liver to carboxylate the glutamyl residues of vitamin K-dependent factors: FII, FVII, FIX, FX, PC, and protein S. Renders them nonfunctional, impairing fibrin formation
- Loss of function is half-life dependent: FVII has the shortest half-life, FII has the longest
- Maintaining a narrow therapeutic range is essential
- INR was developed by the World Health Organization using an international reference plasma (IRP) to which all other thromboplastins can be compared
- INR is used to monitor patients receiving warfarin therapy
  - Recommended that a PT value be expressed as a ratio by normalizing it to the IRP
  - International sensitivity index (ISI) is a measure of the sensitivity & responsiveness of a particular thromboplastin reagent to warfarin-induced reduction of the vitamin K-dependent factors
  - ISI of the IRP = 1.0

$$\text{INR} = (\text{patient's PT}) / (\text{geometric mean of the reference range})_{\text{ISI}}$$

  - Advantages of the INR for monitoring patients receiving oral anticoagulants

ISBN 978-089189-6616

- Minimizes the variation in the PT assay
- Allows comparability of PT results among different laboratories

- Therapeutic ranges
  - INR 2.0-3.0
    - Prophylaxis & treatment of venous thrombosis & PE
    - Prevention of systemic embolism
  - INR 2.5-3.5
    - Mechanical prosthetic valves (high risk)

5.8.2.3 Activated partial thromboplastin time (aPTT)

- Phospholipid and a contact (eg, silica, kaolin) or chemical (elagic acid) activator are added to citrated plasma and incubated; after incubation, Ca^{2+} is added in excess and time to clot formation is measured
- Phospholipid source: Rabbit brain, cephalin, dehydrated rabbit brain, bovine brain, soybean, recombinant sources
- Activated by contact: Silica, ellagic acid, kaolin
- Measures
  - Activation of the contact factors: protein kinase , high-molecular-weight kininogen, FXII, FXI
  - Intrinsic pathway factors: FXII, FXI, FIX, FVIII
  - Common pathway: FI, FII, FV, FX
- Prolonged
  - Deficiencies of all factors except VII and XIII
  - Presence of inhibitors
    - Specific inhibitors: FVIII & FIX
    - Nonspecific inhibitors: LA, heparin, direct thrombin inhibitors
- Shortened
  - Elevated FVIII; acute phase reactants (fibrinogen, vWF)
- Monitors heparin therapy

5.8.2.4 Fibrinogen

- Clauss technique
  - Functional assay; patients' plasma is diluted and excess thrombin is added
  - A reference (standard) curve is prepared using known fibrinogen concentrations with their respective thrombin clotting times
  - Fibrinogen concentration is *inversely proportional* to the thrombin clotting time of diluted plasma
- Detects
  - Quantitative deficiency: Hypofibrinogenemia & hyperfibrinogenemia
  - Qualitative deficiency: Dysfibrinogenemia
- Acute phase protein → elevated in
  - Inflammation
  - Trauma
  - Infection
  - Increases with age
  - Associated with cardiovascular disease & thrombosis
- Low levels suggest bleeding and may be associated with:
  - DIC caused by consumption
  - Thrombolytic therapy resulting in increased levels of fibrin (ogen) breakdown products FDPs (>190 μg/mL)
    - Interfere with fibrin monomer polymerization
- Liver disease due to decreased synthesis or abnormal synthesis
- Heparin (unfractionated) may lead to underestimation

5.8.2.5 Thrombin time (TT) t5.14

- Bovine or human thrombin is added to platelet poor plasma
- Measures the conversion of fibrinogen to fibrin
- Cleaves fibrinopeptides A & B
- Clotting time is measured in seconds
- Sensitive to the presence of heparin

5.8.2.6 Reptilase time t5.14

- Modification of the TT, using reptilase (snake venom isolated from Bothrops atrox)
- Reptilase is added to plasma and the clotting time is recorded in seconds
- Detects the presence of fibrin degradation products (FDP)
- Cleaves fibrinopeptide A only
- Prolonged in disorders of fibrinogen
- Not affected by the presence of heparin & hirudin

t5.14 Comparison of thrombin time & reptilase time

Condition	Thrombin time	Reptilase time
Unfractionated heparin	Prolonged	Normal
warfarin	Normal	Normal
Direct thrombin inhibitors	Prolonged	Normal
Dysfibrinogenemia/ hypofibrinogenemia	Prolonged	Prolonged
Disseminated intravascular coagulation	Prolonged	Prolonged
Liver disease	Prolonged	Prolonged
Neonates	Prolonged	Prolonged

5.8.2.7 D-dimer & FDPs

- Specific product resulting from the degradation of fibrin clots that results from the action of:
  - Thrombin
    - Converts fibrinogen into fibrin clots
  - FXIIIa
    - Cross-links fibrin monomers to stabilize clots
  - Plasmin
    - Cleaves the cross-linked fibrin clot
- FXIII covalently cross-links fibrin by linking 'D' regions of the fibrin molecule; when fibrin is cleaved by plasmin, this results in the formation of various FDPs, including D-dimers
- Increased D-dimers
  - presence of thrombosis, consumptive coagulopathy (DIC) & significant bleeding
  - atrial fibrillation, congestive heart failure & cirrhosis
- D-dimer is useful in the diagnosis of venous thromboembolism (VTE)
  - A normal D-dimer measured with a high-sensitivity assay excludes VTE in selected patients
  - D-dimer assays are most useful in patients with a low or intermediate clinical probability of VTE, based on clinical parameters such as the Well prediction rules
  - A positive D-dimer is relatively nonspecific

5.8.2.8 Mixing study

- Performed on a prolonged prothrombin time (PT) or activated partial thromboplastin time (aPTT) to determine if it is caused by a factor deficiency or an inhibitor
- Equal parts of patient plasma and pooled normal plasma are mixed and the prolonged screening test is repeated
- If the results are corrected, the missing factor has been replaced by the pooled normal plasma and the patient should be worked up for a factor deficiency
- If the result is not corrected, there is something in the patient's plasma that is inhibiting a correction and a workup for an inhibitor should be performed
- There are no recommendations or guidelines to standardize the definition of a correction of a mixing study. The following may be used to define a correction:
  - Based on PT or aPTT upper limit of the normal range
  - Within the limits of 2SD or 3SD of the normal range
  - Within 5 seconds of the 2SD upper limit of the normal range
  - Relative to the value of the pooled normal plasma (NPP)
- Rosner index
  - 1:1 mix

$$\text{index} = \text{CT of 1:1 mix} - \text{CT of NPP} \times 100$$

- Clotting time (CT) of patient
  - Factor deficiency: <15
  - Inhibitor: >15

5.8.2.9 Factor assays (FII, FV, FVII, FVIII, FIX, FX, FXI, FXII)

- Based on a 1-stage clotting assay
- Patient plasma is mixed with a plasma which is deficient in the factor being investigated (eg, FVIII-deficient plasma is used to investigate a patient with a prolonged aPTT and a possible FVIII deficiency)
- Compares the ability of dilutions of a standard/reference plasma, as well as a test plasma, to correct the prolonged PT or aPTT of a plasma that is totally deficient in the factor being tested
  - PT-based factors = FII, FV, FVII & FX
  - aPTT-based factors = FVIII, FIX, FXI & FXII
- The various dilutions of the standard/reference plasma combined with deficient plasma are used to construct the calibration curve
- The concentration of each dilution of a standard of known assay value is plotted against the clotting time of each dilution
- The clotting times of the test plasma in seconds are compared to the clotting times of the known concentrations obtained using the standard plasma
- The calibration curve is used to convert the clotting times to the % activity of the factor being tested
- An inhibitor is suggested if serial dilutions result in an apparent increase in factor activity or nonparallelism is observed
- Results are expressed as percent activity—"normal" plasma contains 100% activity or IU/mL
- With the exception of FVIII, all factors are relatively low in neonates, reaching adult levels by 6 months of age

5.8.2.10 Factor XIII

- Fibrin stabilizing factor, not measured in the coagulation cascade
- Normal PT and aPTT
- Patient will present with delayed bleeding

ISBN 978-089189-6616

- Qualitative screening test
  - Clot solubility test
    - May miss a mild or moderate deficiency:
      - Patient plasma and control form a clot with excess calcium, incubated for 30 minutes
      - Clot is removed and placed in a 5M urea solution and incubated for 24 hours at 37°C (alternatively can use 2% tricholoroacetic acid, or 1% monochloroacetic acid)
    - If clot dissolves, suggests a deficiency of FXIII
    - False positive can occur in patients with low fibrinogen
- Chromogenic FXIII assays
  - Activity based on transglutamase activity
  - Uses a thrombin activated substrate and a chromogenic substrate
  - Color change is proportional to the concentration of FXIIIa

5.8.3 Laboratory evaluation of thrombosis

5.8.3.1 Lupus anticoagulant (LA) testing

5.8.3.1.1 Sensitive vs insensitive aPTT reagent

- aPTT reagents vary in sensitivity based on the type & concentration of phospholipids
- LA presents itself as an antibody to phospholipids in the laboratory
- A reagent that is low in phospholipids is sensitive to the antibody and will result in a prolonged screening test
- An insensitive reagent is high in phospholipids and will mask the presence of LA, resulting in a short or normal aPTT
- Samples for LA testing must be platelet poor; platelets are phospholipids and interfere with testing. The presence of platelets will falsely shorten and mask results

5.8.3.1.2 Dilute Russell viper venom test (DRVVT)

- This test is based on the activation of FX by Russell viper venom (RVV) and varying amounts of phospholipids
- When the LA antibody is present, it binds to the phospholipid and inhibits thrombin generation, prolonging the clotting time
- RVV directly activates FX, as a result, the test is not affected by deficiencies or inhibitors to FVIII, FIX, FXI, or FXII
- The test is performed in 2 parts
  - Screen: The DRVVT screening step uses a reagent with a low concentration of phospholipid which, in the presence of LA, will cause a prolonged result
  - Confirm: The DRVVT confirm step uses a reagent with a high concentration of phospholipid which will mask the LA causing a shortened result
  - The ratio of screen to confirm is calculated. If the ratio is >1.2 the result is positive for LA
- The result can also be normalized using normalized pooled plasma (NPP) to eliminate possible interference of warfarin or a FV or FII deficiency

5.8.3.1.3 Hexagonal phase neutralization

- LA antibodies recognize hexagonal phase phosphatidylethanolamine (HPP) but not those phospholipids that result in a bilayer configuration
- The test consists of an activated partial thromboplastin time (aPTT) performed with the HPP and again without HPP. If the difference in clotting time >8 seconds the result is considered positive

5.8.3.2 Thrombophilia testing

5.8.3.2.1 Antithrombin

- Produced in the liver
- Protease that inhibits coagulation by inhibiting thrombin
- Patients with decreased levels are prone to thrombosis
- Testing for antithrombin is performed with a chromogenic method
  - Excess amounts of FXa are added to the sample
  - In the presence of heparin, a portion of the enzyme is complexed and inactivated by antithrombin in the sample
  - Excess uninhibited Xa cleaves a specific chromogenic substrate, releasing a dye
  - Change is measured by the increase in absorbance

5.8.3.2.2 Protein C

- Vitamin K-dependent glycoprotein synthesized in the liver
- Circulates as an inactive precursor and functions as an anticoagulant after being converted to the serine protease aPC, which then degrades coagulation factors Va & VIIIa
- Decreased levels of PC can result in thrombosis

- PC function can be measured using a clot-based or chromogenic assay
  - Both assays use *Agkistrodon contortrix* venom (Protac) to activate PC
  - Clot-based assays also add PC-deficient plasma, measuring the time to clot and extrapolating the percent activity from a standard curve
  - Substances that interfere with clot-based assays (anticoagulants) will also interfere with a clot-based PC assay. Additionally, increased levels of FVIII can underestimate PC levels
  - PC chromogenic assays measure color using p-nitroaniline released by cleavage of a synthetic chromogenic peptide substrate
  - The chromogenic assay is more specific for PC and less susceptible to interfering substances

5.8.3.2.3 Protein S

- Vitamin K-dependent factor synthesized in the liver
- Cofactor for PC
- Decreased levels of protein S can result in thrombosis
- Functional protein S antigen assays are based on the prolongation of clotting caused by the generation of APC
- Protein S antigen can be measured as a total antigen consisting of protein S bound to C4BP as well as free protein S; the free protein S antigen has functional activity

5.8.3.2.4 aPC resistance

- Measures the aPTT of plasma with or without the addition of exogenous aPC
- In a sample without aPC resistance, the addition of aPC inactivates FVa and FVIIIa and prolongs the clotting time. If a FV Leiden mutation is present, the clotting time shortens
- A ratio (aPTT + aPC)/(aPTT – aPC), patients with a ratio <2.0 are positive for FV Leiden
- If patients have an initial prolongation of the aPTT, results may be inaccurate
- Diluting patients' plasma (1:4) with FV-deficient plasma can reduce interfering substances
- May serve as a screen for the most common FV Leiden mutation

5.8.3.2.5 Molecular testing: FV Leiden, prothrombin mutation

- Factor V Leiden is a single nucleotide polymorphism (SNP) located at exon 10, resulting in a substitution of arginine to glutamine
- FVL mutation causes aPC resistance, leading to thrombosis
- Prothrombin gene testing is performed to detect the G20210A SNP
  - PG20210 mutation leads to increased levels of prothrombin & thrombosis
- Molecular testing for these mutations is used for the assessment of thrombophilia

5.8.3.3 Other testing

5.8.3.3.1 Anti-Xa assay (heparin anti-FXa assay)

- Measures the amount of unfractionated heparin or LMWH present in a sample
- Chromogenic methodology
- When FXa is present in excess along with antithrombin, the inactivation of FXa will be a function of the concentration of heparin
- Reaction:

antithrombin (excess) + heparin [heparin-antithrombin] + antithrombin

- The inactivation of FXa is a function of the concentration of heparin

[heparin-antithrombin] + FXa (excess) → [heparin-antithrombin-FXa] + FXa (residual)

- FXa (residual) that remains should be measured using a chromogenic substrate

FXa + chromogenic peptide substrate—pNA

- The residual FXa cleaves the pNA from the chromogenic substrate and the released pNA is measures at 405 nm
- Proportionate to the concentration of heparin in the patient's plasma

5.8.3.3.2 Bethesda assay (FVIII inhibitor assay, anti-FVIII antibody assay)

- Used to measure antibodies against coagulation factors, most commonly anti-FVIII antibodies
- Procedure:
  - Serial dilutions of patient plasma are made
  - Each is mixed 1:1 with normal plasma and assayed for FVIII activity after a 2-hour incubation
  - The dilution at which the FVIII activity is 50% represents the inhibitor titer
  - The result is expressed in Bethesda units
- One Bethesda unit of inhibition is defined as the amount of inhibitor that will inactivate 50% of the FVIII activity present

ISBN 978-089189-6616

5.9 SARS-CoV-2 & coagulation

- Coronaviruses are RNA viruses and occur among humans, mammals & birds (see also Microbiology 6.6.14)
- They cause respiratory, enteric, hepatic & neurologic diseases

5.9.1 COVID-19 associated coagulopathy (CAC)

- Microthrombi are present in lungs, and alterations of the coagulation cascade can be measured at a systemic level
- Endothelial dysfunction caused by both direct virus cytopathic effect and inflammatory reaction leads to a prothrombotic setting
- Reports of venous thromboembolism (VTE) range in instances from 1.1% in non-ICU up to 69% in ICU patients. Those with more severe disease along with additional risk factors such as older, male, obesity, cancer, history of VTE, and comorbid disease have a higher risk

5.9.2 Cytokine storm

- Combination of the inflammatory nature of the virus and the activation of multiple systems including the immune system which can result in something called a cytokine storm
- Excessive immune response attacks healthy lung tissue leading to acute respiratory distress syndrome and multiorgan failure
  - Blood vessel walls open and allow immune cells into surrounding tissues, but the vessels get so leaky that the lungs may fill with fluid, and blood pressure drops
  - Blood clots circulate throughout the body
  - Untreated cytokine syndrome is usually fatal

5.9.3 Disseminated intravascular coagulation (DIC) & COVID-19

- Patients with COVID-19 may develop sepsis associated with organ dysfunction
- Resulting in the expression of tissue factor and the secretion of von Willebrand disease
- Thrombin circulates, uncontrolled by natural anticoagulation, can activate platelets, and stimulate fibrinolysis
- Levels of D-dimer & fibrinogen degradation products (FDP) are very elevated in all deaths, suggesting both coagulation activation and secondary hyperfibrinolysis

5.9.4 Coagulation testing in COVID-19

- Prolonged prothrombin time (PT) and activated partial thromboplastin time (aPTT)
- Thrombocytopenia
- D-dimer
  - A high D-dimer is because of the wide spread of abnormal coagulation
  - The diagnostic hallmark of COVID-DIC is a rapidly rising D-dimer
  - Patients with D-dimer >1,000 at admission are 20 times more likely to die than patients with lower D-dimer values
  - Fibrinogen is generally elevated
    - However, in extremely severe and late-stage disease, consumption of fibrinogen may occur leading to hypofibrinogenemia

5.10 Selected readings

5.10.1 Books

Keohane EM, Smith L, Otto CN, Walenga JM, eds. *Rodak's Hematology: Clinical Principles and Applications.* 6th ed. Saunders; 2015. ISBN 978-0323530453

Kottke-Marchant K. *An Algorithmic Approach to Hemostasis Testing.* 2nd ed. CAP; 2016. ISBN 978-1941096253

5.10.2 Journals & online

Han H, Yang L, Liu R, et al. Prominent changes in blood coagulation of patients with SARS-CoV-2 infection. *Clin Chem Lab Med.* 2020;58(7):1116-1120. doi 10.1515/cclm-2020-0188

Hoffman M, Monroe DM. Cell based model of hemostasis. *Thromb Haemost.* 2001;85:958-65. doi 10.1055/s-0037-1615947

Isreals SJ. Laboratory testing for platelet function disorders. *Int J Lab Haematol.* 2015;37(suppl 1):18-24. doi 10.1111/ijlh.12346

Khor B, Van Cott EM. Laboratory evaluation of hypercoagulability. *Clin Lab Med.* 2009;29(2):339-66. doi 10.1016/j.cll.2009.03.002

Kreuziger L, Lee A, Garcia D, et al. COVID-19 and VTE/anticoagulation: frequently asked questions. doi 10.1182/asheducation-2015.1.243

Lippi G, Franchini M, Favaloro EJ. Diagnostics of inherited bleeding disorders of secondary hemostasis: an easy guide for routine clinical laboratories. *Semin Thromb Hemost.* 2016;42(5):471-7. doi 10.1055/s-0036-1571311

Mackie I, Cooper P, Lawrie A, et al. Guidelines on the laboratory aspects of assays used in haemostasis and thrombosis. *Int J Lab Hematol.* 2013;35(1):1-13. doi 10.1111/ijlh.12004

Moore GW. Recent guidelines and recommendations for laboratory detection of lupus anticoagulants. *Semin Thromb Hemost.* 2014;2:163-71. doi 10.1055/s-0033-1364185.

NHLBI. The diagnosis, evaluation and management of von Willebrand disease— 2008 clinical practice guidelines. https://www.nhlbi.nih.gov/files/docs/guidelines/vwd. pdf

Smith L. Laboratory diagnosis of the lupus anticoagulant. *Am Soc Clin Lab Sci.* 2017;1:7-14. doi 10.29074/ ascls.30.1.7

Thiagarahan P. Overview of platelet disorders.*http://emedicine.medscape.com/article/201722overview#showall*

Tran H, Joseph J, Young L, et al. New oral anticoagulants: a practical guide on prescription, laboratory testing and peri-procedural/bleeding management. *Intern Med J.* 2014;44(6):525-36. doi 10.1111/ imj.12448

Chapter 6

Microbiology

ISBN 978-089189-6616

6.1 Bacteriology

6.1.1 Patient identification & specimen labeling

- Proper specimen labeling
  - Labels should include patient name, identification number, room number, physician, culture site, date and time of collection
- Requisition form
  - Include patient name, date of birth, gender, room number, physician name and contact information, anatomic site, date and time of collection, diagnosis, antimicrobial agents if given, name of person transcribing orders

6.1.2 Specimen collection

- Blood cultures
  - Disinfect skin with 70%-95% ethanol or isopropyl alcohol and then 2% tincture of iodine or 2% chlorhexidine
  - For conventional blood culture systems, optimal blood to culture medium ratio is 1:5 or 1:10
  - Ideally inoculate each of 2 blood culture bottles (1 set) with 10 mL of blood from adults (20 mL per set), children (5-10 mL per set), newborns (2-4 mL per set)
  - Sodium polyanetholsulfonate (SPS) should be in blood culture bottles. SPS also inactivates neutrophils, certain antibiotics (aminoglycosides, polymyxins), and complement
  - Draw 2-3 sets of bottles in a 24-hour period when each set is a separate venipuncture
  - Incubate 2 bottle sets at 35°C-37°C, with 1 bottle aerobic & 1 bottle anaerobic
- Body fluids (eg, cerebrospinal fluid [CSF], synovial, plural, amniotic, pericardial, ascites)
  - Disinfect skin before aspirating with sterile needle & syringe
- Urine
  - Clean-catch, midstream urine: Clean external genitalia and begin voiding after several milliliters have passed; collect midstream into sterile, screw-cap container
  - Straight catheter: Clean urethral area, insert catheter, collect urine sample after several milliliters have passed into sterile, screw-cap container
  - Indwelling catheter: Disinfect catheter collection port, aspirate urine with needle & syringe, and empty into sterile, screw-cap container
  - Suprapubic: Disinfect skin, aspirate with needle & syringe through the abdominal wall and into the bladder; transport in syringe or sterile screw-capped container
- Respiratory tract
  - Throat: Swab posterior pharynx
  - Nasopharynx: Use smaller wire handle swab and insert up into posterior nasopharynx and hold for 5 seconds. Use of flocked swab for collection is also acceptable
  - Sputum: Patient should cough deeply to expectorate the sample into a sterile, screw-capped cup
  - Induced sputum collected by suctioning and assistance from respiratory therapy. Special procedure collections are done for bronchial washing, bronchial lavage, tracheal aspirate
- Wound/abscess
  - Area should be wiped with alcohol or sterile saline
  - Preferred collection is aspirate with needle & syringe; excess air is expelled from syringe
  - Dacron swab can be used to collect specimen from purulent area of wound
- Stool
  - Collect in clean, leak-proof container and avoid contamination with urine
- Genital: Cervix/vagina/urethra
  - Use swab to collect specimen
- Anaerobes: The following sites usually harbor normal anaerobic flora and should not be cultivated for anaerobes
  - Stool, skin, oropharynx, genital tract

6.1.3 Specimen transport

- Specimens should reach laboratory in a timely manner—30 minutes from time of collection is preferred but no longer than 2 hours after collection
- Blood cultures should be kept at room temperature until arrival in the laboratory
- Body fluids should be kept at room temperature until arrival in the laboratory
- Urine should be refrigerated until arrival in the laboratory, or it can be left at room temperature if arrival at the laboratory occurs within 2 hours of collection
  - Boric acid preservative can be added to urine sample if there is a delay in transport to the laboratory and will maintain specimen up to 24 hours after collection
- Sputum sample should be refrigerated until it can be delivered to the laboratory
- Cultures collected on swabs should be in Stuart or Amies transport systems, except for genital tract specimens
- Stool specimens should be refrigerated until they are delivered to the laboratory or placed in Cary-Blair transport medium
- Inoculate genital specimens for the JEMBEC system for *Neisseria gonorrhoeae* culture and keep at room temperature until delivery at the laboratory

6.1.4 Direct microscopic examination

- Gram staining **t6.1**
  - Routinely performed on certain specimen types, especially those collected from normally sterile sites
  - Gram stain morphology can guide species identification

- Gram-positive organisms have thick peptidoglycan cell wall outer membranes. They retain the purple crystal violet/iodine complex during the decolorizer step **t6.2**
- Gram-negative organisms have thin peptidoglycan cell walls with lipopolysaccharide outer membranes. They lose the crystal violet/iodine complex during the decolorizing step and are visualized using red safranin counterstain; inadequate decolorization results in host cells and bacteria appearing blue

t6.1 Gram stain morphology of selected organisms

Organism	Gram stain morphology
Gram-positive cocci	
Staphylococci	Gram-positive cocci in grapelike clusters
Pyogenic streptococci	Gram-positive cocci in pairs & short chains
Nonpyogenic streptococci	Gram-positive cocci in long chains
Streptococcus pneumoniae	Gram-positive lancet shaped diplococci
Enterococcus spp	Gram-positive cocci, mostly in chains & pairs
Gram-negative cocci	
Neisseria spp	Gram-negative kidney bean shaped diplococci
Gram-positive rods	See **t6.2**
Gram-negative rods	
Vibrio spp	Gram-negative curved, comma shaped short rods
Campylobacter spp	Gram-negative curved, thin, rods (S-shaped, seagull shaped or corkscrew shaped)
Yersinia pestis	Gram-negative rods with bipolar staining ("closed safety pin")
Legionella spp	Gram-invisible in primary smear
Enterics	Gram-negative bacilli, straight rod or coccobacillary
Pseudomonas	Gram-negative bacilli, thin
Haemophilus spp	Gram-negative bacilli, small pleomorphic & coccobacillary

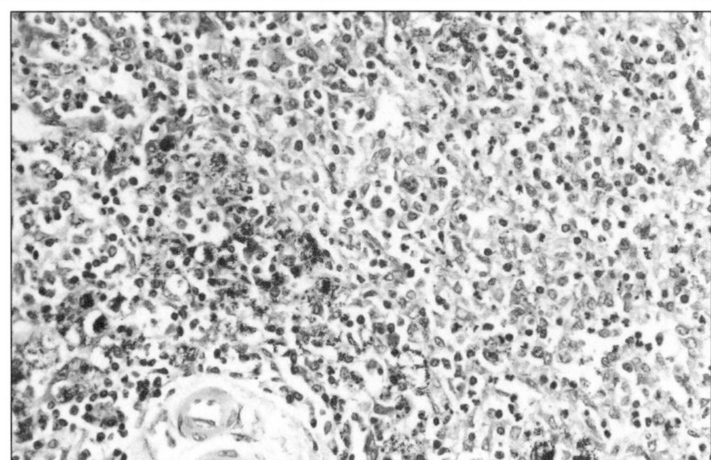

i6.1 Acid-fast stain

- Acid-fast stain
  - For mycobacteria: These bacteria have the cell wall structure of gram-positive bacteria but contain mycolic acids, which repel crystal violet/iodine, thus are usually gram invisible
  - Acid-fast staining uses heat and/or phenol to allow a fuchsin dye to penetrate the hydrophobic barrier and stain the mycolic acids in the cell wall (red stain)
  - The organisms resist decolorization, which is why they are termed "acid-fast" i6.1
  - Ziehl-Neelsen technique: Red carbol fuchsin dye containing phenol is heated to aid penetration of the cell wall; strong acid, 3% hydrochloric acid (HCL), is used for decolorization; methylene blue is counterstain
  - Kinyoun (cold) technique: Higher concentration of phenol and no heat; otherwise same as Ziehl-Neelsen

t6.2 Gram stain morphology: Gram-positive rods

	Short, irregularly shaped, pleomorphic	Regularly shaped, monomorphic		Branching, filamentous
		Small to medium	Large	
Aerobic or facultatively anaerobic	*Corynebacterium* spp	*Listeria* spp	*Bacillus* spp	*Nocardia* spp
	Other coryneforms*	*Erysipelothrix* spp		
	Non-*Nocardia* aerobic actinomycetes†			
Aerotolerant	*Actinomyces* spp‡	Aerotolerant *Lactobacillus* strains		
	Bifidobacterium spp			
Anaerobic, nonspore forming	*Propionibacterium* spp	*Eubacterium* spp		*Actinomyces israelii*
		Lactobacillus spp		
Anaerobic, spore forming		*Clostridium ramosum*	*Clostridium perfringen*(rarely forms spores)	
			Other *Clostridium* spp§	

**Examples include Arcanobacterium spp, Rothia spp & Arthrobacter spp*
†Examples include Rhodococcus spp, Gordonia spp & Tsukamurella spp
‡Examples include Actinomyces neuii, Actinomyces odontolyticus, Actinomyces viscosus
§Examples include Clostridium septicum, Clostridioides difficile, Clostridium sordellii, Clostridium sporogenes & Clostridium bifermentans

 ISBN 978-089189-6616

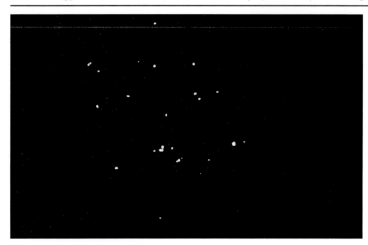

i6.2 Auramine & rhodamine stain

- Fite (modified) acid-fast technique: weaker decolorizing reagent; good for "weakly" acid-fast organisms such as *Nocardia* spp, *Cryptosporidium*, *Cystoisospora bellii* (formerly *Isospora*), *Cyclospora*, *Sarcocystis* & *Legionella micdadei*)
- Fluorescent auramine rhodamine stain for acid-fast bacilli
  - Auramine & rhodamine stain mycolic acids and fluoresce when exposed to ultraviolet light i6.2
- Acridine orange fluorescent stain
  - Detects bacteria & yeasts in smears prepared from blood & body fluids where organisms are in low concentrations

6.1.5 Specimen processing

- Prioritization
  - Level 1 is for immediate processing; examples include blood, CSF, other body fluids, brain biopsy
  - Level 2 includes unpreserved specimens; examples include feces, urine, sputum, tissue, bone, wound
  - Level 3 requires quantitation; examples are urine & tissue
  - Level 4 are preserved specimens; examples are preserved feces, preserved urine, swabs in holding media
- Reasons for specimen rejection
  - Incomplete information on requisition
  - Information on specimen label & requisition do not match
  - Specimen submitted in inappropriate or leaky transport container
  - Inadequate specimen
  - Transport time >2 hours without preservative or appropriate temperature
  - Anaerobic culture submitted from site where anaerobes are indigenous
  - Multiple specimens submitted from same source on same day (except for blood cultures)
  - Direct Gram stain of sputum sample shows <25 white blood cells (WBCs) and >10 squamous epithelial cells per low-power field (lpf)
- Biosafety cabinet & personal protective equipment (PPE)
  - Personal protective equipment (PPE): Gloves, laboratory coats, masks, respirators, face shields, safety glasses. Must never be worn outside laboratory
  - Universal precautions are applied when handling all patient samples; it is assumed that a specimen contains biological agents that correlate with at least a biosafety level 2 (BSL-2)
  - Biosafety cabinets should be used properly to process all specimens. Decontaminate interior work surfaces with 70% ethanol. Do not place items on front intake grill or rear-wall or floor exhaust grills
  - Allow blower to run 15-30 minutes before & 30 minutes after use
  - Turn on UV light to disinfect interior of cabinet when not in use
- Centers for Disease Control and Prevention (CDC) classification of agents of bioterrorism t6.3

t6.3 CDC classification of agents of bioterrorism

Category A (highest priority)	Category B (2nd priority)	Category C (3rd priority; emerging threat agents)
Variola (smallpox)	Encephalitis viruses (α viruses)	Influenza viruses
Hemorrhagic fever viruses	*Brucella* spp (brucellosis)	Nipah virus
Bacillus anthracis (anthrax)	*Burkholderia mallei* (glanders)	Hantavirus
Yersinia pestis (plague)	*Burkholderia pseudomallei* (melioidosis)	Rabies virus
Clostridium botulinum (botulism)	*Chlamydophila psittaci*	Yellow fever virus
Francisella tularensis (tularemia)	*Coxiella burnetii* (Q fever)	Drug resistant TB
	Clostridium perfringens toxin	*Rickettsia conorii*
	Foodborne bacteria (eg, *Salmonella* spp, *Escherichia coli* O157:H7, *Shigella*)	
	Waterborne bacteria (eg, *Vibrio cholerae*, *Cryptosporidium* spp)	
	Rickettsia prowazekii (typhus fever)	
	Staphylococcus aureus enterotoxin B	

- Specimen preparation methods & applications
  - Concentration of large volumes of sterile body fluids is done to increase recovery of bacteria, by using centrifugation & filtration methods
  - Tissue samples are prepared by homogenization

- Digestion & decontamination of respiratory samples is done for recovery of mycobacteria
    - Liquifies sample by digesting proteinaceous material
    - Decontaminates by killing nonmycobacterial agents
    - Agents used: (1) 2-4% NaOH; (2) N-acetyl-L-cysteine; (3) benzalkonium chloride; (4) oxalic acid (specifically removes *Pseudomonas aeruginosa*)

- Types of culture media
  - Nonselective: Adequately supports growth of most microorganisms. (eg, trypticase soy agar) **t6.4**

t6.4 Commonly used nonselective media

Medium	Type	Purpose
Sheep blood agar	Solid	General bacteriology; supports the growth of most bacteria, with important exceptions (eg, *N gonorrhea*, *H influenzae* & *Legionella*)
Chocolate agar	Solid	Cultivation/isolation of fastidious bacteria like *Neisseria* spp & *Haemophilus* spp, but not *Legionella* spp
Buffered charcoal yeast extract (BCYE) agar	Solid	Recovery of *Legionella* spp; contains cysteine & iron supplementation, necessary to support growth of *Legionella* Activated charcoal helps bind & sequester growth inhibitors that may be present in the specimen
Mueller-Hinton agar	Solid	Antimicrobial susceptibility testing of many common bacteria
Thioglycolate broth	Liquid	Cultivation of bacteria, including microaerophilic & obligately anaerobic bacteria; oxygen tension decreases toward bottom of tube, permitting growth of obligate anaerobes & microaerophilic bacteria without incubation in an anaerobic atmosphere

  - Enriched: Growth enhancers such as 5% sheep blood or vitamins are added to nonselective media (eg, 5% sheep blood agar, chocolate agar)
  - Selective: Selects for growth of a group of organisms by adding inhibitory substances such as antimicrobials, dyes, or alcohol. These substances inhibit growth of other organisms. (eg, MacConkey agar selects for growth of most facultative gram-negative bacilli and inhibits growth of gram-positive cocci and bacilli and gram-negative cocci; colistin naladixic acid (CNA) agar selects for growth of gram-positive cocci and bacilli but inhibits growth of gram-negative bacilli & cocci) **t6.5**

t6.5 Commonly used selective media

Medium	Type	Basis for selectivity	Purpose
MacConkey agar (MAC)	Solid	Bile salts & crystal violet inhibit growth of gram-positive bacteria & delicate gram-negative bacteria	Cultivation/isolation of hardy enteric gram-negative rods
Eosin methylene blue (EMB)	Solid	Aniline dyes inhibit growth of gram-positive bacteria	Cultivation/isolation of hardy enteric gram-negative rods
Campylobacter blood agar (Campy-BAP)	Solid	Antimicrobials to which *Campylobacter* spp are resistant (cephalothin, vancomycin, trimethoprim, amphotericin B, polymyxin B)	Recovery of *Campylobacter* spp
Hektoen enteric (HE) agar	Solid	Bile salts & the dyes bromthymol blue & acid fuchsin inhibit the growth of gram-positive organisms & some gram-negative strains	Enhanced recovery of *Salmonella* & *Shigella*, compared with MAC or EMB
Salmonella-Shigella (SS) agar	Solid	Bile salts, sodium citrate & brilliant green dye inhibit gram-positive bacteria & many enterics other than *Salmonella*	Recovery of *Salmonella* & *Shigella*, although *Shigella* strains may be inhibited Not recommended for primary isolation of *Shigella*
Selenite broth	Liquid	Sodium selenite inhibits growth of gram-positive bacteria & many enterics other than *Salmonella*	Recovery & enrichment of *Salmonella*
Thiosulfate-citrate-bile salts-sucrose (TCBS) agar	Solid	Bile salts inhibit gram-positive bacteria Alkaline pH inhibits most enterics & enhances growth of *Vibrio* spp	Recovery of *Vibrio* spp
Cefsulodin-Irgasan-novobiocin (CIN) agar	Solid	Antimicrobials (cefsulodin, Irgasan, novobiocin) & crystal violet inhibit most gram-negative & gram-positive bacteria other than *Yersinia* spp	Recovery of *Yersinia* spp
Anaerobic colistin-nalidixic acid (CNA) agar	Solid	Antimicrobials (colistin, nalidixic acid) inhibit gram-negative bacteria	Recovery of anaerobic streptococci; blood in the agar allows differentiation based on hemolytic reactions
Lim broth	Liquid	Antimicrobials (colistin, nalidixic acid) inhibit gram-negative bacteria	Recovery of group B streptococci (*S agalactiae*)
Regan-Lowe medium	Solid	Antimicrobials to which *Bordetella* spp are resistant (cephalexin)	Recovery of *Bordetella pertussis* & *Bordetella parapertussis*
Thayer-Martin medium	Solid	Antimicrobials to which *Neisseria* spp are resistant (vancomycin, colistin, nystatin & SXT)	Recovery of *Neisseria* spp from nonsterile sites

ISBN 978-089189-6616

- Differential: Supports growth of a group or groups of bacteria AND differentiates within the group (most differential media is also selective). (eg, MacConkey agar selects for growth of most facultative gram-negative bacilli and it also differentiates lactose fermenters & nonlactose fermenters) t6.6

t6.6 Commonly used differential media

Medium	Type	Basis for differentiation	Purpose
MacConkey (MAC) agar	Solid	Lactose fermentation results in pink or red coloration of colonies Lactose nonfermenters form translucent colonies	Differentiating between lactose fermenting & nonlactose fermenting enterics
Eosin methylene blue (EMB)	Solid	Lactose fermentation results in purple-black colonies or colonies with a green metallic sheen Lactose nonfermenters form translucent colonies	Differentiating between lactose fermenting & nonlactose fermenting enterics
Hektoen enteric (HE) agar	Solid	Lactose and/or sucrose fermentation results in yellow or orange coloration of colonies Lactose & sucrose nonfermenters form translucent colonies H_2S production results in black coloration of colonies	Differentiating between lactose and/or sucrose fermenting enterics & nonlactose or nonsucrose fermenting enterics Differentiating between H_2S producing & non-H_2S producing enterics
Salmonella-Shigella (SS) agar	Solid	Lactose fermentation results in pink or red colonies Lactose nonfermenters form translucent colonies H_2S production results in black coloration of colonies	Differentiating between lactose fermenting enterics & nonlactose fermenting enterics Differentiating between H_2S producing & non-H_2S producing enterics
Thiosulfate-citrate-bile salts-sucrose (TCBS) agar	Solid	Sucrose fermentation results in yellow colonies Sucrose nonfermenters form translucent colonies	Differentiating between sucrose fermenting *Vibrios* (eg, *Vibrio cholerae*) & sucrose nonfermenting *Vibrios*
Cefsulodin-Irgasan-Novobiocin (CIN) agar	Solid	Mannitol fermentation results in characteristic "bull's eye" colonies (colorless with red center) Mannitol nonfermenters form translucent colonies	Differentiating between mannitol fermenting *Yersinia* spp (eg, *Yersinia enterocolitica*) & mannitol nonfermenting *Yersinia* spp
Motility test agar	Semisolid	Motile organisms show growth spreading away from the line or inoculation (stab), clouding the agar Nonmotile organisms stay within the stab, leaving the remaining agar clear	Differentiating between motile & nonmotile bacteria

- Inoculation of media
  - Semiqualitative: Specimen is dropped from pipette or swabbed in the first quadrant of media plate. The plate is streaked in the first quadrant to the 2nd, 3rd & 4th quadrants. Growth is graded as 1+, 2+, 3+, 4+ or light, moderate, heavy growth

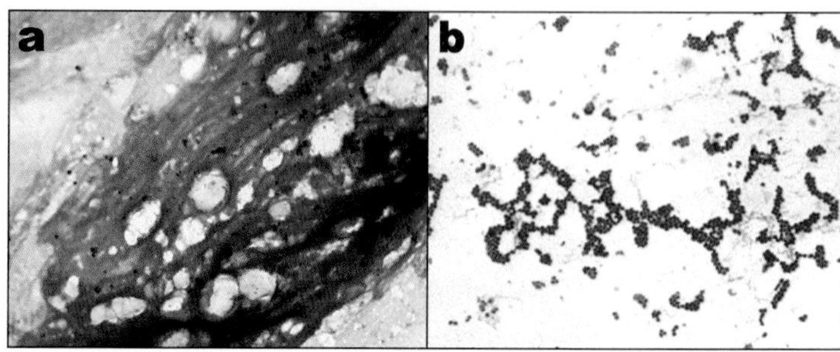

i6.3 Staphylococci: Gram stain morphology

  - Quantitative: For urine cultures, numbers of colonies are counted by using a calibrated inoculation loop that delivers 0.01 or 0.001 mL. Specimen is spread in a routine manner across the entire plate. The number of colonies that grow is multiplied by the dilution factor (eg, if 0.001 mL loop is used, 35 colonies would translate into 35,000 colony-forming units (CFU)/mL
- Incubation of specimens
  - Temperature
    - Most bacterial cultures are incubated at 35°C-37°C
    - *Yersinia enterocolitica* & certain *Pseudomonas* spp (eg, *Pseudomonas fluorescens, Pseudomonas putida*) grow optimally at 25°C-30°C
    - *Campylobacter* spp mostly commonly associated with diarrheal illness (*C jejuni* & *C coli*) grow optimally at 42°C
    - *Listeria monocytogenes* grows optimally at 37°C but displays its characteristic motility only at 25°C, and is notoriously able to multiply at refrigeration temperature (4°C)
  - Atmosphere
    - Aerobic organisms grow in ambient air
    - Anaerobic organisms cannot grow in the presence of oxygen
    - Facultative anaerobes grow in the presence or absence of oxygen
    - Capnophiles require increased concentration of carbon dioxide (CO_2; candle jar or CO_2 incubator)
    - Microaerophiles grow in reduced oxygen & increased CO_2 atmosphere

6.1.6 Specific bacteria

- Note: Many identification methods included in this section; matrix-assisted laser desorption/ionization-time-of-flight mass spectrometry (MALDI-TOF) technology can identify most bacterial isolates

6.1.6.1 Gram-positive cocci

6.1.6.1.1 Staphylococci/Micrococci

- Gram-positive cocci in grapelike clusters & tetrads i6.3

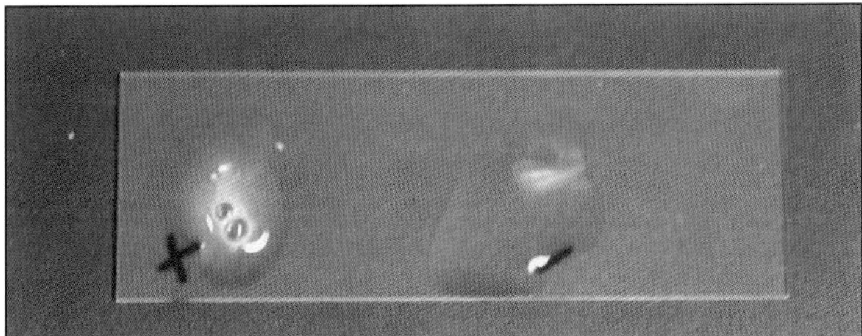

i6.4 Catalase test
Rapid & sustained effervescence (note bubbles on left) after addition of hydrogen peroxide to an isolate indicates the presence of catalase; staphylococci are catalase positive

- In addition to Gram stain morphology, distinguish from streptococci & enterococci using the catalase test (staphylococci/micrococci are catalase positive) i6.4

6.1.6.1.1.1 Coagulase-positive Staphylococci i6.5

- *Staphylococcus aureus*
  - Most clinically significant species causing wound & skin infections, osteomyelitis, pneumonia, toxin-related illnesses that include heat-stable enterotoxin associated with food poisoning
  - Key biochemicals for identification **t6.7** & **t6.8**

t6.7 Key biochemical tests for differentiating some *Staphylococcus* spp

Test	*S aureus*	*S epidermidis*	*S saprophyticus*	*S lugdenensis*
Coagulase (tube)	+	–	–	–
Pyrrolidonlyl arylamidase (PYR)	–	–	–	+
Ornithine decarboxylase	–	±	–	+
Novobiocin	Sensitive	Sensitive	Resistant	Sensitive

t6.8 Key biochemical tests for differentiating Staphylococci & Micrococci

Test	Staphylococci	Micrococci
Catalase	+	+
Coagulase	+	–
Modified oxidase	–	+
Bacitracin (0.4 units)	Resistant	Susceptible
Furazolidone	Susceptible	Resistant

  - Most express β-lactamase, conferring resistance to penicillin, ampicillin & early generation cephalosporins
  - Other penicillins like nafcillin, dicloxacillin, or oxacillin are not inactivated by lactamases
  - Expression of altered penicillin-binding proteins result in methicillin-resistant *S aureus* (MRSA); these carry the *mecA* gene, which allows them to express PBP2A, a penicillin target with little affinity for the drug

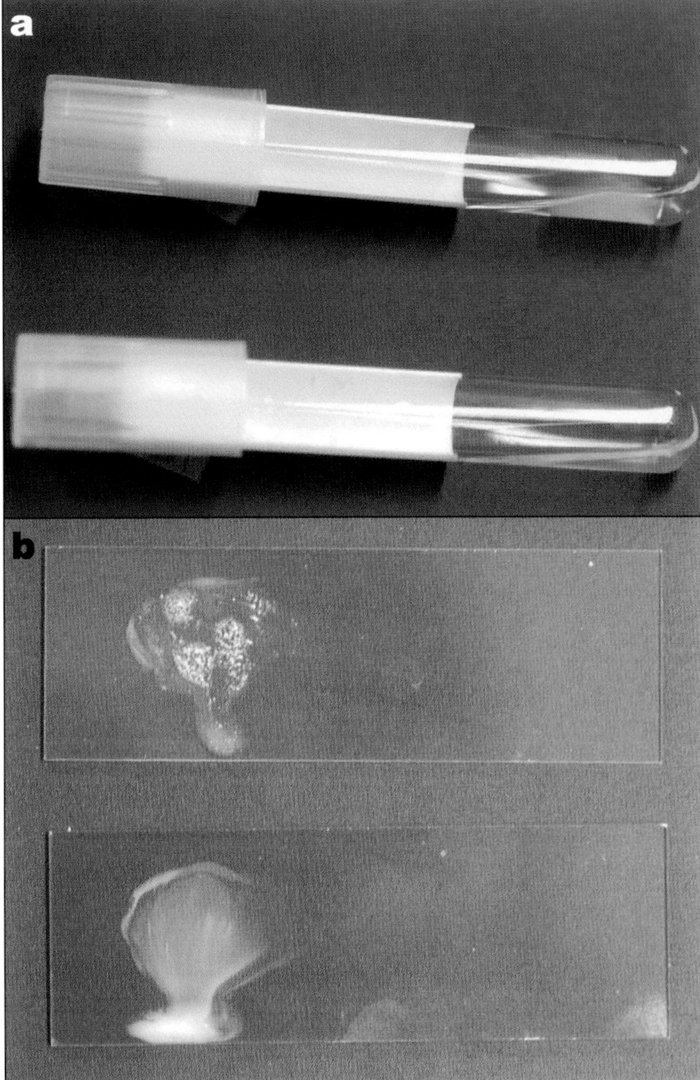

i6.5 The coagulase test is used to presumptively identify *S aureus*
a The tube coagulase test detects free coagulase, producing a coagulum in the presence of plasma (top tube); to avoid false negative reactions, it is necessary to examine the tube at both 4 & 24 hours
b The slide coagulase test detects bound coagulase, producing clumping in the presence of plasma (top slide); the slide test is faster but the tube test is required for confirmation

  - Hospital-acquired (HA)-MRSA is associated with nosocomial infections, healthcare facilities, multiorganism resistance
  - Community-acquired (CA)-MRSA outbreaks seen in daycare centers, contact sports participants, prisoners & military personnel and are often soft tissue infections. CA-MRSA usually more susceptible to antibiotics
  - MRSA identification
    - Routine disk diffusion testing, using cefoxitin as the indicator drug
    - Molecular nucleic acid probes or polymerase chain reaction (PCR) amplification to detect *mecA*

ISBN 978-089189-6616

- Chromogenic agar
- Detection of PBP2A using latex agglutination

- Media for culture or disk diffusion testing must have neutral pH, 2%-4% sodium chloride, 30°C-32°C (no higher than 35°C) incubation for up to 48 hours
- Patients may be screened for MRSA colonization by analyzing a nasal swab using either culture on selective media or PCR-based methods

6.1.6.1.1.2 Coagulase-negative staphylococci t6.7

- *Staphylococcus epidermidis*
  - Skin commensal but can cause endocarditis & infections related to shunts, catheters, intravenous catheters
  - Rarely causes infection in natural tissues, but may cause bloodstream infection related to infected intravascular catheters, prosthetic vascular grafts, or prosthetic cardiac valves
  - Causes prosthetic joint infections or central nervous system (CNS) infection related to ventricular shunts
  - Novobiocin sensitive
- *Staphylococcus saprophyticus*
  - Seen in urinary tract infections (UTIs) in young women of childbearing age
  - Novobiocin resistant
- *Staphylococcus lugdunensis* (SLUG)
  - Skin commensal
  - Causes infections similar in severity to *S aureus*
  - SLUG isolates often positive on slide coagulase test, negative on tube coagulase test, and negative with latex agglutination
  - PYR-positive & ornithine decarboxylase positive

6.1.6.1.1.3 Micrococci t6.8

- Exist in environment & normal flora of skin
- Yellow colonies on sheep blood agar (SBA)
- Catalase-positive; coagulase-positive; sensitive to bacitracin

6.1.6.1.1.4 *Rothia* (formerly *Stomatococcus mucilaginosa*)

- Normal flora of mouth & respiratory tract
- Causes bacteremia, endocarditis, peritonitis in immunocompromised patients
- Large gram-positive cocci in pairs/clusters
- Sticky colonies that adhere to agar
- Weakly catalase positive

6.1.6.1.2 Streptococci & enterococci t6.9

- Initially classified based on hemolytic properties on blood agar plates
  - Complete (β) hemolysis (clear zone surrounding colonies)
  - Incomplete or partial (α) hemolysis (green pigment surrounding colonies)
  - No (γ) hemolysis—red blood cells (RBCs) remain intact; no change in media surrounding colonies

t6.9 Catalase-negative, gram-positive cocci

Hemolysis	Organism	Properties
β	*S pyogenes*	PYR-positive, bacitracin susceptible, expresses Lancefield group A antigens
	S dysgalactiae	PYR-negative, bacitracin resistant (usually), expresses Lancefield group C or G antigens
	S agalactiae	PYR-negative, bacitracin resistant (usually), CAMP factor-positive, hippurate hydrolysis-positive, expresses Lancefield group B antigens
	Some strains of enterococci	PYR-positive, bile esculin-positive, NaCl-positive, bacitracin resistant, expresses Lancefield group D antigens
	Some strains of anginosus group streptococci	PYR-positive, bacitracin resistant, small colonies, butterscotch odor, may express Lancefield group A, C, F or G antigens
α	*S pneumoniae*	Optochin susceptible, bile solubility-positive
	Most viridans streptococci	Optochin resistant, PYR-negative, bile esculin-negative
	Some strains of *S bovis*	Optochin resistant, PYR-negative, bile esculin-positive, NaCl-negative
	Some strains of enterococci (especially *E faecium* strains)	Optochin resistant, PYR-positive, bile esculin-positive, NaCl-positive
Nonhemolytic	Most strains of enterococci	PYR-positive, bile esculin-positive
	Most strains of *S bovis*	PYR-negative, bile esculin-positive, NaCl-negative
	Some strains of viridans streptococci	PYR-negative, bile esculin-negative

6.1.6.1.2.1 β-hemolytic Streptococci

- *Streptococcus pyogenes* (group A streptococci)
  - Causes a wide variety of infections, including pharyngitis, retropharyngeal abscess, bacteremia, several skin & soft tissue infections including impetigo, erysipelas & necrotizing fasciitis
  - Also causes toxin-mediated illnesses, such as toxic shock syndrome & scarlet fever, as well as immune-mediated complications, including acute rheumatic fever (ARF), poststreptococcal glomerulonephritis (PSGN)

Bacteriology>Specific bacteria

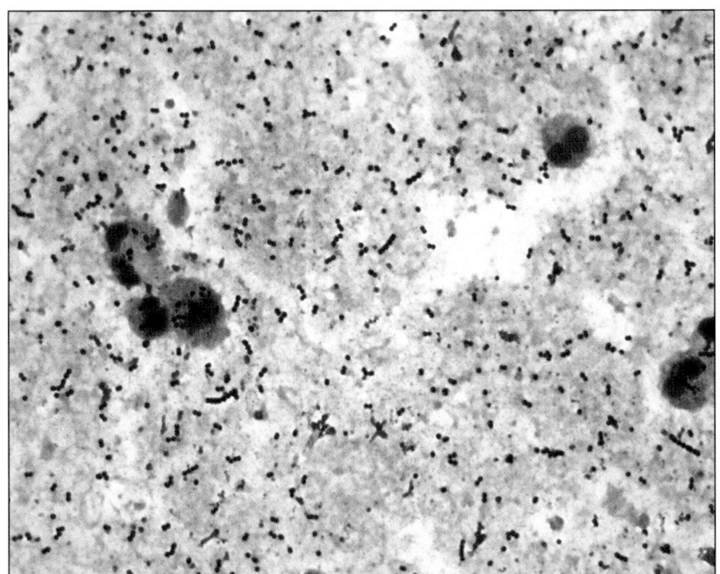

i6.6 Group A streptococci: Gram stain morphology

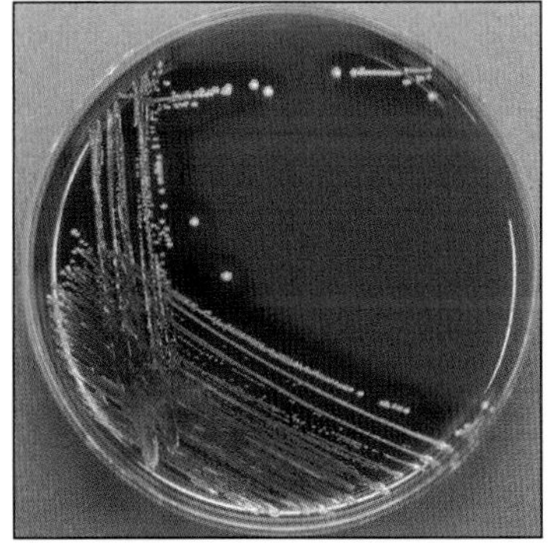

i6.7 Group A streptococci: colony morphology showing a wide zone of β hemolysis on blood agar

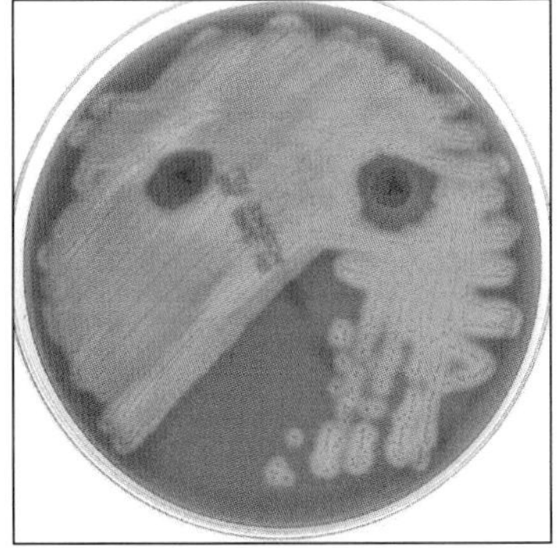

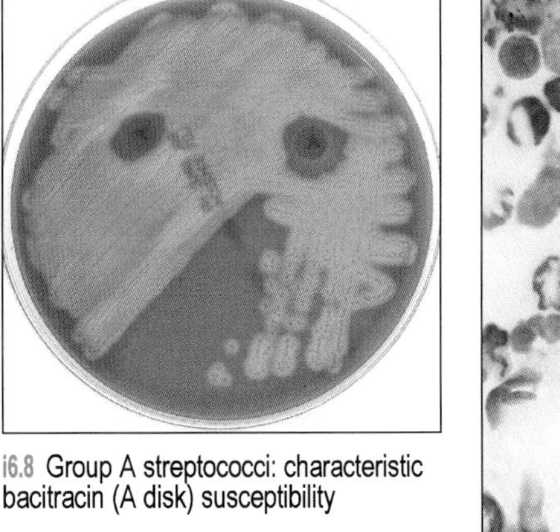

i6.8 Group A streptococci: characteristic bacitracin (A disk) susceptibility

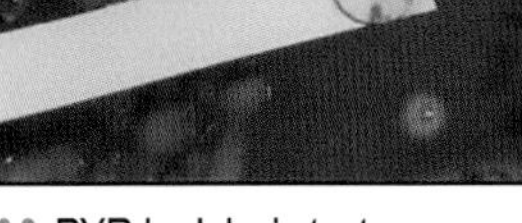

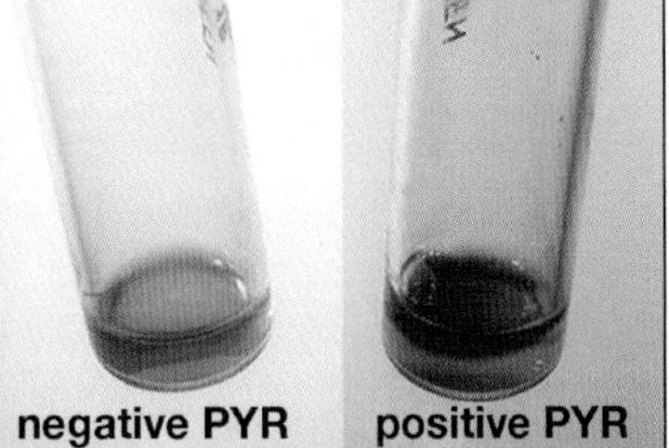

i6.9 PYR hydolysis test

- Gram-positive cocci singly, in pairs & in short chains i6.6
- On blood agar, colonies are large and are surrounded by a wide zone of β hemolyis i6.7
- Susceptible to bacitracin (A disk) i6.8, positive for PYR hydrolysis i6.9, and expresses Lancefield group A antigens i6.10
- Virulence factors include M protein, streptolysin O, streptolysin S, hyaluronidase

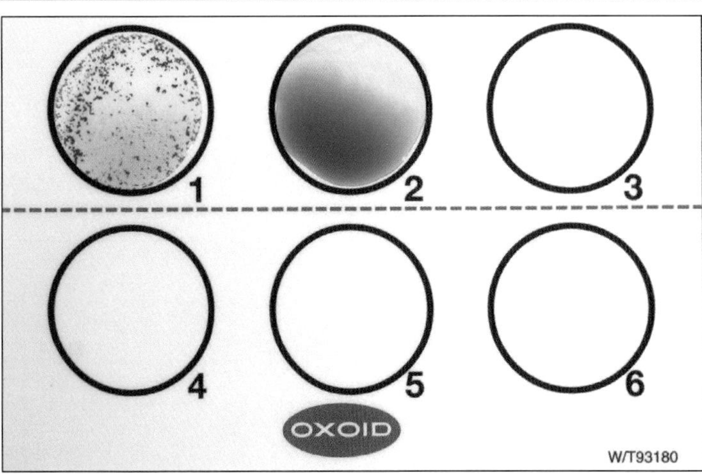

i6.10 A latex agglutination test for the identification of streptococcal groups A, B, C, D, F & G
In well 1, *Streptococcus pyogenes* was agglutinated using Lancefield group A reagent
In well 2, *Streptococcus pyogenes* did not agglutinate using Lancefield group B reagent

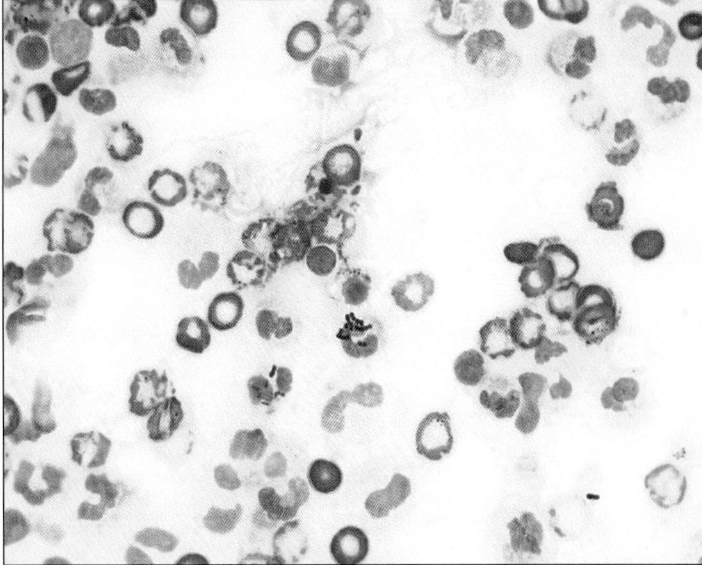

i6.11 Group B streptococci: Gram stain morphology

- *Streptococcus agalactiae* (group B streptococci)
  - Associated with neonatal pneumonia & meningitis, postpartum infections
  - Pregnant women should be screened for GBS colonization at 35-37 weeks' gestation. Screening can be accomplished using culture-based methods, or amplified molecular methods, though in either case, an enrichment broth step (LIM broth) must first be performed. Specimens should be obtained from the vagina & rectum, using a single swab
  - Gram-positive cocci in pairs & short chains i6.11

ISBN 978-089189-6616

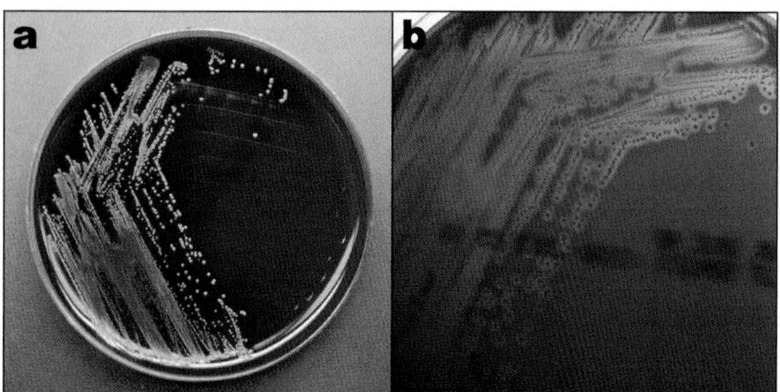

i6.12 Group B streptococci: colony morphology

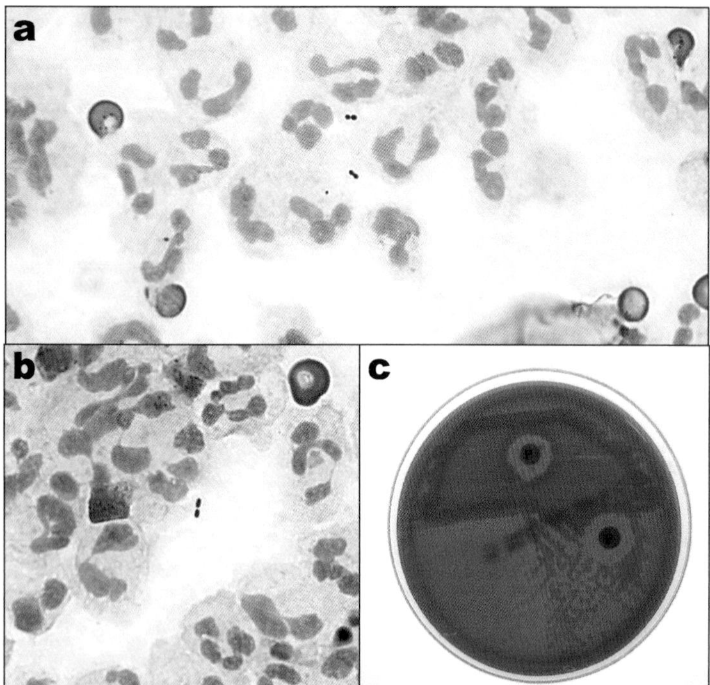

i6.13 *Streptococcus pneumoniae*: a & b Gram stain morphology; c colony morphology & characteristic optochin (P disk) susceptibility

- In culture, forms gray white colonies i6.12a, β-hemolytic with a narrow zone of hemolysis i6.12b
- Positive to both the CAMP (Christie-Atkins-Munch-Peterson) test and hippurate hydrolysis, and express Lancefield group B antigens

6.1.6.1.2.2 α hemolytic, catalase negative, gram-positive cocci

- *Streptococcus pneumoniae*
  - Leading cause of community-acquired pneumonia; may also lead to bacteremia & meningitis; may cause otitis media & sinusitis
  - Lancet shaped, gram-positive diplococci i6.13a, b
  - Bile solubility positive and susceptible to optochin (P disk) i6.13c
  - Strains causing invasive disease have polysaccharide capsule that are mucoid, wet, dome-shaped

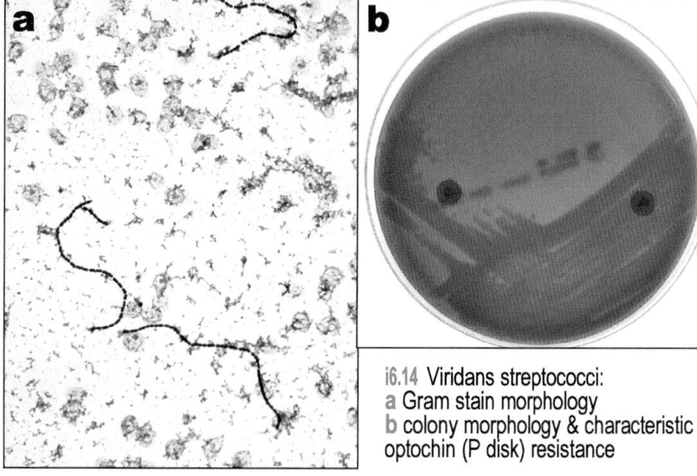

i6.14 Viridans streptococci:
a Gram stain morphology
b colony morphology & characteristic optochin (P disk) resistance

  - Older colonies can autolyse and organisms will die. Colonies have characteristic depressed center
- Viridans streptococci: >30 species
  - Causes subacute bacterial endocarditis, gingivitis, dental carries
  - Long chains of gram-positive cocci i6.14a
  - Optochin resistant i6.14b
  - Colonize the oral cavity; sometimes gastrointestinal (GI) tract or female genital tract
  - Classified into 4 groups: *S mitis* group, *S mutans* group, *S salivarius* group, *S anginosus* group
    - *S mitis* group frequent cause of native valve endocarditis & late-onset prosthetic valve endocarditis
    - *S mutans* group the principal agent of dental caries and can cause endocarditis
    - *S salivarius* group an occasional cause of bacteremia & endocarditis
    - *S anginosus* group cause abscesses at various sites

6.1.6.1.2.3 Nonhemolytic, catalase-negative, gram-positive cocci

- *Enterococcus* spp
  - Normal inhabitants of the lower gastrointestinal tract; cause urinary tract infection (usually nosocomial and related to indwelling catheters), bacteremia, endocarditis, and intraabdominal & pelvic infections
  - Diplococci & short chains i6.15a
  - Small, gray, nonhemolytic colonies on blood agar (can also be α-hemolytic & some can be β-hemolytic) i6.15b
  - Hydrolyze esculin in the presence of bile i6.15c, hydrolyze PYR, and grow in the presence of 6.5% sodium chloride
  - Express Lancefield group D antigens

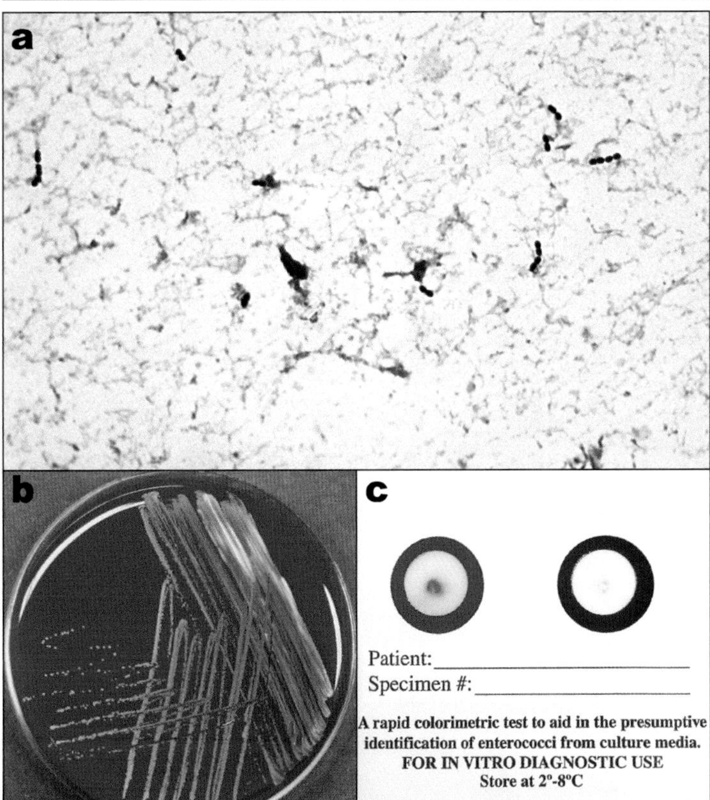

i6.15 Enterococci:
a Gram stain morphology
b colony morphology

- Enterococcus faecalis & Enterococcus faecium account for most clinical isolates
- Resistant to cephalosporins (with a few exceptions), the antistaphylococcal penicillins (eg, methicillin), and the carboxypenicillins (eg, ticarcillin); low level resistance to penicillin & aminoglycosides
- *E faecium* express altered penicillin-binding proteins with little affinity for penicillins, and are frankly resistant to penicillin, the aminopenicillins (eg, ampicillin) & the carbapenems
- Some *E faecium* strains demonstrate vancomycin resistance, in addition to penicillin resistance, conferred by acquisition of the *vanA*, *vanB*, or *vanD* gene clusters

- *Streptococcus bovis* group
  - Colonizes the GI tract, and causes bacteremia & endocarditis
  - Infection by certain subspecies within the *S bovis* group, especially *S gallolyticus* subspecies *gallolyticus*, is associated with colonic malignancy
  - Gram-positive cocci in pairs or short chains i6.16a
  - Gray white, nonhemolytic colonies on blood agar i6.16b
  - Express Lancefield group D antigens
  - Hydrolyze esculin in the presence of bile, PYR negative, cannot grow in 6.5% sodium chloride

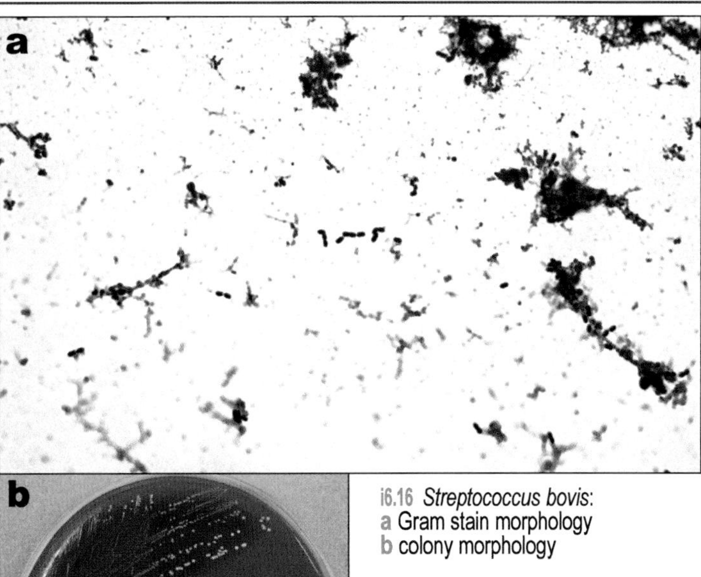

i6.16 *Streptococcus bovis*:
a Gram stain morphology
b colony morphology

6.1.6.1.2.4 *Streptococcus*-like organisms t6.10

- *Abiotrophia* & *Granulicatella*—Nutritionally variant streptococci associated with endocarditis
- *Aerococcus*—Gram stain like staphylococci; grow in 6.5% sodium chloride; resemble viridans streptococci in culture
- *Streptococcus anginosis* group—can cause deep tissue abscesses, bacteremia, endocarditis
- *Pediococcus*—Mimics viridans streptococci and enterococci; hydrolyzes bile esculin, PYR-negative
- *Gamella*—α & nonhemolytic colonies; causes endocarditis & wound infections
- *Leuconostoc*—Resistant to vancomycin; opportunistic pathogen
- *Lactococcus*—α & nonhemolytic colonies

t6.10 Comparison of *Enterococcus*, group D *Streptococcus* & related organisms

	Vanc resistance	Bile esculin	6.5% NaCl	PYR	LAP
Enterococcus	∓	+	+	+	+
Other group D, nonenterococci (*S bovis*)		+	–	–	+
Leuconostoc	+	±	±	–	–
Pediococcus	+	+	±	–	+

LAP, leucine amino peptidase test

ISBN 978-089189-6616

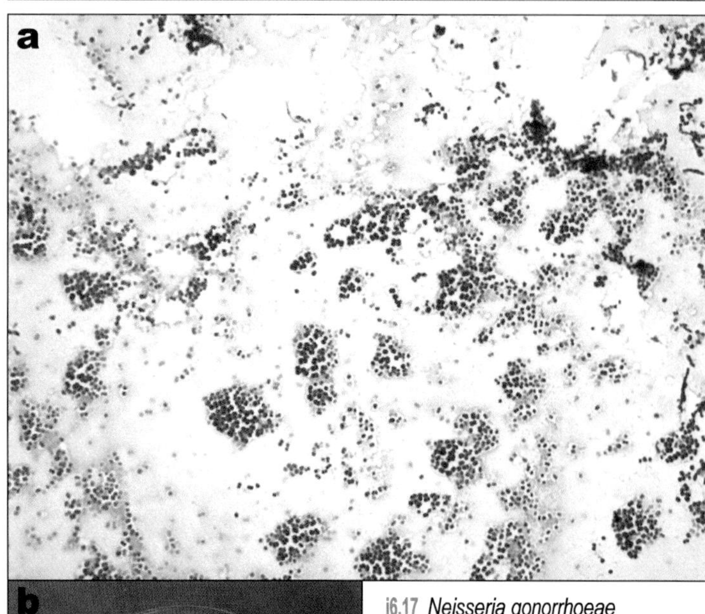

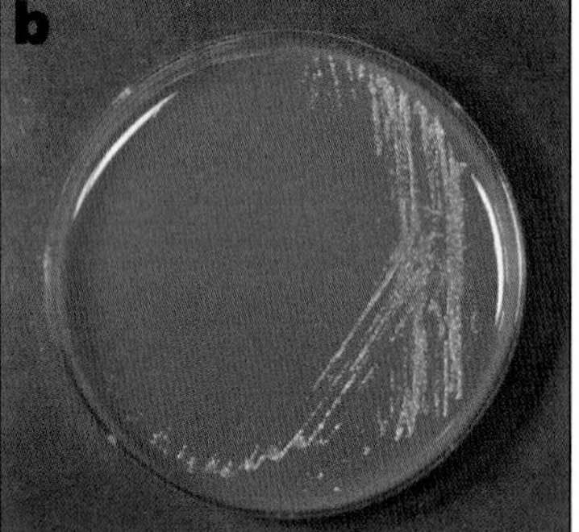

i6.17 *Neisseria gonorrhoeae*
a Gram stain morphology
b colony morphology on chocolate agar

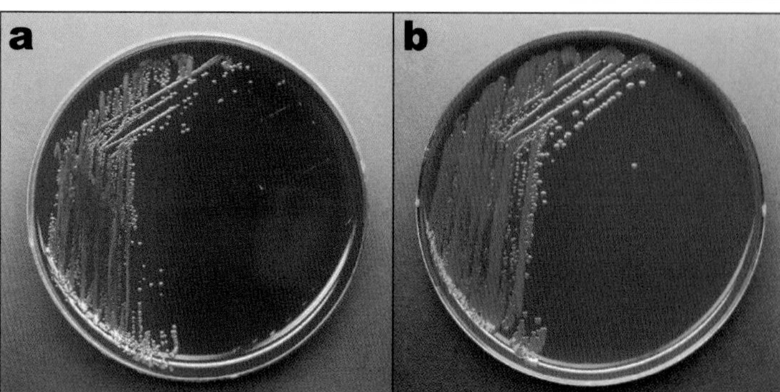

i6.18 *Neisseria meningitidis*: colony morphology on blood agar colony morphology on chocolate agar

6.1.6.2 Gram-negative cocci

- *Neisseria* & *Moraxella* spp
  - *Neisseria* is fastidious and both require incubation in a 3%-5% carbon dioxide environment
  - Oxidase positive **t6.11**
    - They possess the enzyme that oxidizes tetramethyl-phenylenediamine

t6.11 Identification of *Neisseria* spp/*Moraxella catarrhalis* using carbohydrate assimilation

Organism	Glucose	Maltose	Lactose	Sucrose
N gonorrhoeae	+	–	–	–
N meningitidis	+	+	–	–
N lactamica	+	+	+	–
M catarrhalis	–	–	–	–

  - *Neisseria gonorrhoeae*
    - Causes gonorrhea, ophthalmea neonatorum, pelvic inflammatory disease (PID), disseminated gonoccocal infection
    - Culture medium is chocolate agar with antibiotics to inhibit indigenous flora (Thayer-Martin agar, Martin-Lewis, or New York City agar)
    - Clues to identification include classic Gram stain morphology (gram-negative cocci, kidney bean shape) i6.17a, and growth on chocolate agar, no growth on sheep blood agar (SBA) i6.17b
    - Identified using chromogenic enzyme tests, carbohydrate assimilations, the matrix-assisted laser desorption/ionization time-of-flight mass (MALDI-TOF) spectrometry, and direct detection with nucleic acid amplification tests
    - Symptomatic men: Urethral discharge; possible ascending infection causing acute epididymitis; Gram stain showing characteristic gram-negative diplococci provides diagnosis
    - Symptomatic women: Vaginal discharge, pruritis and/or urethritis; possible ascending infection leading to pelvic inflammatory disease (PID); Gram stain is not recommended because normal flora resemble the gonococcus
    - Resistant to penicillins and increasing resistance to ciprofloxacin (a fluoroquinolone); ceftriaxone (a third-generation cephalosporin) is recommended for treatment
  - *Neisseria meningitidis*
    - Agent of meningitis & septicemia
    - Grows on both chocolate & sheep blood agars i6.18a, i6.18b
    - Identified using chromogenic enzyme tests, carbohydrate assimilations, MALDI-TOF mass spectrometry
    - *Neisseria lactamica* mimics *N meningitidis* and lactose assimilation can be delayed. A rapid α-nitrophenyl-β-D-galactopyranoside (ONPG) test will detect lactose in 30 minutes
    - Multiple serogroups defined by capsular polysaccharide antigens; serogroups B, C & Y cause most cases in the United States; serogroup B is not represented in the tetravalent vaccines available but now 2 serogroup B vaccines approved by the Food and Drug Administration (FDA) are now available

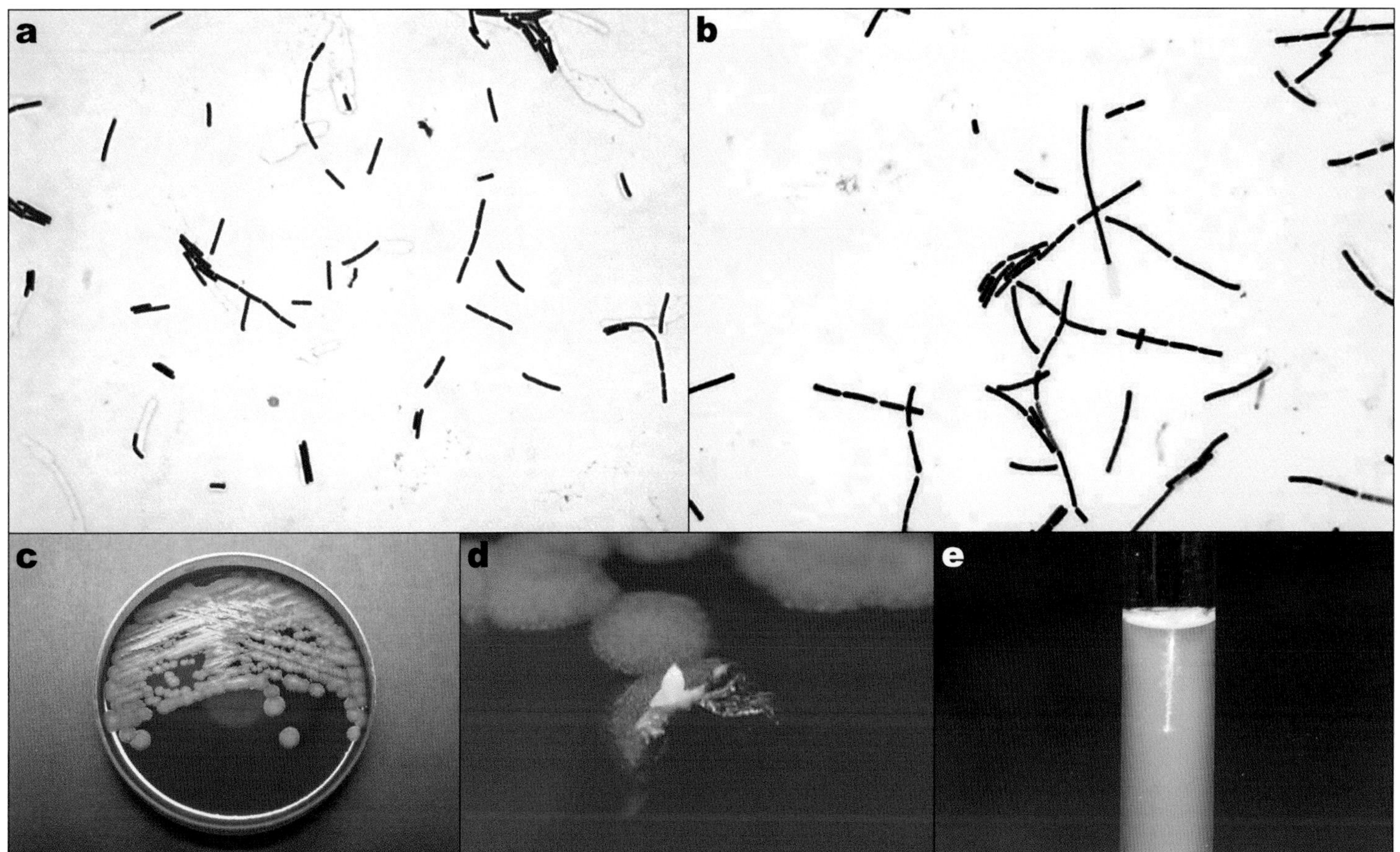

i6.19 *Bacillus* spp: a Gram stain morphology
Bacillus anthracis: b Gram stain morphology; c colony morphology; note ground glass colonies with irregular borders & d tenaciousness; *Bacillus anthracis*: the stab mark is clearly visible & the medium is nonturbid, indicative of nonmotility

- Nasopharyngeal carriage common
- Invasive infection most often takes the form of bacterial meningitis

- Manipulation of suspected sterile body site isolates should be done under biosafety level 2 cabinet to decrease aerosols

- *Moraxella catarrhalis*
  - Common colonizer of the upper respiratory tract and frequent cause of otitis media in children, chronic obstructive pulmonary disease (COPD) exacerbation in older adults
  - Gram stain morphology similar to *Neisseria* spp; can be coccobacillary
  - Grows well on blood agar & chocolate agar; not fastidious; colonies called "hockey puck" because they can be pushed around media and remain intact
  - Oxidase-positive; β-lactamase-positive; butyrate esterase-positive, carbohydrate assimilations (rarely done) **t6.11**

6.1.6.3 Gram-positive bacilli

- Aerobic gram-positive bacilli
  - Spore formation indicates *Bacillus* spp; large rectangular gram-positive rods i6.19a, most of which are motile and catalase positive
  - *Bacillus anthracis*
    - BSL-3 pathogen
    - Forms chains i6.19b & subterminal spores
    - Cutaneous anthrax the most common and least fatal form; acquired by inoculation of spores into a skin wound while handling animals or hides
    - GI anthrax causes ulcerative lesions
    - Inhalational anthrax is typically associated with the processing of contaminated animal hides ("woolsorter disease") but is also the form most commonly caused by the intentional release of purified spores as a terrorist act
    - Presumptive identification
    - Large, nonhemolytic colonies with irregular borders (Medusa head colonies i6.19c) that are tenacious and stand up when teased with a loop i6.19d

ISBN 978-089189-6616

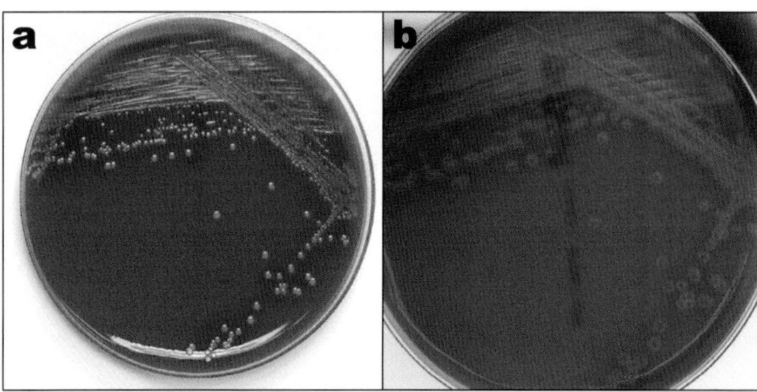

i6.20 *Listeria monocytogenes*: a colony morphology, b reverse

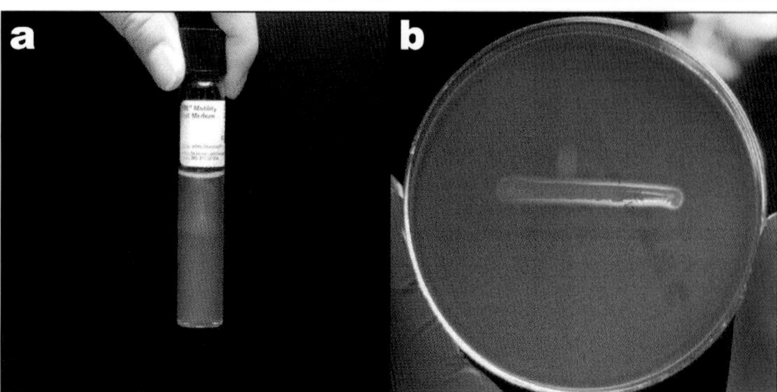

i6.21 *Listeria monocytogenes*:
a umbrella shaped motility
b CAMP test with rectangular zone of hemolysis

- Large, boxcarlike, gram-positive bacilli; oval central to subterminal spores may be present
- Aerobic growth, catalase positive & nonmotile; best demonstrated using semisolid agar (rather than a wet preparation) for safety reasons i6.19e
- Confirmatory identification performed by Laboratory Response Network (LRN)

□ *B cereus*

- Forms chains & demonstrates subterminal spores
- Colonies are large, β-hemolytic & nontenacious, and the organism is motile
- Many foods associated with *B cereus* foodborne illness (Asian rice dishes common cause); common feature is improper storage (lack of refrigeration) after cooking

■ Nonspore formers

□ *Listeria monocytogenes*

- Small colonies in primary culture after 1-2 days i6.20a; β-hemolytic with narrow zone of hemolysis resembling group B streptococci i6.20b
- Gram stain reveals short, nonbranching, gram-positive rods, singly or in short chains
- Catalase positive and demonstrate temperature-dependent tumbling motility in wet mounts (best seen at room temperature; not well demonstrated at 37°C)
- Semisolid agar motility test reveals umbrella shaped motility i6.21a
- Hydrolyzes esculin; CAMP test demonstrates a rectangular zone of enhanced hemolysis i6.21b
- Can grow at 4°C; may contaminate refrigerated foods
- In pregnant women, can seed the placenta causing chorioamnionitis

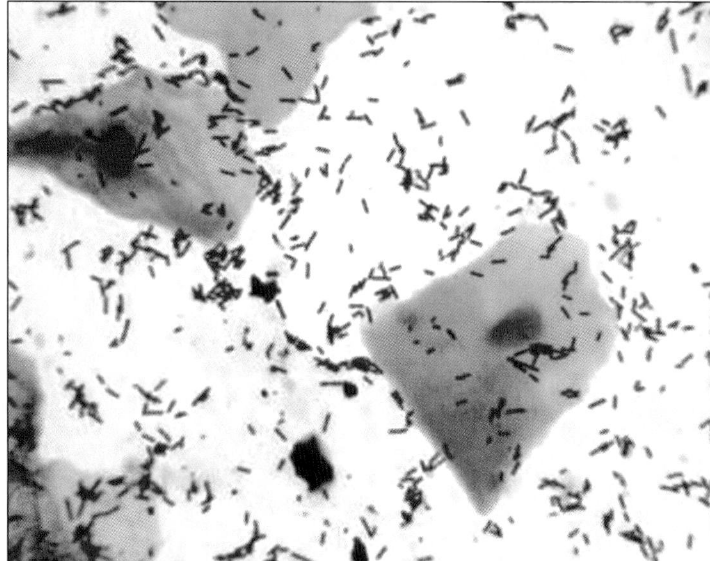

i6.22 *Gardnerella vaginalis*: Gram stain morphology

- Infects neonates who may have granulomatosis infantiseptica
- Other at-risk hosts include patients with compromised cell-mediated immunity, and the elderly, in whom *Listeria* causes bacteremia, meningitis, and/or encephalitis

□ Lactobacilli

- Normal flora in mouth, GI tract, female genital tract (where it protects host from urogenital infections); may grow better anaerobically; often α-hemolytic

□ *Gardnerella vaginalis*

- One of the suspected agents that causes bacterial vaginosis
- Associated with "clue cells" and noticeable lack of lactobacilli
- Short pleomorphic rods that stain gram-variable or gram-negative i6.22

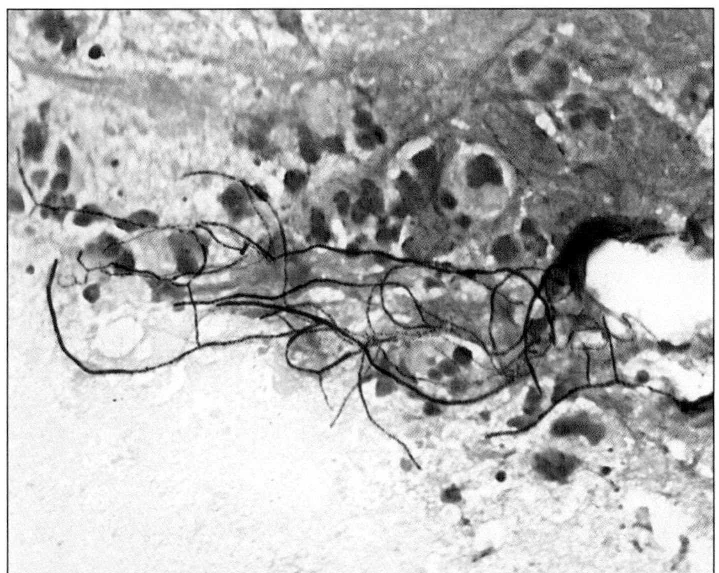

i6.23 *Nocardia*: Gram stain morphology

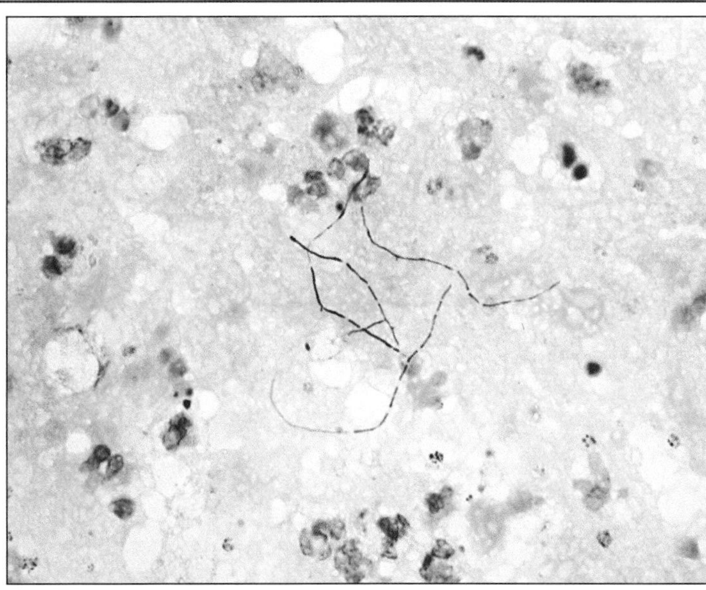

i6.24 *Nocardia*: acid-fast stain

- Direct specimen detection via molecular methods
- Culture rarely performed; grows on V agar, that contains human blood, and are β-hemolytic
- SPS resistant

□ *Erysipelothrix rhusiopathiae*

- Causes erysipeloid, a cellulitis acquired when a wound comes in contact with animal carrying the organism; occupational hazard among anglers, butchers, farmers
- Nonbranching, nonspore forming gram-positive rod
- May be short (coccobacillary) and occur singly and in short chains, or can be long, thin & filamentous
- Nonmotile & catalase-negative; produces H_2S on triple sugar iron (TSI) slants, causing a blackened butt (distinguishes it from *Listeria* & *Lactobacillus*)
- Intrinsically resistant to vancomycin

□ *Nocardia*

- May cause indolent soft tissue infection (mycetoma), forming macroscopic granules similar to the sulfur granules of actinomycosis
- May cause invasive pulmonary infection and disseminated infection, often involving the central nervous system
- Long, thin, filamentous, branching, beaded gram-positive rods i6.23
- Modified acid-fast positive i6.24
- BCYE agar is ideal for primary culture
- Produce chalky, white colonies; become salmon orange pink when mature; "musty basement" odor No hydrolysis of casein, tyrosine, xanthine

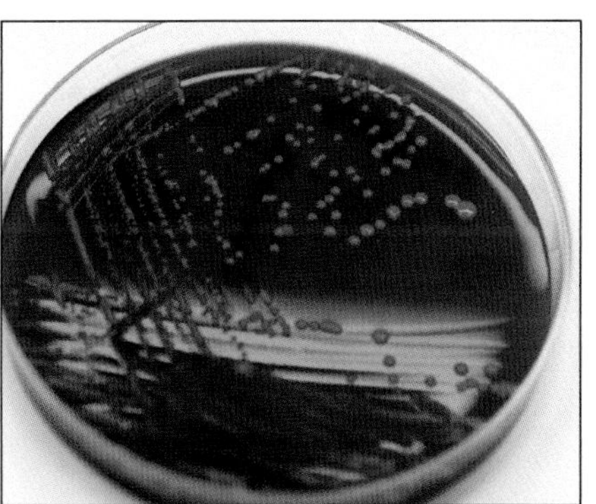

i6.25 *Rhodococcus equi*: colony morphology

□ *Arcanobacterium hemolyticum*

- Causes pharyngitis in older children
- β-hemolytic
- Catalase-negative, nonmotile
- Reverse CAMP (Christie, Atkins, Munch-Petersen): This organism inhibits hemolysis around *S aureus* streak so shows inverted triangle of no hemolysis

□ *Rhodococcus equi*

- Gram-positive cocci, coccobacilli, or coryneform rods
- Often found within histiocytes
- Modified acid-fast positive (like *Nocardia*)
- Colonies are typically salmon colored & slimy i6.25
- Affects immunocompromised patients, most commonly causing pulmonary & bloodstream infections that may go to other locations, eg, lymph nodes, skin

ISBN 978-089189-6616

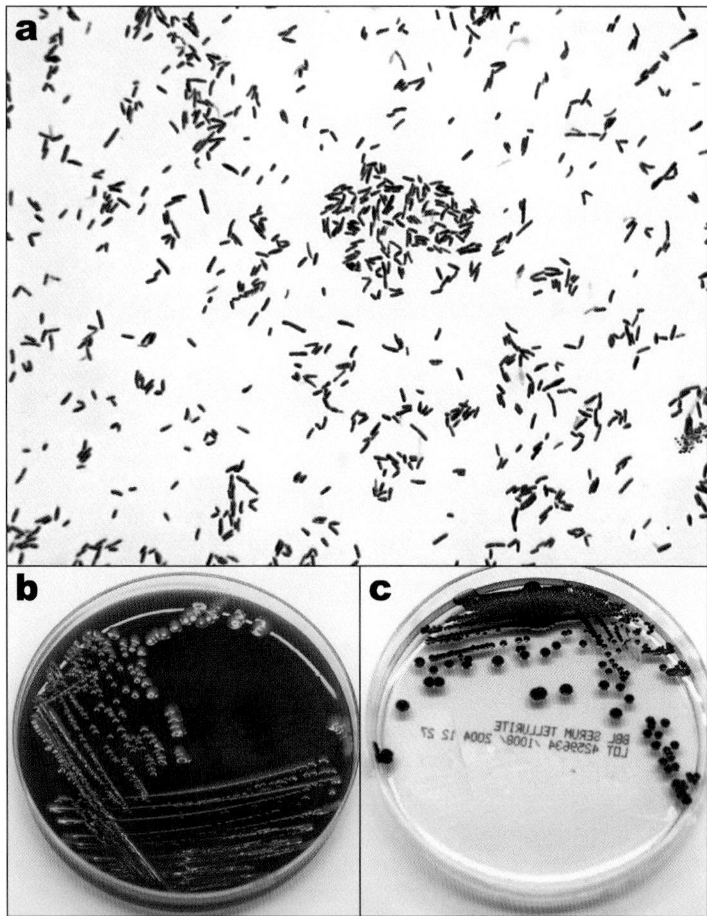

i6.26 *Corynebacterium diphtheriae:*
a Gram stain morphology
b colony morphology
c on agar containing tellurite

- *Corynebacterium diphtheria*
  - Causes diphtheria—fever, sore throat, and development of a white to gray glossy pseudomembrane covering the tonsils and other structures in the oro- & nasopharynx
  - Coryneform or diphtheroid pleomorphic, club shaped, gram-positive rods that tend to palisade & cluster together (best seen from growth on Loeffler medium) i6.26a
  - Grows well on sheep blood agar i6.26b but isolation is improved by using selective media, such as Tinsdale agar
  - Has garlic odor
  - Presumptive identification involves demonstration of the ability to reduce potassium tellurite to metallic tellurite i6.26c
  - Appearance of brown-black colonies surrounded by brown-black halos on Tinsdale agar or cysteine-tellurite blood agar (CTBA). (*Corynebacterium ulcerans* & *Corynebacterium pseudotuberculosis* also form brown halo on CTBA but are urease-positive) is presumptive evidence for *Corynebacterium diphtheria*
  - Diagnosis is made by showing toxin production by immunodiffusion on ELEK plate, enzyme-linked immunosorbent assay (ELISA), or polymerase chain reaction (PCR)
- *Corynebacterium jeikeium*
  - Normal skin flora
  - Causes infections related to catheter lines, prosthetic devices & endocarditis
  - Multidrug resistant
- *Corynebacterium urealyticum*
  - Associated with urinary tract infections (UTIs)
  - Colonies are urease-positive within minutes of inoculating urea slant
  - Multidrug resistant
- Nonpathogenic *Corynebacterium* spp
  - Referred to as "diptheroids"
  - Coryneform or diphtheroid pleomorphic, club-shaped, gram-positive bacilli
  - Frequent isolate and usually considered a commensal or normal flora
- *Tropheryma whipplei*
  - Causative agent of Whipple disease
  - Ubiquitous in the environment; nevertheless, disease develops only in individuals with selective immune deficiency
  - Most affected individuals are older men, with male-to-female ratio of 8-10:1
  - In affected tissues, aggregates of foamy histiocytes are seen; bacillary organisms can be highlighted on periodic acid–Schiff (PAS) stain; they are negative for acid-fast bacilli
  - Cultures not routinely performed
  - Diagnose using microscopic examination of biopsy or molecular methods

6.1.6.4 Gram-negative bacilli

- Includes *Enterobacteriaceae*, oxidase-positive fermenters, nonfermenters, fastidious, miscellaneous

6.1.6.4.1 *Enterobacteriaceae*

- Characterized by aerobic growth on MacConkey, glucose fermentation, oxidase negative, reduce nitrate to nitrite (rare species are oxidase-positive and do not reduce nitrate to nitrite)
- Many are natural inhabitants of the colon
- Nasopharyngeal carriage may occur in hospitalized patients, patients with uncontrolled diabetes mellitus & chronic alcoholics
- Commonly isolated from urine, blood, wounds, abscesses & respiratory tract
- *Salmonella*, *Shigella* spp, Shiga toxin producing *E coli* (STEC) & *Yersinia enterocolitica* are GI pathogens
- Lipid A, a component of LPS, is also called endotoxin
- O or somatic antigen (cell wall) forms the basis for serogrouping
- Antimicrobial resistance common
- *Enterobacteriaceae* includes a large group of organisms **t6.12**
- Hallmark characteristics are reviewed in **t6.13**
- Kligler iron agar & triple sugar iron (KIA/TSI) slants
  - Agar slants that contain proteins, sugars (lactose and glucose, and sucrose (TSI), phenol red indicator, ferrous sulfate and sodium thiosulfate (to detect H_2S)
  - 10:1 ratio of lactose-glucose for KIA, or 10:1 lactose-sucrose & glucose for TSI. Lactose concentration in KIA and lactose and sucrose concentrations in TSI are 10-fold that of glucose (1% vs 0.1%)
  - Phenol red indicator is yellow when the pH is <6.8 and red when >6.8
  - Fermentation evidenced by lowering the pH (yellowing of the indicator)
  - The tubes are interpreted at 18-24 hours **t6.14**

t6.12 Taxonomy of the *Enterobacteriaceae*

Family (tribe)	Genus & species
Escherichieae	*Escherichia: E coli; Shigella: S sonnei, S flexneri, S dysenteriae, S boydii*
Edwardsiellae	*Edwardsiella tarda*
Salmonellae	*Salmonella: S enteritidis, S typhi, S paratyphi, S choleraesuis*
Citrobactereae	*Citrobacter freundii*
Klebsiellae	*Klebsiella: K pneumoniae; K oxytoca; Enterobacter: E aerogenes, E cloacae; Hafnia: H alvei; Pantoea: P agglomerans; Serratia: S marcescens*
Proteae	*Proteus: P vulgaris, P mirabilis; Morganella: M morganii; Providencia: P stuartii*
Yersinieae	*Yersinia enterocolitica*

t6.13 *Enterobacteriaceae*: key characteristics

Reduce nitrate to nitrite	All *Enterobacteriaceae*
Strong lactose fermenters (pink on MacConkey)	*E coli, Klebsiella, Enterobacter*
Hydrogen sulfide (H_2S) positive	*Salmonella, Edwardsiella tarda, Citrobacter freundii, Proteus mirabilis & P vulgaris*
Strongly urease-positive	*Proteus, Morganella, Providencia rettgeri*
Nonmotile	*Shigella, Klebsiella* *Yersinia* grow better at room temperature
Voges-Proskauer (VP) positive	*Klebsiella, Enterobacter, Hafnia, Serratia, Pantoea*
Phenylalanine deaminase (PAD) positive	*Proteus, Morganella, Providencia*
Kligler iron agar & triple sugar iron (KIA/TSI) slants	See **t6.14**

t6.14 KIA slant characteristics

Slant	Butt	Interpretation	Possible organisms	Image
alk/red	alk/red	no fermentation *Enterobacteriaceae* excluded because they all ferment glucose	*Pseudomonas* *Eikenella* *Moraxella* *Campylobacter*	
alk/red	acid/yellow	glucose fermented lactose not fermented	*Shigella* *Serratia* *Providencia* *Yersinia*	
alk/red	Acid/Yellow with H_2S (black)	glucose fermented lactose not fermented H_2S produced	*Salmonella* *Proteus*	
acid/yellow	acid/yellow	lactose fermented	*Escherichia coli*	
acid/yellow	acid/yellow with gas	lactose fermented gas produced	*Klebsiella* *Enterobacter*	

ISBN 978-089189-6616

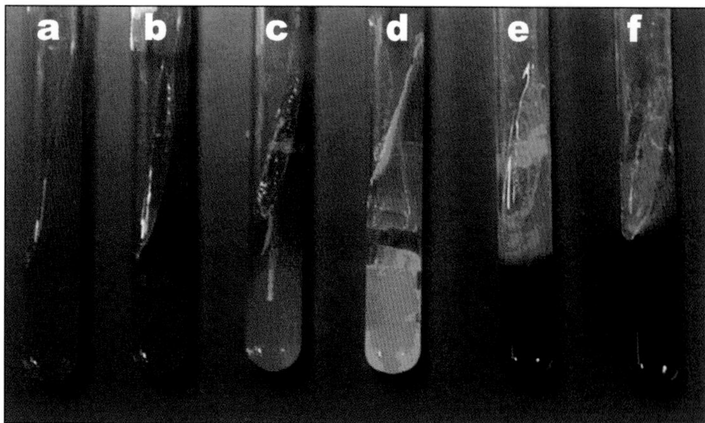

i6.27 Hydrogen sulfide indicator in slants:
a control
b red slant, red butt = no gas, no H_2S
c red slant, yellow butt = no gas, no H_2S
d yellow slant, yellow butt = gas, no H_2S
e yellow slant, yellow butt = no gas, H_2S
f red slant, yellow butt = no gas, H_2S

- Initially, a bacterium that ferments glucose but not lactose will produce an acidic (yellow) slant and acidic (yellow) butt. After the limited quantity of glucose is consumed, the organism will begin oxidative metabolism of proteins, which can only take place in the oxygen-rich environment of the slant; this will turn the slant back to alkaline (red) by 24 hours, while the butt will remain yellow
- Organisms that ferment lactose, which is present in the agar at much higher concentration, will continue to ferment throughout the incubation period, maintaining a yellow slant and butt even after 24 hours
- An H_2S indicator is also present in these slants; H_2S production will result in a black color i6.27

- *Escherichia coli*
  - Normal flora of colon; #1 cause of UTI in the United States, sepsis, meningitis in neonates, diarrhea
  - Lactose fermenting, indole positive, and negative for citrate, urease, Voges-Proskauer (VP), phenylalanine deaminase, and H_2S production
  - Abbreviated ID of specimens other than blood & GI: gnr, oxidase-negative, LF, nonswarming & β-hemolytic on sheep blood agar (SBA); spot indole-positive
  - On eosin-methylene blue (EMB) agar, it produces green, metallic sheen
  - *E coli* can produce ESBL
  - Certain strains are diarrheagenic
    - EHEC (enterohemorrhagic *E coli*) or STEC (Shiga toxin producing *E coli*): Capable of producing Shiga toxin; associated with hemolytic uremic syndrome (HUS), especially serotype O157:H7 (0157:H7 does not ferment sorbitol in sorbitol MacConkey plates)
    - ETEC (enterotoxigenic *E coli*) causes waterborne secretory (watery) diarrhea; main cause of "traveler's diarrhea"; produces choleralike toxins
    - EIEC (enteroinvasive *E coli*) causes dysentery similar to that caused by *Shigella*; produces a Shigalike toxin (T3SS); like *Shigella*, most strains are nonmotile and lactose nonfermenting; Rare in the United States
    - EPEC (enteropathogenic *E coli*) causes dysentery similar to that caused by *Shigella;* does not produce a Shigalike toxin; person-to-person spread
    - EAggEC (enteroaggregative *E coli*) causes infant diarrhea in underdeveloped countries, and chronic refractory diarrhea in human immunodeficiency virus (HIV)–infected patients
- *Klebsiella pneumoniae*
  - Lower respiratory infections, particularly pneumonia; necrotizing and productive brick-red sputum or thin "current jellylike" sputum; UTIs, wound infections, bacteremia
  - Intrinsically resistant to ampicillin & carbenicillin; can produce ESBL
  - Lactose fermenter; colonies show large polysaccharide capsules that are wet & moist
  - Nonmotile, indole negative, citrate-positive, Voges-Proskauer-positive (VP+), ornithine decarboxylase-negative, lysine-positive
  - *Klebsiella oxytoca* infection similar to *K pneumoniae*. It is indole-positive
- *Klebsiella pneumoniae* subspecies
  - Subspecies *K rhinosleromatis*: Chronic disease of nose, oropharynx
  - Subspecies *K ozanae*: Infection of nasal mucous membranes
  - VP-negative, urea-negative
- *Enterobacter cloacae* & *E aerogenes* (now *K aerogenes*)
  - Cause UTIs, wound infections, and blood & CSF infections
  - Frequently resistant to many β-lactam antibiotics including 1st generation cephalosporins
  - *K aerogenes*: Lactose fermenters on Mac, motile, citrate-positive, Voges-Proskauer-positive (VP+), ornithine decarboxylase-positive
  - *E cloacae*: Same as *K aerogenes* except lysine decarboxylase-negative

- *Serratia marcescens*
  - Opportunist pathogen usually seen in health care facilities; causes UTI & respiratory infections
  - Colony has pink/red pigment, but it is a nonlactose fermenter (NLF) on MacConkey agar
  - Produces intracellular DNAse
  - Ferments lactose slowly and is O-nitrophenyl-beta-D-galactopyranoside-positive (ONPG+)
- *Proteus vulgaris* & *Proteus mirabilis*
  - Cause UTIs, wound & ear infections, bacteremia
  - Produces "swarming" colonies on sheep blood agar (SBA)
  - Nonlactose fermenter(NLF) on MacConkey agar
  - Deaminates phenylalanine, urease-positive, produces H_2S
  - Indole: *P mirabilis*-negative; *P vulgaris*-positive
  - Ornithine: *P mirabilis*-positive; *P vulgaris*-negative
  - *P mirabilis* abbreviated ID: swarming on sheep blood agar (SBA), spot indole-negative, ampicillin susceptible
  - *P mirabilis* urease activity is associated with struvite kidney stones
- *Morganella morganii*
  - Causes UTIs, wound infections, diarrhea
  - Nonlactose fermenter (NLF) on MacConkey agar
  - Motile, no swarming, H_2S-negative, ornithine decarboxylase-positive, phenylalanine deaminase-positive, urea-positive
- *Providencia*
  - UTIs
  - Nonlactose fermenter on MacConkey agar
  - H_2S-negative, ornithine decarboxylase-negative, phenyalanine deamination-positive, urea-positive or -negative
- *Citrobacter*
  - Mostly nosocomial infections; UTIs, pneumonia, endocarditis
  - Lactose fermentation-positive or -negative
  - H_2S-positive, urea-positive, lysine decarboxylase-negative (*Salmonella* is urea-negative, lysine decarboxylase-positive)
- *Edwardsiella*
  - Opportunistic and causes bloodstream & wound infections; organism is often of aquatic origin
  - Nonlactose fermenter (NLF) on MacConkey agar
  - H_2S-positive, urea-negative, indole-positive, citrate-negative, lysine decarboxylase-positive
- *Salmonella*
  - Causes gastroenteritis & typhoid fever; some species/serotypes may produce bacteremia: *S cholerasuis*, *S paratyphi* & *S typhi*
  - Source is from eating contaminated foods (poultry, eggs, dairy products)
  - Children with sickle cell disease are prone to *Salmonella* osteomyelitis
  - More than 2500 serotypes in single species, *S enterica*. Common serotypes now written with serotype name capitalized but not italicized (eg, *Salmonella* Typhi)
  - Typhoid fever (enteric fever)
    - *Salmonella enterica* serotype Typhi (major cause)
    - Serotype Paratyphi and Cholerasuis cause paratyphoid fevers that are less severe
    - Bacteria traverse the bowel wall and entrench themselves within reticuloendothelial cells of the liver, spleen & gallbladder
    - Gallbladder a reservoir continually reinfecting the bowel, leading to long-term shedding
  - Nonlactose fermenting (NLF), H_2S-positive (paratyphi-negative), indole-negative, citrate-positive, Voges-Proskauer (VP)–negative, urea-negative, phenylalanine deaminase-negative
  - *Salmonella*: Test with polyvalent A through G, Vi and individual antisera for serogroups A, B, C1, C2, D, E, G
    - If agglutination occurs in Vi only, suspension must be boiled for 10 minutes to inactivate capsular Vi antigen, which can mask the O antigens
    - Then the suspension is retested with A-G antisera
- *Shigella*
  - Humans are the only reservoir; shigellosis is abdominal cramps, diarrhea, fever
  - In the United States, shigellosis most commonly caused by *S sonnei*; in underdeveloped countries, *S flexneri*
  - Requires smallest inoculum of any form of bacterial gastroenteritis—only ~100-200 bacteria
  - *S dysenteriae* produces a Shiga toxin
  - *S flexneri* can lead to postinfectious arthritis in HLA-B27-positive patients
  - Nonlactose fermenting (NLF) on MacConkey agar, H_2S-negative, nonmotile, lysine decarboxylase-negative
  - *S dysenteriae* (serogroup A); *S flexneri* (serogroup B); *S boydii* (serogroup C); *S sonnei* (serogroup D). Remember serogroups by this: "*D*irty *f*ingers *b*ring *s*higella!" Some *Shigella* produce K or capsular antigen that mask the O or cell wall antigens; boiling will remove capsule

- *Yersinia*
  - *Y pestis* causes plague; *Y pseudotuberculosis* produces necrotizing granulomata resembling tuberculosis; *Y enterocolitica* causes enteritis, appendicitis-like illness (most common isolate)
  - Zoonotic; humans are accidental hosts
  - *Yersinia pestis*
    - Biosafety level 3 pathogen
    - Isolate from respiratory specimens, blood & aspirate of bubo
    - LRN protocols for suspicious *Y pestis*: Bipolar staining gram-negative rod; non-spore-forming; very small colonies after 24-hour growth at 37°C on sheep blood agar (SBA); larger colonies if incubated at room temperature; nonlactose fermenting (NLF)
    - Isolate with aforementioned characteristics should be referred immediately to LRN
- *Yersinia enterocolitica*
  - Most common species of *Yersinia* that is isolated; mimics acute appendicitis
  - Isolation at room temperature on selective media (CIN agar)
  - Urease-positive; ornithine decarboxylase-positive; sucrose fermentation
- *Yersinia pseudotuberculosis*
  - Causes disease mostly in animals, with rare human infection involving the mesenteric lymph nodes
  - Urease-positive; ornithine decarboxylase-negative; does not ferment sucrose

6.1.6.4.2 Nonenteric glucose fermenters

- Growth on MacConkey, oxidase-positive
- *Vibrio cholera*
  - Agent for cholera—diffuse diarrhea, "rice-water" stools
  - Cholera organisms are broadly characterized as *V cholerae* O1 & 0139
  - Sucrose positive on selective TCBS agar (yellow colonies); oxidase-positive; string test-positive; 0129 susceptible
  - Does not require sodium chloride for growth
- *V parahemolyticus*
  - Seafood usually source
  - Causes gastroenteritis
  - Requires sodium chloride for growth
  - Sucrose negative on TCBS (green colonies); oxidase-positive; string test-positive; 0129 resistant
- *V vulnificus*
  - Found in coastal waters & estuaries; causes septicemia & wound infections; associated with eating raw oysters; persons with liver problems are more susceptible to organism
  - The gastroenteritis of *V vulnificus* features both vomiting & diarrhea
  - Skin infection may follow trauma, or it may be caused by exposure of already open skin to infected water
  - Requires salt (strict halophile)
  - Sucrose negative on TCBS; oxidase-positive; 0129 susceptible; lactose fermenting (LF) on MacConkey agar; salicin-positive
- *Aeromonas*
  - Found in fresh & brackish water; may be found in hospital or household water (fish tanks)
  - Cause diarrhea & wound infections; not all strains pathogenic; presence in stool culture does not necessarily indicate infection
  - Oxidase-positive; most are lactose fermenting (LF) on MacConkey agar; no growth on TCBS; resistant to O129; do not require sodium chloride; indole-positive
- *Plesiomonas* (now moved to *Enterobacteriaceae*)
  - In soil and estuarine waters in warmer climates
  - Causes gastroenteritis
  - No growth on TCBS; susceptible to 0129; oxidase-positive
- *Campylobacter jejuni*
  - Associated with undercooked beef (hamburgers), poultry; causes diarrhea
  - Tiny curved (seagull shaped) gram-negative rods; recommend using carbol fuchsin for counterstain
  - Growth on selective media (Campy BAP) at 42°C in 10% carbon dioxide (↑CO_2 & ↓O_2 [example: 5% O_2 + 85% N_2 + 10% CO_2]). *C fetus* grows at 37°C and not at 42°C
  - Darting motility
  - Oxidase positive, catalase positive, and positive for hippurate hydrolysis (key to distinguishing *C jejuni* from other *Campylobacter* spp)
  - ELISA testing for antibodies
- *Helicobacter pylori*
  - Causes peptic ulcer/gastric disease
  - Gram-negative, curved bacillus
  - Anti-*H pylori* IgG antibodies detectable after 4 weeks of infection; remains positive after successful treatment
  - Urea breath test used both to diagnose infection & confirm eradication

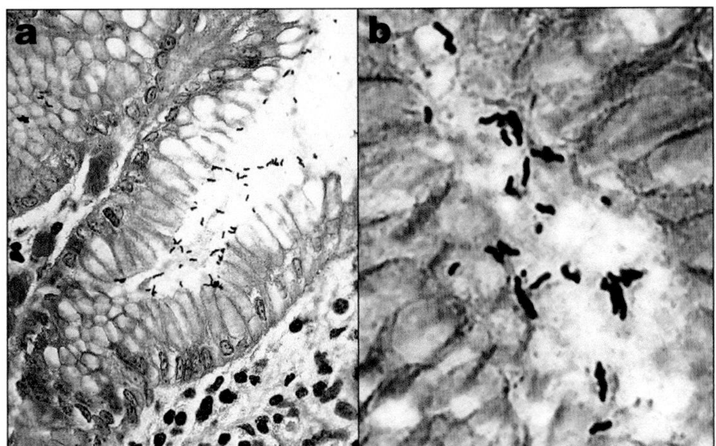

i6.28 *Helicobacter pylori* in Warthin-Starry-stained sections at a low & b high magnification

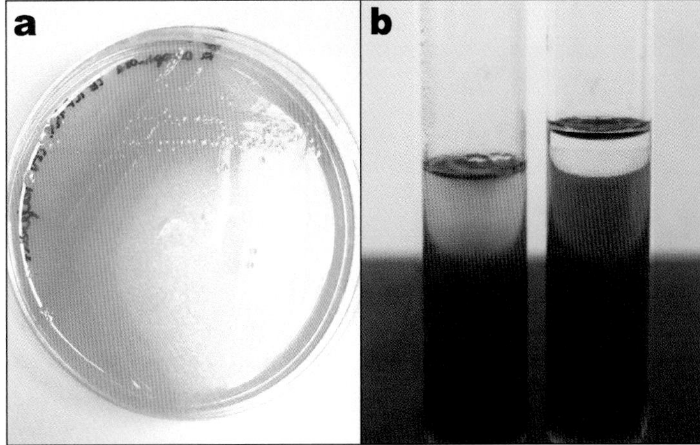

i6.29 *Pseudomonas aeruginosa*:
a pyocyanin pigment
b oxidation/fermentation tube with Hugh-Leifson medium

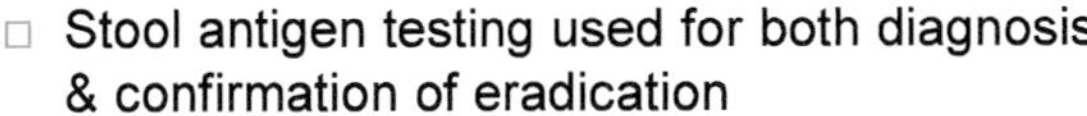

- Stool antigen testing used for both diagnosis & confirmation of eradication
- Histologic examination can be used for diagnosis & confirmation of eradication i6.28

6.1.6.4.3 Nonfermenters

- *Pseudomonas aeruginosa*
  - Associated with nosocomial infections, UTIs, wounds, bacteremia, burn infections, respiratory infections especially in patients with cystic fibrosis
  - Associated with water
  - Endocarditis is encountered in intravenous drug abusers
  - Oxidase positive, gram-negative bacillus that is motile by means of polar monotrichous flagella
  - Colonies often β-hemolytic and produce a grapelike or tortillalike odor; typically produce a water-soluble blue/green pigment (pyocyanin) i6.29a; also can produce yellow-green pigment (pyoverdin), or red (pyorubin) or brown (pyomelanin) pigments
  - Able to grow well at 42°C both in culture and in the environment
  - Cetrimide agar enhances pigment production
  - Glucose fermentation negative; glucose oxidation-positive
  - TSI agar detects fermentation of glucose, lactose, sucrose; is K/K on TSI, showing no fermentation
  - Oxidation/fermentation (O/F) tubes for detection of oxidation/fermentation use Hugh-Leifson medium that contains 1% glucose (or other carbohydrate) and pH indicator bromothymol blue i6.29b
  - Uninoculated media is green and turns yellow in acid environment and blue in alkaline environment
  - 2 tubes are inoculated; one is overlaid with mineral oil and is the anaerobic tube (detects fermentation) and the other has no oil overlay (detects oxidation)
    - If acid is produced in both tubes (yellow throughout tube), the organism is both a fermenter & an oxidizer
    - If acid is produced in anaerobic tube, it is a fermenter
    - If acid is produced in tube with no oil overlay, the organism is an oxidizer
    - If there is no color change in either tube, the organism is asaccharolytic
  - Abbreviated ID: oxidase-positive; recognizable colony morphology on sheep blood agar (SBA) (metallic or pearlescent, flat with rough edges or very mucoid; produce pigment), grape or tortillalike odor
- *Pseudomonas fluorescens*/*Pseudomonas putida*
  - Mostly environmental organisms found in soil, water
  - Do not produce pyocyanin but do produce pyoverdin
  - No growth at 42°C
  - Oxidase-positive
- *Stenotrophomonas maltophilia*
  - Nosocomial pathogen usually in respiratory tract and in immunocompromised patients
  - Oxidase-negative; no pigment production, rapid oxidation of maltose
  - Growth at 42°C; DNAse-positive
  - Inherently resistant to most of the commonly used antipseudomonal antibiotics
- *Acinetobacter* spp
  - Infections related to ventilators, humidifiers, catheters

ISBN 978-089189-6616

- Gram-negative coccobacilli or gram-negative cocci; can also appear as gram-positive cocci in blood culture bottles
- Oxidase-negative
- Growth on MacConkey agar may have purple color that looks like a lactose fermenter
- *A baumanii* resistant to many antibiotics, including fluoroquinolones & carbapenemases
- *A lwoffi* susceptible to most antibiotics

- *Burkholderia cepacia*
  - Seen in patients with cystic fibrosis (CF); resistant to aminoglycosides
  - Nonlactose fermenting (NLF) on MacConkey agar; weak, slow oxidase-positive; lysine decarboxylase-positive
  - *Burkholderia cepacia* selective agar (BCSA) selects for organism and a pink to yellow zone develops around each colony
  - No pigment production
- *Burholderia pseudomallei*
  - Causes melioidosis; usually presents as pneumonia, is aggressive, and forms abscesses in lungs
  - Considered potential bioterrorism agent; can cause laboratory worker-related infections
  - Colonies on sheep blood agar (SBA) are wrinkled, similar to *Pseudomonas stuzeri*
- *Moraxella* spp
  - *Moraxella catarrhalis* discussed with gram-negative cocci
  - Normal flora of upper respiratory & genital tract and can be confused with *Neisseria gonorrhoeae*
  - Coccobacillary; Oxidase-positive
  - Not routinely identified unless from sterile body site
- *Elizabethkingia meningoseptica*
  - Causes pneumonia, endocarditis, wound infections, postoperative bloodstream infections & meningitis in immunosuppressed adults; can cause neonatal meningitis (rare)
  - Filamentous or threadlike gram-negative bacillus
  - Oxidase-positive; light yellow pigment on sheep blood agar (SBA); no growth or weak growth on MacConkey agar
- *Chromobacterium violaceum*
  - Opportunistic pathogen; result of contamination of wound from water or soil
  - Fever, sepsis, skin lesions
  - Can be oxidase-positive but ferments glucose; grows at 42°C
  - Produces violet pigment

6.1.6.4.4 Fastidious gram-negative bacilli

- *Haemophilus* spp
  - Pleomorphic gram-negative bacilli or coccobacilli
  - No growth on sheep blood agar (SBA) or MacConkey agar but small, gray colonies on chocolate agar
  - Require 3%-5% carbon dioxide
  - Require growth factors present in blood: either X factor (hemin) or V factor (NAD) or both. X factor is available in sheep blood agar (SBA) but V factor is not available unless the cells are lysed, as in chocolate agar
  - Classified according to hemolysis & growth requirements **t6.15**
  - Porphyrin test detects ability of *Haemophilus* spp to convert ALA (δ-aminolevulinic acid) into porphrins or porphobilinogen, which are involved in synthesis of X factor. (If an isolate requires the X factor, it will be porphyrin-negative)
    - *H influenzae* porphyin-negative
    - *H parainfluenzae* porphyrin-positive

t6.15 Hemolysis & growth factor characteristics of *Haemophilus* spp

Species	Requires X-factor	Requires V-factor	Hemolysis	ALA
H influenzae	+	+	–	–
H parainfluenzae	–	+	–	+
H haemolyticus	+	+	+	–
H parahaemolyticus	–	+	+	+
H aegyptius	+	+	–	–
H ducreyi	+	–	–	

- *Haemophilus influenzae*
  - Causes invasive disease such as meningitis in children, epiglottitis, septicemia, bronchitis, pneumonia; other diseases are otitis infections, sinusitis, conjunctivitis
  - *H influenza* type B cause most serious infections
  - Isolates should be tested for production of β-lactamase enzyme, showing resistance to ampicillin/amoxicillin & first-generation cephalosporins
  - On sheep blood agar (SBA), *H influenzae* colonies "satellite" around colonies of *S aureus, S pneumoniae,* or *Neisseria* as they provide the V factor (X factor is available in sheep blood agar [SBA])
- *Haemophilus parainfluenzae*
  - Usually considered nonpathogenic and normal flora of upper respiratory tract; rarely causes endocarditis
  - Requires V factor

- *Haemophilus haemolyticus* & *H parahaemolyticus*
  - Considered nonpathogenic
- *Haemophilus aegyptius*
  - Also called Koch-Weeks bacillus and is associated with an acute, contagious conjunctivitis called "pink eye"
  - Requires an enriched chocolate agar supplemented with 1% isovitalex and held for 4 days
- *Haemophilus ducreyi*
  - Causes the sexually transmitted disease (STD) referred to as *chancroid*, which is a genital ulcer disease. It is a "soft chancre" compared to a hard chancre produced by syphilis
  - Requires enriched chocolate agar, incubated in 5%-10% carbon dioxide at 33°C for 7 days
  - Gram stain from lesion shows abundant organisms—"school of fish"
- *Francisella tularensis*
  - Tularemia (rabbit fever, deer fly fever) usually acquired from bite of arthropods or exposure to infected animals; zoonotic infection
  - Ulceroglandular infection and regional lymph node enlargement result from infection
  - BSL-3 organism and must be handled under biological safety cabinet
  - Small gram-negative coccobacilli; direct fluorescent antibody (DFA) stain is useful; PCR has widespread use
  - In vitro growth requires supplementation with sulfhydrylcompounds (eg, cysteine & cystine); also grows on BCYE; poor or no growth on sheep blood agar (SBA); will grow on chocolate in 36-48 hours
  - Biochemicals not recommended for identification because of the highly infectious nature of organism
  - Detects serum antibodies by agglutination
- *Brucella*
  - Causes undulant fever; zoonotic infection
  - Source of infection is livestock, particularly cattle (*Brucella abortus*), goats & sheep (*Brucella melitensis*), and swine (*Brucella suis*)
  - Traditionally an occupational disease among livestock handlers & abattoir workers; now more commonly foodborne (unpasteurized dairy products)
  - Hallmark feature is fever with lymphadenopathy, hepatosplenomegaly & malodorous perspiration; may be a cause of spontaneous abortion, hepatitis (with granulomas in biopsies) & endocarditis (a principal source of mortality)
  - Can be isolated using routine media after extended incubation of 7-10 days in 5%-10% carbon dioxide
  - Gram-negative coccobacillary organisms; bone marrow is specimen of choice; lysis centrifugation and continuous monitoring blood cultures can be used as well
  - This is a Centers for Disease Control and Prevention (CDC) reportable disease
- *Bordetella*
  - *B pertussis* is the etiologic agent of whooping cough; specimen of choice is nasopharyngeal swab collected using a calcium alginate swab
  - Gram-negative coccobacilli; very sensitive to drying
  - Grows in 3-7 days on Bordet-Gengou or Regan-Lowe charcoal media incubated 35°C with supplemental carbon dioxide
  - Colonies are small, smooth & shiny, likened to drops of mercury
  - Can use molecular methods for direct specimen detection or organism ID, direct fluorescent antibody (DFA) for direct specimen detection (must also include culture)
- *Pasteurella*
  - Zoonotic infection; associated with wound infection from cat & other animal bites
  - No growth on MacConkey agar, grows on sheep blood agar (SBA) & chocolate agar; ferments glucose with weak acid production
  - Oxidase positive, catalase positive, and strongly indole positive
  - This gram-negative rod is susceptible to penicillin
- *Legionella*
  - Causes Legionnaire disease & Pontiac fever
  - Infection with *L pneumophila* serogroup 1 (the most prevalent serogroup) can be detected using a urinary antigen test
  - Gram invisible in primary gram-stained smears; Giemsa or silver stain is better stain for tissues
  - Requires L-cysteine supplementation for in vitro culture
  - Whitish colonies in 2-5 days on BCYE
  - Identification can be confirmed on direct fluorescent antibody stain, latex agglutination, matrix-assisted laser desorption/ionization time-of-flight (MALDI-TOF) mass spectrometry & other methods

ISBN 978-089189-6616

- *Capnocytophaga*
  - Causes soft tissue infections after dog or cat bites
  - Spindle shaped or fusiform, thin gram-negative rod
  - Isolation requires carbon dioxide supplementation; isolation from blood is not always possible using routine blood culture media; blind subculture onto chocolate agar (or other enriched media) may be necessary
  - Catalase & oxidase positive
  - Shows gliding motility on agar surface
- *Streptobacillus moniliformis*
  - Causative agent of rat bite fever; isolate from blood, synovial fluid, CSF, skin lesions & abscesses
  - Puffball or cottonball colonies in serum-supplemented thioglycolate broth
  - Culture on media with 10%-20% serum added (brain heart infusion with 20% horse serum)
  - Gram stain shows gram-variable, filamentous rods with moniliform swellings and also can look like string of beads or pearls
  - ID with agglutination testing for serum antibodies
- HACEK group
  - Fastidious gram-negative coccobacilli: *Aggregatibacter* (formerly *Haemophilus*) *aphrophilus*, *Aggregatibacter* (formerly *Actinobacillus*) *actinomycetemcomitans*, *Cardiobacterium hominis*, *Eikenella corrodens* & *Kingella* spp
  - Can cause endocarditis in adults; predominantly seen in young children in whom it causes septic arthritis, osteomyelitis, or occult bacteremia
  - Normal oral flora but seen with poor hygiene or dental work and damaged heart valves
  - Fastidious organisms that require 48-72 hours to grow in an enriched carbon dioxide environment on chocolate agar
  - *Aggregatibacter aphrophilus* (formerly *Haemophilus aphrophilis*)
    - Found in upper respiratory tract infections and associated with dental procedures, abscesses, endocarditis
  - *Aggregatibacter actinomycetemcomitans* is normal flora of mouth but causes subacute bacterial endocarditis and is associated with periodontal disease; colonies have "star shape" with 6 points in center of colony, after 48 hours
  - *Cardiobacterium hominis* is normal mouth, nose, throat flora and infections of the mouth or procedures in the mouth usually are present before endocarditis
  - *Eikenella corrodens*: Associated with human bite wounds; colony can "pit" agar and has a "bleachlike" odor
  - *Kingella* are coccobacillary to short bacilli that cause infections in pediatric population in bones & joints, and also HACEK endocarditis

6.1.6.5 Anaerobes

6.1.6.5.1 Anaerobe specimen collection/ transport/culture media

- Specimen collection & transport
  - Acceptable specimens for culture of anaerobes
    - Aspirates
    - Body fluids
    - Bone
    - Suprapubic urine (no clean catch or catheterized samples)
    - Tissue
    - Wounds, using needle & syringe
    - Transtrachial aspirate or bronchial washings (no expectorated sputum, throat, nasopharyngeal swab, secretions)
    - Feces for toxin detection (eg, *C difficile*)
  - Most infections involving anaerobes are polymicrobic
  - Presumptive evidence of anaerobic infection is presence of foul, putrid odor from tissue specimens and cultures
  - Ideal specimen is whole tissue or aspiration using needle & syringe. After collection with needle & syringe, excess air must be expelled and syringe sealed before transport
  - Swabs are least desirable for sample collection, but must be transported in anaerobic transport system
- Media for culture of anaerobes
  - Media can be reduced to decrease oxygen concentration
  - Nonselective media has agar base with *Brucella*, brain heart infusion, or Columbia with 5% sheep blood (media should contain vitamin K and hemin for recovery of *Prevotella melaninogenica*)
- Selective media
  - Laked blood-kanamycin-vancomycin (LKV) selects for anaerobic gram-negative bacilli, especially *Bacterioides* and *Prevotella* (except *Porphyromonas*, which is inhibited by vancomycin, *Fusobacterium* can be inhibited by kanamycin)
  - *Bacterioides* bile esculin (BBE) agar selects for *Bacteroides fragilis* group. Colonies are black because organism hydrolyzes esculin in media

- Anaerobic phenylethyl alcohol (PEA) or colistin naladixic acid (CNA) agar that select for anaerobic gram-positive cocci & bacilli
- Media must be incubated in anaerobic environment (80%-90% nitrogen, 5% hydrogen, 5%-10% carbon dioxide)
- Once growth detected on anaerobic media, aerotolerance test determines if organism is anaerobe or facultative anaerobe

6.1.6.5.2 Anaerobic gram-positive cocci

- *Peptostreptococcus*, *Finegoldia*, *Peptoniphilus* are commensal flora of the oropharynx, GI tract, vagina & skin
- Associated with endogenous polymicrobial infections, such as abscesses involving the skin, soft tissues, lung, or brain; aspiration pneumonia, necrotizing pneumonia, or empyema; diabetic foot infections, crepitant cellulitis, synergistic gangrene or necrotizing fasciitis; septic abortion or intraabdominal infections
- SPS inhibits *Peptostreptococcus anaerobius*

6.1.6.5.3 Anaerobic gram-negative cocci

- *Viellonella* is only pathogen; found in oral cavity and seen in concert with other organisms in abscesses
- See t6.16 for identification of anaerobic gram-positive and gram-negative cocci, many laboratories identify with a kit (eg, RapidANA) or matrix-assisted laser desorption/ionization time-of-flight (MALDI-TOF) mass spectrometry

t6.16 Differentiation of some anaerobic gram-positive & gram-negative cocci

Organism	Van	Kan	Col	Catalase	SPS susceptibility
Finegoldia magna	S	V	R	–	–
Peptostreptococcus anaerobius	S	R	R	–	+
Peptoniphilus asacharolyticus	S	S	R	–	–
Veillonella spp	R	S	S	V	–

Col, colistin; Kan, kanamycin; R, resistant; S, sensitive; SPS, sodium polyanethylsulfonate; V, variable; Van, vancomycin

6.1.6.5.4 Anaerobic gram-positive bacilli—spore formers

- *Clostridium perfringens*
  - Causes food poisoning, gas gangrene, myonecrosis, bacteremia
  - Large "boxcar shaped" gram-positive rods, often in short chains
  - Double zone of β hemolysis on blood agar
  - Preliminary biochemical identification involves demonstration of lecithinase activity i6.30

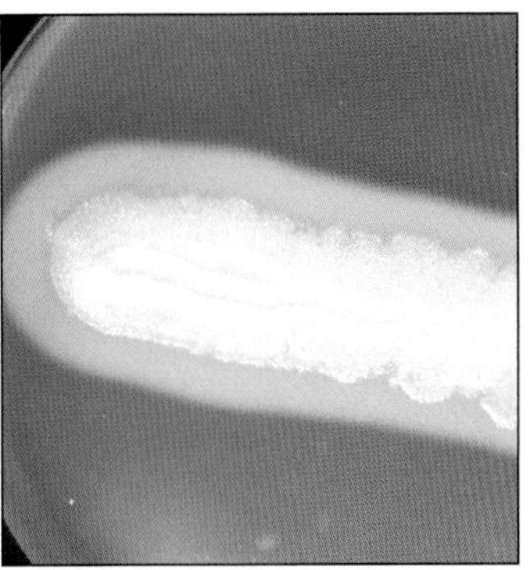

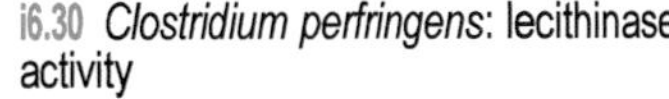

i6.30 *Clostridium perfringens*: lecithinase activity

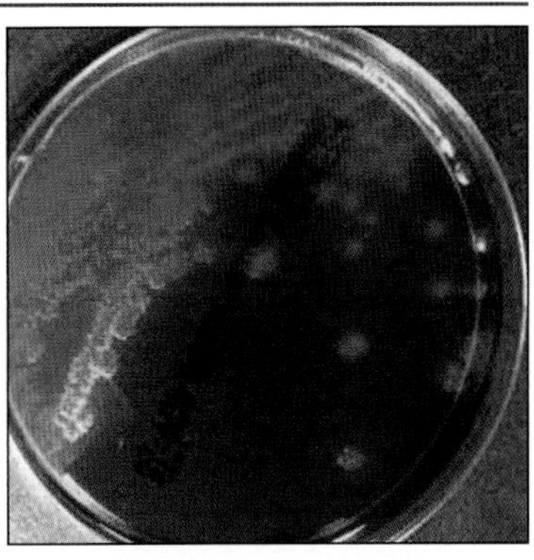

i6.31 *Clostridioides difficile*: colonies on CCFA are yellow, with a ground glass appearance

- *Clostridium septicum*
  - 2nd most common *Clostridium* in clinical specimens
  - Bacteremia can be related to colonic carcinoma or other GI pathology
  - Large gram-positive rod that frequently forms chains
  - Organisms swarm rather than forming discrete colonies; colonies look like "Medusa heads"
- *Clostridium botulinum*
  - Preformed toxin is ingested, associated with home-canned goods
  - Botulism diagnosis usually does not involve isolating the organisms; instead relies on detection of botulinum toxin in serum, stool, vomitus, or food
  - Wound botulism seen when spores enter skin
  - Raw honey a common source of infant botulism
- *Clostridium tetani*
  - Tetanus is a clinical diagnosis; useful laboratory tests for the toxin are unavailable
  - Neurotoxin; spores enter skin through puncture wound
- *Clostridioides difficile*
  - Usually hospital-associated diarrhea that can be severe; occurs after antibiotic usage
  - Culture with selective medium, cycloserine cefoxitin egg yolk fructose agar (CCFA), under strict anaerobic conditions; culture rarely performed
  - Colonies on CCFA are yellow, with a ground glass appearance i6.31, and fluoresce when exposed to UV light
  - Culture of *C difficile* produces "horse manure" odor
  - Gram stain shows thin, regularly shaped gram-positive or gram-variable rods, sometimes with subterminal and free spores
  - Isolation of the organism does not prove *C difficile* colitis, because nontoxigenic *C difficile* strains are common bowel inhabitants

ISBN 978-089189-6616

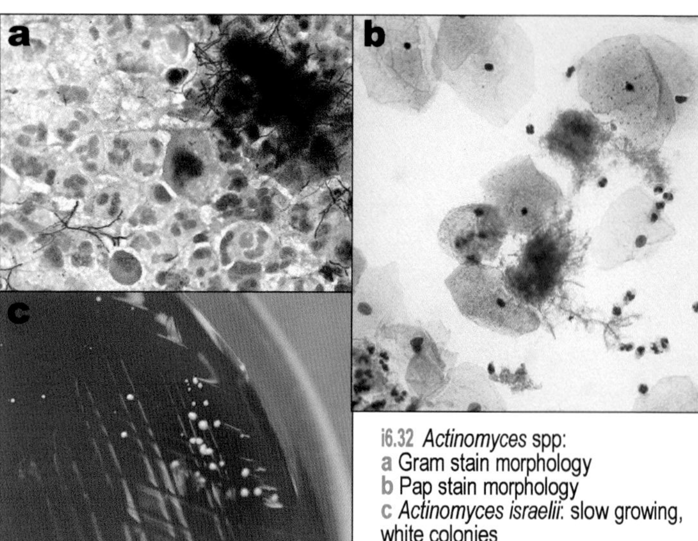

i6.32 *Actinomyces* spp:
a Gram stain morphology
b Pap stain morphology
c *Actinomyces israelii*: slow growing, white colonies

- Cytotoxic culture the gold standard test for detecting toxin production; outdated
- Molecular tests increasingly common; can detect toxin A & toxin B genes
- ELISA for stool toxin relatively insensitive; ELISA for stool glutamate dehydrogenase (GDH), an antigen produced by *C difficile*, somewhat more sensitive than toxin ELISA
- Severe *C difficile* colitis (fulminant colitis, colectomy, or death) increasingly associated with BI/NAP1/027 strain. Newest PCR assays can detect, in addition to toxin-producing strains of *C difficile*, 027 strains

6.1.6.5.5 Anaerobic nonsporeformers

- *Actinomyces* spp
  - Branching, filamentous gram-positive rods i6.32a, b; nearly identical Gram stain morphology to *Nocardia* spp
  - Unlike *Nocardia* spp, *Actinomyces* spp are anaerobes and not acid-fast
  - *Actinomyces israelii* forms white cerebriform (molar tooth) colonies i6.32c
  - Cervicofacial actinomycosis is usually the result of trauma (or surgery)
  - Thoracic actinomycosis usually the result of aspiration
  - Female genital tract actinomycosis associated with intrauterine devices (IUDs)
  - Intraabdominal actinomycosis often related to appendicitis, diverticulitis, or surgery
  - Catalase-negative; indole-negative
- *Propionibacterium* (common isolate *P acnes* is now classified *Cutibacterium acnes*)
  - Skin commensal that can cause infection of prosthetic joints and other foreign bodies (eg, indwelling CSF shunt)
  - Diphtheroid Gram stain morphology
  - Propionic acid production
  - Catalase-positive; indole-positive
- *Bifidobacterium*
  - Normal flora of mouth & intestine; uncommon isolate but can be significant pathogen in dental carries
  - Pleomorphic gram-positive bacillus with ends that may look like a "dog biscuit"
  - Catalase-negative; indole-negative
- *Eubacterium*
  - Most infections associated with mouth & colon
  - Pleomorphic gram-positive bacilli
  - Catalase-negative; indole-negative

6.1.6.5.6 Anaerobic gram-negative bacilli

- *Bacterioides fragilis*
  - Most common anaerobic pathogen, but like the others in this group, is usually a part of a polymicrobial infection
  - Seen in peritoneal infections (eg, ruptured appendix), postabdominal surgery, bacteremia
  - Usually β-lactamase-producing and resistant to penicillin
  - Gram stain morphology is pleomorphic, ranging from bacillary to coccobacillary
  - In Gram stains from liquid media, appear as bacilli with bipolar vacuoles, described as having a "safety pin" appearance
  - On blood agar, forms small, shiny colonies
  - Grows on *Bacterioides* bile esculin (BBE) as black colonies because it hydrolyzes esculin
  - Resistant to vancomycin, kanamycin, colistin; catalase-positive; indole-negative t6.17

t6.17 Differentiation of some anaerobic gram-negative bacilli

Organism	Vancomycin	Kanamycin	Colistin	Bile esculin resistance	Indole	Catalase	Fluorescence
B fragilis	R	R	R	+	–	+	
Fusobacterium spp	R	S	S	–	+	–	chartreuse
Porphyromonas asaccharolytica	S	R	R	–	+	–	red
Prevotella melaninogenica	R	R	V	–	–	–	red

R, resistant; S, sensitive; SPS, sodium polyanethylsulfonate; V, variable

- *Porphyromonas/Prevotella*
  - Normal flora of upper respiratory tract
  - Pleomorphic gram-negative bacilli or coccobacilli
  - Brick red fluorescence when exposed to UV light
  - After several days of growth, the colonies appear brown black in natural light
  - *Porphyromonas* is indole-positive, vancomycin sensitive, pigmented
  - *Prevotella* is indole negative or positive, vancomycin resistant, pigmented
- *Fusobacterium*
  - Normally found in oral cavity
  - *F necrophorum*
    - May colonize the tonsils, is associated with Lemierre syndrome (tonsillitis complicated by septic thrombophlebitis of the internal jugular vein) and with Vincent angina
    - Pleomorphic gram-negative bacilli & coccobacilli
    - Produces lipase on egg yolk agar
    - Colony has rainbow sheen, indole-positive
  - *F nucleatum*
  - Causes infection in oral cavity
  - Long, slender, fusiform gram-negative bacilli on Gram stain
  - Lipase-negative on egg yolk agar; indole-positive
  - Note: Most laboratories identify with kit (RapidANA) or matrix-assisted laser desorption/ionization time-of-flight mass spectrometry (MALDI-TOF)

6.1.6.6 Spirochetes

- Slender, helico or corkscrew-shaped bacteria that are only 0.1-0.5 μm wide and 5-20 μm long

6.1.6.6.1 *Treponema pallidum* subspecies *pallidum* (see Immunology 8.4.1, Blood Banking 1.1.1)

- Tightly coiled organisms that cannot grow in culture but is detected microscopically (darkfield) in serous exudate of lesions
- Causative agent of syphilis
- 3 stages of syphilis
  - Primary: A chancre or ulcer appears at site of inoculation and lasts 1-8 weeks
  - Secondary: Flulike symptoms, sore throat, headache, fever, muscle aches, swollen lymph nodes, rash
  - Tertiary or late stage: 1/3 of untreated patients progress to 3rd stage; lesions (gummas) seen in bone, skin & other tissues; neuro & cardiovascular involvement
- Identification
  - Direct visualization using darkfield microscopy (rarely performed)
  - Nontreponemal are excellent for screening and include RPR & VDRL; not specific for syphilis and produce false-positive
  - Nontreponemal antibodies tend to wane with treatment or in late infection, whereas treponemal antibodies remain positive indefinitely
  - A positive nontreponemal test should be followed with a treponemal test to confirm syphilis diagnosis
  - Treponemal tests detect antibodies specific for syphilis and include fluorescent treponemal antibody absorption (FTA-ABS), *Treponema pallidum* particle agglutination (TP-PA), or various enzyme immunoassay (EIAs)
  - Some laboratories are now using a reverse testing algorithm in which treponemal tests are conducted first and then followed by nontreponemal testing; this presents complexities in interpretation. A treponemal specific test (syphilis IgG by EIA currently recommended by the CDC) results in fewer false-positive results, but positive tests should still be confirmed using a nontreponemal test to confirm disease activity
- *T pallidum* subspecies *pertenue*: Found in Africa, Asia, South America; it causes yaws
- *T pallidum* subspecies *endemicum*: Found in Africa, Asia, Middle East; it causes endemic, nonvenerial syphilis (Bejel)
- *T carateum* causes pinta in South America

6.1.6.6.2 *Borrelia*

- Loosely coiled bacteria with corkscrew motility
- *B burgdorferi* (see Immunology 8.4.3)
  - Causative agent of Lyme disease in North America; *B afzelii* & *B garinii* in Europe
  - In the United States, found in 3 distinct pockets
    - Northeastern states
    - Upper Midwestern states
    - West Coast states (northern California & Oregon)
  - Reservoir is the white footed mouse & deer
  - Vectors are ticks, *Ixodes scapularis* & *Ixodes pacificus*
  - Coinfection with *Babesia* can occur because both organisms use same vector (*Ixodes*)

ISBN 978-089189-6616

- Stages
    - Early: Erythema migrans (EM) at site of inoculation
    - Second stage: Neurologic or cardiac involvement; most commonly facial nerve palsy and/or atrioventricular (A-V) block
    - Third stage: Joints most commonly involved
- Diagnosis: Immunofluorescence assay (IFA) or EIA; confirm with Western blot

- *Borrelia recurrentis*
    - Causes relapsing fever: High fevers that subside after 3-6 days, then return in 1 week

6.1.6.6.3 *Leptospira interrogans*

- Tightly coiled, motile bacteria with hooked ends
- Leptospirosis typically the triad of meningitis, hepatitis, nephritis (Weil disease)
- Humans are infected through contact with the urine of an infected animal, the usual portal of entry being the conjunctiva or abrasions or cuts in the skin
    - In the United States, highest incidence is found in Hawaii
    - Rats are the usual hosts
    - Diagnosis: ELISA

6.1.6.6.4 *Chlamydiae*

- *C trachomatis*
    - Most common sexually transmitted disease in the United States; often infection is asymptomatic
    - Specimens for evaluation include urethra, cervical, urine
    - Often detected from cervical/urethral swab with gonorrhea/chlamydia testing (GC)
    - Manifests as trachoma, lymphogranuloma venereum (LGV), urethritis, epididymitis, prostatitis, proctitis, cervicitis & neonatal infections (inclusion body conjunctivitis, pneumonitis & otitis)
    - Diagnosis: Cell culture (McCoy cells) the gold standard; replaced by nucleic acid amplification tests (NAAT); can be performed on urine, cervical/urethral swab
    - Often detected as part of gonorrhea/chlamydia (GC) direct specimen molecular test
- *C psittaci* (now called *Chlamydophila psittaci*)
    - Causative agent of psittacosis
    - Related to contact with birds
    - Manifests primarily as pneumonitis
    - Diagnose with microimmunofluorescence (MIF)
- *C pneumoniae* (TWAR bacillus, now called *Chlamydophila pneumoniae*)
    - Pneumonia, pharyngitis, sinusitis, bronchitis
    - Diagnose with MIF

6.1.6.6.5 *Rickettsiae* t6.18

- *R rickettsii*
    - Causative agent of Rocky Mountain spotted fever (RMSF)
    - Most common in southeast United States
    - American dog tick, *Dermacentor variabilis*, is the vector of RMSF
    - Early infection causes fever, rash & severe headache; rash begins at the wrists & ankles, progressing proximally
    - Later involvement may manifest as renal failure, disseminated intravascular coagulation (DIC), central nervous system involvement
    - Fulminant disease seen in patients with glucose-6-phosphatase deficiency
    - Diagnose with NAAT, MIF & western blot

t6.18 Rickettsial diseases

Disease	Organism	Vector
Rocky mountain spotted fever	*Rickettsia rickettsii*	Dog tick
Epidemic typhus	*Rickettsia prowazekii*	Louse
Scrub typhus	*Orientia* (previously *Rickettsia*) *tsutsugamushi*	Chigger
Murine typhus	*Rickettsia typhi*	Flea
Cat scratch disease	*Bartonella henselae*	Kitten
Bacillary angiomatosis	*Bartonella henselae*	Kitten
Boutonneuse fever	*Rickettsia conorii*	Tick
Rickettsial pox	*Rickettsia akari*	Mite
Human monocytic ehrlichiosis	*Ehrlichia chaffeensis*	Lone star tick (*Amblyomma americanum*)
Anaplasmosis	*Anaplasma* (previously *Ehrlichia*) *phagocytophilium*	Deer tick
Oroya fever	*Bartonella bacilliformis*	Sandfly
Verruga peruana	*Bartonella bacilliformis*	Sandfly
Trench fever	*Bartonella quintana*	Louse
Brill-Zinsser disease	*Rickettsia prowazekii*	None (recrudescence of epidemic typhus)

- *Coxiella*
  - Obligate intracellular pathogen classified as γ *Proteobacteria*
  - Pleomorphic gram-negative *Coccobacillus*
  - *C burnetii* is the causative agent of Q fever
  - Hosts include livestock, pets, birds, fish & ticks, and these hosts shed organisms in milk, feces & birthing fluids
  - Human infection the result of inhalation during slaughter or while attending a birth; occupational hazard for veterinarians, farmers & abattoir workers
  - Acute Q fever nonspecific in presentation, with 1%-2% fatality, often related to myocarditis
  - Chronic Q fever often takes the form of endocarditis, endovasculitis, or infection of the bone & joint; high mortality
  - Recrudescence of Q fever may occur during pregnancy
  - Diagnosis is based largely on serology (blood) or PCR (affected tissue)
- *Ehrlichia* & *Anaplasma*
  - Found mainly in North America (in midwestern, southeastern & south central states in the United States)
  - Ticks are important vectors
  - Organisms can be seen on Wright-stained blood films within intracellular vacuoles, where they appear as mulberries or morulae
  - Human monocytic ehrlichiosis (HME) caused by *Ehrlichia chaffeensis*; leukopenia, thrombocytopenia, increased serum transaminases
  - Human granulocytic anaplasmosis (HGA) caused by *Anaplasma phagocytophilum*
  - Diagnose both using nucleic acid amplification tests (NAAT) & immunofluorescence assay (IFA)

6.1.6.6.6 *Bartonella* spp

- Trench fever (*B quintana*) transmitted by the human body louse (*Pediculus humanus corporis*)
- Oroya fever & verruga peruana (*B bacilliformis*) transmitted by *Lutzomyia phlebotomine* sandfly; Oroya fever—verruga peruana spectrum has been called *Carrión disease*
- Cat scratch disease & bacillary angiomatosis (*B henselae*)
  - Cat scratch disease: Natural reservoir in cats and is transmitted to humans through a scratch or bite
  - Bacillary angiomatosis: Those with human immunodeficiency virus (HIV) may develop within skin, lymph nodes, or viscera (sometimes called *peliosis*)
- Diagnosis: Serology & molecular methods

6.1.6.6.7 *Mycoplasma* & *Ureaplasma*

- Smallest free-living bacteria; no cell wall, and cell membrane has sterols
- *Mycoplasma pneumoniae*
  - Causes primary atypical pneumonia (walking pneumonia) & tracheobronchitis
  - Associated with autoimmune hemolytic anemia due to cold agglutinins (IgM anti-I antibodies)
  - Identify using PCR & EIA
- *Ureaplasma urealyticum* & *Mycoplasma hominis*
  - Cause nongonococcal urethritis
  - *M hominis* typically produces "fried egg" colonies in culture
  - Identify using PCR or matrix-assisted laser desorption/ionization time-of-flight (MALDI-TOF) mass spectrometry

6.2 Mycobacteria

6.2.1 Laboratory methods

6.2.1.1 Specimen collection & processing

- Bronchial washings & sputum
  - Sodium hydroxide (NaOH) used for decontamination (reduces bacteria in sputum and other nonsterile samples); mycobacteria are resistant because of high lipid content of cell wall
  - N-acetyl-L-cysteine (NALC): Mucolytic agent
  - Centrifuge at >3000*g* for maximum recovery of acid-fast bacilli

ISBN 978-089189-6616

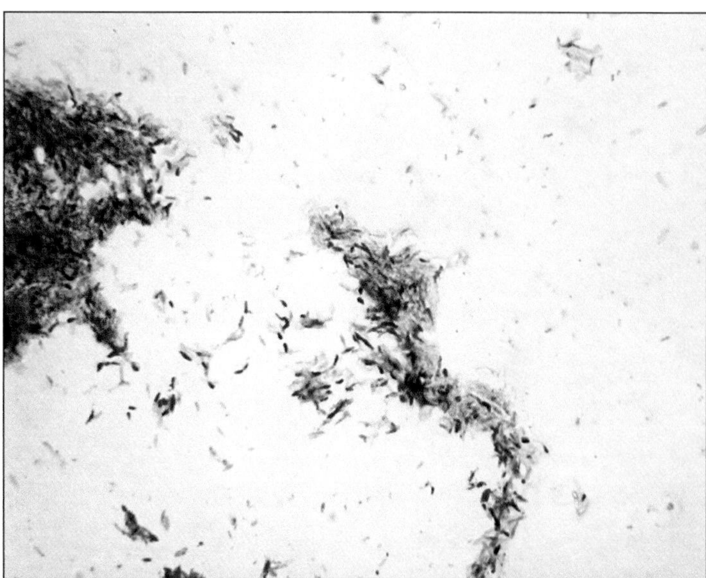

i6.33 Mycobacteria; occasionally, the organisms are visible as gram-positive rods

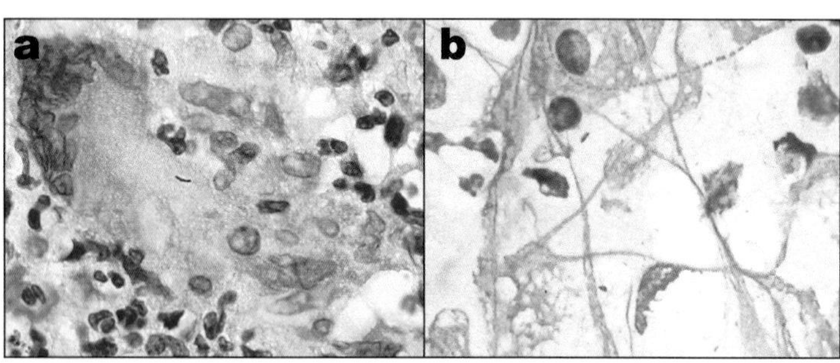

i6.34 Mycobacteria
a AFB-stained tissue section
b AFB-stained BAL specimen

i6.35 Mycobacteria: auramine-rhodamine fluorochrome stain

6.2.1.2 Direct examination

- Gram stain: Gram-positive rods structurally but typically gram-invisible; occasionally visible as weakly gram-positive bacilli i6.33
- Visible by acid-fast stain (Ziehl-Neelsen, Kinyoun); i6.34 or by auramine rhodamine fluorochrome stain i6.35
- Ziehl-Neelsen & Kinyoun
  - For mycobacteria: these bacteria have the cell wall structure of gram-positive bacteria but contain mycolic acids, which repel crystal violet/iodine, thus are usually gram invisible
  - Acid-fast staining uses heat and/or phenol to allow a fuchsin dye to penetrate the hydrophobic barrier and stain the mycolic acids in the cell wall (red stain)
  - The organisms resist decolorization, which is why they are termed "acid-fast"
  - Ziehl-Neelsen technique: red carbol fuchsin dye containing phenol is heated to aid penetration of the cell wall; strong acid, 3% hydrochloric acid, is used for decolorization; methylene blue is counterstain
  - Kinyoun (cold) technique: Higher concentration of phenol and no heat; otherwise same as Ziehl-Neelsen
  - Fite (modified) acid-fast technique: Weaker decolorizing reagent; good for "weakly" acid-fast organisms such as *Nocardia* spp, *Cryptosporidium*, *Cystoisospora bellii* (formerly *Isospora)*, *Cyclospora*, *Sarcocystis* & *Legionella micdadei)*
- Fluorescent auramine rhodamine stain for acid-fast bacilli
  - Auramine & rhodamine stain mycolic acids and fluoresce when exposed to ultraviolet light
  - Rapid growers may not stain with fluorochrome stain

6.2.1.3 Culture

- Gold standard; slow growth
- Required for antimicrobial susceptibility testing
- Primary specimens cultured in liquid (broth) and solid (plate or slant) media
- Grows faster in broth; often augmented by growth monitoring technology; typically, a Middlebrook broth; organisms can be assessed for cording, a characteristic feature of *M tuberculosis* complex
- Solid medium egg based (eg, Lowenstein-Jensen) or agar based (eg, Middlebrook)
  - Some mycobacteria can only be isolated on solid medium; helps to detect mixed mycobacterial infection
  - Middlebrook 7H10 and 7H11 should be refrigerated and stored in dark so formaldehyde does not build up, which is toxic to organism
- First classified as a rapid grower or a slow grower

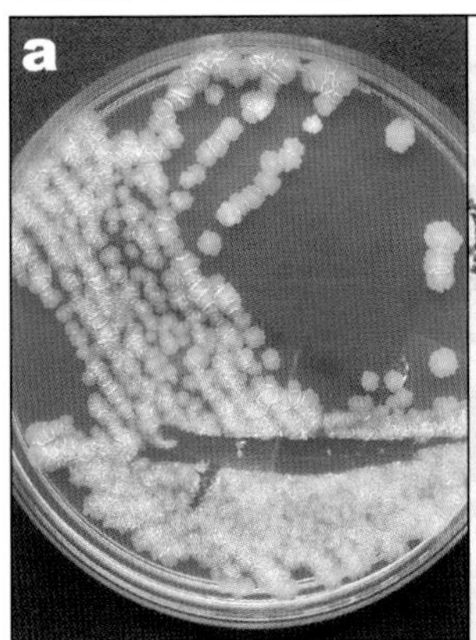

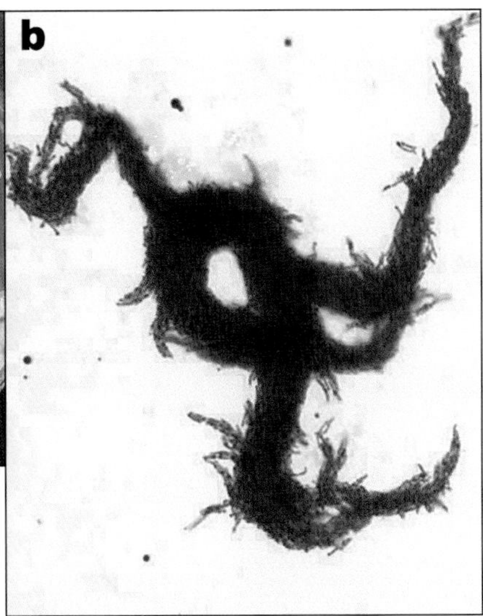

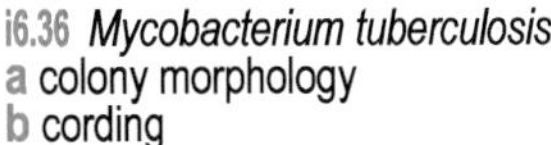
i6.36 *Mycobacterium tuberculosis*:
a colony morphology
b cording

- Further subclassified based on its temperature preference and its colony pigmentation (nonchromogen, scotochromogen, or photochromogen)
  - Nonchromogen: No pigment produced in colonies
  - Scotochromogen: Produce orange or deep yellow pigment in light and dark
  - Photochromogen: Develops pigment when exposed to light and develops no pigment in dark
- Finally classified according to series of biochemical tests; takes days to weeks
- Molecular methods are used in identification
  - Direct nucleic acid amplification assays will detect *M tuberculosis* complex directly from patient specimen
- Automated, continuously monitorting culture systems are available
  - Tubes incubated for 6 weeks
  - Positive tubes stained for AFB

6.2.1.4 Important species t6.19

t6.19 Important mycobacterial species

Site	Most common ***Mycobacterium*** **spp**
Lung	*M avium* complex, *M tuberculosis*, *M kansasii*, *M xenopi*, *M abscessus*
Lymph node	*M avium* complex, *M tuberculosis*, *M scrofulaceum*, *M haemophilum*
Skin & soft tissue	*M fortuitum*, *M chelonae*, *M abscessus*, *M marinum*, *M ulcerans*, *M haemophilum*
GI	*M tuberculosis*, *M avium* complex

6.2.1.5 *Mycobacterium tuberculosis* (MTB)

- Key characteristics
  - Slow growth, forming flat, dry, white, wrinkled colonies on solid media i6.36a
  - Preference for incubation at 37°C; cording in broth i6.36b
  - Slow growth; 2-6 weeks
  - Nonchromogenic & nonpigmented
  - The tuberculin skin test (TST/PPD): Positive test may signify active TB, latent TB, nontuberculous mycobacteria infection, or vaccination with BCG
  - IFN-γ release assays: T cells of persons infected with *M tuberculosis* release interferon γ (IFN-γ) in large quantities; as good as or superior to TST/PPD
  - Same day molecular testing can be done directly on AFB smear-positive respiratory specimens
- Key biochemical for MTB **t6.20**
  - Niacin-positive; nitrate reduction-positive; telluride reduction-negative

t6.20 Differentiation of select *Mycobacterium* spp

Organism	Pigment	Growth rate	Niacin reduction	Nitrate reduction	Tellurite
M tuberculosis	Non	Slow	+	+	–
M avium complex	Non	Slow	–	–	+
M kansasii	Photo	Slow	–	+	–
M marinum	Photo	Slow	–	–	–
M scrofulaceum	Scoto	Slow	–	–	V
M fortuitum	Non	Rapid	–	+	+

Non, nonphotochromogen; Photo, photochromagen; Scoto, scotochromagen; V, variable

- Treatment
  - Must be prolonged for up to 8 months using multiple drugs
  - Drug-resistant strains are significant problem (MDR TB & XDR TB)
  - Some of the TB drugs are isoniazid (NIH), ethambutol, pyrazinamide, rifampin
- Clinical features
  - Tuberculosis may be caused by any of the *Mycobacterium tuberculosis* complex: *M tuberculosis*, *M microti*, *M bovis*, *M africanum* & *M canetti*
  - *M tuberculosis* is the most common pathogen in the complex
  - Spread from person to person by respiratory droplets or aerosols
  - Primary infection pulmonary and may undergo spontaneous eradication; can remain viable/dormant in macrophages for years

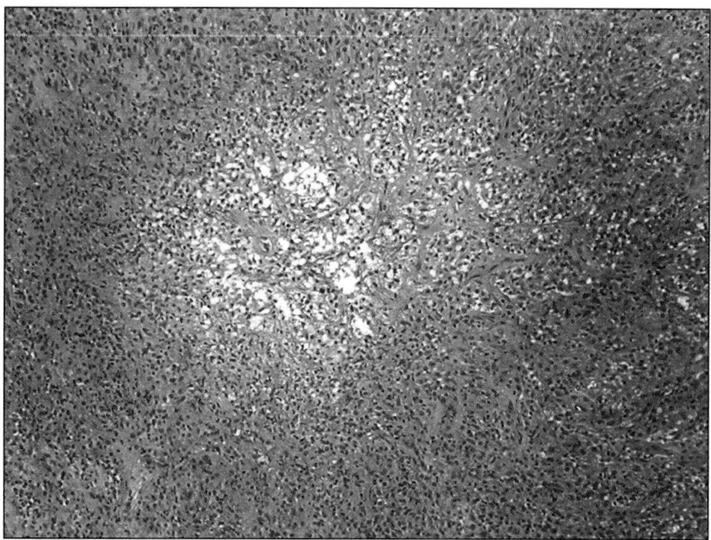

i6.37 *Mycobacterium tuberculosis* (MTB): necrotizing granuloma

- Undergo resolution (latency), forming tubercles (caseating granulomas) usually in upper lobes i6.37
- Produce active disease
- Reactivation presents as active disease
- Thus, active TB may be a feature of acute infection or reactivation infection
- Active TB usually pulmonary but may be extrapulmonary (kidneys, bone, GI tract & meninges)
- BCG strains of *M bovis* have been used for vaccinations against tuberculosis

6.2.1.6 Nontuberculous mycobacteria

- Key features
  - Ubiquitous in the environment; isolation does not necessarily indicate infection
  - True infection more common in patients with compromised immunity
  - Runyon classification of non-*Mycobacterium tuberculosis*
- Slow-growing photochromogens
  - *M kansasii*
  - *M marinum*
- Slow-growing scotochromagens
  - *M gordonae*
- Slow-growing nonpigmented
  - *M avium* & *M intracellulare* complex
- Rapid growers
  - *M fortuitum*
  - *M chelonae*
  - *M abscessus*

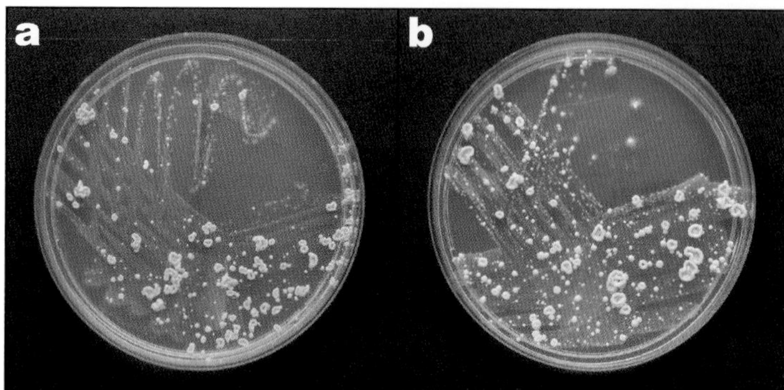

i6.38 *Mycobacterium avium* complex:
a pigmented colony morphology
b nonpigmented colony morphology

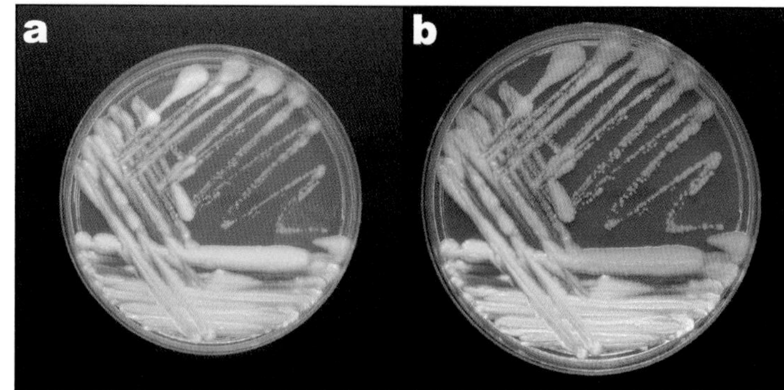

i6.39 *Mycobacterium kansasii*: a colonies are nonpigmented when incubated in the dark, but b produce pigment after light exposure (photochromogenic)

6.2.1.7 *Mycobacterium avium* complex (MAC)

- Includes *M avium* & *M intracellulare*
  - Usually not differentiated but can be done with molecular testing
- Infection may be seen in immunocompromised & immunocompetent individuals
- Amongst the immunocompetent, there are 3 forms of disease
  - One is seen in heavy smokers with upper lobe cavitary disease, resembling classic tuberculosis (TB)
  - Another is called "Lady Windermere syndrome," seen typically in elderly women with weak cough; akin to colonization
  - A third is a hypersensitivity reaction to *Mycobacterium avium* complex after exposure to hot tub water contaminated with the organisms
- *Mycobacterium avium* complex is the most common cause of scrofula in the United States
- In culture, slow growing and usually nonpigmented but may become yellow with age i6.38a, b
- *M kansasii*
  - Infection resembling TB in patients with immunosuppression or underlying pulmonary disease
  - Slow-growing photochromogen i6.39

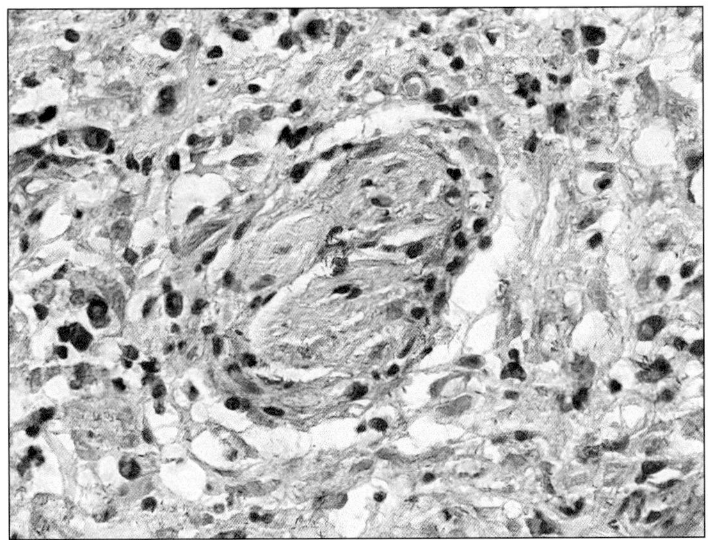

i6.40 *Mycobacterium leprae*: Fite-stained section

- Mycobacteria typically associated with skin & soft tissue infections
  - Includes *M fortuitum* group, *M chelonae*, *M abscessus*, *M marinum*, *M ulcerans* & *M haemophilum*
  - Infection often follows trauma to the skin
- *M marinum* associated with wound exposure to freshwater fish tanks or saltwater, and causes localized cutaneous infection ("fishtank granuloma")
- *M ulcerans* causes indolent, necrotizing, ulcerating cutaneous lesions
- *M scofulaceum* has been associated with cervical lymphadenitis. It is a scotochromagen that looks like *M tuberculosis* on stain
- *M leprae*
  - The cause of leprosy (Hansen disease)
  - In the United States, found in Hawaii, Texas, and Louisiana (where it is harbored by armadillos)
  - Culture cannot be performed on artificial media. In tissue biopsy, it is best visualized using the Fite stain i6.40

6.3 Antimicrobial agents & resistance

6.3.1 Classes of antimicrobial agents

- Antibiotics that inhibit cell wall synthesis (and contain β-lactam ring in structure)
  - Penicillins
    - Natural penicillins: Pen V & Pen G
    - Penicillinase-resistant penicillins, eg, methicillin, nafcillin & oxacillin
    - Aminopenicillins: Ampicillin, amoxicillin
    - Carboxypenicillins: Ticarcillin, carbenicillin
    - Uredopenicillins: Mezlocillin, piperacillin
    - β-lactamase inhibitors (that couple with lactam antibiotics): Clavulanic acid, sulbactam
  - Cephalosporins (eg, from 1st, 2nd, 3rd generation groups)
    - 1st generation: Cefazolin, cephalexin
    - 2nd generation: Cefuroxime, cefaclor, cefoxitin
    - 3rd generation: Ceftazidime, ceftriaxone, cefixime
    - 4th generation: Cefepime
    - 5th generation: Ceftobiprole
  - Carbapenems: Imipenem, meropenem, doripenem, ertapenem
  - Monobactams: Aztreonam
  - Glycopeptides: Vancomycin
  - Lipoglycopeptide: Teicoplanin, daptomycin
- Antibiotics that disrupt cell membrane
  - Bacitracin
  - Polymyxin B & E (colistin)
- Antibiotics that inhibit protein synthesis
  - Aminoglycosides: Gentamicin, tobramycin, amikacin, spectinomycin
  - Tetracyclines
  - Macrolides: Erythromycin, azithromycin, clarithromycin
  - Lincosamide (clindamycin)
  - Oxazolidinone (linezolid)
  - Chloramphenicol
  - Streptogramins (dalfopristin, quinupristin)
- Antibiotics that inhibit nucleic acid synthesis
  - Quinolones: Fluoroquinolones
  - Rifampin
  - Metronidazole
  - Nitrofurantoin
- Antibiotics that inhibit metabolic processes
  - Sulfonamides
  - Para-aminosalicylic acid
  - Trimethoprim
- Antimycobacterial agents
  - Isoniazid
  - Rifampin
  - Ethambutol
  - Pyrazinamide
- Antifungal agents
  - Amphotericin B
  - Azoles: Ketoconazole, itraconazole, fluconazole, voriconazole

ISBN 978-089189-6616

- Capsofungin
- Flucytosine
- Griseofulvin
- Nystatin

6.3.2 Bacterial resistance mechanisms

- Natural (intrinsic) occur naturally in most strains of certain microbes (eg, enterococci resistance to cephalosporins; *Klebsiella pneumoniae* resistant to ampicillin)
- Chromosomal mutations
- Target site changes
- Reduced permeability
- Enzyme production that modifies or inactivates antibiotic
- Plasmid production
- Decreased permeability or uptake, increased efflux
  - Change in number or character of porin channels
  - Increase in ability of organism to pump out cell contents (antibiotics)

6.3.3 Methods for testing susceptibility resistance

- Minimum inhibitory concentration (MIC) is the lowest concentration of antibiotic that inhibits growth of organism
- Minimum bactericidal concentration (MBC) is the lowest concentration of antibiotic that kills ≥99.9% of cells
- Disk agar diffusion (Kirby Bauer)
  - Key points to remember about standardized procedure
    - Inoculum must be equal to 0.5 McFarland standard to give 1.5×10^8 colony-forming units (CFU)/mL (If inoculum is more concentrated, organism will appear to be more resistant)
    - Mueller-Hinton (MH) agar is used in 150 mm plates, 4 mm deep, pH 7.2-7.4
    - Antibiotic disk concentrations are standardized
    - Incubation of MH agar at 35°C for 18-24 hours in ambient air
    - Inoculation of MH agar must be done within 15 minutes of making the organism suspension, and disks must be applied to the MH agar within 15 minutes of media inoculation, and plates should be inverted and incubated within 15 minutes of inoculation (if disks are delayed beyond 15 minute time, zone sizes will be decreased)
    - Zones of inhibition (diameter) are measured using a ruler or caliper and recorded in millimeters
    - To read plate zones, the plate should be held 2-3 inches above a black surface using reflected light
    - Exceptions are with susceptibility of enterococci with vancomycin and staphylococci with oxacillin using transmitted light
    - Swarming over a zone of inhibition should be ignored
    - Zone size is compared to a standard chart to interpret as sensitive, resistant, or intermediate
  - This procedure cannot be used to test slow growing organisms or anaerobes
  - Fastidious organisms such as *Haemophilus*, *Neisseria*, *S pneumoniae* require a modified procedure using specific types of supplemented MH-based medium
- E test
  - Similar to disk agar diffusion and can be used for anaerobes & fastidious organisms
  - A strip is placed on a MH agar plate that has been inoculated with organism suspension. The strip contains gradually increasing concentrations of a specific antibiotic
  - Result is read as a minimum inhibitory concentration (MIC), where the zone of inhibition intersects the strip
- β-lactamase enzyme detection
  - This is performed on isolates of *Staphylococcus*, *Haemophilus*, *N gonorrhoeae*, *M catarrhalis*
  - Chromogenic nitrocefin method is common and produces a pink color if organism has the β-lactamase enzyme that breaks nitrocefin β-lactam ring
  - Iodometric method uses starch solution that is dried on to filter paper. Organism is added to filter paper and then iodine solution is applied. If organisms produces β-lactamase, there is no color change because penicilloic acid binds to iodine
  - Acidic method using a phenol red indicator, a penicillin solution, and the organism. If β-lactamase is produced, the solution turns yellow
- Methicillin-resistant *Staphyloccus aureus* (MRSA) detection
  - Cefoxitin 30 µg disk diffusion test predicts the presence of the *mec*A gene. Cefoxitin is better than oxacillin at inducing the expression of the *mec*A gene
  - Oxacillin 6 ug disk diffusion is used on MH agar with 4% NaCl at 33-35°C in ambient air for up to 48 hours
  - Molecular methods detect the *mec*A gene and can be used on both colonies of the bacteria or direct detection on patient specimens
- Staphylococci and *erm*-mediated inducible clindamycin resistance
  - D zone test will determine if an erythromycin-resistant and clindamycin-susceptible *Staphylococcus* isolate is truly susceptible to clindamycin or if it has an inducible clindamycin resistance because of the *erm* gene
- Vancomycin-resistant enterococci (VRE) detection
  - *E faecium* most common vancomycin-resistant species

- VanA mediated: Inducible, high-level resistance to vancomycin & teicoplanin
- Van B chromosomal mediated: Variable levels of vancomycin resistance and susceptibility to teicoplanin
- Molecular assays (PCR-based) detect VRE

- Extended spectrum β-lactamase (ESBL)
  - Resistance is located on plasmid gene and will inactivate extended spectrum cephalosporin, penicillins, and aztreonam
  - The disk agar diffusion test uses indicator drugs (cefotaxime & ceftazdime) on separate disks and also disks that contain both the indicator drug and clavulanic acid (a β-lactamase inhibitor)
  - If combined disk zone sizes are larger than either disk with indicator drug alone, ESBL is produced by the organism
- Carbapenemases produced by members of the *Enterobacteriaceae* due to expression of bla_{KPC} gene; organisms producing carbapenemase are resistant to all B-lactam antibiotics
  - Hodge test uses disk agar diffusion method in which *E coli* ATCC strain suspension is spread over the MH agar
  - A single imipenem disk is placed in center of agar
  - The organism being tested is then inoculated to MH plate by drawing lines on top of *E coli* suspension, from the edge of the imipenem disk to the agar plate's edge
  - An organism producing carbapenemase will hydrolyze the imipenem and the *E coli* will grow at the edge of the imipenem disk

6.4 Parasitology

6.4.1 Laboratory methods

6.4.1.1 Specimen collection & examination

- Body sites and possible parasites recovered are summarized in **t6.21**
- Stool
  - 3 specimens at least 24 hours apart required to exclude infection
    - Recommendation is 3 stools over a 10-day period
    - Collection container should be clean & dry with tight fitting lid
    - Never collect from a bed pan or toilet bowl
    - Collect before administration of barium enema or antibiotics

t6.21 Most common parasites by body site

Body site	Parasites
Intestinal tract	*Entamoeba* spp, *Iodamoeba butschlii, Endolimax nana, Blastocystis hominis, Giardia lamblia, Chilomastix mesnili, Dientamoeba fragilis, Pentatrichomonas hominis, Balantidium coli, Cryptosporidium* spp, *Cyclospora cayetanensis, Cystoisospora belli,* microsporidia, *Ascaris lumbricoides, Enterobius vermicularis,* hookworm, *Strongyloides stercoralis, Trichuris trichiura, Hymenolepis nana, Hymenolepis diminuta, Taenia saginata, Taenia solium, Diphyllobothrium latum, Dipylidium caninum, Schistosoma* spp (eggs only), *Fasciolopsis buski*
Blood	Erythrocytes: *Plasmodium* spp & *Babesia* spp
	Leukocytes: *Leishmania* spp & *Toxoplasma gondii*
	Whole blood/plasma: *Trypanosoma* spp, microfilariae
Bone marrow	*Leishmania* spp, *Plasmodium* spp
Central nervous system	*Taenia solium* (neurocysticercosis), *Echinococcus* spp, *Naegleria fowleri, Acanthamoeba* spp, *Balamuthia mandrillaris, Toxoplasma gondii,* microsporidia & *Trypanosoma brucei*
Cutaneous ulcer	*Leishmania* spp, *Acanthamoeba* spp
Liver, spleen	*Echinococcus* spp, *Entamoeba histolytica, Leishmania* spp, microsporidia, *Schistosoma mansoni* & *japonicum* (eggs only), *Fasciola hepatica, Clonorchis sinensis*
Muscle	*Trichinella* spp, *Taenia solium* (cysticerci), *Trypanosoma cruzi,* microsporidia
Lungs	*Cryptosporidium* spp, *Echinococcus* spp, *Paragonimus* spp, *Toxoplasma gondii, Strongyloides stercoralis* larvae, microsporidia
Skin & subcutaneous tissue	*Leishmania* spp, *Onchocerca volvulus,* microfilariae, *Sarcoptes scabei, Loa loa* (adult worm)
Urogenital system	*Trichomonas vaginalis, Schistosoma* spp (eggs only), microsporidia, microfilariae
Eyes	*Acanthamoeba* spp, *Toxoplasma gondii, Loa loa, Onchocerca volvulus,* microsporidia

  - Components of a complete stool examination
    - Fresh specimen
      - Specimens should be examined within 1 hour and direct wet mount performed using saline & iodine solutions (note: iodine will kill trophozoites)
      - If specimens cannot be examined within 1 hour, preservatives such as formalin or polyvinyl alcohol (PVA serves as an adhesive to slides) should be used (3 parts preservative & 1 part feces)
      - Artifacts, eg, pollen granules, WBCs, vegetable cells, crystals, can be mistaken for parasite stages
    - Concentration of specimen using formalin ethyl acetate sedimentation or zinc flotation

ISBN 978-089189-6616

- Permanent stains
  - Trichrome
  - Gomori methenamine silver
  - Protozoa that are likely to be missed with routine O&P stains include *Cryptosporidium* spp, *Cyclospora cayetanensis* & *Cystoisospora* (formerly *Isospora*) *belli*; these require modified acid-fast (Kinyoun, DMSO, or auramine-O) or modified safranin stains

- Duodenal contents
  - For the detection of duodenal infections such as *Giardia intestinalis* or *Strongyloides stercoralis*. Collected using direct aspiration during endoscopy or with the Beale string technique
- Cellophane tape preparation or commercial sticky paddle "kit"
  - For detection of *Enterobius vermicularis* (pinworm)

- Blood
  - Parasites that may be detected in blood include
    - *Plasmodium* spp & *Babesia* spp within erythrocytes
      - Giemsa-stained thick & thin blood films are the gold standard method for *Plasmodium* & *Babesia* detection
    - *Leishmania* spp amastigotes & *Toxoplasma gondii* tachyzoites in leukocytes
  - Extracellular *Trypanosoma* spp & the microfilariae (*Wuchereria bancrofti*, *Brugia malayi*, *Loa loa*, *Mansonella* spp) in whole blood/plasma
- Respiratory specimens
  - For the detection of *Paragonimus* spp (lung fluke) eggs, *Strongyloides stercoralis* larvae & hooklets of *Echinococcus* spp from ruptured hydatid cysts
- Cerebrospinal fluid
  - For suspected primary amebic meningoencephalitis (PAM) caused by *Naegleria fowleri* and *Acanthamoeba* in granulomatous amebic encephalitis (GAE)

6.4.1.2 Serology

- Limited role but EIA used to detect parasite antigens in specimens with *Giardia, Cryptosporidium, Entamoeba histolytica*
- Direct fluorescent antibody (DFA) used for detection of *Cryptosporidium* & *Giardia* in specimens
- Prenatal & postnatal toxoplasmosis screening
- Diagnosis of amebic liver abscess due to *E histolytica*

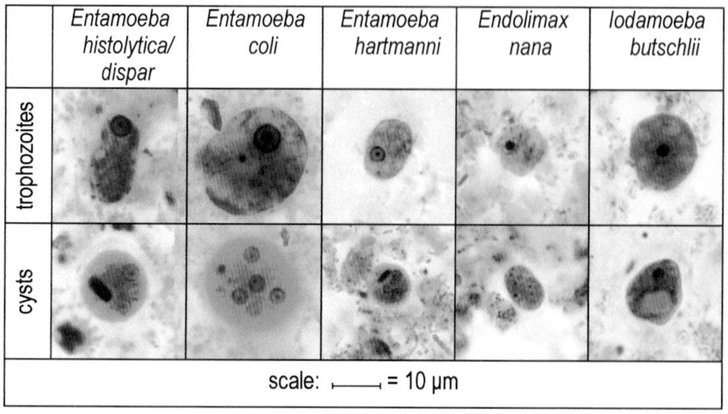

	Entamoeba histolytica/ dispar	*Entamoeba coli*	*Entamoeba hartmanni*	*Endolimax nana*	*Iodamoeba butschlii*
trophozoites					
cysts					
scale: ⟼ = 10 µm					

i6.41 Amebae

6.4.1.3 Culture

- Cultures of parasites are usually not performed
- Some exceptions **t6.22** are the free living amebae (*Acanthamoeba* spp, *Naegleria fowleri*), *Trichomonas vaginalis*, and less commonly, *Leishmania* spp

t6.22 Parasites in culture

Free living amebae	Tap water agar on a bed of *E coli* (for nutrient source)
Leishmania spp & *Trypanosoma* spp	Novy-MacNeal-Nicolle (NNN) medium
Trichomonas vaginalis	Diamond media

6.4.1.4 Molecular methods

- Biofire/multiplex GI panel detects 4 parasites (*Cryptosporidium, Cyclospora, Entamoeba histolytica, Giardia* & 18 other GI pathogens in 1 test)

6.4.2 Protozoa

6.4.2.1 *Amebae* (Sarcodina)

- Unicellular organisms, motile by pseudopodal extension i6.41
- Intestinal amebae: *Entamoeba*, *Endolimax* & *Iodamoeba*
  - *Entamoeba histolytica*
    - Morphologically indistinguishable from the nonpathogenic *Entamoeba dispar*
    - Morphologically similar to *Entamoeba coli* & *Entamoeba hartmanni* **t6.23**

t6.23 Amebae that resemble *Entamoeba histolytica* & *Entamoeba dispar*

Form	Characteristic	*Entamoeba coli*	*E histolytica & E dispar*	*Entamoeba hartmanni*
Trophozoite	Size	20-25 µm	15-20 µm	5-10 µm
	Motility	Nondirectional	Unidirectional	Nondirectional
	Ingested erythrocytes	Absent	Present (*E histolytica* only)	Absent
	Karyosome	Large, eccentric	Small, central	Small, central
	Nuclear chromatin	Clumped along nuclear membrane	Fine, evenly distributed along nuclear membrane	Fine, evenly distributed along nuclear membrane
Cyst	Size	15-25 µm	12-15 µm	5-8 µm
	Nuclei	Up to 8	Never >4	Never >4
	Chromatoidal bars	Frayed ends	Rounded ends	Rounded ends

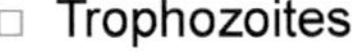

- Trophozoites
  - Measure ~15-20 µm
  - Nucleus has small, central karyosome and fine peripheral chromatin applied evenly to the inner nuclear membrane
  - Cytoplasm appears finely granular and may contain ingested red cells
  - Erythrophagocytosis the only feature that can differentiate *E histolytica* from *E dispar*
  - In wet mounts, progressive directional motility
  - Cysts have up to 4 nuclei, may contain chromatoidal bodies with smooth rounded ends
  - Stool EIA generally superior to microscopic stool examination for diagnosis; multiplex PCR
  - Acquired through ingestion of cysts in fecally contaminated food or water
  - Worldwide distribution
  - Clinical features
    - Ranges from asymptomatic to protracted diarrhea
    - Can invade intestinal wall and disseminates to the liver
    - Amebic abscesses are described as containing anchovy pastelike material
    - Intestinal "flask-shaped" ulcer, usually in the cecum i6.42
- *Entamoeba coli* (see **t6.23**)
  - Larger than *E histolytica*, nondirectional motility, larger eccentric karyosome, clumped peripheral nuclear chromatin, frayed (splintered) chromatoidal bodies, and up to 8 nuclei in cyst forms
  - Nonpathogenic

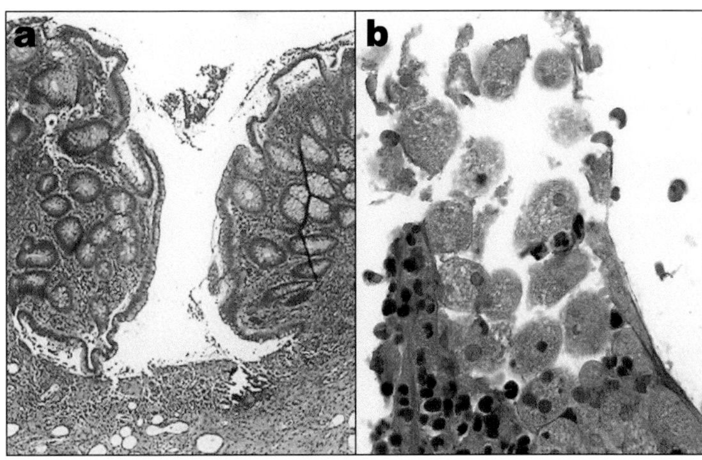

i6.42 H&E stained sections of amebic colitis
a Low magnification shows classic flask shaped ulcer
b Higher magnification reveals trophozoites with ingested RBCs

- *Entamoeba hartmanni*
  - Significantly smaller than *E histolytica*
  - Nondirectonal motility; cytoplasm & trophozoite/cyst structures like *E histolytica*
  - No ingested RBCs
- *Endolimax nana*
  - Small troph & cyst; no peripheral chromatin; cyst has 4 nuclei with karyosomes
  - Troph is nondirectional with single nucleus
  - Nonpathogen
- *Iodamoeba butschlii*
  - No peripheral chromatin
  - Cyst has prominent iodine staining vacuole & large karyosome
  - Trophozoite is nondirectional and has large karyosome
  - Nonpathogen

- Free living amebae
  - Found widely in the environment; rarely opportunistic human pathogens
  - *Naegleria fowleri*
    - Causes primary amebic meningoencephalitis (PAM)
    - Persons who have been swimming or diving in warm stagnant fresh water sources
    - Enters through the nasal cavity and travels to the frontal lobe of the brain via the olfactory nerve running through the cribriform plate
    - Usually fatal

ISBN 978-089189-6616

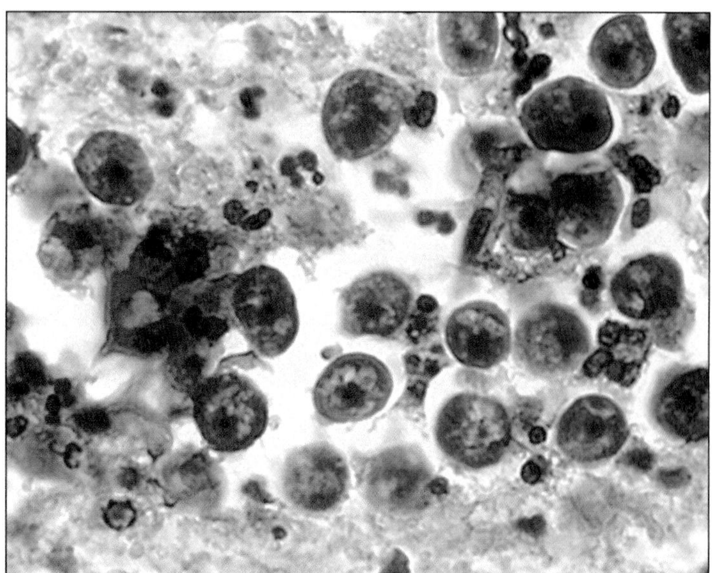

i6.43 *Naegleria fowleri* trophozoite

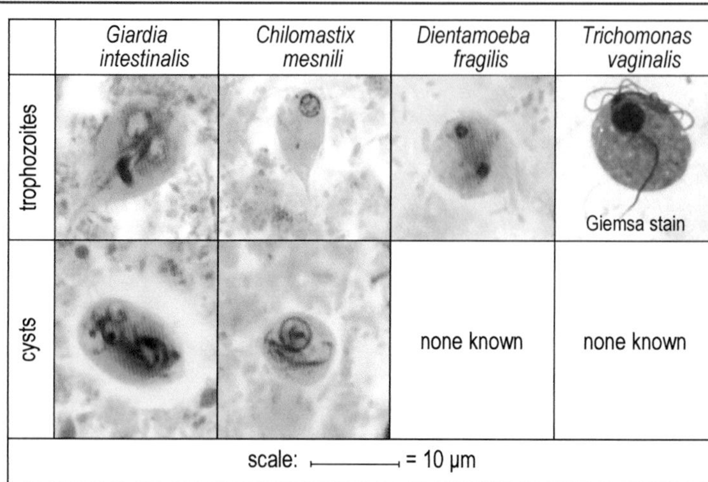

i6.45 Common intestinal & genitourinary flagellates (modified trichrome stain unless indicated)

    - Trophozoites found in CSF or in meninges and surrounding brain tissue i6.43
    - 10-35 µm trophozoites, small nucleus with a large dense central karyosome
    - CSF specimens should not be refrigerated if suspected
  - *Acanthamoeba* spp & *Balamuthia mandrillaris*
    - Both cause granulomatous amebic encephalitis (GAE)
    - Cutaneous or pulmonary i6.44a source
    - Hematogenous dissemination to brain; organisms found in perivascular spaces
    - *Acanthamoeba* spp can also cause amebic keratitis in contact lens wearers
    - Cysts have 2 walls, 1 nucleus, large karyosome i6.44b
    - Trophozoites pleomorphic; small nucleus with a large central karyosome i6.44c
    - Cultures can be performed on lawn of bacteria (*E coli*)

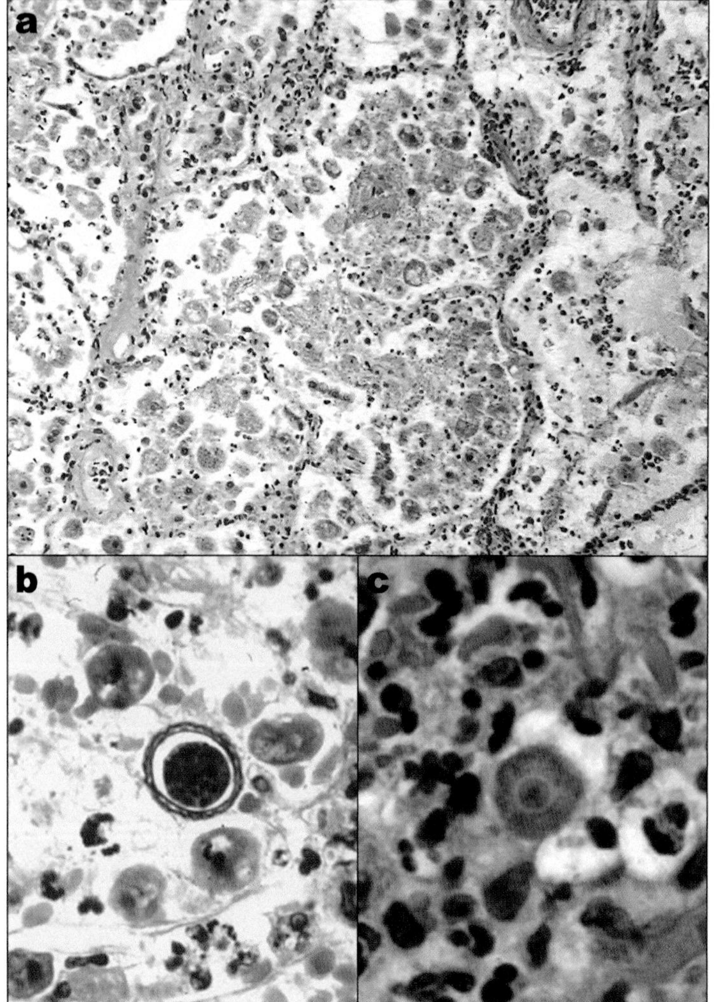

i6.44 *Acanthamoeba*: a free living amebic infection of the lung; b cyst; c trophozoite

6.4.2.2 Flagellates (Mastigophora) i6.45

6.4.2.2.1 *Giardia lamblia* (also known as *G intestinalis*)

- Trophozoites (10-20 µm in length) seen in stool specimens or small bowel biopsies
  - Duodenal aspirate is specimen of choice
  - When viewed from top, kite shaped with central axoneme; 2 nuclei, 1 on either side of centrally located axostyle; 2 parabasal bodies located by axostyle; 2 sucking disks
  - Flagella not easily seen

Parasitology>Protozoa

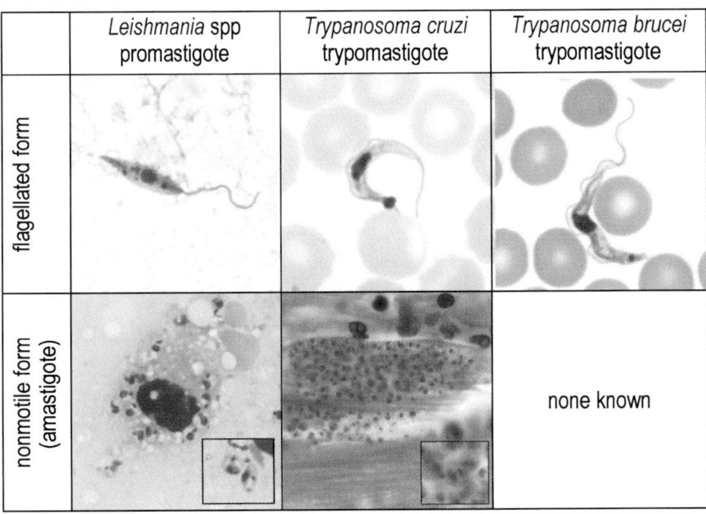

i6.46 Hemoflagellates; images not shown to scale

Leishmania amastigotes | Trypanosoma cruzi amastigotes | Toxoplasma gondii tachyzoites | Histoplasma capsulatum yeasts

i6.47 Intracellular objects

- In wet specimens, characteristic falling leaf motility
- Similar in appearance to *Chilomastix mesnili*: Nonpathogenic; lacks central axoneme, rotary motion; cyst lemon shaped with a single nucleus

- Cysts (8-12 μm) oval and contain 4 nuclei located along central axoneme
  - EIA the preferred method of diagnosis over microscopic methods; DFA; multiplex PCR
  - Most common cause of protozoal gastroenteritis
  - Worldwide distribution
  - Associated with daycare centers, backcountry hiking/camping (drinking contaminated water in streams & ponds)

6.4.2.2.2 *Dientamoeba fragilis*

- Trophozoites round, binucleate; nuclei with "fractured" (fragile) central karyosome
- Internalized flagellum
- Worldwide distribution; diarrhea & anal pruritus
- *Dientamoeba* & *Enterobius vermicularis* (pinworm) coinfection common

6.4.2.2.3 *Trichomonas vaginalis*

- Sexually transmitted; causes vaginitis
- Trophozoites pear shaped with large nucleus at the anterior end of central axostyle
- Undulating membrane that extends about halfway down the organism
- 4 flagella
- Characteristic jerky nondirectional motility

6.4.2.2.4 *Leishmania* spp i6.46

- Best diagnosed on biopsy of infected tissue
- Giemsa-stained smears or hematoxylin & eosin (H&E)-stained sections show tiny 2-5 μm intracellular amastigotes within histiocytes t6.24
- Oval, with small nucleus adjacent to distinct rod-shaped kinetoplast

t6.24 Differential diagnosis for multiple tiny 2-5 μm intracellular organisms i6.47

Organism	Differentiating features	Cell type infected
Leishmania spp	Amastigotes with a small, barlike kinetoplast, GMS-negative	Histiocytes
Histoplasma capsulatum	Small oval yeasts with narrow based budding, pseudocapsule on H&E, GMS-positive	Histiocytes
Toxoplasma gondii	Somewhat curved tachyzoites, mostly extracellular, some in cysts, GMS-negative	Multiple cell types
Trypanosoma cruzi	Amastigotes with a large prominent kinetoplast, GMS-negative	Multiple cell types including heart muscle (classic)

GMS, Gomori methanamine silver

- Acquired from the bite of the sandfly (*Phlebotomus* & *Lutzomyia* genera)
- Most cases found in Algeria, Afghanistan, Saudi Arabia, Syria, Pakistan, Peru, Brazil
- 3 main forms of disease
  - Cutaneous
    - *L tropica*, *L major*, *L aethiopica* (Old World); *L mexicana*, *L braziliensis* (New World)
    - Solitary self-limiting cutaneous lesion at or near the insect bite
    - Seen principally around the Mediterranean
  - Mucocutaneous
    - *L braziliensis* complex
    - Oral/nasal persistent & highly destructive lesions
  - Visceral (kala azar)
    - *L donovani*
    - Hepatosplenic & bone marrow infection

ISBN 978-089189-6616

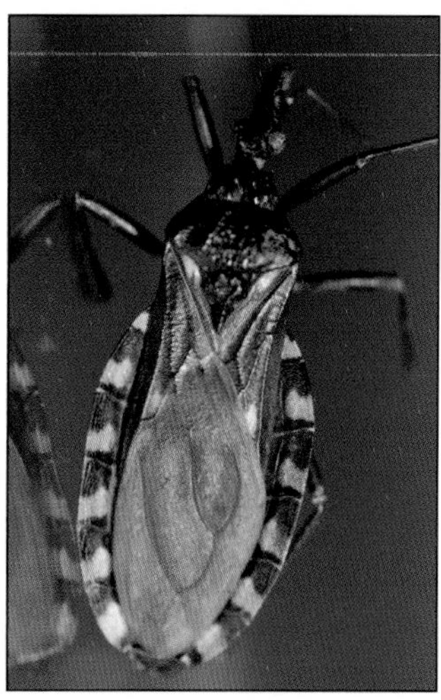

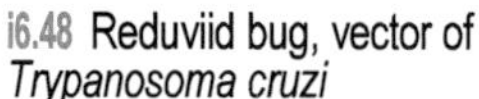

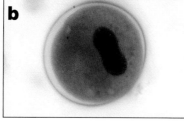

i6.48 Reduviid bug, vector of *Trypanosoma cruzi*

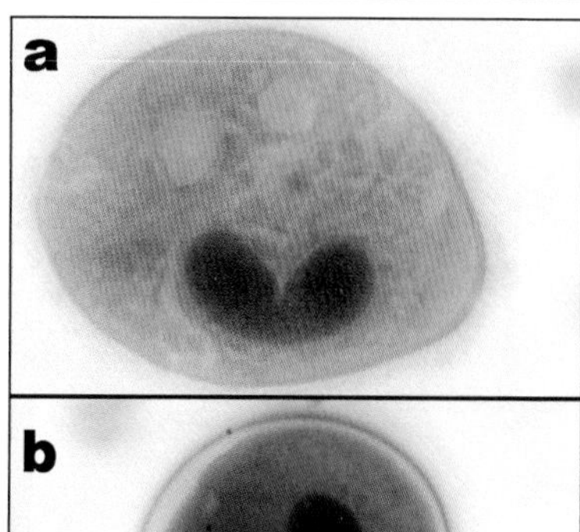

i6.49 *Balantidium coli*; a trophozoite (unstained), b cyst (iron hematoxylin stain)

6.4.2.2.5 *Trypanosoma* spp

- Trypomastigotes can be found in the peripheral blood in acute phase
- *T cruzi* 20 µm and C-shaped with a large posterior kinetoplast
- *T brucei* 30 µm and delicately curved with a small posterior kinetoplast
- Size of kinetoplast the most important feature for differentiating the 2
- Finding peripheral blood trypomastigotes aided by buffy coat examination
- Can be found in heart or other affected organ in chronic phase
- Otherwise, can be diagnosed by serology
- *T cruzi* is the cause of Chagas disease (American trypanosomiasis)
  - Can infect the muscularis of the distal esophagus, resulting in achalasia
  - Can infect myocardium; leading cause of heart failure in South & Central America
- Acquired from reduviid (kissing) bug i6.48
  - Parasite is defecated in feces of reduviid bug when it bites the host
  - Inoculation site (chagoma) often on the face
  - Reduviid bugs found in homes constructed of mud, adobe, and/or thatch
  - Can also be transmitted in other ways: Mother to child, ingestion, transfusion
- *T brucei* is the cause of African sleeping sickness (African trypanosomiasis)
  - Acquired from tsetse (*Glossina*) fly

6.4.2.3 Ciliates (Ciliophora)

6.4.2.3.1 *Balantidium coli* i6.49

- Causes self-limiting diarrhea
- Large trophozoite (up to 200 µm) with cytostome & cilia provide motility
- Thick-walled cyst
- 2 nuclei in both trophozoite & cyst

6.4.3 Apicomplexa

6.4.3.1 Coccidia i6.50

Cystoisospora belli oocysts (25-30 µm maximum dimension)	*Cyclospora cayetanensis* oocysts (8-10 µm diameter)	*Cryptosporidium* spp oocysts (4-6 µm diameter)	*Microsporidia* spp spores (0.8-4 µm maximum dimension)
			(chromotrope 2R stain)
scale: ⟼ = 10 µm			

i6.50 Coccidia & microsporidia (modified acid-fast stain unless indicated)

- *Cryptosporidium parvum* & *Cryptosporidium hominis*
  - Diagnosis
    - Stool samples: 4-6 µm oocysts which are visible with modified acid-fast stain
    - Stool EIA, multiplex PCR, DFA
  - Major cause of protracted watery diarrhea in immunocompromised hosts
- *Cyclospora cayetanensis*
  - Diagnosis
    - Stool samples: Visible with modified acid-fast stain or by autofluorescence; multiplex PCR
    - Infection found principally in Nepal, Peru, Haiti & Guatemala, but has been identified as a source of foodborne disease in the United States from imported soft fruits & vegetables
  - Causes watery diarrhea

- *Cystoisospora* (formerly *Isospora*) *belli*
  - Diagnosis
    - Stool: Oocysts, 25-30 µm, with typical ellipsoidal shape and 1 or 2 sporocysts visible with modified acid-fast stain
  - Causes watery diarrhea
- Sarcocystis
  - May infect intestine and/or striated muscle causing diarrhea and/or myositis
  - Diagnosis
    - Stool: Identification of oocysts (15-20 µm long by 15-20 µm wide) containing 2 sporocysts; will autofluoresce under UV microscopy; weakly acid-fast
    - Skeletal or cardiac muscle: Bradyzoites in tissue specimens
- *Toxoplasma gondii*
  - Diagnosis
    - Tachyzoites are 3-5 µm curved structures with large eccentric nucleus; no kinetoplast; bradyzoites are the intracellular replicative form
    - Serology: IgM positive in congenital & acute infection; rising or very high (>1:1024) IgG also suggests recent infection; low level IgG suggests prior infection and suggests that a pregnant woman is not at risk
    - Polymerase chain reaction
  - Cat is the definitive host
  - Transmitted by ingestion of cat oocyst contaminated feces; ingestion of undercooked meat of animals harboring tissue cysts; blood/organ transplantation; transplacentally
  - Clinical
    - Mononucleosislike syndrome with posterior cervical lymphadenopathy
    - When acquired during pregnancy: in the first trimester, there is risk of fetal loss; in late pregnancy there is risk of fetal CNS infection (periventricular calcification & chorioretinitis)
    - Immunocompromised patients at risk for CNS toxoplasmosis

6.4.3.2 *Microspora* (microsporidia) i6.50

- Spore-forming unicellular & intracellular organisms, now thought to be fungi
- >150 genera, including *Microsporidium*
- Seen in patients with HIV, organ transplantation, elderly persons
- Species
  - Unclassified organisms are called microsporidia
  - *Enterocytozoon bieneusi* (intestinal & hepatobiliary)
  - *Encephalitozoon hellem* (ocular)
  - *Encephalitozoon* (formerly *Septata*) *intestinalis* (intestinal & disseminated)
- Diagnosis
  - Small intestinal biopsy: Numerous oval intracellular organisms in apical aspect of enterocytes
  - Stool samples: 1-3 µm spores that stain deep red with a modified Weber trichrome stain
  - Polymerase chain reaction

6.4.3.3 *Plasmodium* spp

- 4 major species cause malaria: *P falciparum*, *P vivax*, *P ovale*, *P malariae*
  - Human cases of *P knowlesi* also reported in southeast Asia
  - Found in tropics & subtropics worldwide
  - *P ovale* confined to parts of western Africa
- All malarial species are spread by the female *Anopheles* mosquito
  - Sporozoites injected into host go to the liver and proliferate (exoerythrocytic schizogony)
  - Schizonts rupture and release merozoites into bloodstream
  - These infect red cells to initiate erythrocytic schizogony
- Clinical
  - In endemic areas, young children & pregnant women are at greatest risk of death
    - Relative immunity develops in those who survive childhood
    - Outside of endemic areas, all age groups are equally susceptible
  - After inoculation, malaria usually presents in 1-4 weeks
    - The first week is asymptomatic
    - Initial stages of erythrocyte schizogony relatively disorganized and symptoms vague
    - Within weeks schizogony becomes synchronized and produce fever cycles
    - Eventually, symptoms are paroxysmal, with symptomatic periods lasting 6-12 hours and correlating with intermittent intravascular hemolysis

 ISBN 978-089189-6616

	P falciparum	*P malariae*	*P vivax*	*P ovale*
early stage trophozoite (ring form)				
late stage trophozoite	Not usually seen in peripheral blood	band form	ameboid trophozoite	comet form
schizont	Not usually seen in peripheral blood	rosette schizont		
gametocyte	banana form			

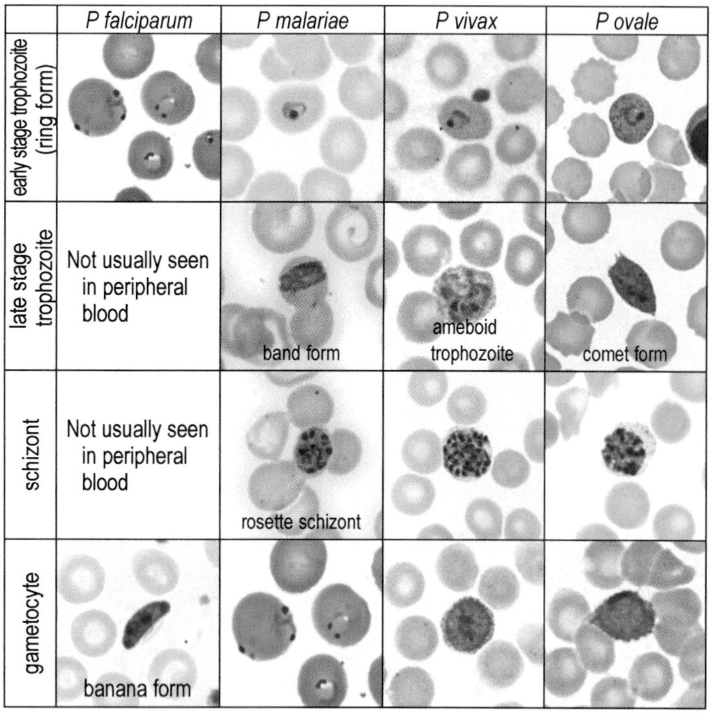

i6.51 Malaria forms

- Some clinical features are species specific
  - Fever spikes every 48 hours (tertian fever): *P ovale*, *P vivax*, *P falciparum*
  - Lethality: *P falciparum* ("malignant tertian malaria")
  - Fever spikes every 72 hours (quartan fever): *P malariae*
  - Nephrotic syndrome: *P malariae*
  - CNS involvement: *P falciparum*
  - Hemosiderinuria, hemoglobinuria & renal failure: *P falciparum* ("blackwater fever")
  - True relapse/recurrence: *P vivax*, *P ovale*
- Reinvasion of RBCs by liver merozoites (from hepatic hypnozoites), after complete clearing of the blood stream by therapy or immunity
- Recrudescence: All
  - Parasitemia rendered low by treatment or immunity increases again
- Infection of young red cells: *P vivax*, *P ovale*
- Infection of old red cells: *P malariae*
- Infection of all red cells: *P falciparum*

- Effect of inherited red cell anomalies
  - Hemoglobin S: Protective against *P falciparum*
  - Thalassemia, hemoglobin C, hemoblobin E, hereditary persistence of hemoglobin F: Thought to be protective
  - Duffy negative blood type: Protective against *P vivax*
  - Glucose-6-phosphate dehydrogenase (G6PD) deficiency: Protective against all species
  - Hereditary ovalocytosis: Thought to be protective against cerebral malaria
- Laboratory diagnosis
  - Wright stains or fluorescent stains such as acridine orange & rhodamine 123
  - Thick blood film for screening
  - Thin blood film for species identification **t6.25**, i6.51, i6.52
  - Ideal time to obtain specimen is before the next anticipated fever spike

t6.25 *Plasmodium* spp

	P vivax & ovale	*P malariae*	*P falciparum*
Infected red cell	Enlarged (reticulocyte), may be fimbriated (*P ovale*)	Small to normal size	All sizes
Ring form trophozoite	≥1/3 the size of red cell, multiple infection not uncommon	Thick, small (1/3 the size of the red cell), bird's eye forms (chromatin dot appears to be detached in center of ring, forming an "eye")	Delicate, small (<1/3 the size of the red cell), may have 2 chromatin dots, appliqué forms, multiply infected RBCs common
Mature trophozoite	*P vivax*: Large amoeboid form that fills red cells *P ovale*: More compact than *P vivax*	Band & basket forms, do not fill red cell, prominent hematin pigment	Rare in peripheral blood
Schizont	*P vivax*: 12-24 merozoites *P ovale*: 6-14 merozoites	6-12 merozoites, often surrounding a clump of hematin pigment ("rosette" form)	Rare in peripheral blood
Gametocytes	Large, oval	Oval, often fills red cell	Banana shaped, distorts red cell
Inclusions	Schüffner dots	–	Maurer clefts
Hematin pigment (brown-black)	+, delicate	+, coarse	+, delicate

  - Examination of at least 100 oil immersion thick film fields or 300 thin film fields is required to achieve the reported sensitivity (5 parasites/μL)
  - Single negative smear insufficient to exclude malaria; 2-3 smears over a 24-hour period are preferred
  - May be aided by flow cytometry, antigen detection & antibody detection
- Species identification
  - Forms found in blood
    - Early trophozoites (ring forms): in early stages occupy <½ the red cell, with 1 or at most 2 nuclei, enlarge, and may take on characteristic features

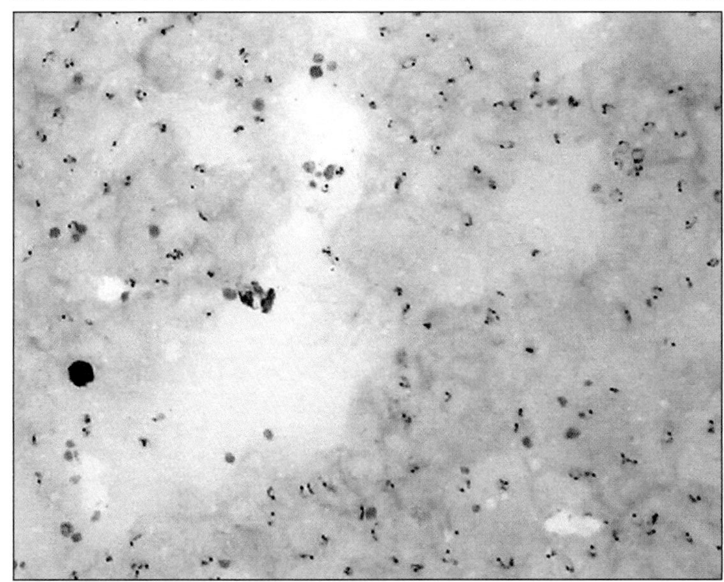

i6.52 Thick blood film showing numerous early trophozoite (ring) forms of *Plasmodium falciparum*

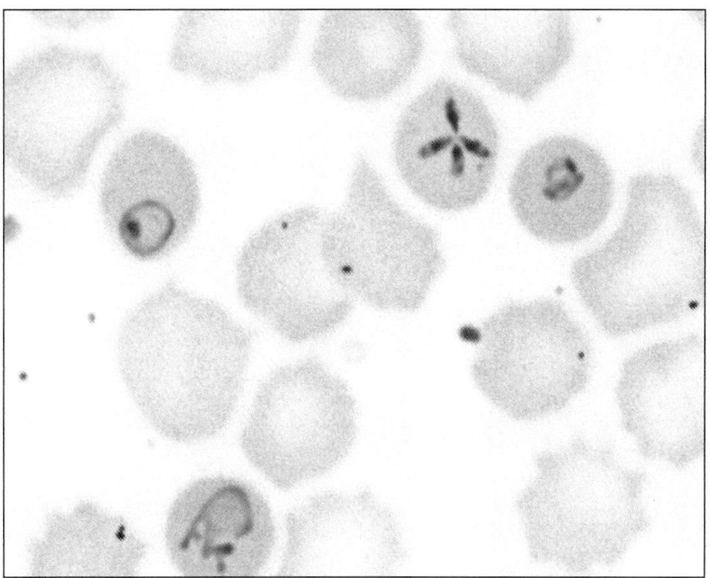

i6.53 *Babesia*

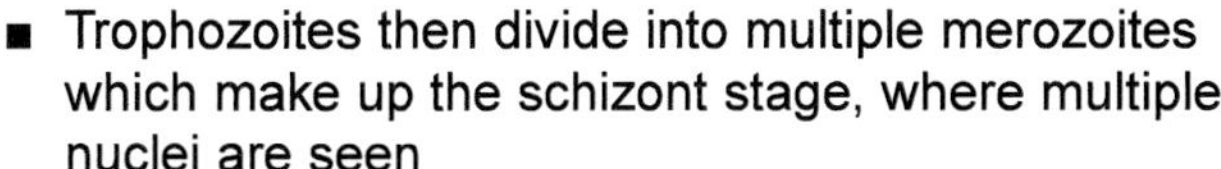

    - Trophozoites then divide into multiple merozoites which make up the schizont stage, where multiple nuclei are seen
    - Schizont ruptures & releases the merozoites to infect other RBCs
    - Some trophozoites also form a gametocyte; a solid mononuclear structure occupying >½ the red cell that is the infective stage for the mosquito
    - Mature stages may contain hematin (brown black) pigment, a heme breakdown product
  - *P falciparum*
    - Only ring forms & gametocytes seen within peripheral blood
    - Erythrocytes with intermediate forms are sequestered in capillaries of the liver, brain, heart & kidneys
    - Ring forms may have double chromatin dots ("headphone forms")
    - Multiple ring forms commonly seen in a single erythrocyte
    - Maurer clefts may be seen: round to comma-shaped red cytoplasmic dots
    - Gametocytes are banana shaped
    - Infected red cells may be of any size
  - *P vivax* & *P ovale*
    - Found in erythrocytes that are slightly enlarged
    - Schüffner dots (stippling) may be present
    - All stages present
    - Schizonts of *P ovale* & *P vivax* have 6-14 & 12-24 merozoites, respectively
    - *P vivax* tends to have more ameboid forms whereas *P ovale* is more compact
    - Erythrocytes infected by *P ovale* are more oval (hence the name) and may be fimbriated
  - *P malariae*
    - Infected erythrocytes of small to normal size
    - No Schüffner dots
    - All stages present
    - Schizonts have 6-12 merozoites
  - Mixed infections: 5% of cases, most often *P falciparum* & *P vivax*
  - Degree of parasitemia (% infected red cells) most important with *P falciparum*
    - >2% parasitemia is considered severe
    - After treatment initiated, transient increase in parasitemia followed by progressive diminution

6.4.3.4 *Babesia*

- Diagnosis (see Immunology 8.4.5)
  - Direct observation in blood smear
    - Trophozoites often multiple in red cells i6.53; may form diads or tetrads (Maltese cross); light blue ring forms with red chromatin dots
    - Extraerythrocytic ring forms often present
    - No pigment or nonring forms seen

- Antibabesial antibodies may be misleading, especially in places with high prevalence
  - Antibody titer, on immunofluorescence assay (IFA), of ≥1:1024 thought to indicate active infection
  - Remote infections typically have a titer of ≤1:64
- Polymerase chain reaction

- Found in United States, Europe, Asia & Africa
  - In the United States, mainly in the northeastern states, usually caused by *B microti*
  - *Babesia divergens* most prevalent species in Europe
- Transmitted by ticks of the genus *Ixodes*
  - In the northeastern United States, *Ixodes scapularis* (formerly *I dammini*) most common
  - Reservoirs are the white-tailed deer & the white-footed mouse
    - White-footed mouse harbors *Babesia divergens* and also:
      - *Borrelia burgdorferi*
      - *Anaplasma phagocytophilum* (human granulocytic ehrlichiosis)
      - *I scapularis* tick may transmit all 3 of these organisms
    - Coinfection with flavivirus has also been noted
- Infection results in a nonperiodic fever & hemolysis
  - Fatal disease occurs mainly in those who have had splenectomies and in immunodeficient hosts

6.4.4 Metazoa

6.4.4.1 Nematodes, intestinal

- *Enterobius vermicularis* (pinworm, oxyuriasis)
  - Adult female has slightly bent & pointed (pinlike) tail
  - Egg is a thin walled 30-50 μm oval with 1 side flattened egg not routinely found in stool; cellophane tape test for collection or use of commercially available sticky paddle i6.54
  - Most common helminthic infection in American children
  - Infection is acquired from ingestion of eggs
  - Mature females inhabit cecum & appendix; nocturnally lay eggs in perianal region
  - Common symptoms are anal pruritus, vaginitis, and/or enuresis
  - Appendicitis is an occasional complication

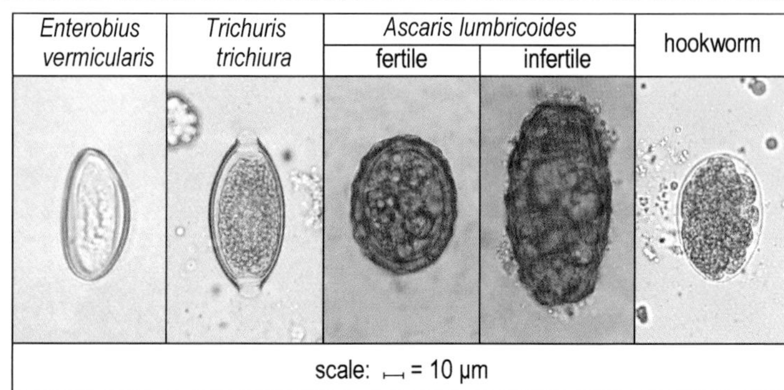

i6.54 Nematode eggs

- *Trichuris trichiura* (whipworm)
  - Adult worm measures up to 5 cm and has a whiplike anterior end
  - Eggs 50× 25 μm, brownish thick shells, barrel shaped with bilateral polar plugs
  - Infection asymptomatic to dysenterylike; rectal prolapse in young children
- *Ascaris lumbricoides* (roundworm)
  - Largest nematode parasitizing the human intestine; adults up to 35 cm
  - Egg 60 μm, bile stained, thick hyaline shell, and rough mammillated surface i6.54
  - Infection results from ingestion of eggs, which hatch to produce larvae
  - Larvae penetrate mucosa, enter bloodstream, and are carried to lungs; may produce transient infiltrates with eosinophilia (Löffler syndrome)
  - Expectorated & swallowed, mature into adults which infect duodenum
  - Asymptomatic or complicated by bowel obstruction, cholangitis, or appendicitis

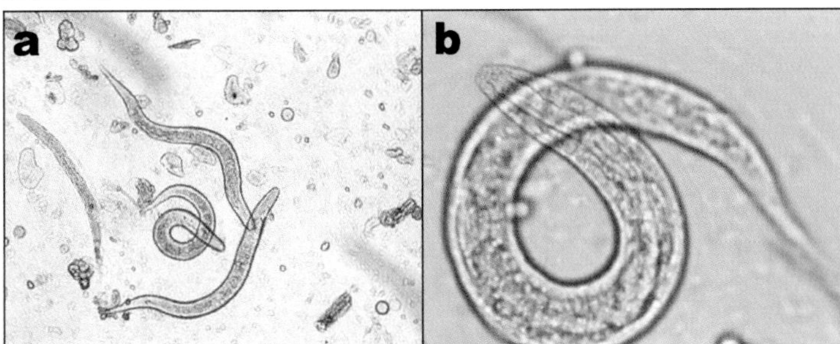

i6.55 a Rhabditiform larvae of *Strongyloides stercoralis*
b The short buccal cavity allows it to be differentiated from hookworm rhabditiform larvae

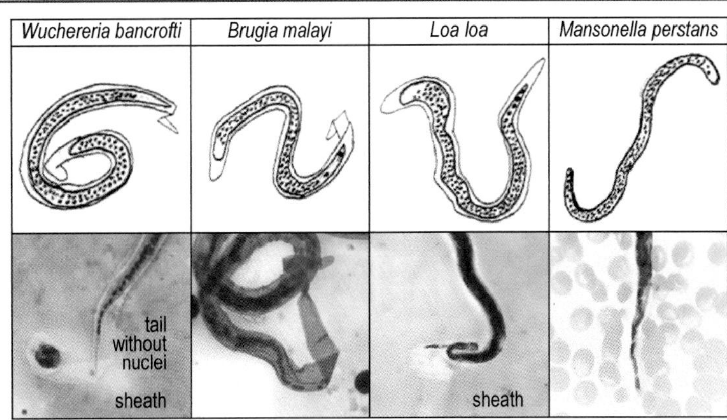

i6.56 Microfilariae found in peripheral blood

- *Necator americanus* & *Ancylostoma duodenale* (hookworms)
  - Adult hookworms measure ~1 cm in length
  - Mouth parts differ: *N americanus* has cutting plates; *A duodenale* has "teeth"
  - Eggs indistinguishable from one another i6.54
    - Thin translucent wall encloses morulalike cluster of spherical embryos
    - Oval, 60×40 µm
  - Found in Asia & sub-Saharan Africa, especially coastal regions
    - *N americanus* (but not *A duodenale*) found in southeastern United States
  - Infection results from penetration of skin by larvae, usually skin of feet
    - Localized pruritic lesion (ground itch)
  - Larvae pass through lungs (Löeffler syndrome) are expectorated and swallowed
  - Adults infest small bowel; may produce iron-deficiency anemia
- *Strongyloides stercoralis* (threadworm)
  - Adult females measure ~3 mm; burrow into intestinal crypts
  - Egg identical to the hookworm egg i6.54 but usually not found in stool
    - Eggs hatch in bowel, and feces contain rhabditoid larvae i6.55
    - Larvae similar to hookworm larvae but have short buccal groove & prominent genital primordium
  - Duodenal aspirate may be helpful
  - Found in:
    - Tropical & subtropical regions throughout the world
    - Also in parts of the southeastern United States
  - Course similar to hookworm: Penetration of skin, migration through lungs, expectorated & swallowed, resulting in duodenal infection
    - In malnourished host, larvae may penetrate bowel wall, circulating through the lungs & reinfecting the duodenum (autoinfection)
    - In immunocompromised host, autoinfection can lead to hyperinfection, a potentially deadly complication in which larvae disseminate widely

t6.26 Microfilariae in blood

Organism	Sheath	Tail nuclei	Periodicity of microfilariae in blood	Adult found in
Wuchereria bancrofti	+	None	Nocturnal	Lymphatics
Brugia malayi	+	2 discontinuous	Nocturnal	Lymphatics
Loa loa	+	Continuous row	Diurnal	Migrating through the subcutis
Mansonella perstans	–	Continuous row	None	Body cavities or subcutis

6.4.4.2 Nematodes, filarial t6.26, i6.56

- Microfilaria found in blood
  - *W bancrofti* & *B malayi* are acquired through the bite of mosquitoes
    - *W bancrofti* & *B malayi* adults infect the lymphatics (elephantiasis)
    - Shed into blood primarily at night (nocturnal periodicity)
    - Highest likelihood of detection is between 10 pm & 2 am
  - *Loa loa* is acquired from the mango (*Chrysops*) fly
    - *Loa loa* adults migrate through subcutaneous & conjunctival locations

ISBN 978-089189-6616

- Causes transient migratory edema (calabar swellings)
- Diurnal periodicity

- *Mansonella perstans* are acquired from the biting midge (*Culicoides*)
  - Inhabit body cavities

- Microfilaria not found in blood
  - *O volvulus* is acquired from the *Simulium* black fly
    - Adults ball up in a subcutaneous nodule (onchocercoma)
    - Release microfilariae into the surrounding skin
    - Microfilariae migrate through the skin & eye
    - Leading cause of blindness (river blindness) in central Africa & Central America
    - Diagnosis is by identifying characteristic larvae in skin snips
- *Dracunculus medinesis* (Guinea worm)
  - Transmitted by ingesting infected fresh water
  - Parasite migrates to skin and grows up to 30 inches; forms blister
  - Worm removed by slowly pulling it around stick (1 inch day)
- *Dirofilaria immitis* (dog heartworm) is acquired from a mosquito
  - Presents as a subcutaneous or pulmonary granulomatous nodule surrounding a degenerating worm

6.4.4.3 Nematodes, zoonotic

- *Trichinella spiralis*
  - Consumption of undercooked meat, especially pork & wild game
  - Infection of the skeletal muscle by encysted larvae, producing myositis & weakness
  - Can be seen on histologic sections of infected skeletal muscle
  - Diagnosis can be made on serology
- *Toxocara canis* (dog roundworm) & *T cati* (cat roundworm)
  - Humans accidentally ingest the eggs
  - Causes of visceral larva migrans (VLM) & ocular larva migrans (OLM)
  - Organism wanders throughout various organs
  - Produces syndrome of hypereosinophilia, hepatosplenomegaly & pneumonitis

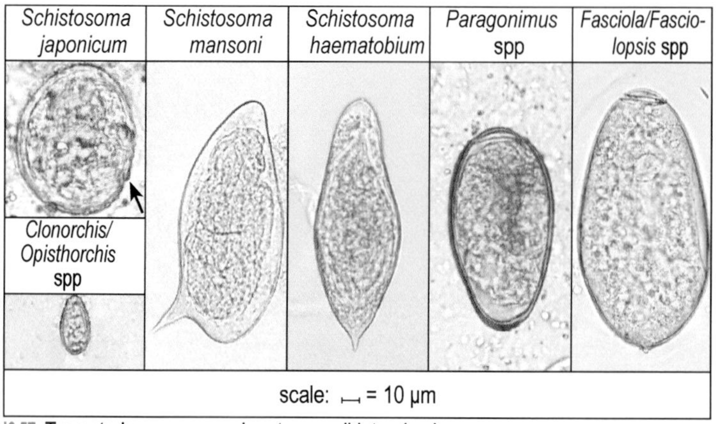

Schistosoma japonicum	*Schistosoma mansoni*	*Schistosoma haematobium*	*Paragonimus* spp	*Fasciola/Fasciolopsis* spp
Clonorchis/Opisthorchis spp				
scale: ⟼ = 10 μm				

i6.57 Trematode ova; arrow denotes small lateral spine

- Anisakiasis
  - Acquired from ingestion of raw or undercooked fish
  - Biopsy may disclose an eosinophil-rich granuloma containing the nematode

6.4.4.4 Trematodes (flukes) t6.27, i6.57

- *Fasciolopsis buski* (intestinal fluke)
  - Acquired by ingestion of freshwater plants (eg, water chestnuts); snail is 1st intermediate host; water plant is 2nd
  - Asia & the Indian subcontinent
  - Infection of duodenum
  - Diagnosis
    - Adult has pointed, but not conical, cephalad
    - Egg 100-150 μm, oval, with thin shell, unshouldered operculum, abopercular knob (identical to *F hepatica*)

t6.27 Operculated eggs

Organism	Shoulder	Size (μm)	Abopercular knob
Clonorchis sinensis	+	30	+
Diphyllobothrium latum (only operculated tapeworm egg)	–	60	+
Paragonimus westermani	+	90	– (abopercular thickening)
Fasciola hepatica *Fasciolopsis buski*	–	120	+

- *Fasciola hepatica* (liver fluke)
  - Acquired by ingestion of freshwater plants (eg, water cress); snail is 1st intermediate host; water plant is 2nd
  - Asia & the Middle East
  - Infection of the bile ducts and hepatic parenchyma with resulting fibrosis/cirrhosis

- Diagnosis
  - Adult has cephalic cone
  - Egg is identical to that of *F buski*

- *Clonorchis sinensis/Opisthorchis* spp (liver fluke)
  - 1st intermediate host is snail; second is freshwater fish
  - Found in parts of Asia
  - Chronic biliary infection
  - Diagnosis
    - Adults have a snoutlike cephalad
    - Egg oval, 30 µm, with shouldered operculum & small abopercular knob
- *Paragonimus westermani* (oriental lung fluke)
  - 1st intermediate host is snail; 2nd intermediate host is freshwater crustaceans (crabs or crayfish)
  - Lung infection with pneumonitis
  - Diagnosis
    - Egg (in sputum or stool) oval, 90 µm, with shouldered operculum
- Schistosomiasis (bilharziasis, blood flukes)
  - Acquired through penetration of the skin (swimmer's itch) by fork-tailed cercariae
    - Found in snail infested water
    - Migrate through the bloodstream to mesenteric & pelvic blood vessels
    - Releases eggs into the bloodstream, which are lodged in small capillaries
    - Eggs can penetrate bowel or bladder wall to be excreted in stool or urine
  - Clinical
    - Acute stage mediated by circulating immune complexes (Katayama fever)
    - Chronic stage reflects local tissue reaction to eggs
  - *S mansoni* found in South America, Caribbean, Africa, Middle East; affects hepatic portal & inferior mesenteric distribution. Eggs can be found in rectal biopsies
  - *S japonicum* found in the Far East; affects liver, leading to cirrhosis; rarely affects CNS
  - *S haematobium* found in Africa, Middle East; affects venous plexus of the bladder, leading to hematuria and irritative bladder symptoms; may result in squamous cell carcinoma of the bladder. Eggs may be seen in urine or bladder biopsies
  - *S intercalatum* closely resembles *S haematobium* but produces intestinal schistosomiasis

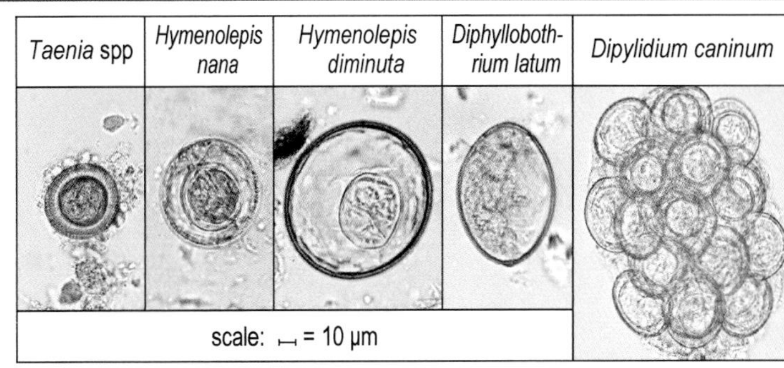

i6.58 Cestode eggs

  - Diagnosis
    - Eggs 75-150 µm and have a single spine
    - *S haematobium* has a terminal spine
    - *S mansoni* has a lateral spine
    - *S japonicum* has small, knoblike spine

6.4.4.5 Cestodes (tapeworms) i6.58

- *Taenia saginata* (beef tapeworm)
  - Diagnosis
    - Egg (identical that of *T solium*) 30-40 µm, spherical, with thick radially striated wall and 3 pairs of hooks
    - Scolex has 4 suckers and a smooth surface (unarmed rostellum)
    - Proglottid longer than it is wide, with >13 lateral uterine branches
  - South & Central America; not found in the United States
  - Acquired by ingestion of encysted organisms (cysticerci) in beef
  - Small bowel infection by adult worm
  - Eggs of *T saginata* not infectious, unlike *T solium*; thus cysticercosis (larval form of disease in humans) due to *T saginata* does not occur
- *Taenia solium* (pork tapeworm)
  - Diagnosis
    - Egg is identical to that of *T saginata*
    - Scolex has 4 suckers and many tiny hooklets on its surface (armed rostellum)
    - Proglottid longer than it is wide, with <13 lateral uterine branches
    - Encysted larval form (cysticercosis) consists of a cyst, roughly 1 cm, with invaginated scolex with a double row of hooklets (acid-fast & birefringent)

ISBN 978-089189-6616

- Occasionally encountered in the United States, usually in recent immigrants
- Intestinal infection results from ingestion of encysted organisms (cysticerci) in "measly" pork
- Cysticercosis results from ingestion of eggs shed in feces of person with intestinal infection; pork ingestion not required

- *Diphyllobothrium latum* (fish tapeworm)
  - Diagnosis
    - Egg 60 µm oval structure with a smooth shell and an unshouldered operculum and small abopercular knob (similar to *P westermani*, which is larger and has a shouldered operculum)
    - Scolex resembles elongated almond with 2 longitudinal sucking grooves
    - Proglottid wider than it is long, with coiled uterus in the shape of a rosette
  - Found in Scandinavia, Russia, Canada, northern United States & Alaska
  - Acquired through ingestion of poorly cooked freshwater fish, resulting in intestinal infection
  - May be complicated by vitamin B_{12} deficiency
- *Hymenolepis nana* (dwarf tapeworm)
  - Diagnosis
    - Egg has thin inner & outer shells; space in between contains 2 pairs of polar filaments; inner shell contains embryo with hooklets
  - Relatively common in the United States
  - Acquired from accidental ingestion of infected arthropods (beetles)
  - Person-to-person spread may occur
- *Dipylidium caninum* (double-pored dog tapeworm)
  - Diagnosis
    - Egg resembles *H diminuta*, except tends to occur in packets of 5-15 eggs
    - Proglottid has a double genital pore, one exiting out of each side
  - Infects cats & dogs; may infects humans after accidental ingestion of fleas
- *Echinococcus* spp
  - Produce cysts containing protoscoleces & hooklets
  - Acquired from food contaminated with eggs from stool of infected dog, the definitive host
  - Common in sheep & cattle raising areas (pastoral infections)
  - Hydatid cyst disease: human ingests eggs and liberated oncosphere migrates to liver and other organs

6.4.4.6 Additional pearls of parasitology t6.28-t6.31

t6.28 Dual infections involving parasites

Ascaris lumbricoides & *Trichuris trichiura*
Pinworm & *Dientamoeba fragilis*
Babesia, Lyme disease & *Anaplasma phagocytophilum*
Lepromatous leprosy or HTLV1 & *Strongyloides stercoralis* hyperinfection

t6.29 Parasitic oculocutaneous infections

Loa loa disease is caused by the adult worm
Onchocerca volvulus disease is caused by the larvae

t6.30 Parasitic infections capable of person to person spread

Enterobius vermicularis
Hymenolepis nana

t6.31 Parasitic infections in immunodeficient patients

Type of immunodeficiency	Susceptibility
T-cell (cellular) immunodeficiency	Many, eg, toxoplasmosis, *Cryptosporidium*, *Cystoisospora*, *Cyclospora*, microsporidia, are more common Others, eg, *Strongyloides*, are more severe
B-cell (humoral) immunodeficiency	*Giardia* more common
Splenectomy	Babesiosis more severe

6.5 Mycology

6.5.1 Laboratory methods

- Direct examination
  - 10%-20% potassium hydroxide (KOH) is a wet mount format
    - Useful for observing fungal elements in hair, skin, nails, tissues by breaking down keratin & skin layers
  - Calcofluor white
    - Fluorochrome stain that binds to cellulose and chitin in fungal cell wall i6.59
    - Can be used with 10%-20% KOH to enhance visualizing fungal elements
    - Appropriate filters on fluorescent scope must be used
  - India ink
    - Presumptive identification of *Cryptococcus neoformans* in CSF but low sensitivity
    - Capsules produced by yeast repel India ink particles that look like a "halo" surrounding the yeast cells i6.60

Mycology>Laboratory methods

- Gomori methenamine silver (GMS) or periodic acid-Schiff (PAS) for identification of fungi in tissue sections
- Giemsa for detection of *H capsulatum* in blood or bone marrow
- Matrix-assisted laser desorption/ionization time-of-flight (MALDI-TOF) mass spectrometry
  - Rapid and sensitive method for identification of yeasts and molds

- Fungal culture
  - Usual media: Brain heart infusion (BHI) agar, Sabouraud dextrose agar & inhibitory mold agar **t6.32** incubated at 25°C-30°C for 4-6 weeks
  - Special media **t6.33**

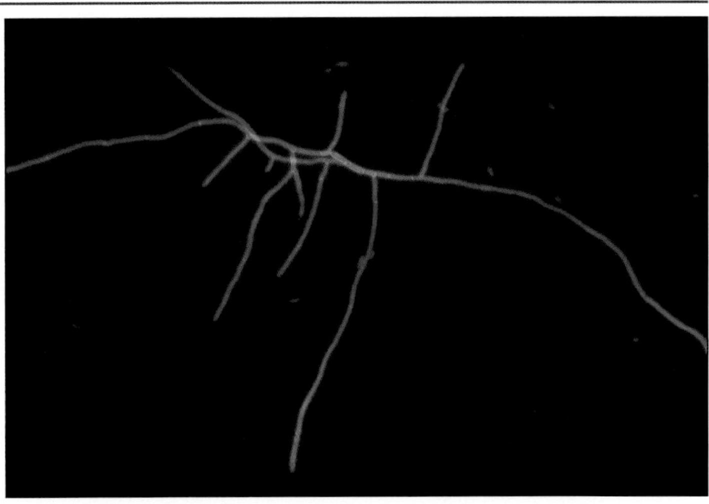

i6.59 Fungal hyphae stained with calcofluor white, viewed under UV light

t6.32 Fungal media

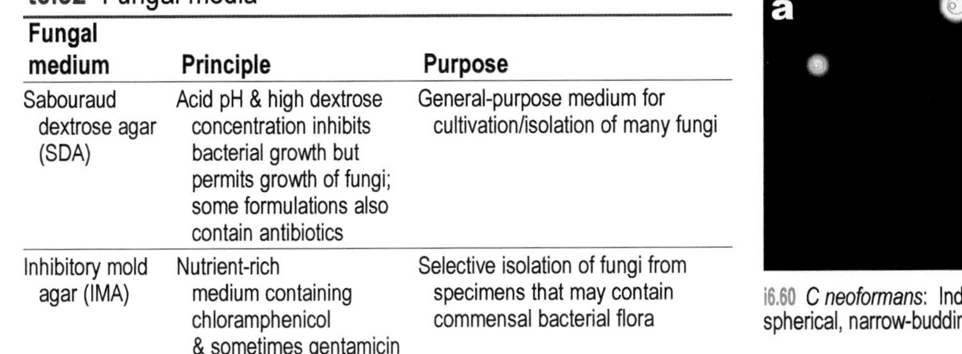

Fungal medium	Principle	Purpose
Sabouraud dextrose agar (SDA)	Acid pH & high dextrose concentration inhibits bacterial growth but permits growth of fungi; some formulations also contain antibiotics	General-purpose medium for cultivation/isolation of many fungi
Inhibitory mold agar (IMA)	Nutrient-rich medium containing chloramphenicol & sometimes gentamicin or ciprofloxacin; chloramphenicol suppresses the growth of many bacteria	Selective isolation of fungi from specimens that may contain commensal bacterial flora
Brain heart infusion agar (BHI)	Nutrient-rich medium containing brain/meat infusion, peptone & dextrose Chloramphenicol & gentamicin can be added for selectivity	The nonselective formulation is a general-purpose medium used in the cultivation/isolation of bacteria, yeasts & molds When supplemented with chloramphenicol & gentamicin, it is used for selective isolation of fungi from specimens that may contain commensal bacterial flora
Cycloheximide-containing media	Cycloheximide inhibits the growth of many saprophytic fungi, while permitting growth of most (but not all) pathogenic fungi Chloramphenicol & gentamicin can be added to inhibit bacteria	Selective isolation of slow-growing pathogenic fungi that may be overgrown by rapidly growing saprophytic fungi Notably, cycloheximide also inhibits the growth of certain pathogenic fungi, including *C neoformans*, many *Candida* spp, *Aspergillus* spp & the zygomycetes, among others It is frequently used to target dermatophytes or thermally dimorphic fungi
CHROMagar	Chloramphenicol inhibits bacteria; chromogenic mix selects for yeasts & differentiates by color formation	Presumptive ID for *C albicans* *C albicans:* Light to medium green colonies *C tropicalis:* Dark blue colonies *C krusei*: Flat, pink colonies

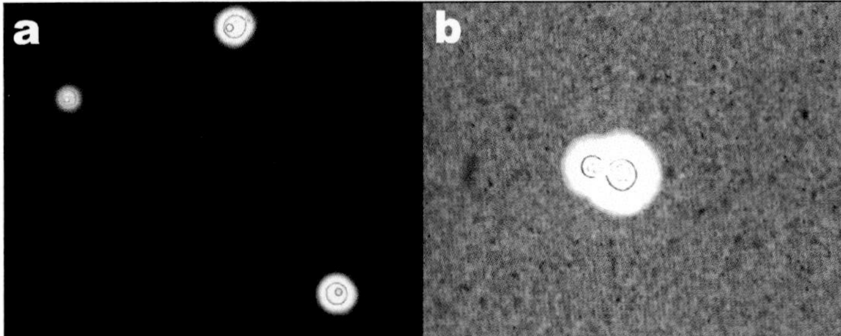

i6.60 *C neoformans*: India ink preparation at a low & b high magnification show spherical, narrow-budding yeasts with thick capsule

t6.33 Specialized fungal culture media

Medium	Purpose
Cornmeal or potato dextrose agar	Promotion of characteristic reproductive structures & pigmentation useful for morphologic identification of mold isolates, when general purpose media prove inadequate for a particular isolate
Cornmeal or rice agar with Tween 80	Promotion of characteristic structures (eg, chlamydospores, arthroconidia) useful for morphologic identification of yeast isolates, when more routine identification methods prove inadequate
Sabouraud dextrose agar, Dixon medium, or Leeming-Notman medium overlaid with sterile olive oil	Isolation/cultivation of *Malassezia* spp, all of which (except *M pachydermatis*) require lipid supplementation for growth
Trichophyton agars	Differentiation between species of *Trichophyton*, which can be difficult to speciate based on morphology alone
Bird seed (Niger seed) agar	Demonstration of phenol oxidase activity in *Cryptococcus neoformans* isolates

- Initial classification of a fungal isolate **t6.34**
  - Colony morphology
    - Yeasts form creamy or mucoid colonies; molds make fuzzy or filamentous colonies
    - Dimorphic fungi grow as yeast at 37°C and as molds at 25°C-30°C

ISBN 978-089189-6616

t6.34 Classification of fungi based on morphology

	Yeast			Mold			Thermally dimorphic
Morphology	Blastoconidia only	Blastoconidia with pseudohyphae	Arthroconidia	Septate hyphae		Pauciseptate hyphae	
				Hyaline/Brightly colored molds (hyphae & other structures are nonmelanized)	Dematiaceous molds (hyphae and/or conidia are darkly pigmented with melanin)		
Important examples	*Cryptococcus* *Candida glabrata* *Rhodotorula* *Malassezia*	*Candida* spp (except *C glabrata*) *Saccharomyces cerevisiae*	*Trichosporon* *Geotrichum*	*Aspergillus* *Penicillium* *Fusarium* Dermatophytes (*Epidermophyton, Microsporum, Trichophyton*)	*Alternaria* *P boydiil,S boydii,* *Scedosporium prolificans,* *Curvularia*	*Zygomycetes* (eg, *Rhizopus, Mucor, Cunninghamella, Rhizomucor*)	*Histoplasma capsulatum* *Blastomyces dermatitidis* *Coccidioides immitis & posadasii** *Paracoccidioides brasiliensis* *Sporothrix schenkii* *Penicillium marnefii*

**In routine culture, Coccidioides produces the same structures (septate hyphae & arthroconidia) whether grown at 25°C or 37°C; it can technically be considered thermally dimorphic, because the structures it produces in tissue (spherules) can be induced in culture at 37°C using special media*

t6.35 Summary of dimorphic fungi

Species	Yeast form characteristics	Mold form characteristics	Route of infection	Common sites of disseminated infection
H capsulatum var *capsulatum*	2-4 µm, narrow based budding	Septate hyphae with tear shaped microconidia & thick walled, tuberculate macroconidia	Inhalation	Reticuloendothelial system, mediastinum
B dermatitidis	8-15 µm thick walled, broad based budding	Septate hyphae with lollipoplike conidia atop unbranched conidiophores	Inhalation	Skin, mucous membranes
C immitis	10-100 µm spherules containing 2-5 µm (nonbudding) endospores	Barrel shaped arthroconidia alternating with empty cells	Inhalation	Skin, bone, joints
P brasiliensis	10-50 µm mariner's wheel (circumferential budding)	Septate hyphae with intercalary & terminal chlamydospores	Inhalation or traumatic inoculation	Skin, mucous membranes, bone marrow, lymphatics
S schenckii	4-6 µm elongated (cigars) with narrow based budding	Rosettes of microconidia at the apex of swollen, delicate conidiophores	Traumatic inoculation	Regional lymphatics
P marneffei	3-5 µm ovoid, divide by fission	Colonies producing diffusible red pigment	Inhalation	Bone marrow, skin

- Yeasts
  - Colony morphology
    - *Cryptococcus* spp may produce mucoid colonies
    - *Candida albicans* may form "feet" or starlike projections
  - Yeasts further classified by biochemical testing, matrix-assisted laser desorption/ionization time-of-flight (MALDI-TOF) mass spectrometry or morphologic classification after growth on special yeast morphology medium
  - Molds
    - Hyaline septate molds have hyphae with frequent septations
      - Surface of colonies may be white or colored
      - Reverse side of the plate is usually light
    - Dematiaceous molds: Septate molds that produce melanin
      - Surface & reverse side of the plate are both dark
    - Zygomycetes: aseptate or pauciseptate
      - Rapidly growing (lid lifters)
      - May be pigmented, but do not make melanin (reverse side of the plate is light)
    - Dimorphic fungi: Septate hyphae at 25°C-30°C; yeasts when incubated at 37°C
    - Molds further classified by examination of conidia or spores

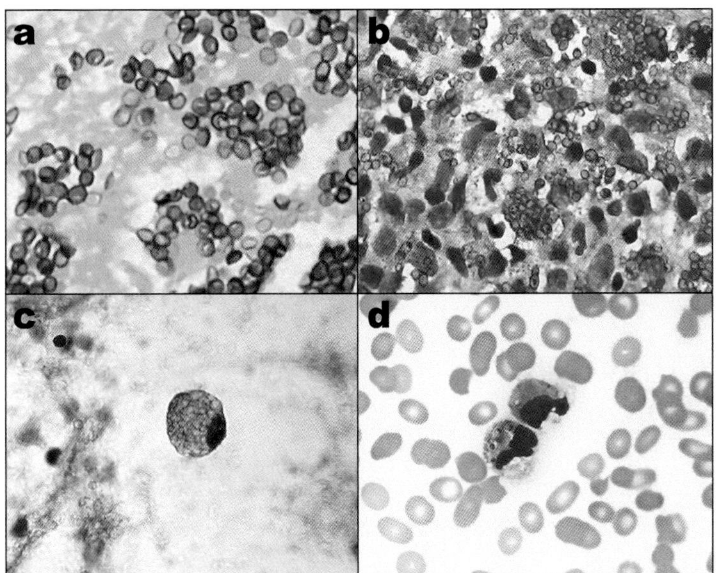

i6.61 *Histoplasma capsulatum*
a GMS-stained, b PAS-stained tissue sections demonstrate small yeasts with narrow based budding; c H&E-stained, d Wright-stained smears demonstrate intracellular yeast forms

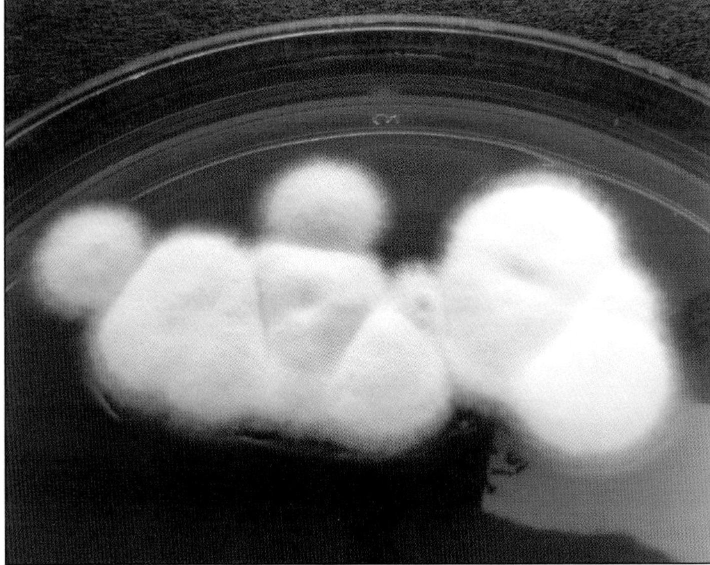

i6.62 *Histoplasma capsulatum* cultured at 25°C-30°C colony morphology—powdery or cottony white mold

6.5.2 Thermally dimorphic fungi t6.35

6.5.2.1 *Histoplasma capsulatum*

- Diagnosis
  - In clinical specimens i6.61
    - Typically found within histiocytes
    - 2-4 µm ovoid yeast with narrow based budding
    - *H capsulatum var duboisii* differs from *H capsulatum var capsulatum* **t6.36**
  - Cultures
    - Slow-growing cottony white mold i6.62 at 25°C-30°C

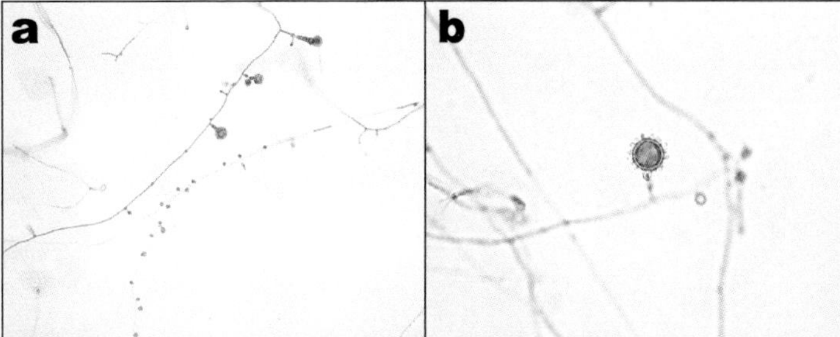

i6.63 *Histoplasma capsulatum*; in mold form, demonstrates a septated, hyaline hyphae with intermittent small (2 µm), smooth, microconidia & b large (7-15 µm), thick walled, spiny macroconidia

    - Septate hyaline hyphae with intermittent small (2-5 µm), smooth, microconidia and large (7-15 µm), thick-walled, spiny macroconidia i6.63
    - Undergo yeast conversion at 37°C (difficult to convert)
  - Urine or serum histoplasma antigen test; molecular testing
- Histoplasmosis caused by *H capsulatum var capsulatum*
  - Ohio & Mississippi River valleys; throughout Latin America & Spain
    - In soil contaminated by droppings from chickens or bats (high nitrogen content)
  - Primary infection is pulmonary
  - Disseminated infection affects reticuloendothelial system
- *H capsulatum var duboisii*
  - Central & western Africa

t6.36 *Histoplasma capsulatum* varieties compared

	var *capsulatum*	var *duboisii*
Geography	Worldwide, but most common in North & Central (Latin) America; eastern United States represents the area of highest endemicity	Central & western Africa, especially Nigeria, Senegal, the Congo & Angola
Disease	Pulmonary, with or without dissemination to the reticuloendothelial system	May be localized or disseminated; most frequently involves skin, subcutaneous tissue & bone
Culture	Slowly growing, white cottony colonies; microscopic examination reveals hyaline, septate mold with smooth microconidia & thick walled, tuberculate (spiked) macroconidia	Colony & microscopic morphology is indistinguishable from *var capsulatum*
Tissue	Often intracellular within histiocytes or reticuloendothelial cells; oval, small (2-4 µm) yeast bud on a narrow base	Often intracellular within giant cells or macrophages Round to oval, thick walled yeast measuring 7-15 µm Bud on a narrow base, unlike *Blastomyces dermatitidis,* the yeast of which is similar in size

ISBN 978-089189-6616

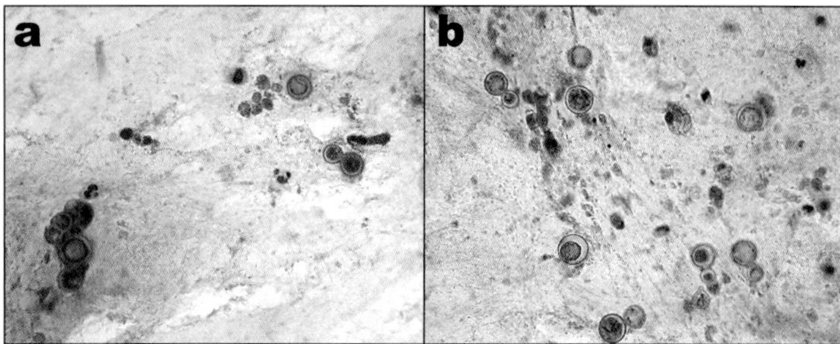

i6.64 *Blastomyces dermatitidis*
a & b Smears demonstrate uniform, large (8-15 μm) yeasts with broad based budding; the yeast cell walls are thick & double contoured

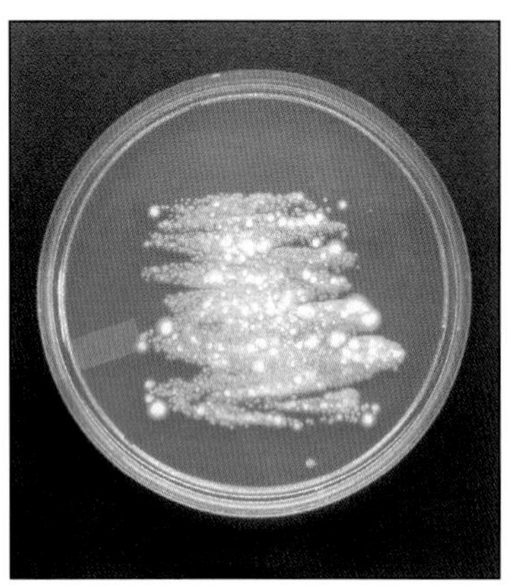

i6.65 *Blastomyces dermatitidis*; the mold form has a cottony white surface that darkens to tan with age

6.5.2.2 *Blastomyces dermatitidis*

- Diagnosis
  - In clinical specimens i6.64: Uniform, large (8-15 μm) yeasts with broad based budding. The yeast cell walls are thick & double contoured
  - Cultures
    - Slow-growing mold with a cottony white surface that darkens to tan with age i6.65 at 25°C-30°C
    - Septate hyaline hyphae with short, unbranched conidiophores producing single, pyriform to round, smooth conidia that measure 2-10 μm (lollipops)
    - Morphology similar to the nondimorphic mold *Chrysosporium*
    - Conversion to yeast at 37°C
- Blastomycosis
  - Mississippi & Ohio River valleys; also in the southeastern United States & in areas bordering the Great Lakes
  - Found in soil, acquired through inhalation
  - Primary infection pulmonary
  - Disseminated infection, if it occurs, affects skin, mucous membranes & bone

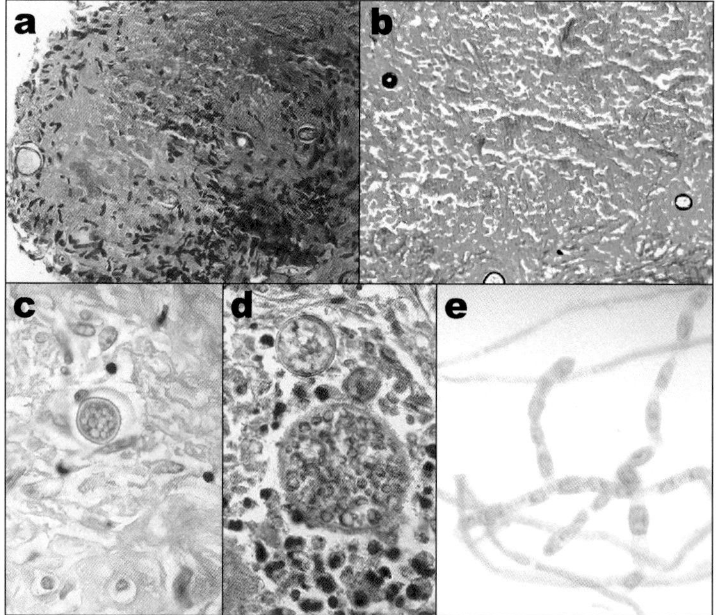

i6.66 *Coccidioides immitis*
a, c-d In tissue sections stained with H&E, it appears as large (10-100 μm) spherules with thick, hyaline walls that enclose numerous tiny (2-5 μm) endospores, which do not bud
b The spherules are highlighted by GMS stain
e In culture, mature arthroconidia are barrel shaped & alternate with empty cells

6.5.2.3 *Coccidioides immitis* & *posadasii*

- Diagnosis
  - In clinical specimens i6.66a-d: Large (10-100 μm) spherules with thick, hyaline walls that enclose hundreds of tiny (2-5 μm) endospores
    - Spherules are not yeasts
  - Culture
    - At 25°C-30°C, grows rapidly (3-5 days) with white, tan, or gray colonies that are cottony when mature
    - Hyaline, septate hyphae & arthroconidia; mature arthroconidia are barrel shaped & alternate with empty cells i6.66e
    - Immature arthroconidia may resemble the arthroconidia of *Malbranchea* spp
- Coccidioidomycosis
  - *Coccidioides immitis* found in the San Joaquin Valley of California; *C posadasii* found in southwestern United States, Mexico & Central America
  - Infectious arthroconidia are present in soil; acquired through inhalation (arthroconidia in laboratory also highly infectious)
  - Primary infection is pulmonary
  - Disseminated infection, if it occurs, affects skin & bone

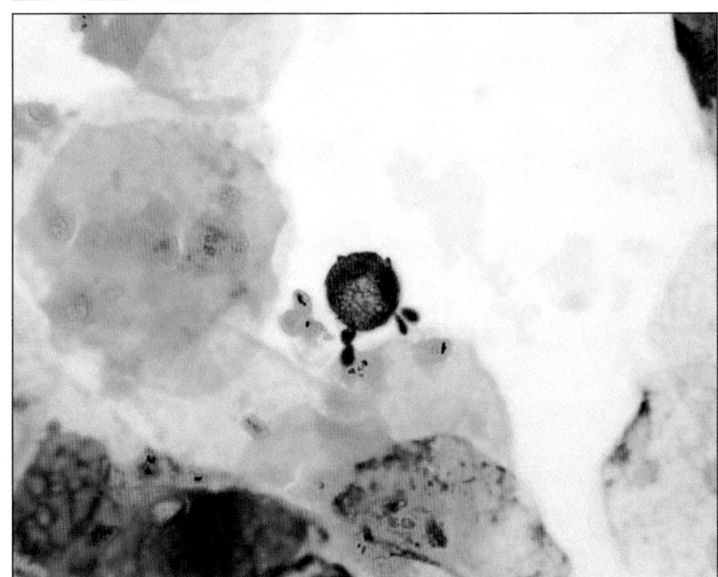

i6.67 *Paracoccidioides brasiliensis* yeast form with circumferential budding

6.5.2.4 *Paracoccidioides brasiliensis*

- Diagnosis
  - In clinical specimens, round, large (10-50 µm) yeast with circumferential budding; mariner's wheel i6.67
  - Culture
    - At 25°C-30°C, slow-growing mold with a white to tan surface & variable texture
    - Hyaline septate hyphae with terminal & intercalary chlamydospores, and infrequent, pear-shaped microconidia arranged along the hyphae
    - At 37°C, converts to yeast form
- Paracoccidioidomycosis
  - Rainforests of Central & South America
  - Primary infection pulmonary
  - Dissemination, if it occurs, to skin, mucosa, reticulo-endothelial system

6.5.2.5 *Sporothrix schenckii*

- Diagnosis
  - In clinical specimens, 4-6 µm elongated ("cigar shaped") yeasts with narrow-based budding
  - Culture
    - At 25°C-30°C grows rapidly; develops moist, white to gray or gray-orange colonies that become leathery and turn brown to black with age i6.68a
    - Delicate, hyaline, septate hyphae producing conidiophores topped by clusters of microconidia ("rosettes") i6.68b

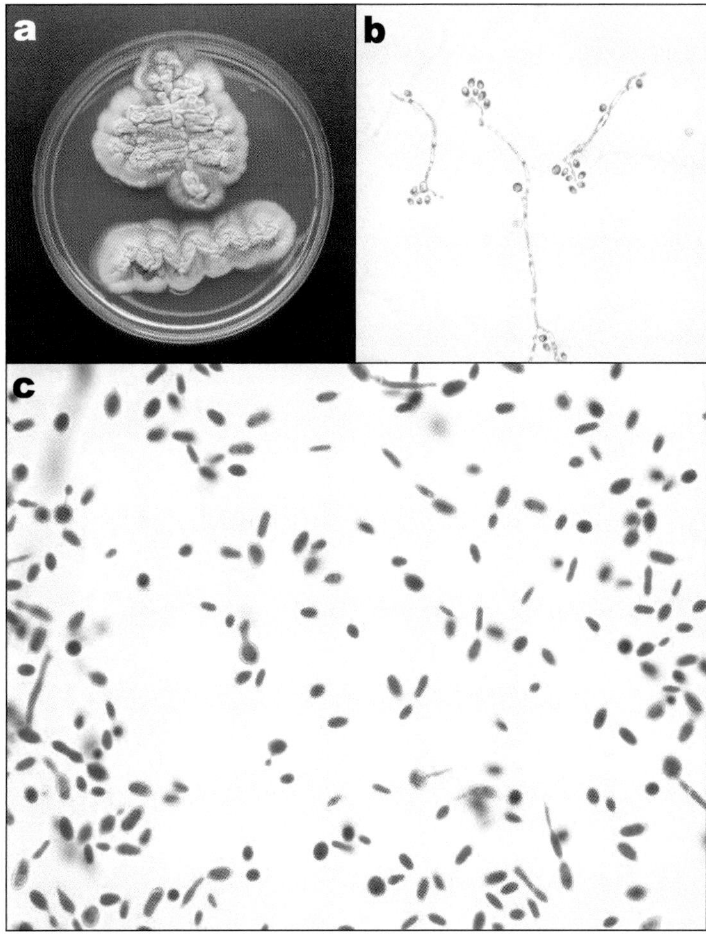

i6.68 *Sporothrix schenckii*: a mold colonies cultured at 25°C-30°C
b mold form; conidiophores topped by clusters of microconidia ("rosettes")
c yeast form; "cigar bodies"

    - Conversion to the yeast at 37°C, appearing as oval or long and thin ("cigar bodies") that bud on a narrow base i6.68c
- Sporotrichosis
  - Worldwide
  - Acquired by penetrating injury from contaminated plant ("rose gardener disease")
  - Lymphocutaneous infection, with nodular, ulcerative lesions that follow the lymphatics

6.5.2.6 *Talaromyces* (formerly *Penicillium*) *marneffei*

- Diagnosis
  - In clinical specimens, ovoid 3-5 µm yeast that divide by fission
  - Culture
    - At 25°C-30°C, rapidly growing tan colonies that are initially powdery or velvety on the surface, and become green aerial hyphae and reddish-brown vegetative hyphae with maturity

ISBN 978-089189-6616

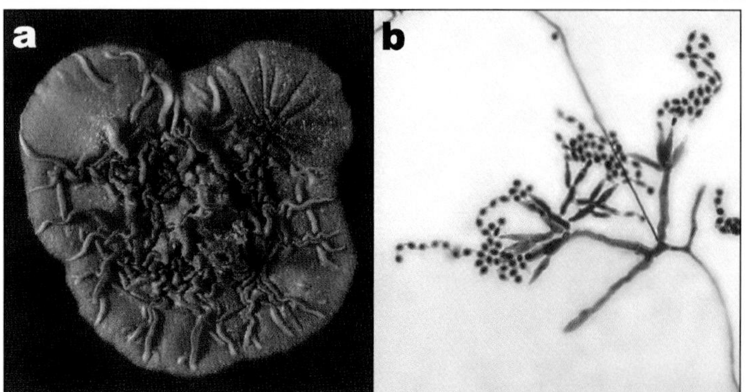

i6.69 *Talaromyces marneffei*:
a red pigment diffused into the agar around colonies
b oval conidia at the terminal ends of the phialides

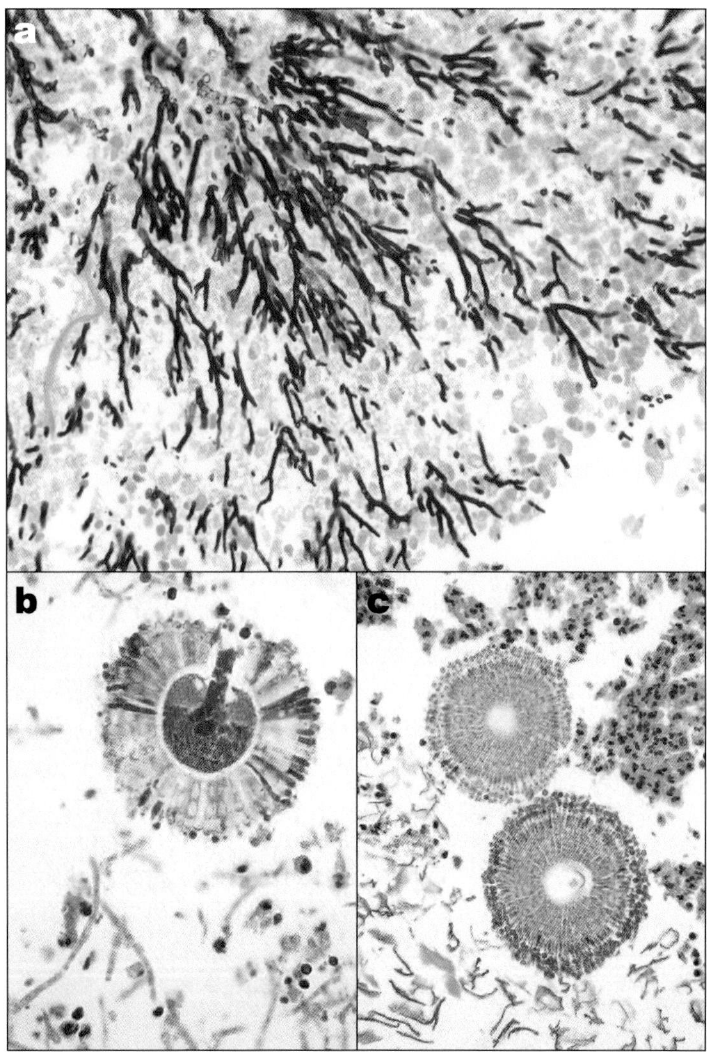

i6.70 *Aspergillus* spp:
a in tissue, narrow septate hyphae with acute angle dichotomous evenly spaced branching is characteristic but not genus specific
b, c when growing in an air filled space (in this case a paranasal sinus) may demonstrate the formation of fruiting heads; in this case, *A niger*

- Red pigment diffuses into the agar around colonies i6.69a
- Hyaline septate hyphae with conidiophores and metulae producing brushlike clusters of phialides. Chains of small, oval conidia form at the terminal ends of the phialides i6.69b
- Yeast conversion at 37°C: Yeasts 3-5 µm, oval, with fission; yeast cells resemble those of *Histoplasma capsulatum*

- Talaromycosis (formerly known as penicilliosis or penicillosis): Endemic in southeast Asia & not found elsewhere; seen in immunocompromised persons

6.5.3 Hyaline/brightly colored molds (opportunistic)

6.5.3.1 *Aspergillus* spp

- Diagnosis
  - In clinical specimens
    - Hyaline, septate hyphae with 45° dichotomous, evenly spaced (arboreal) branching i6.70a
    - This appearance is not specific
    - Fruiting heads may be seen in air-filled tissue pockets i6.70b, c
  - Culture
    - Rapidly growing; identified based on colony morphology & microscopic morphology of swollen vesicle ("aspergillum") at ends of conidiophores
    - *A fumigatus*: Colonies blue green with white apron i6.71a and light reverse i6.71b; conidiophores terminate in a swollen vesicle having a single row of phialides (uniseriate) that cover only the top 2/3 of the vesicle. Each phialide gives rise to a chain of small (2-4 µm), round conidia i6.71c
    - *A flavus*: Yellow green to olive colonies i6.72a with light reverse i6.72b; circumferential phialides i6.72c, some strains uniseriate & others biseriate
    - *A niger*: Dark brown to black colonies i6.73a with light reverse; vesicles with 2 rows of phialides (biseriate) covering the entire surface of the vesicle i6.73b. Phialides produce chains of rough, round, dark conidia
    - *A terreus*: Colonies are cinnamon brown on the surface i6.74a, with a yellow or orange reverse i6.74b; phialides cover only the top 2/3 of the vesicle but in contrast to *A fumigatus*, *A terreus* is biseriate and typically has longer chains of conidia
  - ELISA assay for the serum marker galactomannan and/or 1-3-β-D-glucan or matrix-assisted laser desorption/ionization time-of-flight (MALDI-TOF) mass spectrometry

Mycology>Hyaline/brightly colored molds (opportunistic)

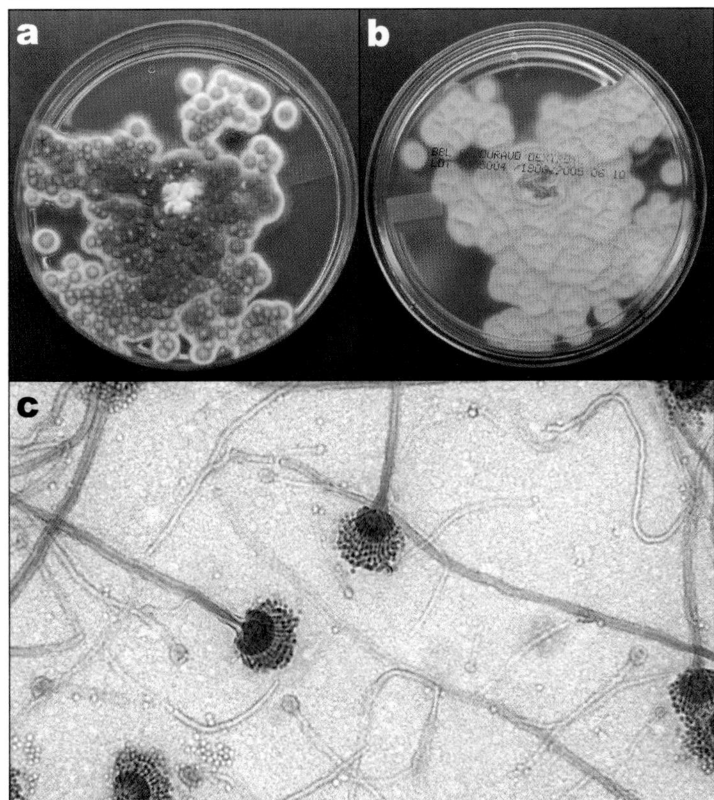

i6.71 *Aspergillus fumigatus*: a colonies are blue-green with a distinct white apron & b a light reverse
c swollen vesicles with single row of phialides (uniseriate) that cover only the top 2/3 of the vesicle

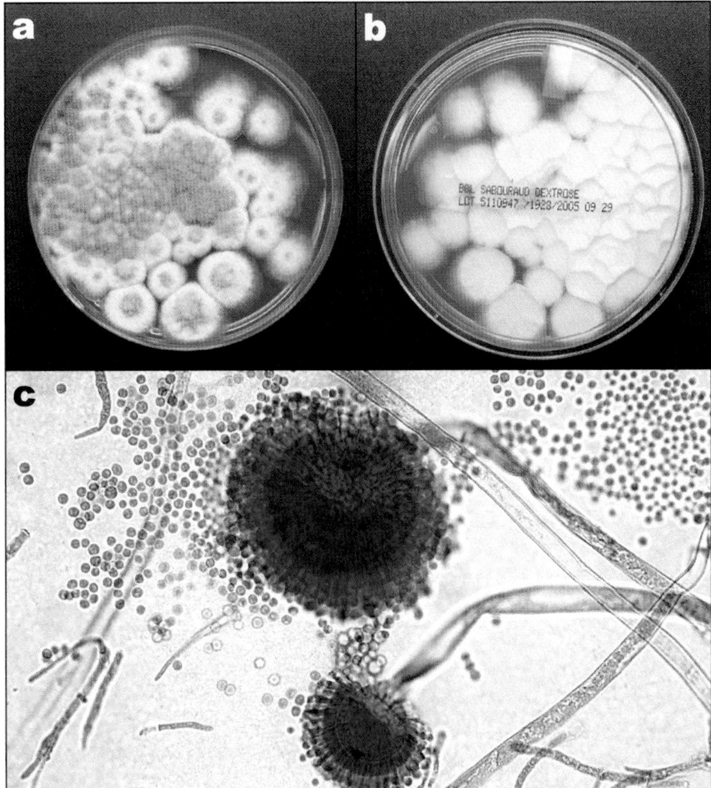

i6.72 *Aspergillus flavus*: a colonies are yellow-green to olive with b a light reverse
c circumferential phialides

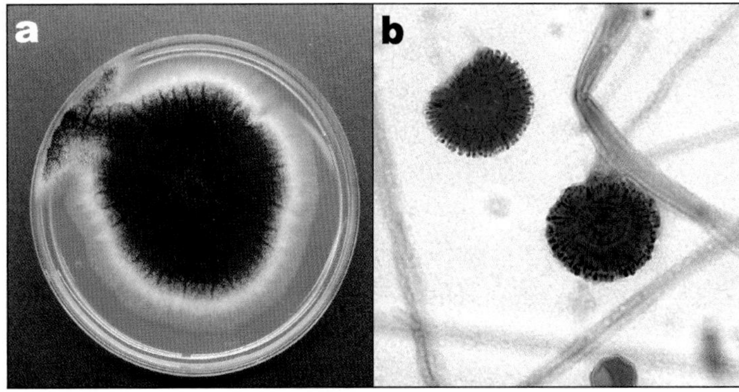

i6.73 *Aspergillus niger*: a colonies are dark brown to black; the reverse side is light
b circumferential biseriate pigmented phialides

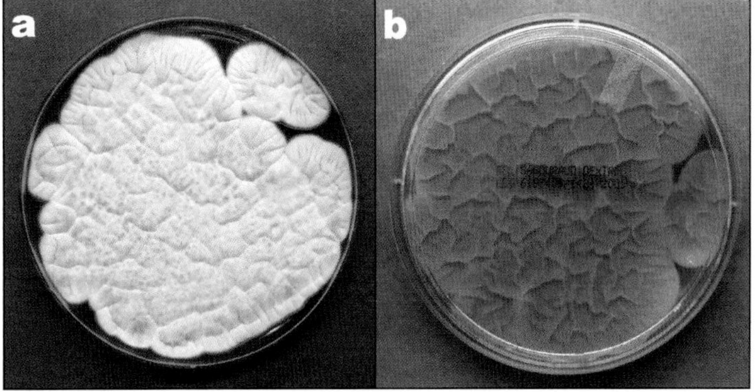

i6.74 *Aspergillus terreus* colonies a are cinnamon brown on the surface with b a yellow or orange reverse

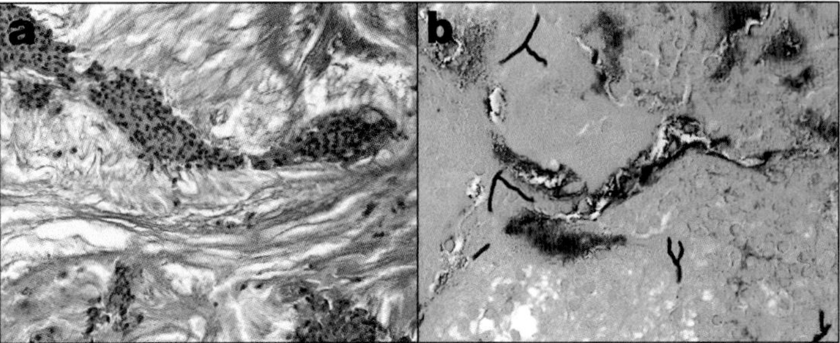

i6.75 Allergic fungal sinusitis
a A clue is eosinophil permeated mucin containing b fungal hyphae on GMS stained sections

- Aspergillosis
  - Ubiquitous in soil & on decaying vegetable matter
  - Most commonly affects the respiratory tract
  - Immunocompetent host with cavitary lung disease: aspergilloma (fungus ball)
  - Atopic host: Allergic bronchopulmonary aspergillosis or allergic fungal sinusitis i6.75
  - Immunosuppressed host: Invasive bronchopulmonary aspergillosis (IBPA) or invasive fungal sinusitis

ISBN 978-089189-6616

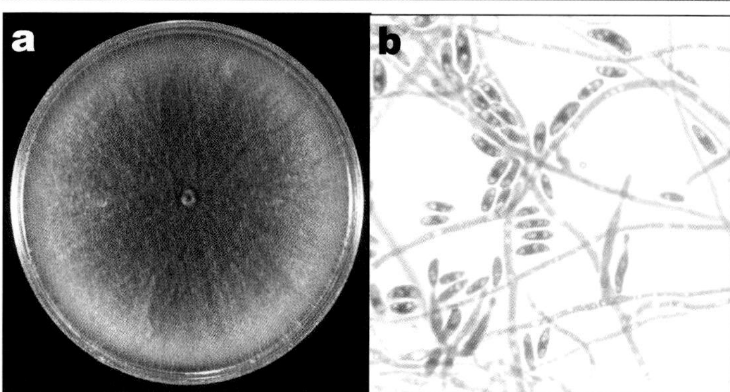

i6.76 *Fusarium*: a colonies are violet
b canoe-shaped, multicellular macroconidia

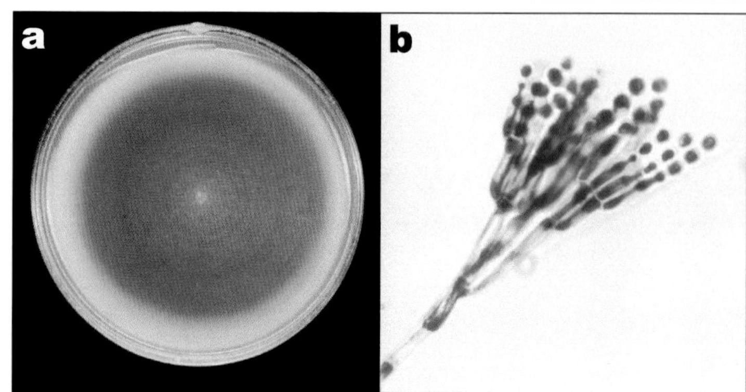

i6.79 *Penicillium*: a powdery bluish green colonies
b flask-shaped phialides give rise to unbranching chains of microconidia

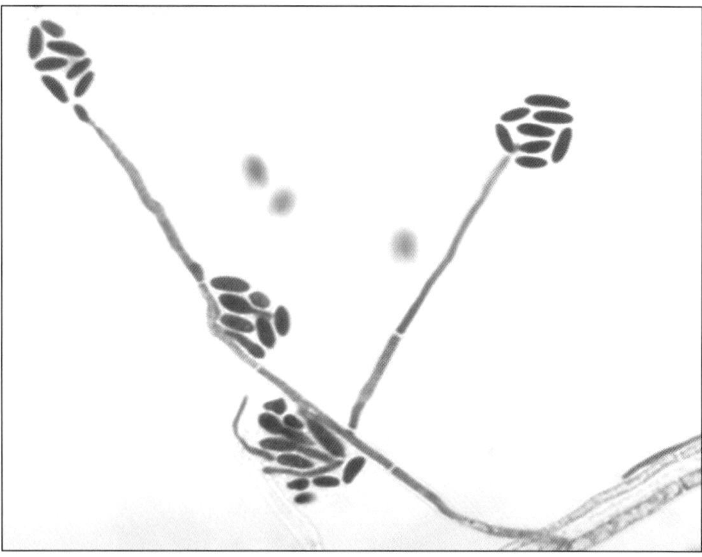

i6.77 *Acremonium* unbranched phialides

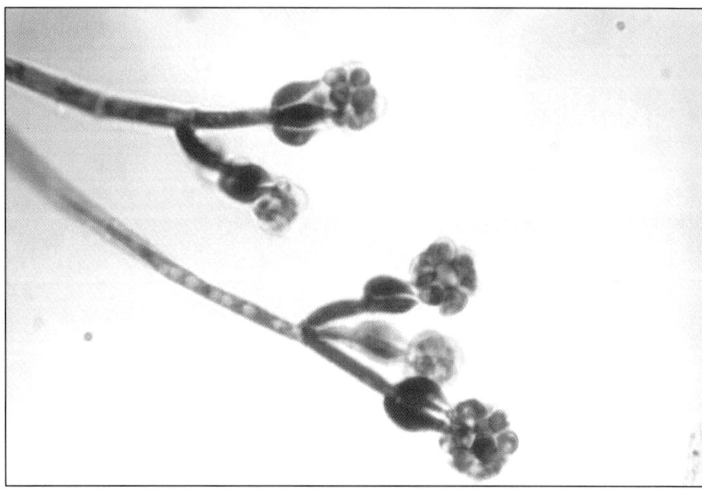

i6.78 *Gliocladium* with numerous floral like, spore-bearing conidiophores clustered in a ball. The thin-walled, hyaline conidiophores are branched

- When *A flavus* contaminates food, it may produce aflatoxins, carcinogens for hepatocellular carcinoma
- *A niger* pulmonary infection associated with oxalosis (calcium oxalate tissue deposition)
- *A terreus* resistant to amphotericin B

6.5.3.2 Other hyaline/brightly colored molds

- *Fusarium* spp
  - Causes infections similar to *Aspergillus* spp, in addition to fungal keratitis and opportunistic infection in burn wounds
  - Colony is usually violet i6.76a
  - Canoe-shaped, multicellular macroconidia with 3-6 cells each, often clumping together i6.76b
- *Acremonium* spp
  - Can cause mycetoma
  - Colonies can be gray, white, yellowish, or pale rose
  - It produces long, narrow, unbranched phialides bearing clusters of single or 2-celled microconidia i6.77
- *Gliocladium* spp
  - Considered a contaminant
  - Center of colony becomes dark green for most isolates
  - Branching conidiophores bearing flask-shaped phialides resembling *Penicillium*. However, microconidia do not chain but rather cluster in a ball, resembling a golf ball held at the end of outstretched fingertips i6.78
- *Penicillium* spp
  - Usually considered contaminant; has been associated with cutaneous, respiratory, external ear infections
  - Colony surface is powdery bluish green with white border i6.79a
  - Brushlike arrangement of flask-shaped phialides give rise to unbranching chains of microconidia i6.79b

Mycology>Hyaline/brightly colored molds (opportunistic)

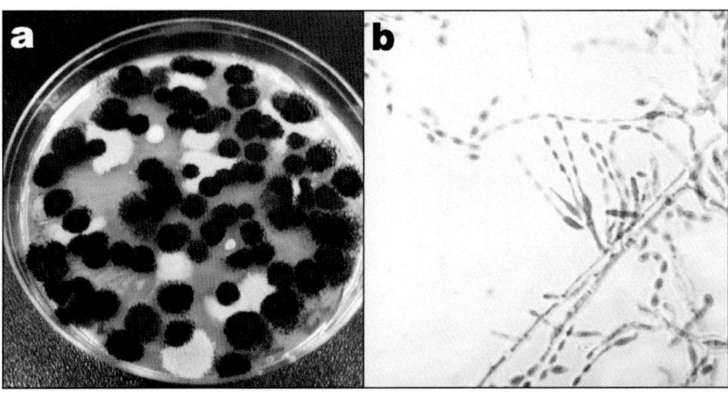

i6.80 *Paecilomyces*: a colonies may be yellowish brown, pink, white, yellow-green b chains of oval or spindle-shaped microconidia emanate from the phialides

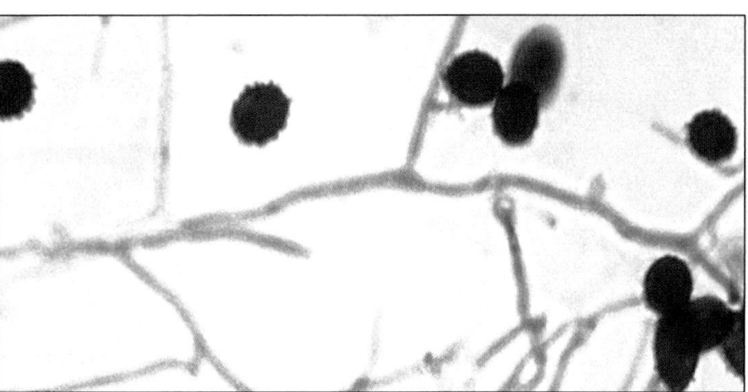

i6.82 *Chrysosporium* microconidia on conidiophores

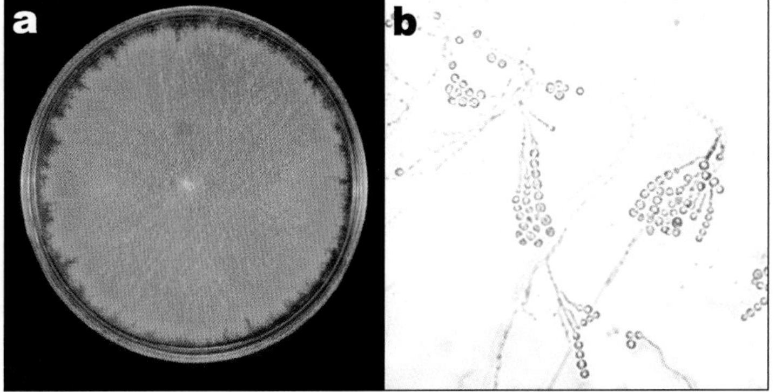

i6.81 *Scopulariopsis*: a colonies are light brown or tan b conidia are rough & "lemon drop" shaped

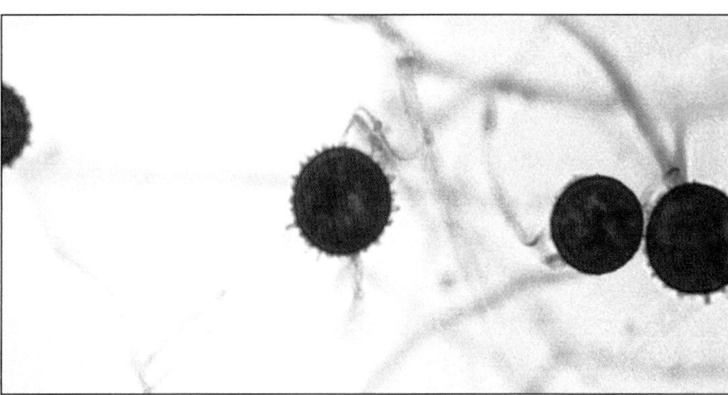

i6.83 *Sepedonium* conidiophores

- *Paecilomyces* spp
  - Usually considered a contaminant; also seen in sinusitis & eye infections
  - Colony surface is yellowish brown, pink, white, yellow-green but never bright green or blue-green i6.80a
  - Branching conidiophores with elongated, flask-shaped phialids arranged in pairs or brushlike groups. Long chains of oval or spindle-shaped microconidia emanate from the phialides i6.80b
- *Scopulariopsis* spp
  - Common contaminants but also cause nail infections
  - Colony is powdery light brown or tan i6.81a
  - Single or branched conidiophores that give rise to annellides (similar to phialides); conidia are rough & "lemon drop" shaped i6.81b
- *Chrysosporium* spp
  - Considered a contaminant
  - Colony morphology varies but is usually lighter in color—white, yellow, or tan
  - Single, cutoff microconidia directly on hyphae or on the tips of simple conidiophores i6.82
  - Will look like *Blastomyces* mold form
- *Sepedonium* spp
  - Considered a contaminant
  - Colonies are often yellow with age
  - Singly borne, hyaline conidia at the ends of branched or unbranched conidiophores. The conidia are large, thick walled, and echinulate, resembling the macroconidia of the mold form of *H capsulatum* i6.83

ISBN 978-089189-6616

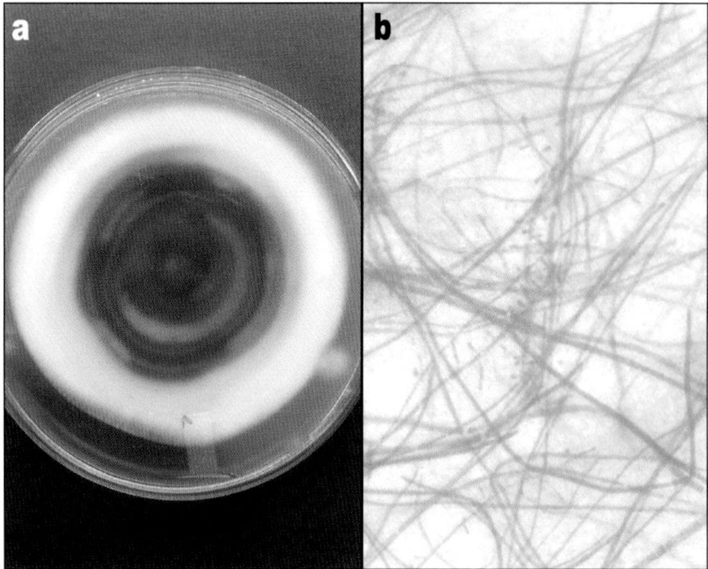

i6.84 *Trichophyton rubrum:* a red reverse; b birds on a wire

6.5.3.3 Dermatophytes

- Clinical
  - Infection of superficial, keratinized structures such as hair, nails & the stratum corneum of skin
  - Diseases are referred to as athlete's foot, ringworm (tinea capitus, tinae corporis, tinea barbae) onychomycosis (nail infection)
- Diagnosis
  - Potassium hydroxide (KOH) preparation or calcofluor white preparation of skin scrapings, nail clippings & hair samples
  - Observe colony morphology and microscopic morphology of conidia production
  - Matrix-assisted laser desorption/ionization time-of-flight (MALDI-TOF) mass spectrometry
- *Trichophyton rubrum*
  - Infects skin & nails; most frequently isolated dermatophyte infecting humans worldwide
  - Colony surface is white to buff; red pigment causes the reverse side of the plate to appear red i6.84a
  - Tear-shaped microconidia form singly along the hyphae, giving a "birds on a telephone wire" appearance; pencil-like macroconidia may be present i6.84b
  - Does not perforate hair in vitro and is urease-negative (7 days)

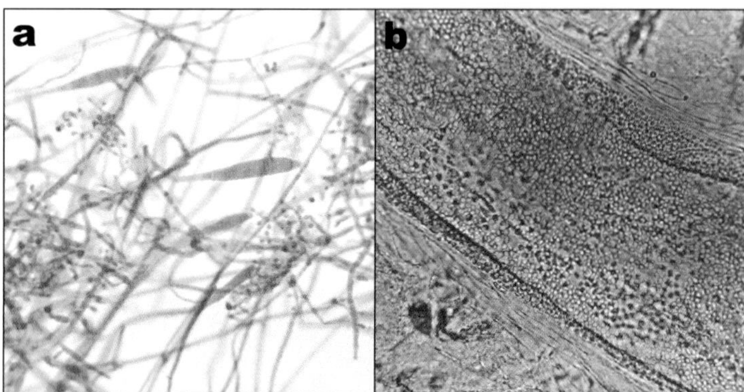

i6.85 Trichophyton mentagrophytes: a larger, elongated macroconidia, and the tiny, round microconidia; b fungal organisms are present on the outside of the hair shaft, known as an ectothrix, as well as on the inside of the hair shaft, known as an endothrix

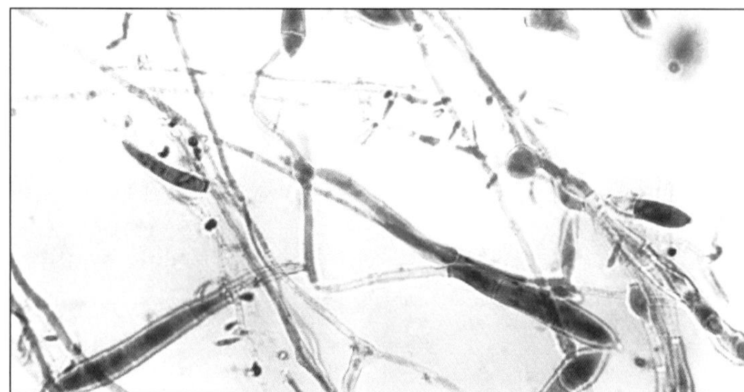

i6.86 *Trichophyton tonsurans*: teardrop-shaped microconidia, attached to, and branching perpendicularly from the filamentous, elongated hyphae & larger, elongated, septate macroconidia, also emanating from these same hyphae

- *Trichophyton mentagrophytes*
  - Invades hair, skin & nails and is common cause of athlete's foot
  - Morphology varies; surface may be buff or white or yellowish and reverse can be colorless, yellow, tan, or red
  - Microconidia are very round and arranged in clusters, and occasional spiral hyphae may be seen; macroconidia may be seen and are cigar shaped i6.85a
  - Penetrates hair shafts in vitro i6.85b, unlike *T rubrum*, which can appear morphologically similar. It is urease-positive (7 days)
- *Trichophyton tonsurans*
  - Major pathogen for ringworm of the scalp
  - Morphology varies; reverse is usually reddish brown, yellow, or colorless
  - Microconidia display marked size & shape variability—teardrop, club shaped, balloon shaped, round; macroconidia are rare & irregular i6.86
  - Urease-positive, no in vitro hair penetration, 4+ growth on medium with thiamine, and ± or 1+ on medium without thiamine

Mycology>Hyaline/brightly colored molds (opportunistic)

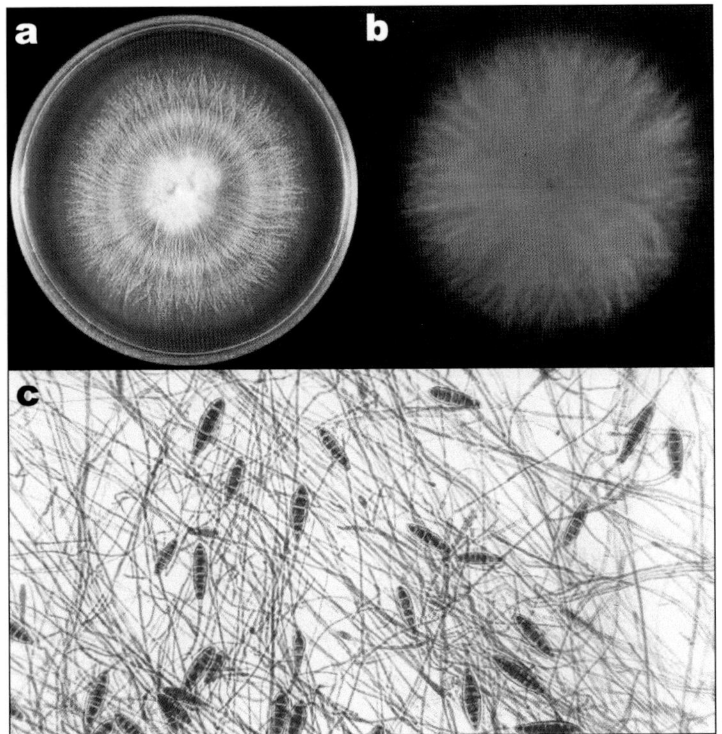

i6.87 *Microsporum canis*:
a characteristic, cream-colored surface that was streaked with numerousd radial grooves emanating from the colony's center
b reverse with characteristic, bright yellow-orange to golden coloration
c spindle-shaped macroconidia with a roughened surface dispersed amongst a meshwork of the filamentous hyphae

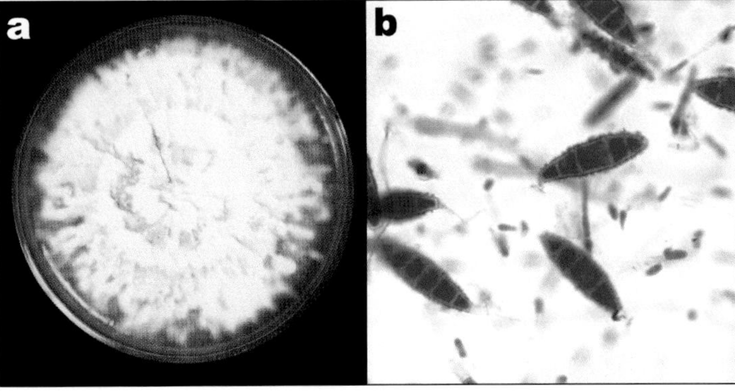

i6.88 *Microsporum gypseum*:
a characteristic cream-colored, suede-textured, ruffled surface
b oblong-shaped macroconidia

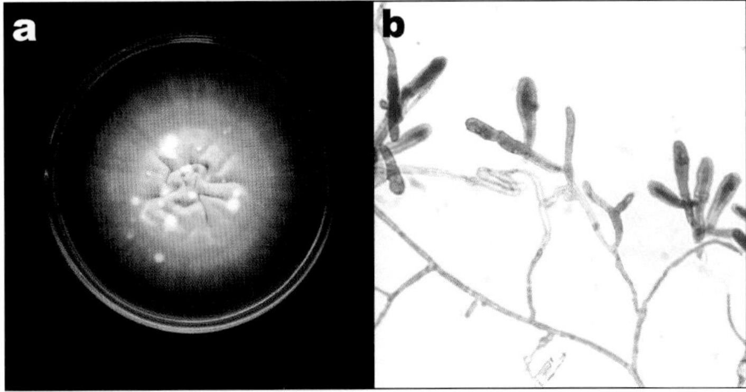

i6.89 *Epidermophyton floccosum*: a characteristic colonial morphology with suede-like texture, raised, folded central region, and white punctate regions, composed of pleomorphic mycelial tufts
b macroconidia branched from the organism's filamentous hyphae

- *Microsporum canis*
  - Infects the scalp & skin; usually acquired from infected dogs or cats
  - Surface is white with yellow pigment at edge i6.87a; reverse is deep yellow i6.87b
  - Macroconidia are spindle shaped & rough (echinulate), and taper to a knoblike end; each macroconidium contains >6 cells, separated by transverse septae i6.87c. Microconidia may be seen but do not help with identification
- *Microsporum gypseum*
  - May infect scalp & skin but more often infects animals
  - Colony surface is powdery to granular, buff, tan, or cinnamon i6.88a. Reverse will vary in color
  - Macroconidia are oval-shaped, rough-walled, with rounded ends and transverse septae. Each macroconidium contains no more than 6 cells i6.88b. Microconidia can be seen but do not help with identification
- *Microsporum audouinii*
  - Former cause of tinea capitis epidemics in children
  - Colony surface is gray, tan, or white; reverse is salmon color
  - Terminal chlamydospores on hyphae that often have comblike appearance
  - Macroconidia & microconidia seldom seen
- *Epidermophyton floccosum*
  - Infects skin & nails
  - Colony surface is yellow to olive-gray or khaki and reverse can be orange to brown i6.89a
  - Macroconidia are smooth, club-shaped structures with rounded ends, which may be found singly or in characteristic clusters; each macroconidium contains 2-6 cells, separated by transverse septae i6.89b
  - Microconidia never produced

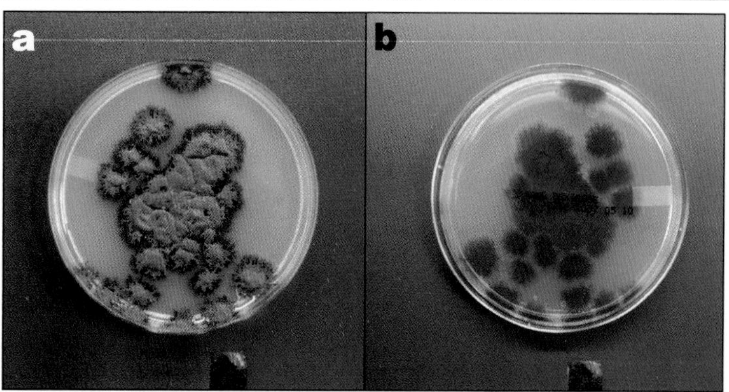

i6.90 Dematiaceous molds are typically pigmented a on the surface & b reverse side of the plate

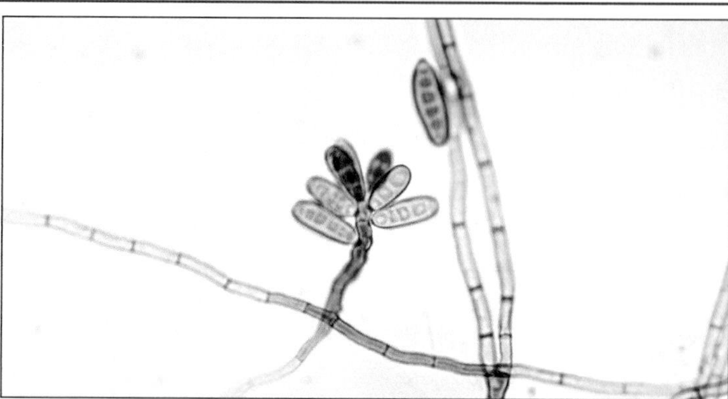

i6.92 *Bipolaris*: septate hyphae, septate, geniculate conidiophore topped by a cluster of 3- to 6-celled conidia, referred to as poroconidia

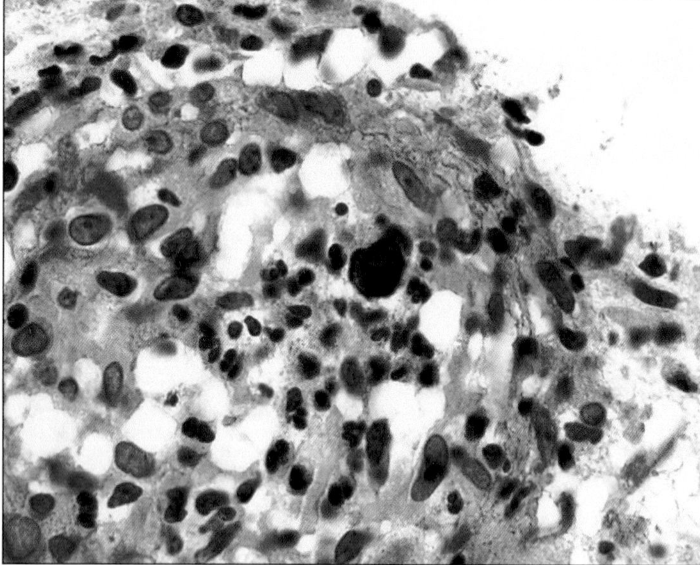

i6.91 Chromoblastomycosis, demonstrating muriform bodies (sclerotic bodies having internal septations in more than one plane)

6.5.4 Dematiaceous molds

- Characterized by production of melanin pigment
  - Colonies often darkly pigmented on the surface and reverse side of the plate, because both their hyphae and conidia are melanized i6.90
  - In tissue, intrinsic pigmentation is a clue to the presence of a dematiaceous mold
- Clinical: Dematiaceous molds may produce 3 types of infection
  - Chromoblastomycosis
    - Subcutaneous mycosis associated with prominent pseudoepitheliomatous hyperplasia
    - In tissue, pigmented hyphae & sclerotic (muriform) bodies i6.91
    - *Fonsecaea pedrosoi*, *Phialophora verrucosa* & *Cladophialophora carrionii* are principal agents (not inclusive)
    - Found in tropical & subtropical areas
    - Gain entrance through puncture wounds; infections on the lower extremities
- Mycetoma (Madura foot or maduromycosis)
  - Subcutaneous infection with draining sinus tracts
  - Can be caused by bacteria (actinomycotic mycetoma) or molds (eumycotic mycetoma)
  - Eumycotic mycetoma usually caused by dematiaceous molds
  - Subcutaneous nodule contains granules (mold within a proteinaceous matrix)
  - Usually the result of a puncture wound
  - Eumycotic principle causes: *Madurella*, *Exophiala*, *W angiella*, *P boydii*/ *S boydii*
  - Actinomycotic: Aerobic actinomycetes, such as *Nocardia* spp
  - Phaeohyphomycosis
  - Infections by dematiaceous molds that can be cutaneous, subcutaneous, or systemic (eg, *Exophiala, Phialophora, Alternaria, Bipolaris*)
- Dematiacious rapid growers
  - *Bipolaris*
    - Contaminant but also causes allergic sinusitis and infections of eye, skin, lung, etc
    - Colony surface is gray, brown, or black and reverse is dark brown to black
    - Oval, transversely septate conidia arise from bent (geniculate) conidiophores. Production of germ tubes from both ends of the conidia in saline mounts incubated for 12-24 hours. Each conidum contains 3-5 septations i6.92

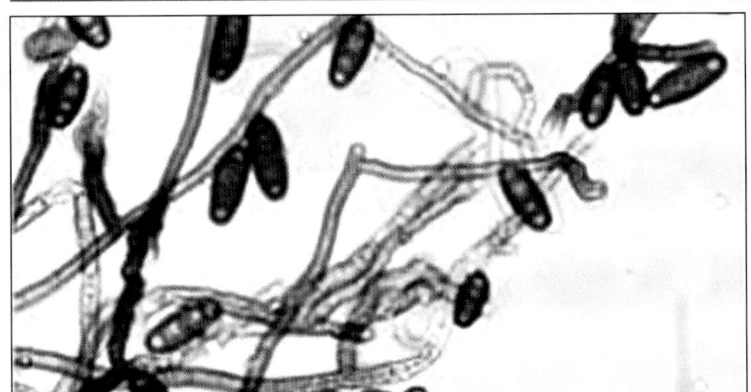

i6.93 *Drechslera* with germ tubes along the sides of the conidia

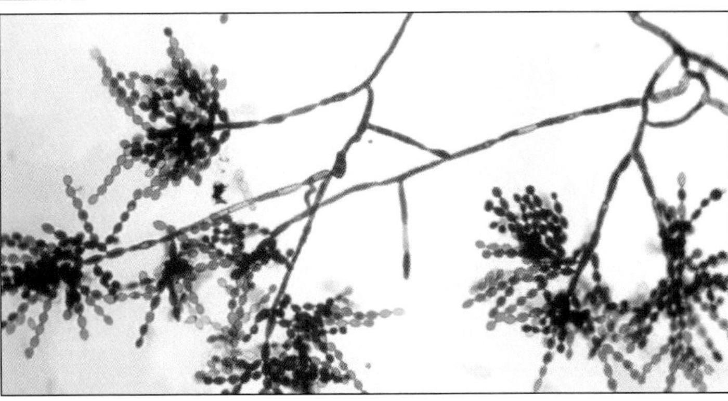

i6.94 *Cladosporium*: chains of conidia, emanating from septate conidiophores, which in turn, branched from the organism's septate hyphae

- *Drechslera*
  - Considered a contaminant; conidia similar to *Bipolaris* but is distinguished by its lack of production of bipolar germ tubes in saline incubation; instead, germ tubes along the sides of the conidia i6.93
- *Cladosporium*
  - Considered a contaminant
  - Colony surface is greenish brown or black with black reverse
  - Short branching conidiophores that have "shield cells" that bear short chains of conidia i6.94
- *Exserohilum*
  - Causes phaeohypomycosis, usually in the sinuses, skin, tissue & cornea
  - Surface is black or dark gray and reverse is black
  - Resembles *Bipolaris*, except that its conidia are longer & thinner, and have more septations (7-11) i6.95
- *Helminthosporium*
  - Considered a contaminant
  - Colony surface is black or dark gray and reverse is black
  - Large, thick-walled conidia are club shaped and arranged with the broader end of the conidia attached to the conidiophores i6.96
- *Curvularia*
  - Opportunisitic, causing sinus & corneal infections, mycetoma & phaeohyphomycosis
  - Surface is olive-green, brown, or black with dark reverse
  - Transversely septated condia with 4 cells; curve distinctly when mature due to swelling of a central cell i6.97

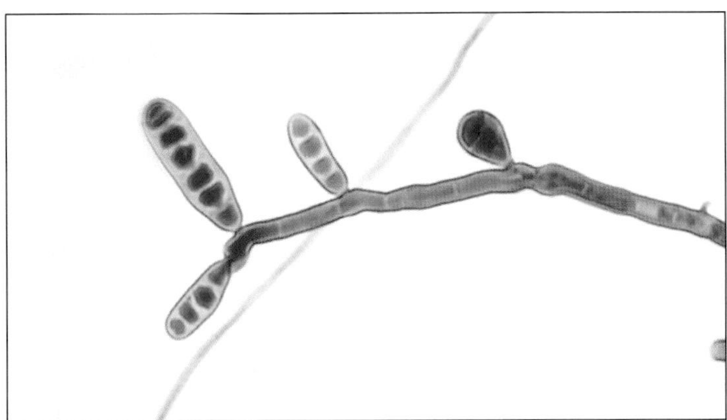

i6.95 *Exserohilum*: fine branching septate hyphal filament in the background, septate conidiophore, and septate, ellipsoid macroconidia, branching from the conidiophore in a geniculate manner

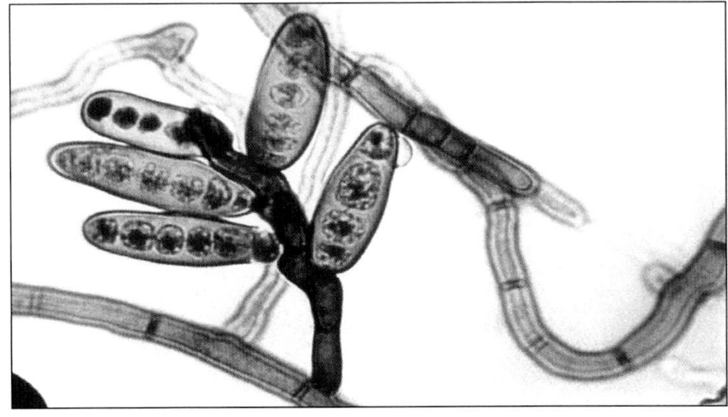

i6.96 *Helminthosporium*: darkly stained conidiophore, topped with 5 oblong multicellular conidia. Note how the conidiophore had branched the septate hypha

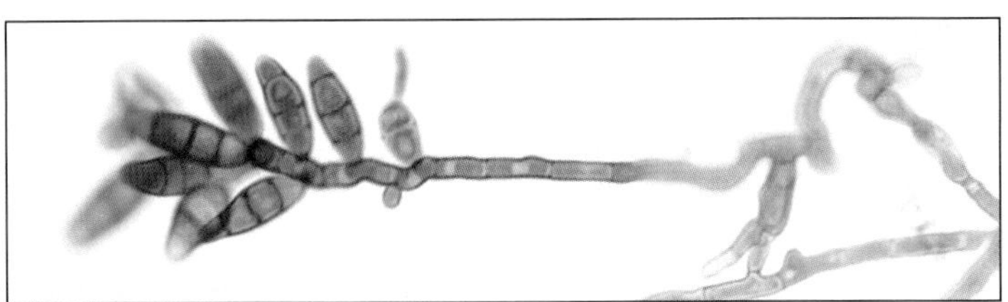

i6.97 *Curvularia*: a solitary conidiophore topped by a number of 4-cell conidia

ISBN 978-089189-6616

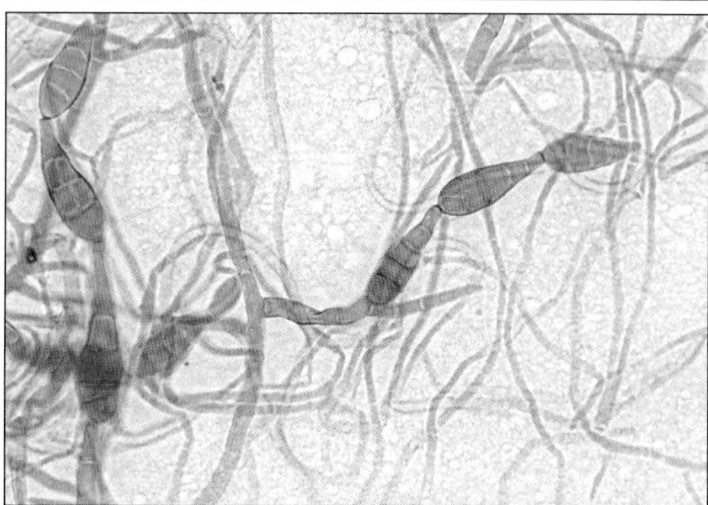

i6.98 *Alternaria* spp form chains of conidia with transverse & longitudinal (muriform) septations; one end of each conidium is blunt & the other pointed

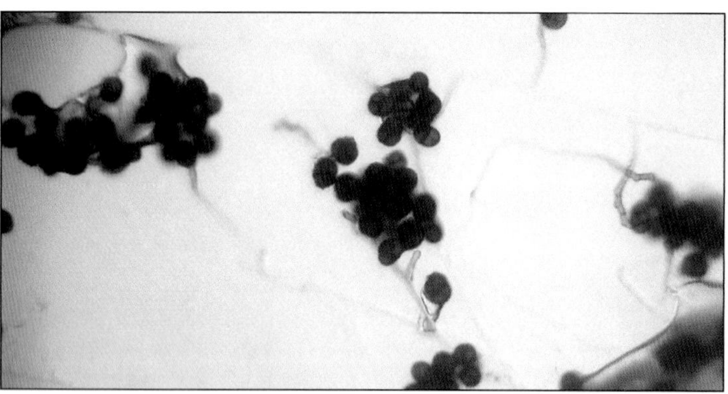

i6.99 *Ulocladium*: oval conidia borne singly on geniculate conidiophores

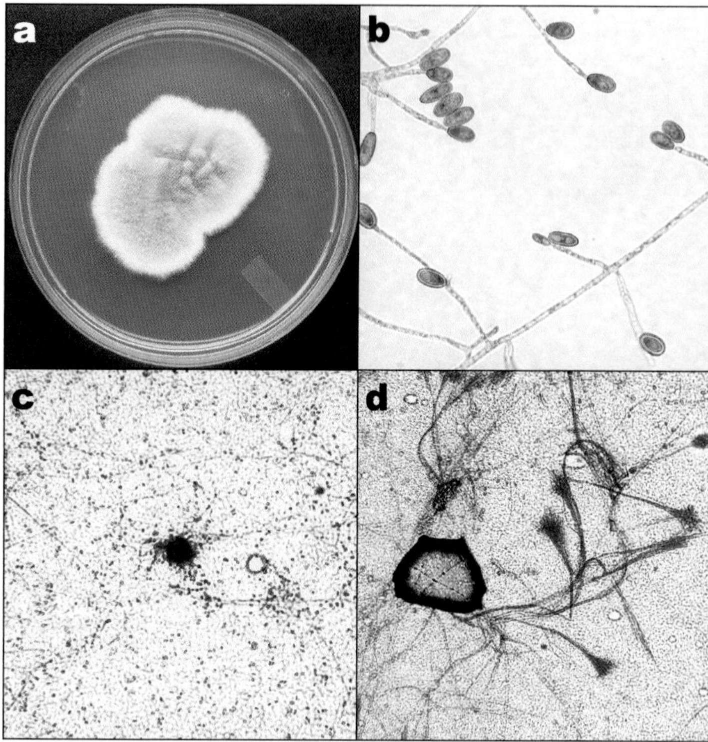

i6.100 *Pseudallescheria boydii* & *Scedosporium boydii* complex
a forms a mold colony with a light brown melanized surface
b oval, truncated, melanized microconidia with nonmelanized hyphae
c in the sexual state, the mold produces large dark cleistothecia
d the alternative asexual form, Graphium, characterized by thick mats of long conidiophores stuck together side by side, resembling the bristles of a broom

- *Alternaria*
  - Considered a contaminant but may cause disease in tissue, nails, sinuses
  - Colony surface is brown or greenish black and reverse is black
  - Chains of club-shaped conidia with transverse & longitudinal septations in the conidia and have alternating blunt & pointed ends i6.98
- *Ulocladium*
  - Considered a contaminant
  - Colony is dark brown to black with a black reverse
  - Smooth or rough oval conidia borne singly on bent (geniculate) conidiophores i6.99

- Slow-growing dematiaceous molds
  - *Pseudallescheria boydii* & *Scedosporium boydii* complex
    - *P boydii* is sexual state & *S boydii* is asexual state
    - Common cause of mycetoma
    - Light gray or brown surface i6.100a, owing to melanization of its oval, truncated microconidia i6.100b
    - Hyphae are hyaline (nonmelanized), resulting in a light reverse
    - In its sexual state, produces large (50-200 μm), dark cleistothecia i6.100c
    - Asexual state does not form cleistothecia but produces conidiophores that bear conidia singly or in small groups. They resemble mold phase of *Blastomyces dermatitidis*
    - Alternative asexual form produces *Graphium* type conidiation; it is characterized by thick mats of long conidiophores stuck together side by side, resembling the bristles of a broom i6.100d
    - *P boydii* & *S boydii* complex resistant to amphotericin B, but usually susceptible to triazoles such as voriconazole & posaconazole

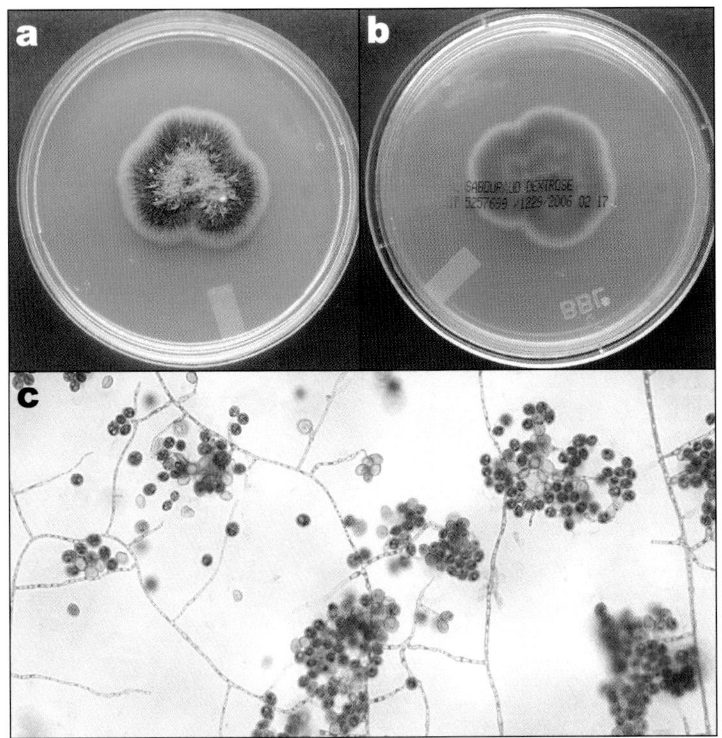

i6.101 *Scedosporium prolificans* has a gray or black a surface & b reverse c microconidia are oval & truncated, forming clusters at the end of annellides, which have swollen bases & thin necks

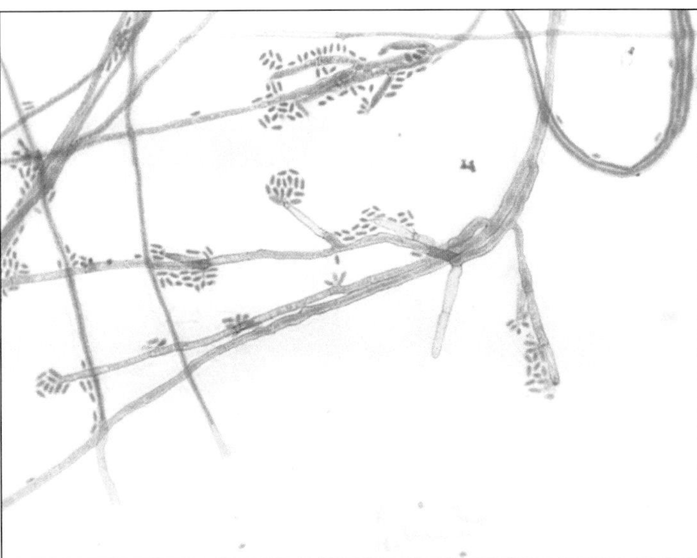

i6.102 *Exophiala jeanselmei*: short, peg-like conidiophore topped by elongated, cigar-shaped conidia, with characteristic torulose hyphae, which exhibit a vacuolated appearance

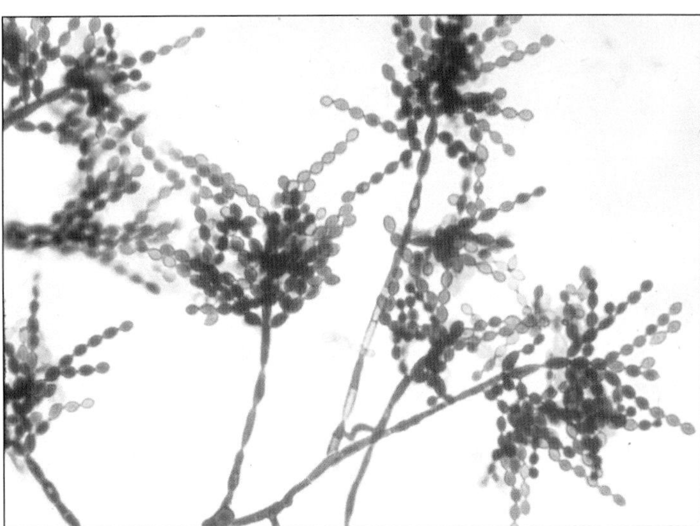

i6.103 *Cladophialophora carrionii*: branching chains of oval conidia

- *Scedosporium prolificans*
  - Causes invasive infections in both immunocompromised & immunocompetent hosts
  - Colony may be yeastlike when young, turning dark gray to black. Gray or black surface and reverse i6.101a, b
  - Microconidia are oval, forming clusters at the end of annellides (conidiogenous cells) i6.101c
  - The annellides have swollen bases & thin necks
  - Resistant not only to amphotericin B, but also to the azoles & echinocandins, making antifungal therapy ineffective
- *Exophiala jeanselmei* complex
  - Causes mycetoma & phaeohyphomycosis
  - Colony surface is brown to green black with black reverse
  - Young colony produces many yeastlike cells; with age, the conidiophores are slender, with narrow & elongated tips. Conidia are oval and are in clusters at end of a conidiophore i6.102
- *Cladophialophora carrionii*
  - Agent of chromoblastomycosis
  - Colony has gray, gray-green, or brown surface with black reverse
  - Conidiophores have long, branching chains of oval conidia i6.103

ISBN 978-089189-6616

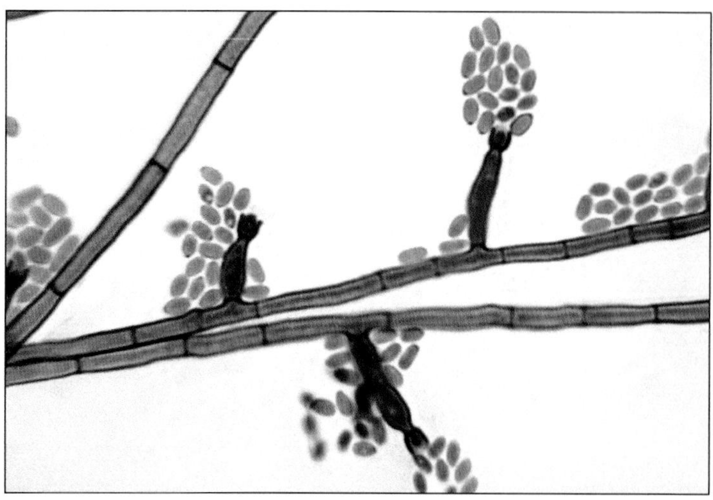

i6.104 *Phialophora verrucosa*, including its vase-shaped phialides with their darkly stained, cup-shaped collarettes, topped with its respective cluster of smooth-walled conidia

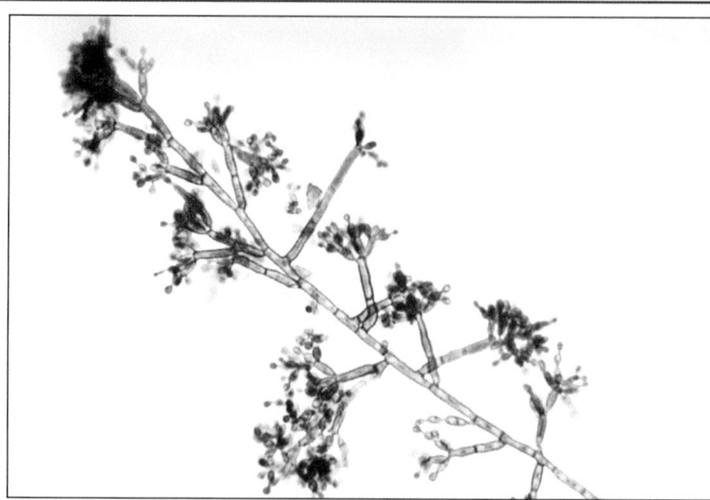

i6.105 *Fonsecaea pedrosoi* conidiophores

- *Phialophora verrucosa*
  - Agent of chromoblastomycosis & phaeohyphomycosis
  - Colony surface is dark green to black with black reverse
  - Phialides look like vases with a flared cuplike collarette; round or oval conidia gather at the end of the phialid, looks like a "vase of flowers" i6.104
- *Fonsecaea pedrosoi*
  - Common cause of chromoblastomycosis
  - Colony surface is dark green, gray, or black with black reverse
  - Four types of conidiation can develop on conidiophore i6.105
    - *Fonsecaea* type: "Denticles" on conidiophore bear oval conidia; short chains develop
    - *Rhinocladiella* type: Oval conidia are born at tip and along the side of conidiophore
    - *Cladosporium* type: "Shield"-shaped conidia on short, branching chains of oval conidia
    - *Phialophora* type: Vase-shaped phialides have cuplike structure at the end (vase of flowers) with accumulation of conidia

6.5.5 Zygomycetes

- Have broad hyphae & usually nonseptate
- Clinical
  - Several forms of invasive infection: Rhinocerebral, pulmonary, gastrointestinal & cutaneous
  - Hosts typically immunocompromised
  - Risk factors: Uncontrolled diabetes (especially ketoacidosis), stem cell or solid organ transplantation, neutropenia, corticosteroid therapy, or severe burns
  - Like *Aspergillus* spp, zygomycetes characteristically invade vessel walls
  - Can be seen in routine H&E-stained sections
  - In clinical specimens, hyphae are broad with few or no septations; branching infrequent
  - Culture: Rapid growth typical and can fill lid of petri dish

Mycology>Zygomycetes

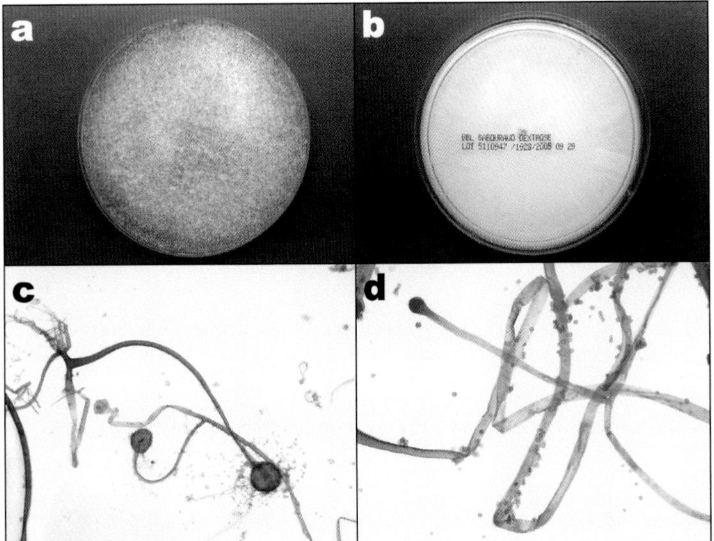

i6.106 *Rhizopus* spp:
a, b in culture: colonies are rapidly growing (lid lifters) & quickly cover the entire agar surface; they are initially cottony & white, turning light brown with sporulation
c, d rhizoids & unbranched sporangiophores that arise directly over the rhizoids; their sporangia are prominent spherical structures that tend to collapse when mature, resembling a collapsed umbrella; their sporangiophores lack an apophysis

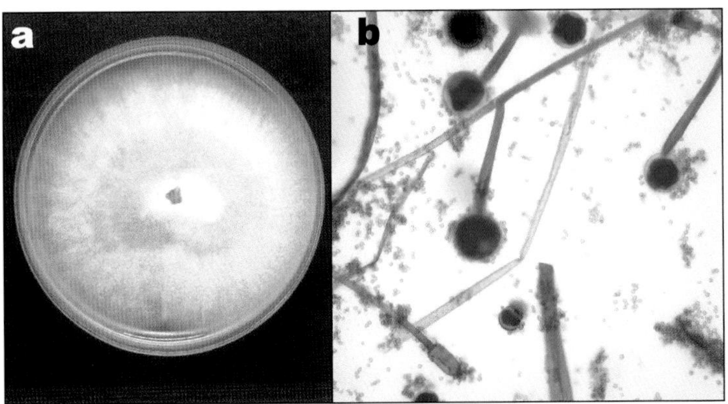

i6.107 *Mucor* spp:
a colonies are rapidly growing (lid lifters), fluffy & become pigmented with the development of sporangia
b note the absence of rhizoids; sporangiophores can be branched or unbranched, but lack an apophysis; their sporangia are large spherical structures that tend to fall apart, releasing their numerous spores

- *Rhizopus* spp i6.106: Rhizoids & unbranched sporangiophores that arise directly over the rhizoids. Their sporangia (sacklike structures that contain spores) are prominent spherical structures full of tiny spores, which tend to collapse when mature, resembling a collapsed umbrella. Sporangiophores lack an apophysis
- *Mucor* spp i6.107: Do not produce rhizoids. Sporangiophores can be branched or unbranched but lack an apophysis. Their sporangia are large spherical structures that tend to fall apart, releasing their numerous spores

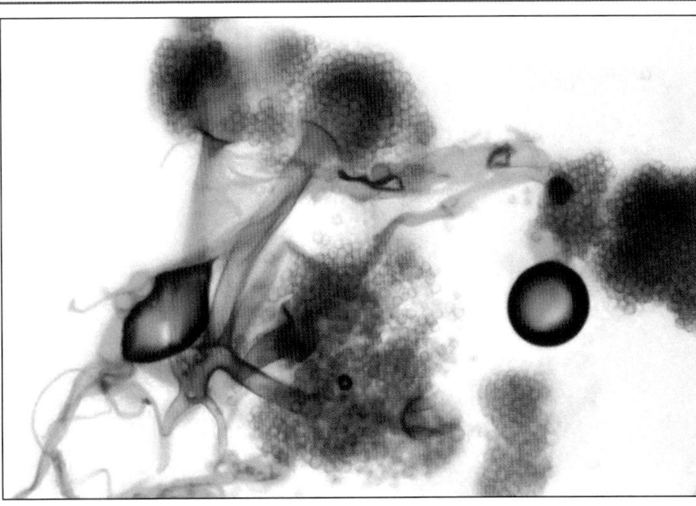

i6.108 *Lichtheimia* (formerly *Absidia*) branched sporangiophores form a conical apical apophysis

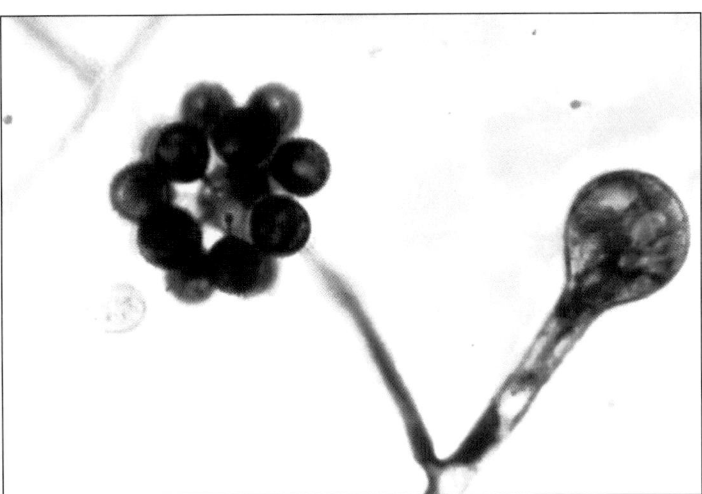

i6.109 *Cunninghamella* conidiophores

- *Lichtheimia* (formerly *Absidia*): Produce rhizoids but the sporangiophores arise at points between rhizoids, rather than over the rhizoids. Sporangiophores are branched and form a conical apophysis at the top i6.108
- *Cunninghamella* spp: Branched sporangiophores are topped by large vesicles. The vesicles are covered with spines (denticles), each of which supports a single spore contained within a round sporangiolum i6.109

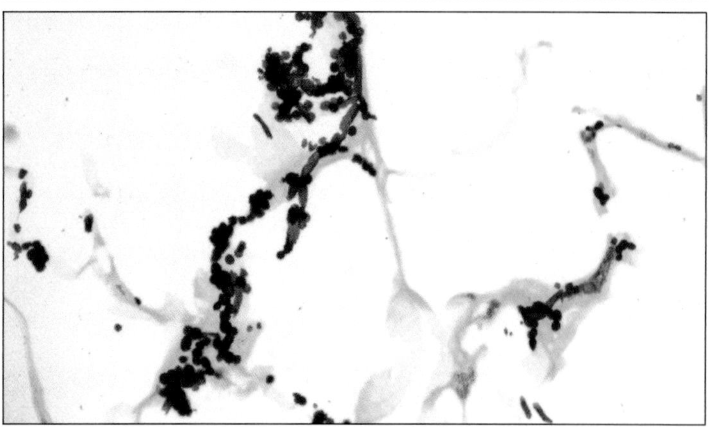

i6.110 *Candida* pseudohyphae seen in a GMS stained section

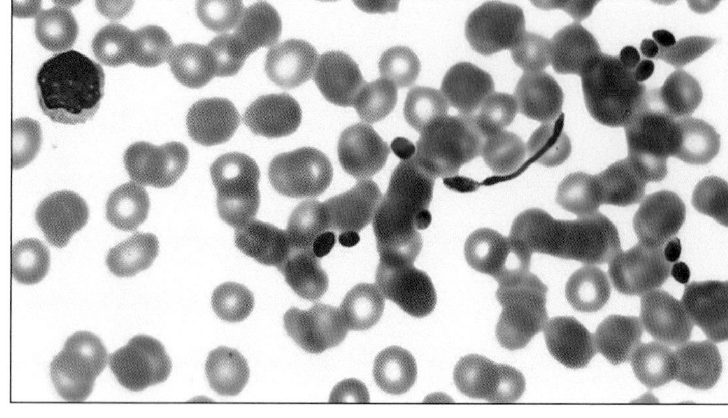

i6.111 Pseudohyphae: note the pale constriction between the yeast & the hyphal structure

6.5.6 Yeasts & yeastlike fungi

6.5.6.1 Diagnosis

- Presumptive identification
  - Chromagar: Agar plates that are selective for yeast, allowing for differentiation between some common *Candida* spp on the basis of colony color
    - *Candida albicans*: Light to medium green colonies
    - *Candida tropicalis*: Dark blue colonies
    - *Candida krusei*: Flat, pink colonies
  - Germ tube test: Presumptively identifies *C albicans*
    - Yeast are incubated in serum at 37°C for up to 3 hours. A wet mount is prepared and examined for the formation of germ tubes (hyphae with no constriction at the juncture with the yeast cell)
    - *C albicans* yeasts produce true hyphae without a constriction between the mother cell and the hyphal element (most species produce only pseudohyphae, with a constriction) i6.110
    - *C dubliniensis* also produces germ tubes within 3 hours
  - Rapid trehalose assimilation: Presumptively identifies *C glabrata*
    - Yeast isolate is inoculated into broth containing trehalose and a pH indicator. After a short (3 hour) incubation at 42°C, fermentation of the substrate causes a color change, indicating a positive result
  - Urease test: Presumptively identifies *Cryptococcus* spp
    - Urease enzyme activity distinguishes ascomycetous yeasts (no urease activity) from basidiomycetous yeasts (urease activity)
    - Urea disks can detect urease activity by a color change within a few hours; somewhat longer testing required by urea agar slants
    - Other common basidiomycetous (urease positive) yeasts: *Rhodotorula* spp & *Trichosporon* spp
  - Phenol oxidase test: Presumptively identifies *Cryptococcus neoformans*
    - *C neoformans* is able to oxidize diphenolic compounds such as caffeic acid, dopamine, and dopa to produce darkly pigmented melanin or melanin precursors
    - Classic phenol oxidase test involves performing a culture of a yeast isolate on bird seed agar, a natural source of caffeic acid (growth of brown pigmented colonies supports the presumptive identification of *C neoformans*, nonpigmented colonies indicate a negative result)
    - Rapid method involves the use of caffeic acid disks, which are inoculated with a yeast isolate and can demonstrate brown pigment production within a few hours
- Definitive identification
  - Assimilation & other biochemical tests
  - Matrix-assisted laser desorption/ionization time-of-flight (MALDI-TOF) mass spectrometry
  - Kit & automated identification systems
  - Demonstration of specific morphology using specialized media
    - Certain media, especially rice or cornmeal agar supplemented with Tween 80, will reliably induce formation of characteristic yeast structures such as blastoconidia, pseudohyphae, true hyphae, arthroconidia, or chlamydospores (chlamydoconidia)

6.5.6.2 Notes on specific yeasts

- *C albicans*
  - Most common *Candida* spp isolated from humans, regardless of site
  - 3-5 µm budding yeast with accompanying pseudohyphae i6.111 and occasional true hyphae

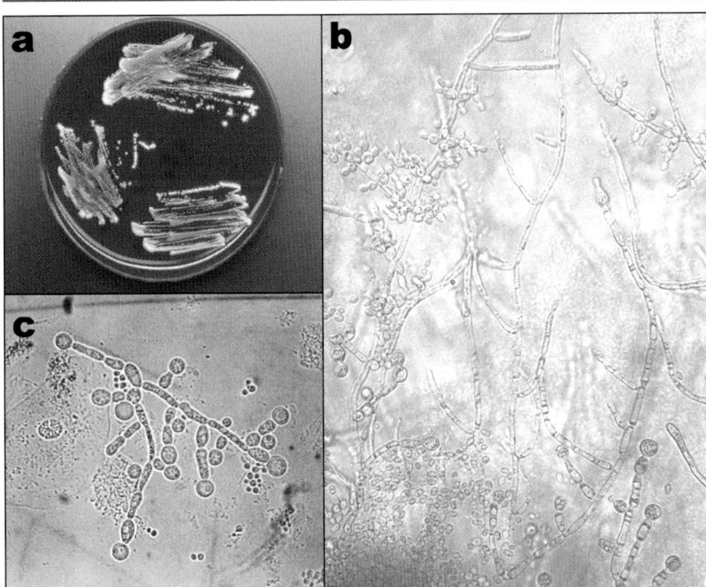

i6.112 *Candida albicans:* a colonies frequently form filamentous extensions ("feet") around the edges
b on yeast morphology medium, pseudohyphae are seen with clusters of blastoconidia at septations & single terminal chlamydospores
c true hyphae, pseudohyphae, clamydospores, blastospor

- Colonies grown on solid medium frequently form filamentous extensions ("feet") around the edges i6.112a; not seen in nonalbicans species
- When cultures performed on yeast morphology medium (cornmeal or rice agar with Tween), pseudohyphae are formed with clusters of blastoconidia at the septations i6.112b; also, terminal chlamydospores seen i6.112c
- Positive germ tube test
- Forms green colonies on chromogenic agar
- Most clinical isolates are susceptible to azole agents, echinocandins & amphotericin B

- *Candida dubliniensis*
  - Oral candidiasis in HIV-infected patients
  - Similar to *C albicans*: Germ tube positive, darker green colonies on CHROMagar, terminal chlamydospores produced
  - No growth at 42°C (C albicans is positive for growth)
- *Candida auris*
  - Emerging pathogen associated with outbreaks in healthcare facilities (eg. in patients with lines or tubes for breathing, feeding, central venous catheters)
  - Causes serious invasive infection
  - Multidrug resistant
  - Difficult to ID using traditional, kit, and some instruments; MALDI-TOF
- *Candida glabrata*
  - Frequently isolated from blood & urine

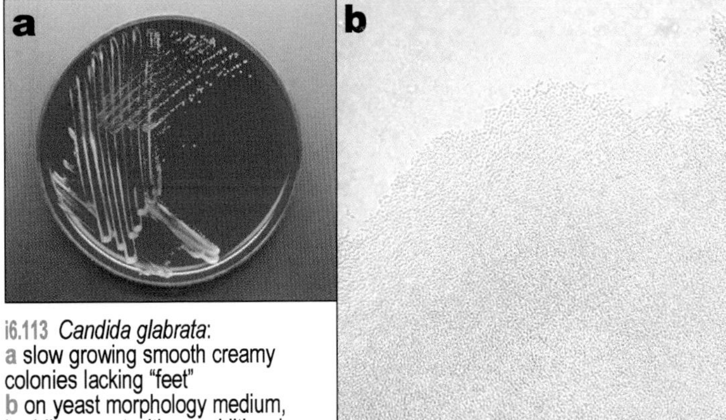

i6.113 *Candida glabrata*:
a slow growing smooth creamy colonies lacking "feet"
b on yeast morphology medium, budding yeast with no additional structures formed

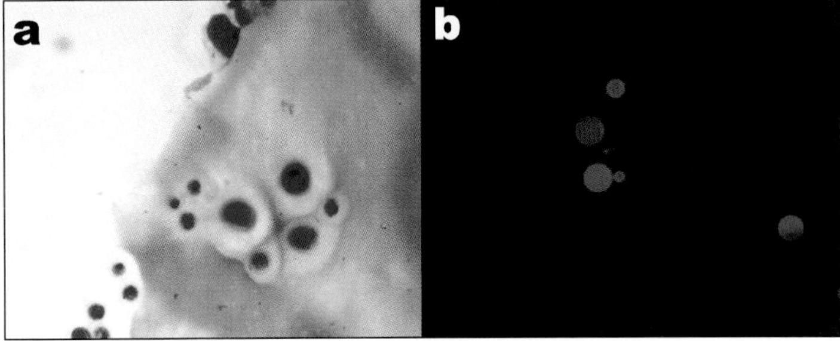

i6.114 *Cryptococcus neoformans*: a Wright stain & b calcofluor white show spherical, narrow budding yeasts that vary greatly in size

  - 2-4 µm budding yeast (blastoconidia), without pseudohyphae
  - Grow more slowly than other *Candida* spp; may take an extra day for mature colony formation i6.113a
  - Yeast morphology medium does not induce structures other than budding yeast i6.113b
  - Positive on the rapid trehalose assimilation test
  - Frequently reduced susceptibility to azole agents (both imidazoles & triazoles), but most isolates are susceptible to echinocandins & amphotericin B
- *Cryptococcus* spp
  - Main human pathogens are *C neoformans* & *C gattii*
  - *C neoformans* is the cause of most infections in the United States
  - *C gattii* largely confined to tropical zones but emerging in northwestern United States
  - *C neoformans*: Soil containing bird excreta (pigeon, chicken)
  - *C gattii*: Associated with eucalyptus trees
  - 3-15 µm narrow budding yeasts that vary in size i6.114
  - Encapsulated (although rare capsule-deficient strains exist), highlighted in wet mounts using India ink i6.115a, b
    - India ink wet mount is not a sensitive test

ISBN 978-089189-6616

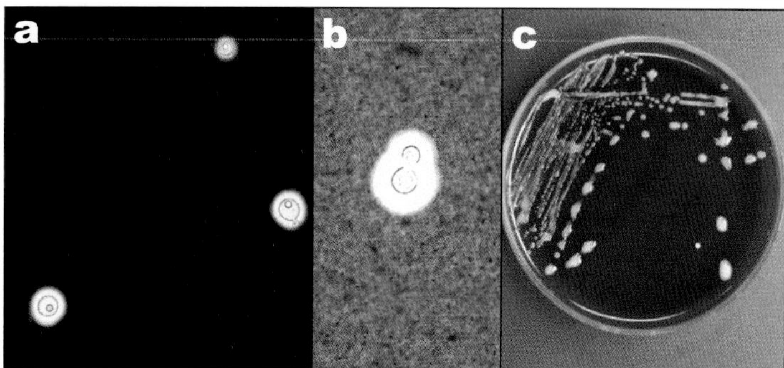

i6.115 *C neoformans*: India ink preparation at a low & b high magnification show spherical, narrow-budding yeasts with thick capsule
c mucoid colonies on solid agar

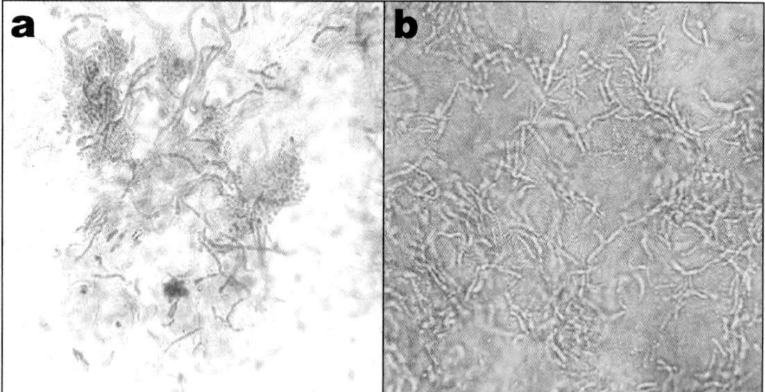

i6.116 *Malasezzia*:
a CSB (Chicago sky blue) stain showing short & angular hyphae with clusters of spherical/flask-shaped yeasts, giving the characteristic spaghetti and meatball appearance
b KOH wet mount reveals clusters of spherical yeasts seen as refractile elements

  - Colonies frequently mucoid i6.115c, owing to the capsular material
  - Never forms other structures like pseudohyphae
  - Cryptococcal capsular polysaccharide antigen can be detected in either serum or body fluids (usually CSF)
- *Malasezzia furfur*
  - Causes tinea versicolor & disseminated infection in infants who receive lipid replacement therapy
  - Skin colonizer that requires lipids for growth
  - Identify using potassium hydroxide (KOH) wet mount showing budding yeasts & hyphae—"spaghetti & meatballs" appearance i6.116a, b (more visible with special stain)
  - Overlay culture media with olive oil to get growth
- *Pneumocystis jiroveci*
  - Formerly known as *P carinii*
  - In vitro cultures cannot be performed
  - Major pathogen in immunodeficient hosts
    - In HIV-infected patients with acquired immunodeficiency syndrome (AIDS) with CD4 count <200 cells/mL

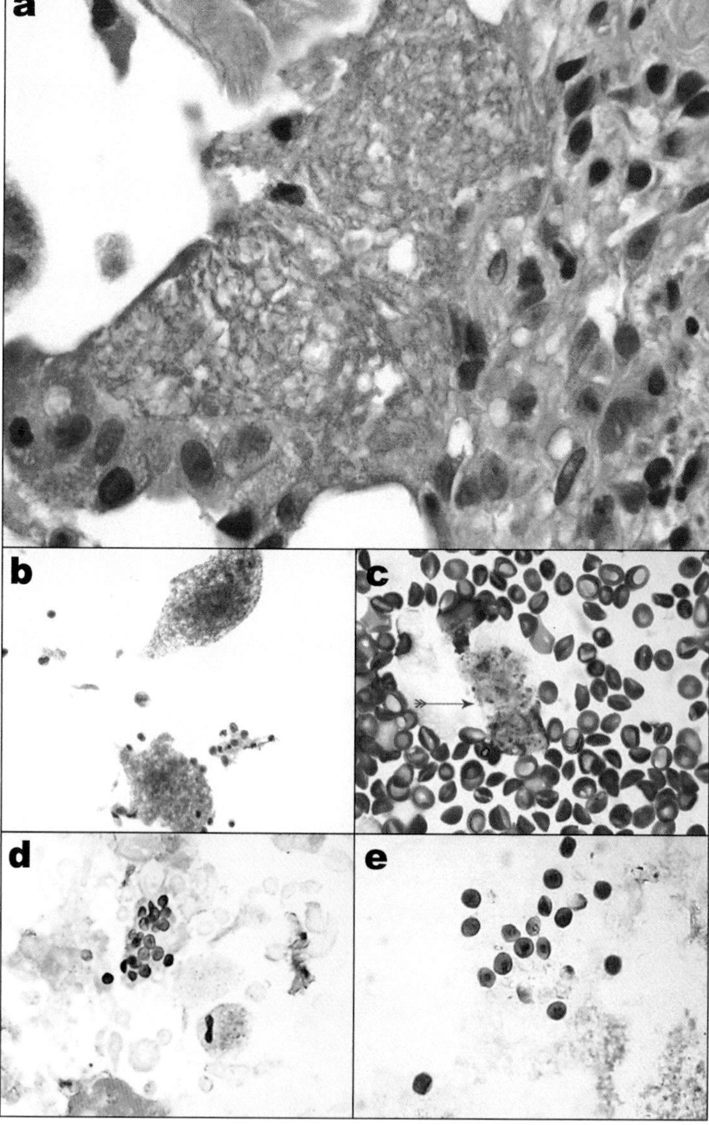

i6.117 *Pneumocystis*: characteristic exudative material is seen within alveolar airspaces on a an H&E stained lung section & b on Pap stained & c Wright stained sputum smears; note the central dot visible within the empty spaces on the Wright stained preparation
In GMS stained preparations at d low & e high magnification, the organisms are approximately the size of yeast but do not bud; they tend to cluster & have a central dark staining dot when stained with silver stains; cyst forms are round or cup shaped & have been likened to crushed ping pong balls

    - Infected patients typically present with respiratory symptoms
    - Serologic testing is not helpful
    - Respiratory samples show typical exudate i6.117, and organisms easily seen on Papanicolaou-stained, Giemsa-stained & Gomori methenamine silver (GMS)-stained preparations
    - Immunofluorescent staining with anti *Pneumocystis* monoclonal antibodies can provide greater specificity

6.5.6.3 Antifungal agents

- Amphotericin B: Kills most yeasts & molds but side effects are nephrotoxicity, fever, chills, myalgias
- Azoles
  - Ketoconazole: Yeasts & dimorphic fungi, but less effective than other agents and does have side affects
  - Fluconazole: Specific for yeast infections but *C krusei* is intrinsically resistant and *C glabrata* has decreased susceptibility
  - Itraconazole: For yeast & mold infections
  - Porconazole: For yeast & mold infections
  - Voriconazole: For yeast & mold infections
- Capsofungin: For *Candida* spp & *Aspergillus*
- Flucytosine: For yeasts
- Griseofulvin: For dermatophytes
- Susceptibility testing is limited and usually done by reference laboratories

6.6 Virology

6.6.1 Specimen collection & transport

- Viral shedding is highest in early stages of infection and decreases rapidly a few days after acute symptoms
- Aspiration of secretions is the preferred specimen
  - If swabs are used, they must be Dacron or rayon
  - Calcium alginate & wood shafted swabs can interfere with some molecular testing and also inhibit some viral replication
  - Viral samples can be put in saline, tryptic soy broth (TSB), or transport medium (eg, albumin, gelatin, fetal-bovine serum, and has antifungal & antimicrobial agents with buffered isotonic solution)
  - Process viral sample immediately OR store at 4°C. If specimen must be stored for >4 days before processing, freeze at −70°C (−20°C causes ice crystals to form)
  - Specimens for transport medium: Swabs & tissue samples, respiratory samples
  - Specimens that should not be put in transport medium: Blood, CSF, urine, amniotic, pleural, pericardial fluids

6.6.2 Laboratory methods

- Cell culture
  - Cell culture is now seldom used in routine clinical microbiology laboratories. The outline will not include detection of viruses using cell culture methodology
  - It is the gold standard method for isolating live viruses to show active infection
  - Cell cultures observed for presence of cytopathic effect (CPE) **t6.37**, which is identified when the tissue monolayer shows evidence of disruption

t6.37 Viral CPE

Enterovirus	CMV	Adenovirus	RSV	HSV
Tear shaped cells	Focal plaques in HDF	Grapelike clusters	Syncytial cells	Sweeping, globular cells

  - Viruses have their own distinct patterns of CPE
- Serology
  - Measures host response to virus; detects circulating antibody
  - Paired sera, taken 7-10 days apart (acute & convalescent), showing a 4-fold or greater rise in IgG titer is generally considered diagnostic of infection
  - Positive IgG antibody may indicate current or past infection
  - Positive IgM antibody indicates current infection
- Direct antigen detection
  - Enzyme-linked immunosorbent assay (EIA)
  - Latex agglutination
  - Direct fluorescent antibody (DFA)
- Molecular techniques
  - Nucleic acid amplification tests (NAAT)
  - Film array
  - Reverse transcription (RT)
  - Signal amplification
  - Target amplification (nucleic acid sequence-based amplification [NASBA] & transcription-mediated amplification [TMA])
- In-situ hybridization used for the cytologic or histologic ID of virus DNA or RNA present in tissue cells of patients (eg, human papillomavirus [HPV] in cervical samples, cytomegalovirus [CMV] in lung biopsy, herpes simplex virus [HSV] in skin biopsy, or parvovirus B19 in marrow)

- Histology
  - Light microscopy useful for viruses with characteristic inclusions t6.38
  - Immunohistochemistry may be applied to histologic in-situ hybridizaton

t6.38 Viral histology

Virus	Nuclear inclusions	Cytoplasmic inclusions	Syncytia	Notes
RSV	–	–	+	
HSV	+	–	+	Cowdry type A ("owl eye") bodies in **m**ultinucleated cells; nuclei are **m**olded & chromatin is **m**arginalized (3 Ms of HSV infection)
Adenovirus	+	–	–	"Smudge cells"
CMV	+	+	–	"Owl eye" inclusion, not multinucleated
Measles	+	+	+	Warthin-Finkeldey giant cells
Rabies	–	+	–	Negri bodies

6.6.3 Classification t6.39

t6.39 Virus classification

	DNA viruses		RNA viruses	
	Single stranded	Double stranded	Single stranded	Double stranded
Nonenveloped	Parvoviridae Bocavirus	Adenoviridae Papillomaviridae Polyomaviridae	Picornaviridae (poliovirus, enteroviruses), hepatitis A, rhinovirus) Calciviridae (norovirus) Hepeviridae (hepatitis E)	Reoviridae: rotavirus
Enveloped		Herpesviridae Hepadnaviridae (HBV) Poxviridae	Flaviviridae (HCV, yellow fever, dengue, WNV, St Louis & Japanese encephalitis) Togaviridae (rubella, EEE, Zika) Retroviridae (HIV, HTLV) Orthomyxoviridae (influenza) Paramyxoviridae (RSV, hMPV, parainfluenza, mumps, measles) Rhabdoviridae (rabies) Coronaviridae Arenaviridae Bunyaviridae (hantavirus, California encephalitis) Deltavirus (hepatitis D) Filoviridae (Marburg, Ebola)	

6.6.4 Human herpesviruses (HHV) t6.40

6.6.4.1 Herpes simplex virus (HSV)

- HSV type 1
  - Mouth & lips infected, herpes labialis (cold sores), pharyngitis, hand/finger (herpetic whitlow), genital infection & herpes encephalitis/meningitis
  - Transmitted by saliva. Primary infection usually occurs before puberty
  - Virus infects & achieves dormancy within the nuclei of trigeminal ganglia HSV type 2
- HSV type 2
  - Genital herpes, occasional skin infections, oropharyngeal infection, herpes meningitis (does not typically cause encephalitis), neonatal herpes
  - Dormancy in sacral ganglia
- Diagnosis
  - Enzyme immunoassay (EIA) & direct fluorescent antibody (DFA)
  - Direct DNA probes & polymerase chain reaction (PCR) becoming more widespread

t6.40 Human herpesviruses

Herpes virus	Latency	Clinical disease: Acute	Clinical disease: Reactivation
HSV1	Dorsal root ganglia	Acute gingivostomatitis Pharyngitis Skin infection of hand/finger (herpetic whitlow) Genital herpes (less commonly)	Herpes labialis Herpes encephalitis Less likely to cause recurrent genital herpes lesions than those caused by HSV2
HSV2	Dorsal root ganglia	Genital herpes Skin infection (herpetic whitlow) Acute gingivostomatitis (less commonly)	Genital herpes Herpes meningitis
CMV	Histiocytes, endothelial cells, T lymphocytes	Mononucleosislike syndrome; disseminated infection in neonates & immunocompromised hosts	Disseminated infection
VZV	Dorsal root ganglia	Varicella (chicken pox)	Zoster (shingles)
EBV	B cells Burkitts lymphoma, NP carcinoma	t6.41	t6.41
HHV6	T cells	Roseola (exanthem subitum)	Reactivation in immunocompromised hosts
HHV7	Lymphocytes	Roseola (occasionally)	Reactivation in immunocompromised hosts
HHV8	B lymphocytes, endothelial cells	Unknown	Kaposi sarcoma Primary body cavity lymphoma

CMV, cytomegalovirus; EBV, Epstein-Barr virus; HHV, human herpesvirus; HSV, herpes simplex virus; VZV, varicella zoster virus

6.6.4.2 Varicella zoster virus (VZV) (see Immunology 8.4.6.4)

- Primary VZV
  - Generally benign, causing childhood varicella (chicken pox)
  - May be complicated by life-threatening pneumonia in adolescents & adults
  - Pregnant women & immunocompromised individuals are at risk for serious disseminated infection
- Reactivation of VZV
  - Causes zoster (shingles), a painful dermatomal vesicular rash
  - Pain may persist long after the rash clears (postherpetic neuralgia)
- Congenital varicella
  - Congenital varicella diagnosed when there is:
    - Evidence of maternal varicella infection during pregnancy
    - Skin lesions on the newborn
    - Serologic evidence of infection in the newborn (either IgM or persistent IgG beyond 7 months)
- Diagnosis: Serology (positive IgM or 4-fold rise in IgG), direct antigen detection (DFA of skin scrapings), PCR (especially useful for diagnosis of CNS involvement)

6.6.4.3 Cytomegalovirus (CMV) (see Immunology 8.4.6.6)

- Primary CMV infection
  - Transmitted in breast milk, sexual contact, organ & blood transfusions, close contact
  - Usually either asymptomatic or a mononucleosislike syndrome in immunocompetent host
  - In immunocompromised persons (transplant recipients) & neonates, can cause serious infections; rare congenital involvement
- CMV colitis
  - Immunosuppressed patients
  - May present as inflammatory bowel disease (Crohn disease or ulcerative colitis) exacerbation
- Identification
  - Identification of viral cytopathic effect (CPE) by light microscopy is usually possible **t6.37**
  - Diagnosis: ELISA is most common serologic test, PCR is most common molecular test
  - MRC-5 cell line requires 30 days to develop cytopathic effect (CPE) while shell vial is 48 hours

6.6.4.4 Epstein-Barr virus (EBV) (see Immunology 8.4.6.5)

- Primary infection is infectious mononucleosis: Sore throat, fever, lymphadenopathy, splenomegaly, hepatomegaly, malaise **t6.41**
- Enters body through the pharyngeal mucosa; "kissing disease"
- Infects B lymphocytes
- CD8-positive T lymphocytes proliferate and are responsible for the peripheral blood atypical lymphocytosis that is seen

t6.41 Clinical syndromes caused by EBV

Disease	Stage of infection	Notes
Infectious mononucleosis	Primary	Mainly in adolescents & young adults
X-linked lymphoproliferative disease (Duncan disease)	Primary	Mainly males affected (usually boys); patients with this disorder mount an overactive immune response to EBV, resulting in fulminant infectious mononucleosis, B-cell lymphoma, aplastic anemia & dysgammaglobulinemia
Burkitt lymphoma	latent	Endemic, sporadic & immunodeficiency associated forms; nearly 100% of endemic Burkitt lymphoma in African children & 25% of sporadic & immunodeficiency associated cases
Hodgkin lymphoma	Latent	EBV in 50% of cases
Primary effusion lymphoma	Latent	EBV in 70% of cases (HHV-8 in 100%)
Lymphomatoid granulomatosis	Latent	Systemic angiodestructive lymphoproliferative disease
Posttransplant lymphoproliferative disorder	Latent	>95% EBV-positive
Oral hairy leukoplakia	Latent	In HIV infection; EBER-negative
Nasopharyngeal carcinoma	Latent	Nearly 100% EBV-positive in Chinese & Inuit populations; 75% EBV-positive in United States

EBV, Epstein-Barr virus; EBER, EBV-encoded RNA; HHV, human herpesvirus

- Diagnosis
  - The monospot test is based on the frequent presence of heterophile antibodies in EBV infection; in particular, antibody with strong affinity for beef erythrocyte that is uninhibited by adsorption with guinea pig kidney antigen (the differential absorption test)
    - Monospot is fairly specific but insensitive, being present in 80% of infected teens & adults, 40% of all infected children, and 20% of infected children <4 years old

ISBN 978-089189-6616

- CDC does not recommend using the monospot test because it produces both false-positive & false-negative results
- Viral capsid antigen (VCA)
  - Anti-VCA IgM appears early in infection and disappears in 4-6 weeks
  - Anti-VCA IgG appears in acute phase of EBV and peaks at 2-4 weeks after onset, declines slightly & persists for lifetime
- Anti-early antigen (EA) IgG appears in acute phases of illness and decreases significantly after 3-6 months. Its presence is sign of active disease but 20% of healthy population can have antibodies for years
- Anti-Epstein Barr nucleic antigen (EBNA) appears slowly 2-4 months after onset of symptoms and persists for the rest of a person's life
- Primarily serologic **f6.1**, **t6.42**

t6.42 EBV serology

Stage	Heterophile	IgM anti-VCA	IgG anti-EA	IgG anti-VCA	Anti-EBNA
Uninfected	–	–	–	–	–
Early acute	–/+	+	–	+	–
Acute	±	+	+	+	–/+
Convalescent	–	–	+	+	+
Remote	–	–	+	–/+	+

EA, early antigen; EBV, Epstein-Barr virus; EBNA, Epstein-Barr nucleic antigen; VCA, viral capsid antigen

6.6.4.5 Human herpesvirus 6 (HHV-6)

- Primary infection
  - Usually asymptomatic or nonspecific febrile illness
  - May present as roseola infantum (Sixth disease) in infants
  - Highly neurotropic; may cause viral encephalitis
  - Responsible for a significant proportion of childhood febrile seizures
- Reactivation
  - Primarily affects immunocompromised hosts
  - Occurs in ~1/2 of bone marrow transplant recipients and 1/3 of solid organ transplant recipients
- Diagnosis
  - EIA, PCR, clinical presentation

6.6.4.6 Human herpesvirus 7 (HHV-7)

- Closely related to HHV-6; also causes roseola

6.6.4.7 Human herpesvirus 8 (HHV-8)

- Also known as Kaposi sarcoma-associated herpesvirus (KSHV)
- Rare in immunocompetent persons
- Diagnosis: Molecular methods, immunohistochemical staining, or serology

6.6.5 Adenovirus

- Clinical features
  - Infections are self-limiting and include respiratory tract, GI tract, eye (other areas in low incidence)
- Diagnosis
  - Serology (positive IgM or 4-fold rise in IgG)
  - Fluorescent antibody (FA), EIA, molecular tests (PCR)

6.6.6 Parvovirus

- Parvovirus B19 (genus *Erythrovirus*)
  - Erythema infectiosum (red rash or "slapped cheek disease"; Fifth disease)
  - Aplastic anemia
  - Primary maternal infection during gestation can lead to hydrops fetalis
  - Infection in persons with chronic hemolytic anemia (eg, sickle cell disease) can cause an aplastic crisis
  - Identification with immunohistochemistry (IHC), fluorescence in situ hybridization (FISH), or polymerase chain reaction (PCR)
- Human bocavirus
  - A respiratory virus that, at this time, is detectable only on polymerase chain reaction (PCR)

6.6.7 Papillomavirus

- Clinical features
  - Linked to cervical cancer and one of most common sexually transmitted diseases (STDs)
  - Human papillomavirus (HPV) causes proliferative epithelial lesions, warts
  - Vaccine protects women, men/boys from cancer and transmission of virus to women
  - Identified with PCR
  - No viremic phase associated with the virus. Women will not present with symptoms, can only be detected on cervical Pap smear, and molecular testing performed from Pap collection

6.6.8 Poxviridae

- Poxviruses cause vesicular skin eruptions
- Variola
    - Causes smallpox, a vesicular eruption similar to chickenpox with fever
    - WHO declared world free of smallpox in 1980, with stocks of virus still maintained in some laboratories
    - Considered an agent of possible bioterrorism
    - Vaccination lasts up to 10 years, which means most of the worlds' population is susceptible
- Vaccinia virus
    - A laboratory-derived virus related to variola that is used in the smallpox vaccine

6.6.9 Hepatitis viruses t6.43

t6.43 Hepatitis viruses

Virus	Transmission	Incubation	Chronicity	Comments
HAV	Fecal-oral	15-30 days	0%	Most common viral hepatitis in United States; Abrupt onset
HBV	Parenteral	15-150 days, average 60-90 days	2%-10% of everyone 30%-90% of children <5 years	Usually insidious; mortality: ~1%
HCV	Parenteral	30-150 days	60%-85%	~10,000 deaths annually
HDV	Parenteral	21-49 days	5% of coinfections ≤80% of superinfections	Exists as a co-infection with HBV
HEV	Fecal-oral	15-60 days, average 40 days	0%	20%-30% fatality rate in pregnancy
HGV	Parenteral	Unknown	Unknown	Significance of infection unknown

HAV, hepatitis A virus; HBV, hepatitis B virus; HCV, hepatitis C virus; HDV, hepatitis D virus; HEV, hepatitis E virus; HGV, hepatitis G virus

6.6.9.1 Hepatitis A virus (HAV)—Picornavirus

- Fecal oral transmission; hepatitis associated with water- & food-related outbreaks or via close personal contact with infected persons
- Causes sudden, acute disease with fever, chills, fatigue, aches, possible jaundice

- Diagnosis of acute infection (see Immunology 8.4.9.1)
- Clinical features
    - Demonstration of IgM anti-HAV using ELISA or radioimmunoassay
    - IgG anti-HAV may indicate acute or past infection; persists for life
- Vaccination to HAV is available

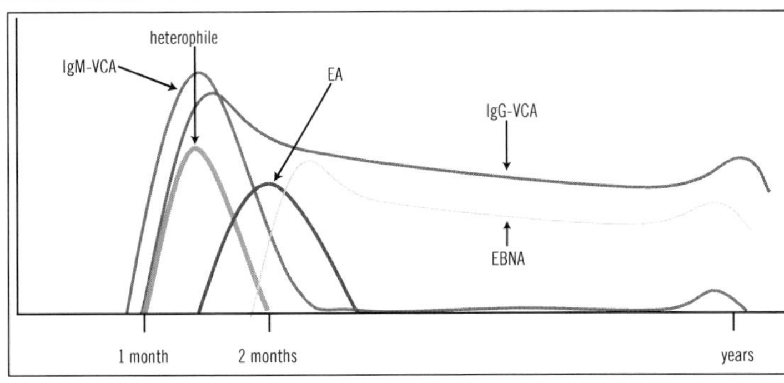

f6.1 EBV serology in primary infection & reactivation

6.6.9.2 Hepatitis B virus (HBV)—Hepadnavirus

- Clinical features (see Immunology 8.4.9.2)
    - Bloodborne pathogen is transmitted in blood, semen, other body fluids (saliva, breast milk, vaginal secretions, amniotic fluid)
    - Transmitted by sexual contact, sharing needles & syringes, mother-to-infant transmission at birth
    - Causes acute or chronic symptoms
    - Symptoms include fever, fatigue, nausea, vomiting, abdominal pain, jaundice
- DNA virus; intact virion is called the Dane particle, which is very stable
    - Virus has hepatitis B core antigen (HBcAg), hepatitis B surface antigen (HBsAg) & hepatitis Be antigen (HBeAg)
- HBV viral markers
    - Hepatitis B surface antigen (HbsAg; Australia antigen)
        - Indicates active disease, acute carrier state of virus, or incubation period in patient
    - Hepatitis B e antigen (HBeAg)
        - Indicates acute disease with active viral replication
        - Only produced when the virus is in replicating form
    - Antibody to hepatitis B core antigen (anti-HBc)
        - Present throughout the lifetime of somebody who has been infected with HBV
        - Shows acute & chronic infection
        - Hepatitis B core IgM present during the acute infection
    - Antibody to hepatitis B e antigen (anti HBe)
        - Found when HBe becomes negative
        - Does not imply resolved infection or immunity
        - Indicates chronic infection
    - Antibody to surface antigen (HBsAb)
        - Indicates resolution of infection and confers immunity to disease
        - Also indicates vaccination

ISBN 978-089189-6616

- Acute hepatitis B infection **f6.2**, **t6.44**
  - Serologic markers begin to emerge 2-10 weeks after exposure
  - HBsAg appears first, followed by HBeAg and IgM anti-HBc
  - HBV DNA is detectable in serum before HBsAg
  - Emergence of antibodies (anti-HBs, anti-HBc) coincides with emergence of symptoms
  - In most patients, there is complete resolution of acute HBV infection
  - This is heralded by the emergence of anti-HBe & anti-HBs
  - Some patients develop chronic infection; HBsAg remains positive
- Chronic hepatitis B infection
  - Defined by persistence of HBsAg for >6 months **t6.44**
  - Persistent HBsAg without clinical hepatitis is called the chronic carrier state
  - Chronicity develops in:
    - 5% of healthy infected adults
    - 10% of immunocompromised adults
    - 90% of neonates infected transplacentally
  - Chronic HBs antigenemia can be associated with polyarteritis nodosum (PAN)
- Molecular assays
  - There are 3 major applications of molecular assays in HBV
    - Making initial diagnosis of HBV
    - Replicative vs nonreplicative chronic HBV: Those with $>10^5$ copies of HBV DNA/mL are considered replicative
    - Response to therapy: Undetectable HBV DNA is considered a virologic response

t6.44 Hepatitis B (HBV) serology

Clinical status	HBsAg	Anti-HBc	Anti-HBs
Neither prior infection nor immunization	–	–	–
Prior immunization	–	–	+
Acute HBV	+	+ (IgM)	–
Chronic HBV	+	+	–
Resolved HBV	–	+ (IgM & IgG)	+

6.6.9.3 Hepatitis C virus (HCV)—Flavivirus

- Clinical features (see Immunology 8.4.9.4)
  - Most common cause of transfusion associated viral hepatitis: Exposure to infected blood
  - Long incubation period (years)

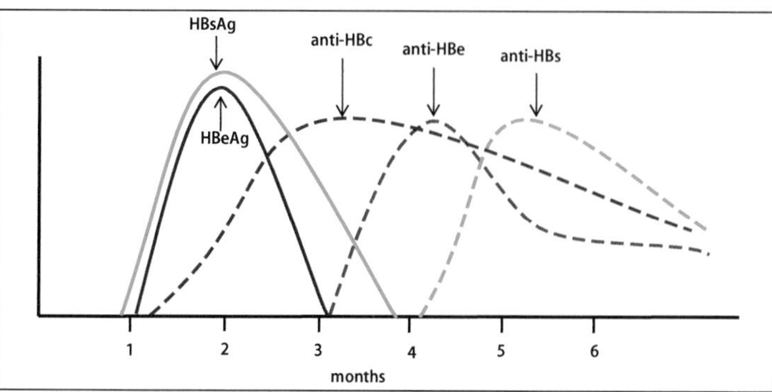

f6.2 Serologic patterns in acute HBV with resolution of infection

  - At first, person is asymptomatic or mildly symptomatic
  - Disease symptoms include fever, fatigue, dark urine, abdominal pain, nausea, vomiting, jaundice, joint pain
    - 60% of those infected develop chronic HCV
    - 15% of those with chronic HCV develop cirrhosis
    - 5% of those with cirrhosis develop hepatocellular carcinoma
- No vaccine available
- Diagnosis **t6.45**
  - Enzyme immunoassay (EIA)-based assays for anti-HCV antibodies
  - Chemiluminescence immunoassay for anti-HCV antibodies
  - Polymerase chain reaction (PCR)

t6.45 Possible HCV results

Anti-HCV EIA	RIBA	HCV RNA	Interpretation
–	–	+	Very early HCV infection (<3 mo)
+	+	+	Current HCV infection, acute or chronic
+	–/indeterminate	–	False positive anti-HCV EIA
+	+	–	Cleared/resolved prior HCV infection

EIA, enzyme immunoassay; HCV, hepatitis C virus; RIBA, recombinant immunoblot assay

6.6.9.4 Hepatitis E virus (HEV)

- Clinical features
  - Liver infection uncommon in the United States
  - Fecal oral spread
  - Affects young adults, peaking between 15 and 35 years of age
- Diagnosis
  - Rule out hepatitis A, B, C & other hepatotropic viruses
  - Molecular testing

6.6.9.5 Other viruses causing hepatitis

- EBV, CMV, HSV, VZV & yellow fever

6.6.10 Orthomyxovirus (see Immunology 8.4.6.11)

6.6.10.1 Influenzae A

- Clinical features
  - Annual outbreaks, usually during cold weather—November to April
  - Seasonal subtypes include H3 & H1
  - Spread by aerosols
  - Severe morbidity results from complications of acute infection
    - Influenza pneumonia, secondary bacterial pneumonia (most common cause of death), Reye syndrome, myositis, myocarditis & Guillain-Barré syndrome
- Virus undergoes regular antigenic changes that prevent lifelong immunity
  - Antigenic drift (minor changes) results from point mutation in H&N genes
    - Drift produces annual outbreaks & epidemics
  - Antigenic shift (major changes) result from genetic reassortment between strains
    - Shift produces worldwide outbreaks (pandemics) every 10-20 years
- Surface antigens
  - Hemagglutinin (H) & neuroaminidase (N) antigens continually change (eg, HINI, H5NI subtype of influenza A and agent of avian or bird flu)
- Diagnosis
  - Preferred specimens include nasopharyngeal swabs or washings and bronchoalveolar lavages, placed directly into viral transport medium
  - Do not freeze specimens
  - Perform a culture of the traditional gold standard (being replaced by polymerase chain reaction [PCR])
  - Rapid antigen tests, eg, direct fluorescent antibody (DFA), enzyme immunoassay (EIA)
  - Rapid molecular testing (reverse transcriptase-PCR [RT-PCR])
  - Nucleic acid detection (NAT), detection of influenza viral RNA using polymerase chain reaction (PCR)

6.6.10.2 Influenza B

- Seasonal and only infects humans
- Does not undergo antigenic shift

6.6.11 Paramyxoviruses

6.6.11.1 Parainfluenza virus

- Parainfluenza 1 is the most common causes of croup in children
- Diagnosis based on antigen detection (immunofluorescent assays) or polymerase chain reaction (PCR)

6.6.11.2 Measles (morbillivirus)

- The cause of classic measles (rubeola)
  - Classic prodrome of cough, coryza, conjunctivitis with or without Koplik spots (lesions on oral mucosa)
  - Descending rash beginning on the head
  - Immunizations drastically reduce the number of cases in the United States
- Diagnose using enzyme immunoassay (EIA), immunofluorescence (IF), molecular tests

6.6.11.3 Mumps virus (rubulavirus) (see Immunology 8.4.6.9)

- Cause of parotitis (swelling primarily of parotid glands)
- Virus shed in saliva & urine
- Vaccine protection incomplete and outbreaks have occurred in the United States
- Diagnosis made with enzyme immunoassay (EIA) & other serologic methods, immunofluorescence (IF)

6.6.11.4 Respiratory syncytial virus (pneumovirus)

- Clinical features
  - Most common cause of lower respiratory tract infection (pneumonia & respiratory bronchiolitis) in infants & toddlers
  - Localized outbreaks, such as in daycare centers, with nearly 100% attack rate
  - Same time as flu season (November-March/April)
  - Can be a serious infection in older patients where pneumonia develops
- Diagnosis
  - Nasopharyngeal swabs & washes for specimen collection; do not freeze
  - Rapid direct fluorescent antibody (DFA) shows large, multinucleated cells (syncytial), enzyme immunoassay (EIA) techniques, polymerase chain reaction (PCR)

6.6.12 Picornaviruses

- Small RNA viruses; pico = small

6.6.12.1 Enteroviruses

- Spread via aerosols, fecal-oral route, fomites; most common cause of viral meningitis (aseptic meningitis)

 ISBN 978-089189-6616

  - Poliovirus: Causes poliomyelitis; vaccine available
  - Coxsackie A: Hand-foot-and-mouth disease (HFMD); aseptic meningitis
  - Coxsackie B: Myocarditis & pericarditis; aseptic meningitis
  - Echovirus: Aseptic meningitis
  - Hepatitis A
- Diagnose with molecular methods

6.6.12.2 Rhinovirus

- Most common cause of the common cold
- Transmit via respiratory aerosols & secretions on fomites
- Diagnose using molecular methods; no vaccine

6.6.13 Family *Bunyaviridae*

- Along with a few other families, such as *Togaviridae*, includes many of the agents previously classified as arboviruses (arthropod borne). Not all agents in these families are arthropod borne
- Hantavirus
  - Acquired through aerosolized rodent excreta
  - Causes hantavirus pulmonary syndrome and also affects the kidneys
  - A newer hantavirus discovered in New Mexico and spread by deer mice is Sin Nombre (no name) virus
  - Use enzyme immunoassay (EIA) & molecular methods to diagnose
- Bunyavirus (eg, California encephalitis)
- Nairovirus (eg, Crimean Congo hemorrhagic fever virus)
- Phlebovirus (eg, Rift Valley fever virus)

6.6.14 Family *Coronaviridae*

- Large family of viruses causing mild to moderate upper respiratory tract illnesses
- Three cause serious infection in humans
  - Severe acute respiratory syndrome (SARS-CoV)
  - Middle East respiratory virus (MERS)
  - SARS-CoV-2 (COVID-19)—cause of a global pandemic

6.6.15 Family *Togaviridae*

- Rubella virus (see Immunology 8.4.6.7)
  - Clinical features
    - Person-to-person spread via respiratory droplets; collect nasopharyngeal specimens or secretions from infected infant
    - Causes a febrile illness with rash (German measles)
    - Generally benign but may have consequence for developing fetus if there is maternal infection
    - Booster vaccination for children as part of measles-mumps-rubella (MMR) vaccine. Booster given before children start school
    - Booster vaccination recommended in nonimmune women of childbearing age
- Equine encephalitis viruses—mosquito-borne; birds are natural reservoir; humans & horses are infected from mosquito bites

6.6.16 Family *Flaviviridae*

- Hepatitis C virus, dengue, yellow fever, St Louis encephalitis, West Nile virus
- Dengue & yellow fever transmitted most commonly by *Aedes* spp mosquitos
- Dengue fever (breakbone fever—bone pain) and yellow fever cause fever, chills, backache, jaundice & hemorrhage in severe cases
- Yellow fever is viscerotropic for the heart, kidney, GI tract & liver; the most characteristic lesion of yellow fever is in the liver
- St Louis encephalitis transmitted by mosquitoes; asymptomatic, mild, or severe encephalitis
- West Nile virus (WNV) (see Immunology 8.4.6.10)
  - Bird virus multiplies in avian host and female *Culex* mosquito is vector
  - Humans are incidental hosts
- Zikavirus
  - Epidemic in Brazil in infants; causes microcephaly
  - Diagnose with molecular methods

6.6.17 Family *Reoviridae*

- Rotavirus
  - Most common cause of viral gastroenteritis in children & infants
  - Transmission via fecal-oral route
  - Vomiting, diarrhea, fever, respiratory symptoms

6.6.18 Family *Rhabdoviridae*

- Rabies
  - Clinical features
    - In poorly controlled areas, dogs & cats transmit 90% of rabies
    - In areas with good control, most cases are the result of exposures to bats, wolves, coyotes, foxes, skunks & raccoons

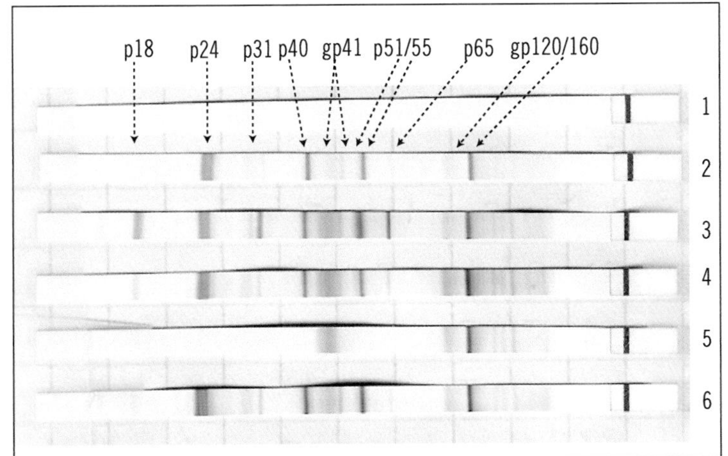

f6.3 HIV western blot
Lane 1 is negative control
Lane 2 is weak positive control & lane 6 is the strong positive control
Lanes 3-5 are positive patient samples

- The bite of an infected animal deposits virus into soft tissues
- Mental changes occur: Irritability, depression, seizures, paralysis, coma, death

- Vaccine available for those who might be exposed and to those who have high risk of exposure (veterinarian, cave explorers)
- Diagnose by testing brain tissue of infected animal

6.6.19 Family *Arenaviridae*

- These viruses infect rodents and are shed in feces, urine, saliva
- Lymphocytic choriomeningitis virus (LCM)
  - Only one of *Arenaviridae* found in United States
  - Carried by mice & hamsters
- Lassa fever virus
  - Most well-known of this family
  - Spreads by contact with secretions from a specific rat
  - Seen more in West African countries

6.6.20 Family *Retroviridae*

- Human T-cell leukemia/lymphoma virus (HTLV1)
  - Endemic in southern Japan, the Caribbean, parts of Africa
  - Transmitted parenterally (intravenous drug use, transfusion), sexual contact & transplacentally
  - Virus infects CD4+ T lymphocytes
  - Diagnostic similar to HIV—Screening enzyme-linked immunosorbent assay (ELISA), confirmatory Western blot, or polymerase chain reaction (PCR)
- HIV1 & HIV2
  - Agent for AIDS; HIV2 is mostly in West Africa
    - Transmitted in blood, semen, vaginal secretions
    - Not transmitted by casual contact (touching, hugging, coughing, via water or food, swimming pools
    - Opportunistic infections occur, along with malignancies such as Kaposi sarcoma
    - High-risk populations are sexually active gay and bisexual men, sexual activity with multiple partners, IV drug users, newborns of HIV+ mothers
    - Begins asymptomatic, then flulike symptoms, then progresses to significant immunosuppression (AIDS)
  - Laboratory tests
    - ELISA, a test for anti HIV1/2 antibodies to recombinant antigens and peptides, is the principal method for HIV screening
      - Sensitivity is >99%
      - Anti-HIV antibodies detectable within 6-8 weeks of infection (window period)
      - p24 protein detectable by 2-3 weeks
      - 4th generation tests detect antibody & antigen; by detecting antigen, early infections are identified before antibody produced
    - Western blot is used for confirmatory testing **f6.3**
      - A sample with known HIV proteins is subjected to gel electrophoresis. The gel is then transferred (blotted) onto nitrocellulose paper, to which patient serum is added. After staining, visible bands reflect antibodies within patient serum
      - The CDC has defined a positive HIV1 Western blot as the presence of any 2 of the following bands: p24, gp41, gp120/160
      - If no bands are present, the test is considered negative
      - If ≥1 bands are present but not in a combination that meets criteria for positivity, then the test is considered indeterminate. Repeat test within 6 months. Those who are repeatedly indeterminate over 6 months and who have no risk factors can be considered negative. Otherwise, a nucleic acid based test is advised
    - The sensitivity of HIV RNA in acute infection is essentially 100%. However, the specificity is not 100%, and some false positives occur; as soon as feasible, a positive HIV RNA should be confirmed with ELISA & Western blot
    - PCR testing for HIV proviral DNA is the recommended test in the diagnosis of neonatal HIV infection, but HIV RNA may be equally good. Umbilical cord blood should not be tested
    - CD4 count, determined by flow cytometry, was the earliest index of disease progression

ISBN 978-089189-6616

- AIDS is diagnosed when CD4 T-cell counts are <200/μL with virus load >75,000 copies/mL
- CD4 count still used in making treatment decisions
- Viral load
  - This is the primary variable used to determine when to initiate highly active antiretroviral therapy (HAART), and it is the viral load that determines the efficacy of this treatment
  - Quantification of circulating HIV RNA also used to monitor treatment & disease progression

6.7 Clinical syndromes

- (NOTE: For organism etiology, transmission, virulence, identification, see specific bacterial sections)

6.7.1 Urinary tract infection (UTI)

- Lower UTI: Bladder (cystitis) & urethritis
- Upper UTI: Kidney (pyelonephritis) & ureters

6.7.1.1 Common pathogens

- *Enterobacteriaceae* (*E coli* is most common)
- *Staphylococcus saprophyticus*
- *Enterococcus*
- *Pseudomonas* spp
- *Streptococcus agalactiae*
- *Candida* spp (yeast)
- Focus points on pathogens
  - *Escherichia coli* is the most common cause; 85% of all community acquired UTIs, especially UPEC (uropathogenic) strains
  - *Staphylococcus saprophyticus* common in young sexually active women
  - Other *Enterobacteriaceae*—especially *Klebsiella* spp & *Enterobacter* spp
  - *Enterococcus* common agent of UTI
  - Culture negative UTI often due to *Ureaplasma urealyti cum*, *Chlamydia* spp, or *Mycoplasma hominis*
  - Fungal UTI is mainly caused by *Candida* spp and associated with indwelling catheters or recent antibiotic therapy

6.7.1.2 Specimens

- Midstream clean catch: once several ml of urine has been voided, the patient collects urine sample in sterile container
- Catheterization
  - Straight catheter: Catheter is inserted into bladder, several milliliters of urine passes from the catheter, and then a sample is collected in sterile container
  - Indwelling catheter: Using a sterile needle & syringe, several milliliters are aspirated from the collection port on the catheter tubing
    - Do not sample collection bag because of presence of colonizing organisms
  - Suprapubic aspiration: Needle is inserted into lower abdominal wall into bladder, using aseptic technique. This can also be used to culture for anaerobes
  - Unacceptable specimens: Urine catheter tips, pooled urine samples, sample >2 hours old and left at room temperature; sample from catheter bag
  - Preservative: Specimens should be refrigerated if cannot be processed within 2 hours of collection *OR* can be held at room temperature for 24 hours if sample is put in boric acid preservative
  - Specimen processing
    - A calibrated loop is used to inoculate media
      - 0.001 mL loop used for most specimens
      - 0.01 mL loop used for catheter or suprapubic specimens

6.7.1.3 Asymptomatic bacteriuria

- Bacterial colonization without clinical symptoms
- >100,000 colony-forming units (CFU)/mL in patients with no symptoms
- Usually requires no treatment
  - Exceptions: Pregnant women & patients undergoing urologic instrumentation
- Diagnosis
  - Asymptomatic women: 2 consecutive clean catch voided urines, with isolation of the same species, $\geq 10^5$ CFU/mL)
  - Asymptomatic men: Single clean catch voided urine specimen with isolation of a single species, $\geq 10^5$ CFU/mL
  - Any patient: Single catheterized urine specimen or suprapubic sample or when patient has taken antibiotics, single bacterial species, $\geq 10^2$ CFU/mL
  - Multiple uropathogens (3 or more): Probable contamination

6.7.1.4 Symptomatic bacteriuria

- Adults: Symptoms of uncomplicated UTI of lower urinary tract include dysuria, frequency, urgency
- Adults: Acute, complicated UTI show same symptoms of lower UTI with flank pain, fever, chills, vomiting, nausea (pyelonephritis)
- Diagnosis
  - >100 to <100,000 CFU/mL single organism
  - >100,000 CFU/mL single organism

- Any patient: Single catheterized urine specimen or suprapubic sample or when patient has taken antibiotics, single bacterial species, ≥10^2 CFU/mL
- If >2 types of bacteria are found, contamination is suspected, unless pyuria is present or if the patient has long-term catheterization, and possible if 1 organism is predominant. A repeat culture is recommended
- Multiple uropathogens (≥3): Probable contamination

6.7.1.5 Laboratory approach

- Culture of collected urine sample, as outlined above
- Gram stain can provide information but not done routinely; stain performed on uncentrifuged urine that shows ≥1 bacterial cells/oil immersion field (OIF) correlates with 100,000 CFU/mL
  - Very useful for diagnosis in neonates and/or infants suspected of having UTI
- Urine dipstick leukocyte esterase: sensitivity 70%-95% and specificity 70%
- Urine dipstick nitrite: positive with organism capable of reducing nitrate to nitrite, such as coliforms. Specificity 95%, sensitivity 50%. Negative in the presence of *Staphylococcus saprophyticus*, enterococci & non-nitrate reducing gram-negative bacilli
- Automated urine screening: photometry methods, flow cytometry, particle filtration

6.7.2 Gastrointestinal tract

6.7.2.1 Major bacterial pathogens

- Noninflammatory (watery, without fever): *Vibrio cholera*, enterotoxigenic *E coli* (ETEC), *C perfringens*, *S aureus* & *B cereus*
  - ETEC produces choleralike toxin. Most common cause of traveler's diarrhea
  - Cholera
    - Severe voluminous watery diarrhea with flecks of white mucus (rice water stool)
    - Caused principally by serogroup O1 & serogroup O139
    - Commonly acquired from shellfish
- Inflammatory (dysenteric): *Shigella*, *Campylobacter*, *Salmonellae*, *enterohemorrhagic E coli* (EHEC), *Clostridioides difficile*, *Aeromonas*, *Yersinia* & *Vibrio* (noncholera)
  - Enterohemorrhagic *E coli* (EHEC)
    - Produces Shiga toxin; acquired through the ingestion of undercooked processed (ground) beef and contaminated milk, fruit & vegetables
    - *E coli* 0157:H7 is the most common strain
    - Associated with hemolytic uremic syndrome (HUS)
      - Bloody stools
      - Antibiotics should not be given
  - Enteroinvasive *E coli* (EIEC)
    - Rare in the United States
    - Dysentery illness similar to *Shigella* infection
  - *Salmonella*
    - Contracted with animal contact—either live or in the form of food (milk, raw chicken & eggs)
    - Morbidity derives from bacteremia, with a potential for seeding of bone, joints, vascular walls, heart, or brain. The very young & very old are at greatest risk for bacteremia, in addition to those with immunodeficiency, malignancy, diabetes, HIV infection, sickle cell disease, and indwelling prostheses
  - *Campylobacter jejuni*
    - Most common cause of bacterial enteritis in the United States
    - Ingestion of contaminated food (chicken) or water
    - Associated with Guillain-Barré syndrome
  - *Clostridium perfringens*
    - Spores found within food that is inadequately cooked
    - Sporulation/enterotoxin production produces vomiting and watery diarrhea that, like *S aureus* food poisoning, may present within 8 hours of consumption
  - *Clostridioides difficile*
    - Most common cause of antibiotic-associated diarrhea
    - Culture may give misguiding results, since hospitalized inpatients are rapidly colonized with *C difficile*; it is toxin production that is diagnostic of *C difficile* colitis
    - Reference method is the cytotoxicity assay
    - Antigenic toxin assays (ELISA) have limited sensitivity, varying from 60%-80%
    - PCR, using real time assays for toxin genes (*tcdA* for toxin A, *tcdB* for toxin B, and *tcdC* toxin A/B regulator gene), has sensitivity and specificity of 95%-100%
  - *Shigella*
    - May be foodborne but person-to-person spread and spread by insects (houseflies) also occurs, because of very small inoculum required for infection

ISBN 978-089189-6616

6.7.2.2 Viral pathogens

- Viruses are the most common cause, especially noroviruses (rotavirus, Norwalklike virus, enteric adenoviruses)
- Rotavirus outbreaks occur during the cold weather months ("winter vomiting disease")
  - It is common in daycare centers
  - There is severe fluid loss
  - It is most common in pediatric populations
  - Vaccines have resulted in significant decline in cases
- Norovirus is foodborne but can be transmitted from person to person
  - Requires a very small inoculum
  - Common cause of cruise ship-acquired diarrhea & vomiting

6.7.2.3 Parasite pathogens

- With the exception of *Giardia*, *Entamoeba* & *Cryptosporidium*, parasite pathogens of the GI tract are uncommon in developed countries
- *Entamoeba histolytica* should be considered in prolonged diarrhea or in a recent traveler (or immigrant) who presents with bloody diarrhea
- Stool microscopy has only ~50% sensitivity for *E histolytica* (and specificity is limited by the morphologically identical but nonpathogenic *E dispar*), but stool EIA has very high sensitivity & specificity

6.7.2.4 Laboratory approach for bacterial pathogens

- Stool microscopy has 2 purposes: To determine if leukocytes & RBCs are present (low clinical value)
- Assays for stool lactoferrin (a product of neutrophils) can substitute for a microscopic search for leukocytes
- Molecular panels (FilmArray) detect most common bacterial, viral & parasitic pathogens in 1 test system
- Routine stool culture is capable of isolating a limited range of organisms including *Salmonella* spp, *Shigella* spp, *E coli 0157:H7*, *Campylobacter* spp, *Yersinia enterocolitica* & *Vibrio* spp
- Most laboratories routinely test for *E coli* O157:H7 with culture, enzyme immunoassay (EIA), and/or polymerase chain reaction (PCR)-based tests, and many laboratories now routinely test for *C difficile* in community-acquired diarrhea (and always in hospital-acquired cases) using glutamate dehydrogenase (GDH) screen, enzyme immunoassay (EIA), or polymerase chain reaction (PCR)-based tests
- Serotyping: Confirmation must be done on *Salmonella*, *Shigella*, enterohemorrhagic *E coli* when the isolate's biochemical properties identify it as one of these
  - *Salmonella*: Test with polyvalent A through G, Vi, and individual antisera for serogroups A, B, C1, C2, D, E, G
    - If agglutination occurs in Vi only, suspension must be boiled for 10 minutes to inactivate capsular Vi antigen, which can mask the O antigens
    - Then the suspension is retested with A-G antisera
  - *Shigella*: Serotype for identification
    - Group A: *S dysenteriae*
    - Group B: *S flexneri*
    - Group C: *S boydii*
    - Group D: *S dysenteriae*
  - *E coli* 0157:H7: Serotyping and also chromogenic media and ELISA used for identification

6.7.3 Upper respiratory tract

- Common normal flora of oropharyngeal area
  - *Streptococcus*—α & nonhemolytic
  - Streptococcus pneumonia
  - Group B *Streptococcus*, not group A
  - *Neisseria* spp
  - Diphtheroids
  - *Micrococcus*
  - Coagulase-negative *Staphylococcus*
  - Anaerobic organisms (gram-positive cocci, gram-negative rods, gram-positive rods)
  - *Haemophilus* spp
  - *Eikenella*
- Bacterial pathogens in upper respiratory tract specimens **t6.46**

t6.46 Upper respiratory tract sites & bacterial pathogens

Disease	Specimen	Common Bacterial Pathogens
Pharyngitis	Swab of tonsillar area & posterior pharynx	*S pyogenes*
		Streptococcus, groups C & G
		C diphtheriae (if symptoms)
		Arcanobacterium
		N gonorrhoeae (if history suggests)
		(viruses, eg, rhinovirus, influenza)
Sinusitis	Aspiration of sinus	*S pneumoniae*
		H influenzae
		S aureus
		S pyogenes
		Anaerobes
		Moraxella catarrhalis
		(viruses, eg, rhinovirus)
Otitis media	Usually sample not collected unless therapy failure; culture by tympanocentesis	*S pneumoniae*
		H influenzae
		S pyogenes
		Moraxella catarrhalis
		Pseudomonas aeruginosa
Epiglottitis	Swab when airway is secure; blood cultures	*H influenzae*
		S pneumoniae
		S pyogenes
		S aureus
		M catarrhalis
Nasopharyngitis	Nasopharyngeal swab	*Bordetella pertussis*
		Bordetella spp
		(viruses, eg, rhino, xoronavirus, respiratory syncytial virus, influenza)

- Direct detection & molecular methods for identification of 3 major upper respiratory tract pathogens
  - *Streptococcus pyogenes*
    - Throat culture
    - Rapid antigen detection using enzyme immunoassay (EIA)
    - Latex agglutination
    - polymerase chain reaction (PCR)
  - *Bordetella pertussis*
    - polymerase chain reaction (PCR)
    - Direct fluorescent antibody (DFA) not used as confirmatory but as a complementary test along with polymerase chain reaction (PCR)
  - *Corynebacterium diphtheriae*
    - Polymerase chain reaction (PCR) for *tox* gene
    - Elek immunoprecipitation test to detect diphtheria toxin

6.7.4 Lower respiratory tract

- Lower respiratory tract bacterial infections/site/pathogens **t6.47**

t6.47 Bacterial infections of the lower respiratory tract

Disease	Specimen	Bacterial pathogens
Community-acquired pneumonia	Sputum	*S pneumoniae*
		H influenzae
		Mycoplasma pneumoniae
		S aureus
		Chlamydophila pneumoniae
		Legionella pneumophila
		Mycobacterium tuberculosis
		(viruses & fungi also)
Hospital-acquired pneumonia	Sputum or transtracheal aspirate	*S aureus*
		Klebsiella & other *Enterobacteriaceae*
		Pseudomonas aeruginosa
		Acinetobacter spp
		Legionella pneumophila
		Stenotrophomonas maltophilia
Aspiration pneumonia	Sputum or transtracheal aspirate	*S aureus*
		Enterobacteriaceae
		Mixture of anaerobic & aerobic bacteria
Cystic fibrosis	Sputum or transtracheal aspirate	*Pseudomonas aeruginosa*
		Burkholderia cepacia
		H influenzae
		S aureus
Chronic pneumonia	Early morning sputum	*Mycobacterium tuberculosis*
		Fungi
Bronchitis	Bronchial wash or bronchial alveolar lavage Tissue biopsy	*H influenzae*
		M catarrhalis
		Mycoplasma pneumoniae
		Chlamydophila pneumoniae
		S pneumoniae
		Bordetella pertussis
Empyema	Pleural fluid	*S pneumoniae*
		S aureus
		Klebsiella
		H influenzae
		Pseudomonas
		Anaerobes

- Screening of sputum cultures
  - Direct Gram stain examination evaluates specimen quality, whether the sample is from the lower respiratory tract or only from the upper respiratory tract
    - Acceptable specimen shows ≤10 squamous epithelial cells (SEC) and ≥25 WBC/low-power field (lpf) (mostly neutrophils)
    - Unacceptable specimen shows ≥25 SEC/lpf OR the presence of more SEC than WBCs
    - Samples with ≥25 WBC/lpf usually are considered acceptable, even with ≥10 SEC/lpf

ISBN 978-089189-6616

- Quantitative culture of bronchial alveolar lavage (BAL)
  - Use a .01 L or .001 μL calibrated loop for delivering specimen to media
  - There should be low numbers of upper respiratory tract normal flora and higher numbers of pathogen(s)
- Common normal flora of upper respiratory tract that can "contaminate" lower respiratory tract specimens (list not inclusive)
  - *Streptococcus*—α & nonhemolytic
  - *Streptococcus pneumoniae*
  - β-hemolytic *Streptococcus* spp, not group A
  - *Neisseria* spp
  - Diphtheroids
  - *Micrococcus*
  - Coagulase-negative *Staphylococcus*
  - Anaerobic organisms (gram-positive cocci, gram-negative rods, gram-positive rods)
  - *Haemophilus* spp
  - *Eikenella*
- Notes to remember
  - *Streptococcus pneumoniae* (Pneumococcus)
    - Most common cause of community-acquired pneumonia
    - Lobar pneumonia
    - Often associated with bacteremia
    - 5%-10% of adults have pharyngeal colonization
    - Positive urinary antigen test
  - *Staphylococcus aureus*
    - Major cause of hospital-acquired pneumonia
    - Necrotizing pneumonia with cavitation
  - *Mycoplasma pneumoniae*
    - Walking pneumonia or atypical pneumonia and bronchitis
    - Low-grade fever, malaise, headache, and dry, nonproductive cough
  - *Haemophilus influenzae*
    - Bronchopneumonia
    - Chronic obstructive pulmonary disease (COPD) a major risk factor. Together with *Moraxella catarrhalis*, a major cause of acute exacerbation of COPD
  - *Legionella pneumophila*
    - Exposure to aerosolized particles—construction-associated dust, hot tub, cooling systems
    - Severely affected patients usually have underlying smoking history, chronic obstructive pulmonary disease (COPD)
    - Legionnaires' disease: Atypical pneumonia with high fever
    - Positive urinary antigen test for serogroup 1
    - Pontiac fever: Flulike illness without pneumonia
  - *Pseudomonas aeruginosa*, *Serratia marcescens*, *Acinetobacter baumannii* have similar features
    - In community-acquired pneumonia, tend to afflict those with underlying bronchiectasis, cystic fibrosis & advanced malignancy
    - Significant causes of hospital-acquired pneumonia, particularly ventilator-associated pneumonia
  - Remember the viruses that cause lower respiratory tract infections, even though bacterial pathogens are the focus of these sections
  - Major pathogens are influenza virus, respiratory syncytial virus (RSV), parainfluenza viruses, rhinovirus, adenovirus, and the recently described agents hantavirus, metapneumovirus, severe acute respiratory syndrome (SARS)-associated coronavirus
  - Hantavirus pulmonary syndrome (HPS)
    - Emerged in "4 corners" region of New Mexico
    - Sin Nombre virus
    - Deer mouse sheds virus in urine & feces
    - Flulike prodrome followed by acute respiratory distress syndrome (ARDS)
  - Parainfluenza virus: Most common cause of croup
  - Respiratory syncytial virus (RSV): Most common cause of bronchiolitis in children
  - Severe acute respiratory syndrome (SARS)
    - Emerged in China
    - SARS coronavirus (SARS-CoV)
    - Flulike prodrome followed by ARDS

6.7.5 Bacterial diseases of the blood

- Definition of terms
  - Bacteremia: Presence of bacteria in bloodstream and may or may not indicate infection
    - Transient: Bacteria are temporarily in bloodstream and then removed by immune system
      - Examples are brushing teeth, draining abscess, colonoscopy
      - Can lead to endocarditis

- Intermittent: bacteria seed into blood stream periodically from primary infection site
  - Examples are pneumonia, UTI, tissue infection where the pathogen gets into the bloodstream
- Continuous: Bacteria constantly in the bloodstream of patient with intravascular infections (eg, endocarditis)

- Sepsis: Bacteria in bloodstream with symptoms (fever, chills, hypotension) of bacterial invasion and toxin production
  - Laboratory values that count among markers of sepsis
    - Respiratory alkalosis
    - Hypoxemia
    - Abnormal WBC count
    - Increased C-reactive protein (CRP)
    - Increased interleukin 6 (IL-6)
    - Increased procalcitonin (PCT)
    - Increased lactate
    - Hyperglycemia
    - Altered coagulation parameters
    - Thrombocytopenia
    - Hyperbilirubinemia

- Specimen collection guidelines for blood cultures
  - Preparation of skin for venipuncture
    - Decontaminate skin with 70%-95% ethanol or isopropyl alcohol
    - Apply 2% tincture of iodine or 2% chlorhexidine to area and leave on for at least 30 seconds
    - Remove disinfectant with alcohol pad
    - NOTE: Do not draw from indwelling catheter line or arterial line
  - Volume of sample
    - Adults: Recommend 10-20 mL per set; for 2-bottle system, half of sample goes into an aerobic bottle and the other half into an anaerobic bottle
    - Children
      - 10 mL per set for child up to 36 kg (80 lbs)
      - 6 mL per set for child up to 12 kg (27 lbs)
    - Newborn
      - 2 mL per set from an infant <1 kg (< 2.2 lbs)
      - 4 mL per set from an infant up to 2 kg (4.4 lbs)
  - Inoculation of blood culture media
    - Decontaminate top of blood culture bottles and use syringe to inoculate blood culture broth
    - Broth should have sodium polyanethole sulfonate (SPS) included (ethylene tetraacetic acid [EDTA], heparin, sodium citrate can inhibit bacterial growth)
- Common skin contaminants of blood cultures
  - Coagulase-negative *Staphylococcus*
  - *Micrococcus*
  - Diphtheroids (*Corynebacterium*)
  - *Propionibacterium*
- Bacteria that cause bacteremia/septicemia
  - Coagulase-negative *Staphylococcus* (in multiple cultures; have same antibiotic patterns)
  - *Staphylococcus aureus*
  - *Streptococcus pneumoniae*
  - *Enterococcus*
  - Viridans group, streptococci
  - β-hemolytic streptococci
  - Nutritionally variant *Streptococcus* (*Abiotrophia*)
  - *Enterobacteriaceae* (eg, *E coli, Klebsiella, Enterobacter*)
  - *Pseudomonas*
  - *Bacteroides*
  - *Clostridium*
  - In neonates: *E coli* & group B *Streptococcus*
- Bacteria that cause endocarditis
  - Viridans group, streptococci
  - Coagulase-negative *Staphylococcus*
  - *Staphylococcus aureus*
  - *Enterococcus*
  - Nutritionally variant *Streptococcus* (*Abiotrophia*)
- Identification of bacterial pathogens in blood
  - Manual: 2-bottle system with both aerobic & anaerobic cultures
  - Continuous monitoring systems
    - In most laboratories, these have replaced the manual system
    - Biphasic system uses 2 blood culture bottles, aerobic & anaerobic
    - Signal system uses 1 bottle that supports both aerobic & anaerobic organisms and detects carbon dioxide production of bacteria
    - Lysis: Centrifugation system uses tube that lyses blood and then centrifugation concentrates the sample; pellet contains WBCs, RBCs & bacteria; pellet is inoculated to media
  - Automated systems: Allow detection of positive blood cultures in 6-24 hours; some incorporate antimicrobial removal device that absorbs any antibiotic present in patient's blood

ISBN 978-089189-6616

- Rapid ID of organisms from blood culture
  - Gram stain provides basic yet critical information for physician; therapy can be started based on stain results
  - Direct tube coagulase; performed when gram-positive cocci in clusters seen on Gram stain of blood culture
  - Oxidase
  - Modified Kinyoun stain
  - Fluorescence in situ hybridization
  - Nucleic acid amplification (PCR)

6.7.6 Central nervous system/meningitis

6.7.6.1 Meningitis

- Infection of the meninges (consists of dura mater, arachnoid membrane, pia mater)
- Most common infection of CNS
- Potentially life-threatening
- Acute or purulent meningitis
  - Usually bacteria are pathogens
  - Symptoms are fever, headache, stiff neck, irritability, lethargy, coma
- Chronic meningitis
  - Slow onset over weeks
  - Often caused by fungi, mycobacteria, and occasionally protozoa
- Aseptic meningitis
  - Absence of bacteria or fungi
  - Viruses are usually the pathogens (enteroviruses most common in all age groups)
  - Often self-limiting

6.7.6.2 Encephalitis

- Usually viral: Arbovirus (most common), herpes simplex type 1 (HSV1), HHV6, mumps virus, measles virus & varicella zoster virus

6.7.6.3 Specimen collection by lumbar puncture & transport of CSF specimens

- Ideally collect 3 tubes of CSF in sterile tubes, 1-2 mL fluid in each
  - Typically, tube 2 or 3 should be sent to microbiology laboratory for Gram stain & culture (culture should be performed on sample that is least likely to be contaminated)
  - Tube 3 is usually tested for glucose, protein, cell counts
- Transport to laboratory and process immediately
  - If delay in processing, keep CSF specimen at room temperature for up to 24 hours
  - If viruses expected, store in refrigerator up to 48 hours and −70°C for >48 hours

6.7.6.4 Bacterial pathogens of acute meningitis **t6.48**

t6.48 Common bacterial pathogens of acute meningitis

Patient Age	Bacterial Pathogens
Newborns (<1 mo)	Group B *Streptococcus, E coli*
	Listeria monocytogenes
Infants & children	*Haemophilus influenza* type B
	Neisseria meningitidis
	Streptococcus pneumoniae
Adults(including elderly & imunocompromised)	*S pneumoniae*
	N meningitidis
	L monocytogenes

6.7.6.5 Laboratory diagnosis of bacterial meningitis

- Gram stain: Microscopy provides critical information to physician
- CSF analysis **t6.49**

t6.49 CSF analysis: acute & aseptic meningitis

Disease	WBCs/mm^3	Predominant WBC	Glucose mg/dL	Protein mg/dL
Normal	0-5	Lymphocytes & monocytes	50-75	15-45
Acute	>1000	Neutrophils	↓ (0-40)	↑ (100-500)
Aseptic	100-500	Lymphocytes	normal to slight ↓	normal to ↑

- Direct antigen detection
  - Designed to detect antigens of *Haemophilus influenzae* type B, *Neisseria meningitidis* serogroups A, C, Y, W135, *Streptococcus agalactiae, Streptococcus pneumoniae, E coli* serotype KI
  - Limited value due to false-positive results, so most laboratories no longer perform this
- India ink
  - Detects polysaccharide capsule of *Cryptococcus neoformans* (yeast)
  - Low sensitivity
  - No longer recommended for direct specimen testing
- Latex agglutination for *C neoformans*—More sensitive than India ink
- Molecular methods

6.7.7 Other body fluids

- Pleural, peritoneal, pericardial, synovial, amniotic, and vitreous & aqueous humor
- Normal skin flora that are potential contaminants in body fluids
  - Coagulase-negative *Staphylococcus*
  - Diphtheroids (*Corynebacterium*)
  - *Propionibacterium*
- Pleural fluid
  - Sterile fluid that is between 2 membranes covering the lungs
  - Symptoms same as for pneumonia
  - Common pathogens
    - *Streptococcus pneumoniae*
    - *Staphylococcus aureus*
    - *Klebsiella*
    - *Haemophilus influenzae*
    - *Pseudomonas*
    - *Mycobacterium tuberculosis*
    - Anaerobes
  - Collect by needle & syringe
    - Centrifuge fluid for direct Gram stain & inoculation to media
- Synovial fluid
  - Diagnose septic arthritis based on pain, fever, tenderness, swelling
  - Bacteria that cause septic arthritis
    - Neonate (<1 mo): *Staphylococcus aureus*, group B *Streptococcus*, enteric gram-negative rod
    - 1 mo-4 y: *S aureus*, group A *Streptococcus*, *Streptococcus pneumoniae*, *Neisseria meningitidis*, *Haemophilus influenzae*
    - 4-16 y: *Staphylococcus aureus*, group A *Streptococcus*
    - 16-40 y: *Neisseria gonorrhoeae*, *Staphylococcus aureus*
    - >40 years: *Staphylococcus aureus*
  - Aspirate fluid with sterile needle
  - Direct Gram stain & culture
- Other sterile body fluids
  - Peritoneal fluid covers most organs of abdomen
    - Common pathogens: *Staphylococcus*, *Streptococcus*, *Haemophilus influenzae*, *M tuberculosis*, *Enterobacteriaceae*
  - Pericardial fluid surrounds the heart
    - Pathogens: Often viral pathogens (eg, *Enterovirus*), *Streptococcus pneumoniae*
  - Amniotic fluid is in the amniotic sac
    - Pathogens: *E coli*, group B *Streptococcus*, anaerobic bacteria
  - Vitreous & aqueous humor is fluidlike substance in eye
    - Pathogens: Coagulase-negative *Staphylococcus*, *Staphylococcus aureus*, *Streptococcus*, *Enterococcus*, gram-negative rod, viruses (HIV-1)
  - Perform direct Gram stain & culture

6.7.8 Bacterial skin, soft tissue, bone infections

- Normal flora of skin that can cause disease or contaminate specimens
  - Coagulase negative *Staphylococcus*
  - Diphtheroids
  - *Micrococcus*
  - *Propionibacterium*
  - Gram-negative rod
  - Yeast (in moist areas)
- Types of skin infections & common pathogens
  - Impetigo: Highly contagious; pustules form & rupture, releasing a thick, yellow discharge; forms crusty layers
    - *Streptococcus pyogenes* (nonbullous)
    - *Staphylococcus aureus* (bullous)
  - Erysipelas: Superficial cellulitis typically appearing on face as bright red to crimson color
    - *Streptococcus pyogenes*
  - Erysipeloid: Superficial soft tissue associated with animals, hides, poultry, fish & introduced by trauma into skin
    - *Erysipelothrix rhusiopathiae*
  - Cellulitis: Infection of superficial skin & subcutaneous tissues
    - *Streptococcus pyogenes*
    - *Staphylococcus aureus*
    - Methicillin-resistant *Staphylococcus aureus* (MRSA), both hospital & community acquired
  - Folliculitis: Infection of hair follicle
    - *Staphylococcus aureus*
    - *Pseudomonas aeruginosa* (from contaminated swimming pools or hot tubs)
    - Gram-negative rod
  - Furuncles: Boils & abscesses
    - *Staphylococcus aureus*

ISBN 978-089189-6616

  - Carbuncle: Infection goes deeper into subcutaneous tissues, often with multiple abscesses
    - *Staphylococcus aureus*
  - Burn wounds
    - *Staphylococcus aureus*
    - *Pseudomonas aeruginosa*
    - *Streptococcus pyogenes*
    - *Enterococcus*
  - Bite wounds
    - Human bite wounds
      - *Staphylococcus aureus*
      - *Staphylococcus anginosus*
      - *Eikenella corrodens*
      - Anaerobes
  - Dog & cat bite wounds
    - *Pasteurella multocida*
    - *Staphylococcus*
    - Anaerobes
  - Soft tissue wounds
    - β-hemolytic streptococci, groups A, C, G
    - *Staphylococcus aureus*, MRSA
    - *Clostridium perfringens* (gas gangrene)
    - Mixed: Enterics & anaerobes
- Mycetoma (subcutaneous infection; sinus tracts form and pus drain from site)
  - *Nocardia*
  - *Actinomadura*
  - Anaerobes
  - Also caused by fungi
- Bone (osteomyelitis)
  - *Staphylococcus aureus* & other *Staphylococcus* spp
  - Streptococci
  - Pseudomonas
  - Enterics (*E coli*, *Proteus*)
  - *Kingella*
  - Organisms associated with bite wounds
  - ID by bone scan, biopsy, or aspiration; blood cultures
- Zoonotic infections with skin manifestations
  - Rickettsiosis: Skin rash; Rocky Mountain spotted fever (RMSF)
  - Bartonellosis: Pustule; *Bartonella henselae* causes cat scratch disease
  - Rat bite fever: Petechial or pustular rash; *Streptobacillus moniliformis*
  - Tularemia: Painful ulcer on skin; *Francisella tularensis*
  - Lyme disease: Erythema migrans (a skin lesion that forms at site of tick bite and has a "target" appearance); *Borrelia burgdorferi*
  - Leptospirosis: Rash; *Leptospira interrogans*
  - Bubonic plague: Vesicle or ulcer forms on skin at site of flea bite; *Yersinia pestis*
  - Cutaneous anthrax: Vesicle forms; *Bacillus anthrasis*
- Specimen collection & processing
  - Aspirates or biopsies are recommended over swabs for obtaining culture material
  - Abscesses & deep wounds: aspirate for Gram stain & culture (remember anaerobes)
  - Cellulitis & erysipelas: Clinically diagnose unless abscesses or bullae form, then aspirate, direct Gram stain smear & culture
  - Erysipeloid: Clinically diagnosis or biopsy, Gram stain, culture
  - Fasciitis: Tissue biopsy, Gram stain, culture

6.7.9 Genital tract bacterial infections

- Normal flora vs pathogens **t6.50 & t6.51**
- Cervicitis/urethritis
  - Purulent discharge or asymptomatic
  - *Chlamydia trachomatis* is most common reported STD in the United States
  - *Neisseria gonorrhoeae* is 2nd most common reported STD
  - Untreated infection can cause pelvic inflammatory disease (PID), ectopic pregnancy, and infertility
  - Co-infections with both organisms are common so diagnostic testing and treatment should cover both organisms
  - Gram stain of male urethral exudate can be diagnostic if WBCs and intracellular gram-negative diplococci seen
  - ID with enzyme immunoassay (EIA), direct fluorescent antibody (DFA), molecular testing
- Candidiasis (yeast)
  - Genital itching or burning and discharge of watery to thick, white, "cottage cheeselike" discharge
  - Not considered a true sexually transmitted disease (STD)
  - *Candida* are normal flora in low numbers
  - Wet mount of discharge using 10% potassium hydroxide (KOH) shows budding yeast
  - ID of candidiasis is usually a clinical diagnosis (most cases caused by *Candida albicans*)

Clinical syndromes>Genital tract bacterial infections

t6.50 Normal bacterial flora of genital tract

Site	Normal flora
Urethra	Coagulase-negative staphylococci
	Corynebacteria
	Obligate anaerobes
Vagina	Lactobacilli
	Corynebacteria
	Staphylococci
	Streptococci
	Enteric gram- rods
	Anaerobes
	Yeasts (fungus)
Cervix	Usually not colonized with normal flora

t6.51 Bacterial pathogens of the genital tract

Site	Pathogen
Urethra	*Neisseria gonorrhoeae*
	Chlamydia trachomatis
	Ureaplasma
	Mycoplasma
Epididymitis in men	*N gonorrhoeae*
	C trachomatis
Vagina	Group B *Streptococcus*
	Trichomonas vaginalis (parasite)
	Candida albicans (yeast)
	Gardnerella vaginalis & anaerobes
	Staphylococcus aureus
Cervix	*N gonorrhoeae*
	C trachomatis
Pelvic inflammatory disease	Seen in untreated cases of *N gonorrhoeae* & *C trachomatis*
Genital ulcers	*Haemophilus ducreyi* (chancroid)
	Treponema pallidum

- *Trichomonas vaginalis* (parasite)
  - Causes greenish discharge, strong & foul odor
  - May be asymptomatic
  - pH of discharge is >5 (3.8-4.5 is normal pH)
  - Wet mount of discharge shows flagellated parasite with twitching, nervous movement
- Bacterial vaginosis (associated with *Gardnerella vaginalis*)
  - Homogenous, yellow discharge with "fishy" odor and pH of 5.0
  - "Whiff test" positive when 10% potassium hydroxide (KOH) added to saline wet prep of discharge; fishy aroma occurs because of volatilization of amines in sample
  - Vaginal squamous epithelial cells (SEC; clue cells) coated with gram-variable *G vaginalis* seen on wet mount or Gram stain
- Bacteria causing genital ulcers
  - Chancroid (soft chancre)
    - Sexually transmitted disease (STD) caused by *Haemophilus ducreyi*
    - It is very difficult to perform a culture compared to other *Haemophilus* spp
    - GC agar base with hemoglobin, isovitalix, fetal calf serum *OR* Mueller-Hinton agar with chocolatized horse blood and isovitalex
    - ID by enzyme immunoassay (EIA); molecular testing pending
  - Syphillis
    - Sexually transmitted disease (STD) caused by *Treponema pallidum*
      - Primary: A chancre or ulcer appears at site of inoculation and lasts 1-8 weeks
      - Secondary: Flulike symptoms, sore throat, headache, fever, muscle aches, swollen lymph nodes, rash
      - Tertiary or late stage: One third of untreated patients progress to 3rd stage; lesions (gummas) seen in bone, skin, and other tissues; neuro- & cardiovascular involvement
    - Direct visualization using darkfield microscopy (rarely performed)
    - Nontreponemal are excellent for screening and include rapid plasma regain (RPR) & venereal disease research laboratory (VDRL); not specific for syphilis and produce false-positive results
    - Nontreponemal antibodies tend to wane with treatment or in late infection, whereas treponemal antibodies remain positive indefinitely
    - A positive nontreponemal test should be followed with a treponemal test to confirm syphilis diagnosis
    - Treponemal tests detect antibodies specific for syphilis and includes fluorescent treponemal antibody absorption (FTA-ABS), *Treponema pallidum* particle agglutination (TP-PA), or various EIAs
    - Some laboratories are now doing a reverse testing algorithm in which treponemal tests are first conducted, followed by nontreponemal testing. This presents complexities in interpretation. A treponemal specific test (syphilis IgG by enzyme immunoassay (EIA) currently recommended by the CDC) results in fewer false-positive results, but positive tests should still be confirmed using a nontreponemal test to confirm disease activity
- NOTE on genital tract infections: Remember viruses that are sexually transmitted diseases (STDs), such as HIV, CMV, papillomavirus, hepatitis B, HSV-2, HSV-1

ISBN 978-089189-6616

6.8 Vectors

- Diseases that art transmitted by vectors are listed in t6.52

t6.52 General information on disease vectors

Vector	Disease	Organism
Mosquitoes		
Anopheles spp	Dog heartworm	*Dirofilaria immitis*
	Malaria	*Plasmodium* spp
	Lymphatic filariasis	*Brugia malayi*
	Lymphatic filariasis	*Wuchereria bancrofti*
Aedes spp, most commonly *A aegypti* & *A albopictus*	Arboviral disease	Including: Dengue virus, yellow fever virus & Chikungunya virus
Culex spp	Arboviral disease	Including: West Nile virus, Saint Louis encephalitis virus, Japanese encephalitis virus
	Lymphatic filariasis	*Wuchereria bancrofti*
	Lymphatic filariasis	*Brugia malayi*
Ticks		
Ixodes spp Most common: Eastern United States: *I scapularis* Western United States: *I pacificus* Europe: *I ricinus*	Lyme disease	*Borrelia burgdorferi*
	Babesiosis	*Babesia* spp
	Anaplasmosis	*Anaplasma phagocytophilum*
	Tickborne encephalitis	Tickborne encephalitis virus (TBEV)
Lone Star tick—*Amblyomma americanum*	Ehrlichiosis	*Ehrlichia* spp
	Tularemia	*Francisella tularensis*
	Southern tick-associated illness (STARI)	Unknown etiology
Dermacentor spp Most common: Southern & western United States: *D andersoni* Southern & eastern United States: *D variabilis*	Rocky Mountain spotted fever	*Rickettsia rickettsii*
	Tularemia	*Francisella tularensis*
	Colorado tick fever	Colorado tick fever virus
Ornithodoros spp (soft ticks)	Relapsing fever	*Borrelia* spp
Flies		
Deer fly—*Chrysops* spp	Tularemia—"deerfly fever"	*Francisella tularensis*
	Loiasis	*Loa loa*
Dung fly—*Musca sorbens*	Trachoma	*Chlamydia trachomatis*
Sandfly (*Phlebotomus* & *Lutzomyia* spp)	Leishmaniasis	*Leishmania* spp
	Bartonellosis; carrion disease	*Bartonella bacilliformis*
	Arboviral disease	Vesicular stomatitis virus, toscana & sicilian virus
Black fly—*Simulium* spp	Onchocerciasis; river blindness	*Onchocerca volvulus*
Tsetse fly—*Glossina* spp	African trypanosomiasis	*Trypanosoma brucei*
Fleas		
Rat fleas	Plague	*Yersinia pestis*
	Murine typhus	*Rickettsia typhus*
Dog & cat fleas	Double pored dog tapeworm	*Dipylidium caninum*
Lice		
Body lice—*Pediculus humanus*	Epidemic typhus	*Rickettsia prowazekii*
	Liceborne relapsing fever	*Borrelia recurrentis*
	Trench fever	*Bartonella quintana*
Mites		
Mite (*Liponyssoides sanguineus*)	Rickettsial pox	*Rickettsia akari*
Chigger (Trombiculid mite)	Scrub typhus	*Orientia tsutsugamushi*
Others		
Midges—*Culicoides* spp	Filariasis	*Mansonella* spp
Reduviid bug—*Triatominae*	American trypanosomiasis; Chagas disease	*Trypanosoma cruzi*

6.9 Postanalytical (see Chapter 7 Laboratory Operations)

6.9.1 Documentation practices

- Equipment must have log sheets that record calibration checks, maintenance, upgrades, repairs
- Media & reagents must have defined criteria that ensure they will perform correctly
  - Sterility
  - Ability to support growth of microorganisms
  - Ability to give correct reactions
  - Dates are recorded, showing date opened & date of expiration
- Personnel must have documentation of competency
  - Continuing education required for yearly certification maintenance program (American Society for Clinical Pathology [ASCP]). This is not required for those who were grandfathered in before the Credential Maintenance Program (CMP) was in place
  - Competency evaluations: Observations, simulated specimens, external quality assessment programs

6.9.2 Urgent/critical value reporting

- Verbally provide the result and have the physician/ primary care practitioner repeat the information; document with date/time/practitioner name
- Examples of results must be communicated immediately to unit, physician/primary care practitioner, and possibly, infection control group

- Positive blood culture
- Positive CSF
- Positive acid-fast smear
- *Mycobacterium tuberculosis* ID
- *Plasmodium falciparum*
- *Streptococcus pyogenes* from normal sterile site
- *Streptococcus agalactiae* from genital site of pregnant woman
- Herpes simplex from genital site of pregnant woman
- Positive result on influenza or RSV testing of infant

6.9.3 Result review & correction reports

- Each result must be reviewed by a qualified laboratorian every day
- Corrected reports are necessary to document issues in result reporting
  - Example of correction report
    - Date
    - Problem defined
    - Evaluation of problem
    - Corrective action
    - Outcome
    - Signature of person submitting report

6.9.4 Reporting to infection control & public health

- Infection control surveillance—goal is to prevent spread of infection
  - Data on statistics collected on existing infections, for both total & targeted surveillance data
    - Helps recognize outbreaks, trends, and outcomes of preventions
    - Laboratory provides surveillance information every day for hospital infection control group
    - Daily review of culture results provides infection control with current information
    - Data mining is done using LIS with a sophisticated date review system
  - Other information provided to infection control group
    - Specimen contamination rates
    - Number of isolates per site
    - Types of pathogens isolated
    - Prevalence of pathogens
    - Resistant strains
- Public health reporting
  - Federal and/or state regulations require laboratories to repost the ID of suspicious or certain infectious disease pathogens
- Laboratory Response Network
  - LRN-B: Biological test samples for potential biological terror threats
  - LRN-C: Chemical test samples for potential chemical terror threats
  - Network of laboratories
    - Sentinel laboratoriesmost hospital-based microbiology facilities
      - Recognize possible bioterrorism agent
      - Perform basic testing to rule out
      - Refer suspicious specimens or isolates to LRN-B facilities
    - Reference laboratories: >150 facilities in the United States, mostly state public health facilities
      - Perform confirmatory testing
    - National laboratories (3 total): Centers for Disease Control and Prevention (CDC), United States Army Medical Research Institute, Naval Medical Research Center
      - BSL4 facilities for most dangerous microorganisms
      - Provide definitive identification
  - Diseases of major public health concern that need immediate notification
    - Anthrax
    - Botulism
    - Diphtheria
    - Plague
    - Rabies
    - Smallpox
    - Cholera
    - Meningococcal meningitis
    - Measles
    - Yellow fever
    - Tularemia
  - Other diseases of public health concern that must be reported within 1 day to 1 week of ID
    - Hepatitis A
    - Legionnaires' disease
    - Foodborne outbreaks
    - Pertussis
    - Tuberculosis
    - Syphilis

- Typhoid fever
- Tetanus
- Vancomycin-intermediate *S aureus* (VISA) & vancomycin-resistant *S aureus* (VRSA)
- Brucellosis
- Giardiasis
- Hepatitis B & C
- Rocky Mountain spotted fever (RMSF)
- Lyme disease
- Trichinosis
- Gonorrhoeae & chlamydia

- Reporting to hospital committees
  - Hospital infection control committees need laboratory data that include:
    - Blood culture contamination rates
    - Organisms isolated from patients in specific units
    - Organisms isolated from specific sites
    - Antiobiogram information

- Antimicrobial susceptibility stewardship
  - Definition of antimicrobial stewardship: Medical laboratory scientist's responsibility to participate in the healthcare team, provide a systematic approach to the use of antimicrobial agents in achieving optimal outcomes, and help minimize toxicity & emergence of resistance
  - Antimicrobial susceptibility testing is performed only on bacteria likely to cause infection and that have published, standardized testing protocols
  - Selection of antimicrobials to test against an organism is influenced (determined) by isolation site, patient population, antimicrobial administration (ie, oral vs intravenous vs intramuscular), hospital/institution formulary and Clinical & Laboratory Standards Institute (CLSI) recommendations
  - Control organisms from American Type Culture Collection (ATCC) are used for testing antimicrobials, media, inoculum
  - Correct storage of media, disks & other supplies is required
  - Documentation of zone sizes, minimum inhibitory concentration (MIC) values is done daily
  - Data are collected on antibiograms from specific organisms, which are shared with physicians, hospital pharmacy & infectious diseases department
  - Physicians & infectious diseases department are notified when resistance occurs (eg, vancomycin-resistant *Enterococcus* (VRE), methicillin-resistant *S aureus* (MRSA), carbapenem resistance)
  - Some laboratories publish the hospital/institution antimicrobial susceptibility data for common organisms as a guide for treatment, in the form of a cumulative antiobiogram
  - Expected antimicrobial susceptibility pattern examp
    - *Staphylococcus* spp—penicillin R
    - *Streptococcus pyogenes*—penicillin S
    - Enterococci—cephalosporins R
    - *Klebsiella pneumoniae*—ampicillin R
    - *Enterobacter cloacae*—ampicillin & first-generati cephalosporin R
    - *Proteus mirabilis*—nitrofurantoin R & tetracycline
    - MRSA is resistant to commonly used β-lactam agents (eg, ampicillin, cephalosporins, β-lactam/β-lactam inhibitor combination, imipene regardless of in vitro test results. However, new β-lactams have been developed to treat MRSA

6.10 Selected readings

6.10.1 Books

Carroll KC, Pfaller MA, Landry ML, McAdam ML, Patel R, Richter SS, Warnock DW. *Manual of Clinical Microbiology*. 12th ed. AS Press. 2011. ISBN 978-1555814632

Kiser K, Payne WC, Taff TA. *Clinical Laboratory Microbiology, A Practical Approach*. Pearson. 2011. ISBN 978-0130921956

Leber A, ed. *Clinical Microbiology Procedures Handbook*. 4th ed. ASM Press. 2016. ISBN 978-1555818807

Larone DH. *Medically Important Fungi: A Guide to Identification*. ed. ASM Press. 2011. ISBN 978-1555816605

Murray PR, Rosenthal KS, Pfaller MA. *Medical Microbiology*. 7th Elsevier. 2013. ISBN 978-0323091244

Mais, DM, ed. *Quick Compendium of Clinical Pathology*. 4th ed. ASCP Press. 2018. ISBN 978-0891896678

Mahon CR, Lehman DC. *Textbook of Diagnostic Microbiology*. 6th ed. Elsevier. 2018. ISBN 978-0323613170

Procop GW, Church DL, Hall GS, Janda WM, Koneman EW, Schreckenberger PC, Woods GL. *Koneman's Color Atlas and Textbook of Diagnostic Microbiology*. 7th ed. Jones & Barrett Learning. 2019. ISBN 978-1284322378

Tille PM. *Bailey & Scott's Diagnostic Microbiology*. 14th ed. Elsevi 2016. ISBN 978-0323354820

6.10.2 Journals & online

CLSI M100 S27: 2017. *Performance Standards for Antimicrobial Susceptibility Testing 27e*. Available at: https://clsi.org/educatio microbiology

Centers for Disease Control and Prevention at www.cdc.gov. Diseases and Conditions; Public Health Image Library; DPDx

Chapter 7

Laboratory Operations

7.1 Legislation & regulation, agencies & oversight

7.1.1 Clinical Laboratory Improvement Amendment of 1988 (CLIA)

- CLIA '88 was enacted as an amendment to the Clinical Laboratory Act of 1967.
- The Centers for Medicare and Medicaid Services (CMS) have been charged with enforcing CLIA requirements which apply to facilities performing clinical testing on "materials derived from the human body" for the purposes of diagnosis, care and treatment of patients
- CLIA does not apply to research testing
- CMS has granted deeming status to multiple agencies that are authorized to inspect and accredit medical laboratories if the laboratory meets specific requirements and predetermined standards
    - Accrediting agencies may enforce additional requirements for accreditation which must be at least as stringent as CLIA's requirement
- A laboratory is classified according to the highest complexity testing it performs
    - A new laboratory must apply for a CLIA license and accreditation certification and receive a certificate of registration before patient testing begins
    - Nonwaived testing sites must be inspected by CLIA/CMS or accrediting agencies with "deemed" status such as College of American Pathologists (CAP), The Joint Commission (TJC) & Commission on Accreditation of Laboratories (COLA) every 2 years to renew & maintain accreditation

7.1.1.1 Test complexity

- The Food & Drug Administration (FDA) is responsible for classifying laboratory tests and test systems by complexity based on 7 criteria described in the CLIA regulations
- Waived tests
    - There is no specific educational requirement beyond a high school diploma and no specific training requirements for individuals who perform waived tests
    - Sites that perform only waived testing must have a CLIA certificate of waiver and follow the manufacturer's instructions; other CLIA requirements do not apply to these sites
    - Waived tests are simple and accurate enough to be largely error free and pose no reasonable risk of harm to the patient if the test is performed incorrectly. Examples include the common urine dipstick tests, fecal occult blood testing, urine pregnancy tests, home glucose monitoring tests, spun hematocrit
    - The only requirement of those conducting waived testing are that they follow manufacturers' instructions
- Nonwaived (moderate & high complexity)
    - A scoring system is applied to nonwaived tests to determine whether they are of moderate or high complexity; in general, most automated tests are considered moderate, while those that have a significant manual component are high complexity (eg, parasite identification)
    - If a test of moderate complexity is modified, it generally is considered a high complexity test
    - Requirements include qualified laboratory director & testing personnel, test method validation, written procedures to ensure proper specimen collection & procedure performance, the testing of positive & negative controls each day patient samples are tested, enrollment in proficiency testing, stipulations regarding record keeping & biennial (every other year) inspection
    - Requirements of moderate & high complexity testing differ mainly in the personnel requirements
- Provider-performed microscopy (PPM)
    - PPM is a subcategory of moderate complexity testing
    - To be regarded as PPM, a procedure must be performed by a physician, dentist, or midlevel practitioner under physician supervision, and it must be performed during the patient visit when the specimen is collected
    - The primary instrument for performing the test must be a bright field or phase contrast microscope
    - PPM examinations include direct wet mounts, potassium hydroxide (KOH) preparations, pinworm examinations, fern tests, examinations of urine sediment
    - Other CLIA requirements for nonwaived testing sites
        - Written or electronic requisitions to document laboratory test orders from individuals authorized by law
        - Written technical testing procedures (as opposed to manufacturer's instructions)
        - Defined quality control practices
        - Minimum requirements stipulated for result reporting (must be reported with a statement of the reference range on a form that properly identifies the patient)
        - Records required and materials to be retained for specified durations
        - Participation required in proficiency testing (PT) programs or the use of alternate PT methods when commercial PT is not available; acceptable performance criteria must be defined
            - PT vendors must be approved by CMS, and once a laboratory selects a vendor, it must remain with the same vendor for 1 full year before switching to another

7.1.2 Medical devices & biologics

- The FDA is responsible for regulating companies who manufacture, repackage, relabel or import medical devices sold in the United States
- Medical devices are defined as "any instrument, apparatus, or other article that is used to prevent, diagnose, mitigate, or treat a disease or to affect the structure or function of the body, with the exception of drugs"
- Laboratory instruments, reagent kits, blood collection devices & blood irradiators are examples of medical devices
- Medical devices are classified from class 1 to class 3
  - Each class has defined regulatory requirements that increase with the level of classification
- Laboratory users have a duty to report medical device malfunction
- FDA is responsible for ensuring the safety of the nation's blood supply and is responsible for regulating biological products, including blood and blood components, starting with donors to appropriate handling and distribution of blood products for patient use
- The Center for Biologics Evaluation and Research (CBER) is the subdivision of the FDA responsible for ensuring the safety & efficacy of the biological products

7.1.2.1 Analyte-specific reagents (ASRs) & laboratory-developed tests (LDTs)

- ASR is defined as "antibodies, both polyclonal and monoclonal, specific receptor proteins, ligands, nucleic acid sequences, and similar reagents which, through specific binding or chemical reactions with substances in a specimen, are intended for use in a diagnostic application for identification and quantification of an individual chemical substance or ligand in biological specimens" (in contrast to general purpose reagents that are nonspecific)
- Whether an antibody is or is not an ASR depends on its labeling: Those labeled as "for in vitro diagnostic use" are not ASRs
- A reagent developed by a manufacturer for sole use in its test system (ie, reagent not separately marketed by the manufacturer) is not an ASR
- The FDA considers ASRs to be medical devices and therefore subject to its regulation; under this authority, it published "the ASR rule" in 1997
  - Classifies ASRs, imposes restrictions on their sale and use, and delineates labeling requirements
  - Reports of test results must include the statement, "This test was developed, and its performance characteristics determined by (laboratory name). It has not been cleared or approved by the US Food and Drug Administration"
  - The ASR must be labeled "Analyte Specific Reagent." Analytical and performance characteristics are not established. (if a manufacturer wishes to make performance claims, then the ASR must be submitted through the usual premarket approval process)

7.1.3 Medicare, Medicaid & the prospective payment system

- The Social Security Act of 1965 established Medicare & Medicaid, currently referred to Centers for Medicare & Medicaid Services (CMS)
- Medicare is administered by CMS and provides health care benefits to 3 groups:
  - Individuals aged ≥65 years
  - Individuals with certain disabilities
  - Individuals with end-stage renal disease (permanent kidney failure requiring dialysis or kidney transplantation)
- Medicare part A helps cover inpatient medical care
  - Inpatient services are reimbursed a fixed sum according to diagnosis-related groups (DRGs) regardless of the services provided
  - Laboratory testing performed during the 3 calendar days before, during, and within 14 days after hospitalization is bundled into the DRG payment, ie, cannot be billed to Medicare separately
  - Most people do not pay a premium for part A
- Medicare part B helps cover outpatient services & inpatient physician services according to a fee schedule (fee for service).
  - Premium payments are automatically deducted from social security payment for those individuals who enroll in part B
- Prescription drug coverage is paid under part D
- Health care providers are required to give patients who are covered by original Medicare an advance beneficiary notice (ABN) of noncoverage in advance if the service is not likely or certainly to be covered by Medicare
- A laboratory must have a current CLIA certificate to submit claims to Medicare or Medicaid
  - Medicare claims are usually processed by nongovernmental contractors referred to as "fiscal intermediaries," who process part A claims, and "carriers," who process part B claims
- Medicaid is a federal program that is administered by states
  - States set eligibility requirements & fee schedules
  - Intended to extend benefits to low-income families

ISBN 978-089189-6616

7.1.4 Billing & reimbursement

- Medical billing codes are used to classify a patient's treatment, diagnosis, and associated medical supplies
- Required for a health care provider to submit claims to receive reimbursement for services
- The primary codes used for laboratory claims include:
    - International Coding or Classification of Disease (ICD): Specific to diagnosis or a medical problem used to establish medical necessity
    - Current procedural terminology (CPT): Describes procedure(s) performed
    - CPT modifiers: Added to a CPT code to describe a special circumstance
    - Health Care Procedural Coding System (HCPCS): Describes blood products, medical goods, or services
    - Revenue codes are 3-digit or 4-digit numbers used on hospital insurance claim forms (UB-04) that describe where a patient received treatment or the type of item a patient received

7.1.5 Corporate compliance programs

- Compliance programs are designed to promote adherence to applicable federal & state laws & regulations that govern health care
- The program uses effective controls and workforce education to prevent fraud, waste & abuse of health care dollars wherever possible
- The False Claims Act prohibits the submission of false or fraudulent claims for medical services to a federal government health care program
- People who report false or fraudulent claims are protected from retaliation

7.1.5.1 Fraud, waste & abuse

- Definitions
    - Fraud is an intentional deception or misrepresentation made by a person with the knowledge that the deception could result in some unauthorized benefit to himself or herself or some other person or entity. It includes any act that constitutes fraud under applicable federal or state law
    - Waste refers to practices that result in unnecessarily increased costs because of mismanagement or overuse of medical services
        - Unlike fraud, waste is usually caused by mistake rather than intentionally wrongful actions
    - Abuse means provider practices that are inconsistent with sound fiscal, business, or medical practices, and result in unnecessary costs to a health care program or other third-party payers, or in reimbursement for services that are not medically necessary
- Examples of potential health care fraud that should be reported
    - Billing for a service not provided or not ordered by an authorized individual
    - Billing for a service that is not documented in the medical record
    - Billing for services separately when they should have been billed together as a single charge (metabolic panel)
    - Duplicate bills or charges for the same service
    - Not refunding overpayments

7.1.5.2 Billing errors and other compliance issues

- Many billing errors are simply unintentional mistakes
    - Ignoring mistakes, choosing not to fix them, and failing to prevent them from recurring could be considered a false claim by government payers such as Medicare and Medicaid
    - When an organization submits a fraudulent or false claim to Medicare or Medicaid, the health care organization risks the loss of funding from these programs and significant financial penalties
    - Individuals involved run the risk of losing their license or being excluded from Medicare and Medicaid programs
- The Anti-Kickback Statute is a federal law to protect patients from providers making decisions based on the influence of anything of value
    - Anyone who knowingly receives or pays anything of value to influence patient referral can be criminally prosecuted
- Physician Self-Referral (Stark) Law states that any financial relationship between a provider of designated health services & a physician who does not fall within an exception called "safe harbor" is prohibited
- Patient Protection & Affordable Care Act (also known as health care reform) makes compliance programs mandatory
    - If overpayments are received from a government payer, it must be returned in a specified time or it is considered a false claim

7.1.6 Packaging & shipping of specimens

- Department of Transportation (DOT); United States Post Office (USPS); International Air Transport Association (IATA) all have different requirements for packaging & shipping of biological specimens, infectious materials & hazardous materials

7.1.7 Freedom of Information Act

- FOIA generally provides public access to federal agency records or information in the possession of a government agency unless the information is protected from disclosure by an exemption or a category that is specifically excluded

7.1.8 Health Insurance Portability and Accountability Act (HIPAA)

- The Health Insurance Portability and Accountability Act was developed in 1996 and became part of the Social Security Act
- The primary purpose of the HIPAA rules is to protect health care coverage for workers who lose or change jobs
- HIPAA strengthened & expanded health care privacy requirements
- The Privacy Act (1974): Protects records that can be retrieved by personal identifiers and prohibits disclosures without written consent unless a specified exception applies
- The Privacy Rule (1996): HIPAA, a federal law designed to provide privacy standards to protect patients' medical records and other health information provided to health plans, doctors, hospitals, and other health care providers. The Privacy Rule defines "protected health information" (PHI) and "covered entities"
    - Protected health information (PHI) refers to any individually identifiable health information; health information includes demographic data, health condition, or the fact that health care was provided
    - Sharing of PHI is permitted for the purposes of diagnosis, treatment, payment, or for laboratory operations
    - Sharing of PHI may be required (notifiable infections); however required release of PHI must be tracked
- Covered entities (CE) include 3 basic groups: Health care providers, health plans, and health care clearinghouses
    - CEs must limit the sharing of information and must proactively secure information to prevent unauthorized access, including encryption of data & shredding of paper containing PHI
        - If a CE engages a business associate to help carry out its health care activities and functions, the CE must have a written business associate agreement or other arrangement with the business associate that:
            - Establishes specifically what the business associate has been engaged to do
            - Requires the business associate to comply with HIPAA
- The Security Rule (1996) established security standards for the protection of electronic health information by operationalizing the protections described in the Privacy Rule by addressing technical and nontechnical safeguards that covered entities must put in place to secure electronic PHI

7.1.9 The Occupational Safety & Health Administration (OSHA)

- The Occupational Safety and Health Act of 1970 was passed to protect workers from workplace hazards
- Employers are required to follow OSHA regulations and OSHA-approved state regulations (must meet or exceed federal OSHA standards for approval)
- Incident reports must be filled for all incidents, including near misses and those that cause serious temporary or permanent harm or illness

7.1.9.1 Hazardous chemicals

- OSHA requires that laboratories create & execute a hazardous chemicals hygiene plan that:
    - Specifies the use of personal protective equipment and procedures to ensure that protective equipment (eg, fume hoods) is functioning correctly
    - Describes the provisions for postexposure evaluation
    - Specifies a chemical hygiene officer and describes the recordkeeping requirements
    - Includes employee training
- OSHA requires employers to ensure that employee exposures remain at or below personal exposure limits (PELs) established by OSHA

7.1.9.2 Bloodborne pathogens

- OSHA requires that laboratories create & execute an exposure control plan that:
    - Specifies use of personal protective equipment and universal precautions (standard precautions)
    - Specifies provision of hepatitis B vaccination by the employer
    - Considers engineering & process controls to minimize risk of exposure as well as procedures for identifying exposures, postexposure evaluation, and investigation

7.1.10 National Labor Relations Act

- Congress enacted the National Labor Relations Act ("NLRA") in 1935 to:
    - Protect the rights of employees & employers
    - Encourage collective bargaining

ISBN 978-089189-6616

  - Curtail certain private sector labor & management practices, which can harm the general welfare of workers, businesses & the US economy

7.1.11 Civil rights & employment

7.1.11.1 Outlaws discrimination based on race, color, religion, sex, or national origin

7.1.11.2 Discrimination & employment law

- There are four theories of employment discrimination that have emerged since the enactment of Title VII of the Civil Rights Act
  - Disparate treatment
  - Disparate impact
  - Harassment
  - Retaliation
- Federal employment discrimination laws enforced by the U.S. Equal Employment Opportunity Commission (EEOC) protect employees against discrimination and unfair treatment in the workplace
- These laws exist at the federal, state and local levels and cover numerous employer activities including hiring, employee relations and management
- These laws make it illegal to retaliate against a person because the person complained about discrimination, filed a charge of discrimination, or participated in an employment discrimination investigation or lawsuit
- Employers must reasonably accommodate applicants' and employees' rights under these laws, unless doing so would impose an undue hardship on the operation of the employer's business

7.1.11.2.1 Title VII of the Civil Rights Act of 1964 (Title VII)

- It is illegal to discriminate against someone on the basis of race, color, religion, national origin, sex, sexual orientation, or gender identity
- The law requires that employers reasonably accommodate applicants' and employees' sincerely held religious practices

7.1.11.2.2 The Pregnancy Discrimination Act

- Amends Title VII to make it illegal to discriminate against a woman because of pregnancy, childbirth, or a medical condition related to pregnancy or childbirth

7.1.11.2.3 The Equal Pay Act of 1963 (EPA)

- It is illegal to pay different wages to men and women if they perform equal work in the same workplace.

7.1.11.2.4 The Age Discrimination in Employment Act of 1967 (ADEA)

- People who are 40 or older are protected from discrimination because of age

7.1.11.2.5 Title I of the Americans with Disabilities Act of 1990 (ADA)

- It is illegal to discriminate against a qualified person with a disability in the private sector and in state and local governments.
- The law requires that employers reasonably accommodate the known physical or mental limitations of an otherwise qualified individual with a disability who is an applicant or employee

7.1.11.2.6 Sections 102 & 103 of the Civil Rights Act of 1991

- Amends Title VII and the ADA to permit jury trials and compensatory and punitive damage awards in intentional discrimination cases

7.1.11.2.7 Sections 501 & 505 of the Rehabilitation Act of 1973

- It is illegal to discriminate against a qualified person with a disability in the federal government.
- The law requires that employers reasonably accommodate the known physical or mental limitations of an otherwise qualified individual with a disability who is an applicant or employee

7.1.11.2.8 The Genetic Information Nondiscrimination Act of 2008 (GINA)

- It is illegal to discriminate against employees or applicants because of genetic information
- Genetic information includes information about an individual's genetic tests and the genetic tests of an individual's family members, as well as information about any disease, disorder or condition of an individual's family members (ie, an individual's family medical history)

7.1.11.3 Diversity, equity & inclusion (DE&I) in the laboratory

- Laboratory leaders should develop engagement strategies incorporating effective, inclusive communications that articulate and promote the value of each team member to the success of laboratory outcomes and in benefit to patients

- Guidance to a team is offered for assuring DE&I. If/when DE&I gaps or challenges present, it is essential to be inclusive of a high-functioning team that is well-resourced with customized education and resources to positively move DE&I forward
- Laboratory orientation and mentorship programs should include elements of DE&I training and engagement
- Inclusive community-based engagement is beneficial to a diverse laboratory team and elevates the laboratory's visibility and value

7.1.11.3.1 Hiring: diverse workforces

- Diversity = the "what", meaning the demographics of the workforce
- Reduce bias in hiring
- Remove biased language from job descriptions
- Utilize structured and unstructured interviews
- Use multiple interviewers per candidate
- Develop skill assessments
- Provide salary range and do not ask for salary history
- Post and source recruits more intentionally and widespread

7.1.11.3.2 Retention: inclusive workforces

- Inclusion = The "how", meaning the culture of the workforce
- Creating equal opportunities for all employees
- Establish mentorship programs
- Foster a sense of belonging in which uniqueness is encourages, appreciated, and respected
- Develop ongoing inclusion behaviors, policies, practices, discussions, and trainings

7.1.11.3.3 Professional development

- Development opportunities are inclusive, equally provided, and elevates contributions from team members
- Professional development plans are relevant and timely for DE&I learnings with team engagement in related initiatives
- DE&I advisory groups and teams may be developed to enhance and assure DE&I priorities throughout laboratory medicine and pathology practices
- Subteams can offer insight into specific opportunities to assure DE&I, while also creating meaningful activities and outcomes

7.1.11.3.4 Creating inclusive educational content for those with vision and/or auditory considerations

- Use high-contrast coloring of text
- Avoid using colors to emphasize or convey meaning
- Use simple, easily readible fonts
- Use bullets and numbering
- Provide written summaries, presentation slides, and/or closed captioning on educational videos

7.1.11.3.5 Create & foster inclusive policies

- Ensure equal access to opportunities
- Establish organizational flexibility and agility
- Foster diverse representation at all levels of a team, department, and organization
- Create behavioral standards and hold people accountable
- Train everyone on DE&I topics, such as implicit bias, micro-aggressions, and more
- Accept and honor multiple religious holidays and practices
- Create inclusive maternity and paternity leave practices
- Establish whistleblower systems to report inappropriate behaviors, actions, and statements
- Establish fair and unbiased performance management evaluations and systems

7.2 Financial considerations in the laboratory

7.2.1 Types of costs & calculation of the breakeven point

- Laboratory costs can be considered either fixed or variable depending on volume f7.1
  - Fixed costs (eg, instrument purchase, laboratory information system, management labor) are not affected by the number of tests performed
  - Variable costs such as reagents & technologist pay correlate with the number of tests performed
- Some costs are direct & some indirect
  - Direct costs are incurred directly from the performance of the test
  - Indirect costs are not (information technology [IT] support, rent, utilities, cleaning services)
- Actual cost is the sum of direct, indirect, and overhead costs incurred performing testing
- Unit cost is the cost incurred in performing 1 test (cost per reportable or cost per billable test)

ISBN 978-089189-6616

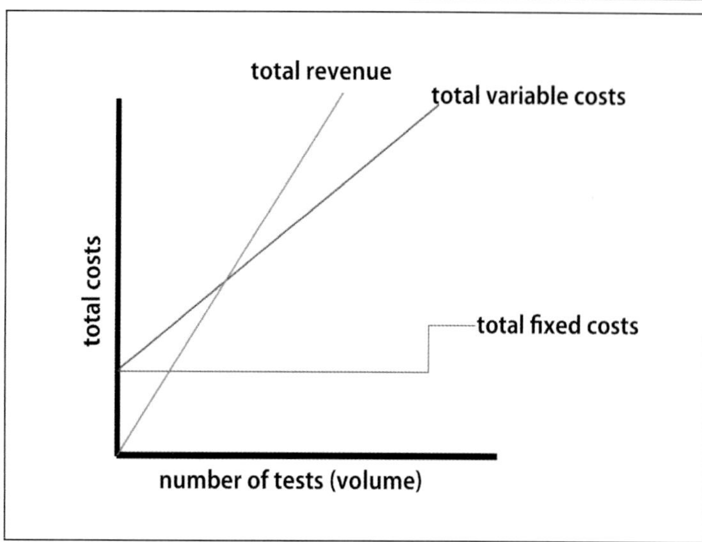

f7.1 Types of costs

net income = revenue (R) – fixed cost (FC) – variable cost (VC)

so, we seek the point at which net income is 0, or the point at which

$0 = R - FC - VC$

if Z is the number of tests performed, then the point we seek is

$0 = R \times Z - FC - VC \times Z$

this can be rearranged to

$FC = R \times Z - VC \times Z$ or

$FC = (R - VC) \times Z$

then rearranged to

$Z = FC \div (R - VC)$

so, if we assume we will charge \$9 per test, then $Z = \$500 \div (\$9 - \$5) = 125$ tests

f7.2 Calculation of the breakeven point

- Determined by adding the fixed & variable costs involved in performing the test
- Note that variable costs per unit are the same regardless of the number of tests performed
- Breakeven point is the number of tests needed to reach a zero net income f7.2
- Fixed costs per unit decrease as the number of tests performed increases t7.1

t7.1 Relationship of total cost to unit cost

Assumptions: fixed cost is \$500, variable cost is \$5/test

Tests performed	100	200	300
Total cost	\$500 + \$500 = \$1000	\$500 + \$1000 = \$1500	\$500 + \$1500 = \$2000
Unit cost	\$1000 ÷ 100 tests = \$10/test	\$1500 ÷ 200 tests = \$7.50/test	\$2000 ÷ 300 tests = \$6.66/test

7.2.2 Budgeting

- For laboratories, there are generally 4 major parts of the budget: capital, personnel, operating & allocation (overhead)
- Capital budget is for "big ticket" items such as laboratory instruments/equipment whose return on investment may be achieved over multiple years
  - Reagent/lease or reagent/rental agreements are an alternative to purchasing instrumentation as capital expenditures where the cost of the instrument is rolled into the reagent cost
  - Reagents are purchased at a set cost per test, which varies with volume
  - Reagent/rental agreements allow the flexibility to switch to a new instrument platform as technology changes
- Personnel budget is the projection of personnel needs, generally expressed in full time equivalents (FTEs)
  - A full-time employee salary is based on working 2,080 hours a year (40 hours a week)
  - Labor-related expenses (salaries & benefits) typically consume the highest proportion of budget dollars compared to all other expense categories
- Operating budget considers the following:
  - All the costs of day-to-day operations, including reagents and other consumables
  - The cost of reference laboratory tests
  - The costs of transfusion service blood
  - Professional fees
  - Depreciation, maintenance & nonconsumable equipment costs ("small ticket" items such as computer monitors)
- Workload recording is a tool used to monitor productivity, strategic planning, and to project future budget needs
  - Ideally, the workload recording units are weighed to reflect the labor & medical supply expense associated with each test performed
  - Performed tests or billed tests are often used, but are not weighted measures

7.3 Statistical considerations in the laboratory

7.3.1 Definitions

7.3.1.1 Gaussian distribution, estimates of central tendency & estimates of variation

- *Gaussian* refers to a distribution of data symmetrically around the mean, with most values closest to the center
- Estimates of central tendency: Mean, median & mode

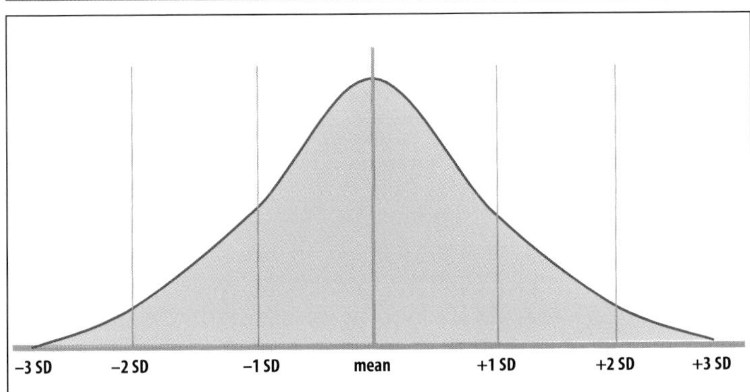

f7.3 Gaussian curve

- In a perfect Gaussian distribution, mean, median & mode are identical
  - Mean is the arithmetic average. Mean = $\Sigma x^i/n$
  - Median is the middle value of a range of values
  - Mode is the most frequently occurring value in a range of values
- Some datasets are non-Gaussian—skewed positively or negatively
  - Skews alter the mean & median but do not affect the mode
  - In a positively skewed set of data,

$$\text{mean} > \text{median} > \text{mode}$$

- Estimates of variation
  - The standard deviation (SD) is a reflection of variation
  - The SD is the average distance of an individual value from the mean

$$SD = \sqrt{\Sigma(xi - \text{mean})^2/(n - 1)}$$

- In the ideal Gaussian distribution, 68.2% of the population falls within –1 SD and +1 SD, 95.5% falls within –2 SD and +2 SD, and 99.7% fall within –3 SD and +3 SD **f7.3**
- Confidence interval (CI) is a range of values that we are fairly sure our true value lies in, typically 95% CI with a normal distribution ±2 SD around a mean (–2.5% to 97.5%). The CI is calculated from observations (statistical sampling, ie, measurements)

7.3.1.2 Reliability: Analytic accuracy & precision

- Imprecision & inaccuracy result from random error & systematic error, respectively
- Total analytical error is the sum of random & systematic error
  - Analytic accuracy is the extent to which a test result approximates the "true" value

	disease	**no disease**
positive test	true positive (TP)	false positive (FP)
negative test	false negative (FN)	true negative (TN)

f7.4 Punnett square

  - Accuracy has no numerical value, but is reflected in the correlation coefficient of bias plots
  - Analytic accuracy is controlled through regular calibration
  - Diagnostic accuracy (clinical accuracy) refers to the ability of a test to discriminate among patient groups
- Precision refers to the reproducibility of a result
  - Imprecision is reflected in dispersion; it is expressed in terms of the coefficient of variation (CV)

$$CV = SD/\text{mean} \times 100$$

  - Because the CV is a function of the mean, it refers to the precision at a specific analyte concentration
  - Precision is controlled through regular testing of QC reagents
  - As a rule of thumb, desirable precision for most analytes is <10%

7.3.1.3 Clinical sensitivity & specificity

- Clinical or diagnostic sensitivity
  - The ability of the test to detect disease when present
  - Positivity in the presence of disease **f7.4**

$$\text{sensitivity} = TP/(TP + FN)$$

- Clinical or diagnostic specificity
  - The ability of the test to detect only the disease sought
  - Negativity in the absence of disease **f7.4**

$$\text{specificity} = TN/(TN + FP)$$

- The clinical sensitivity & specificity should be distinguished from the analytical sensitivity & specificity, which refer to the ability of the assay to detect small quantities of the analyte (analytical sensitivity) and its ability to accurately measure the analyte in the presence of other substances (analytical specificity)

ISBN 978-089189-6616

7.3.1.4 Predictive value

- Positive predictive value (PPV)
    - Probability of disease when the test result is positive **f7.4**

$$PPV = TP/(TP + FP)$$

- Negative predictive value (NPV)
    - Probability of no disease when the test result is negative

$$NPV = TN/(TN + FN)$$

    - The prevalence of the disease in the population affects predictive value
    - When disease prevalence is low, the PPV declines and the NPV increases
    - Note that sensitivity & specificity are not influenced by prevalence

7.3.1.5 Percent change

- Percent change is calculated by subtracting the old value from the new value, dividing the result by the old value
    - For example, the percent change from 5 to 7 is: 2/5 = 0.4 or 40%

7.3.1.6 Relative risk

- Relative risk is the ratio of the risk in the presence of a factor to the baseline risk
- It is the risk of an outcome "Y" in the presence of condition "X" as compared to the general population

$$\text{relative risk} = \frac{(\text{\# with X who develop Y})/(\text{\# with X})}{(\text{\# in population who develop Y})/(\text{\# in population})}$$

7.3.1.7 Diagnostic accuracy

- *Diagnostic accuracy* refers to the ability of a test to distinguish between groups of patients (disease vs no disease)
- Distinct from *analytical accuracy*, which refers to the ability of a test to correctly measure analyte

7.3.1.8 Reference intervals

- Reference ranges or reference intervals are established based on where 95% of healthy individuals would fall
    - Reference intervals are a useful guide and can be a critical decision management tool used for the appropriate interpretation of laboratory test results
    - Reference intervals must be stratified based on population-dependent variables such as age, sex, and in some cases, ethnicity
- Laboratories are required to report a reference interval with every test result
- Each laboratory is required by CLIA to "verify that the manufacturer's reference intervals are appropriate for the laboratory's patient population" or determine reference intervals for laboratory-developed tests (LDTs)
- The laboratory must either verify such reference intervals or establish its own, at the discretion of the medical director, and document how its reference interval was established

7.3.1.9 Establishing & adopting reference intervals

- Establishing reference intervals
    - A reference population is a group of healthy individuals demographically comparable to the patient population
    - CLSI recommends testing at least 120 such individuals, applying exclusion criteria as appropriate, and controlling preanalytical variables
    - The reference interval may be taken as the central 95% of values or as all values falling within +2 SD and –2 SD
    - Some analytes (eg, serum prostate specific antigen) have no relevant lower limit
- Adopting reference intervals
    - Laboratories usually *adopt* reference intervals rather than establish them
    - The source of the reference interval may be literature, manufacturer, or the laboratory's own previously established reference interval (when a new instrument or method is being implemented)
    - Adopted reference intervals should be verified within the laboratory
    - CLSI recommends testing at least 20 healthy individuals
    - If 20 tests are conducted, at least 18 should fall within the established reference range under consideration

7.4 Implementation of new methods

7.4.1 Overview

- When a new method or new instrument is introduced to the laboratory a process is undertaken that includes assessment of performance, writing a procedure, integration into the information system, training, and education

- The extent of method performance assessment depends on the status of the method—whether FDA approved or not, and if approved, whether waived or not. Assays that do not have FDA approval require formal validation, whereas FDA-approved tests may require only verification
- Validation vs verification
  - Method validation is a much more extensive process than method verification
    - Method verification consists of experiments performed to confirm that, within the laboratory, a test performs as the manufacturer claims
    - Method validation consists of experiments to prove both the clinical value of a test and performance characteristics
    - Validation has all the components of verification but has (1) greater statistical power (usually involves larger sample numbers), and (2) assessment of additional parameters (clinical sensitivity, clinical specificity, and PPV)
    - Validation is required when implementing a laboratory-developed test, a non-FDA cleared test, or any modification of an FDA-approved test
    - Validation is not required when FDA-approved tests are used within the scope for which they were approved and without modification
  - Method verification
    - Usually involves the following elements:
      - Precision
      - Accuracy
      - Reportable range
      - Reference intervals
      - Analytical sensitivity
      - Analytical specificity
    - CLIA specifically mandates elements 1-4 for all tests and 1-6 for laboratory-developed test (LDTs)
    - CLIA does not specify how these elements are to be done or what is considered acceptable
    - The medical director is responsible for outlining a verification plan t7.2
    - The verification experiment samples may be derived from patient samples, samples obtained from healthy subjects (laboratory technologist blood), quality control (QC) materials, or proficiency testing samples

t7.2 Validation plan checklist

Calibration & calibration verification
Precision verification & establishment of quality control ranges
Establishment of reference intervals & critical values (if any)
Determination of analytical sensitivity
Determination of analytical specificity
Determination of accuracy/interferences
Method comparison (primary)
Method comparison (secondary), if any
Carryover tests
Establishment of analytical measurement range & clinical reportable range
Establishment of parameters for calibration & quality control
Determination of specimen stability
Verification of interfaces & reports
Procedure written & approved by medical director
Application for proficiency testing
Training of laboratorians & competency assessment
Notification of clinicians

7.4.2 Elements of method verification

7.4.2.1 Calibration & calibration verification

- Calibration is the process of adjusting the instrument to read out the known actual concentration of a calibrator
- Calibration verification involves the use of several specimens with known concentrations (patient samples, commercial calibrators, proficiency testing material, controls) to ensure the validity of the calibrator over a wider range of results
- Calibration is analogous to "zeroing" a scale, and calibration verification is analogous to then testing the scale using a series of known weights
- Calibration verification must be carried out at least once every 6 months and more frequently under some circumstances, eg, after major preventive maintenance

7.4.2.2 Precision & establishment of quality control ranges

- *Precision* refers to the reproducibility of a result; imprecision is reflected in the degree to which repeated measurements disperse in relation to the mean
- Precision is verified by replicating measurements on the same specimens, both simultaneously (within run precision) and consecutively (between run precision)
- The mean & standard deviation of these measurements can be used to establish QC ranges for statistical QC
- The "rule of thumb" is 20 samples for most experiments

7.4.2.3 Accuracy, inaccuracy (bias) & method comparison

- Accuracy refers to the correctness of a result, as compared to a known "true" value
- This can be verified in 2 ways

ISBN 978-089189-6616

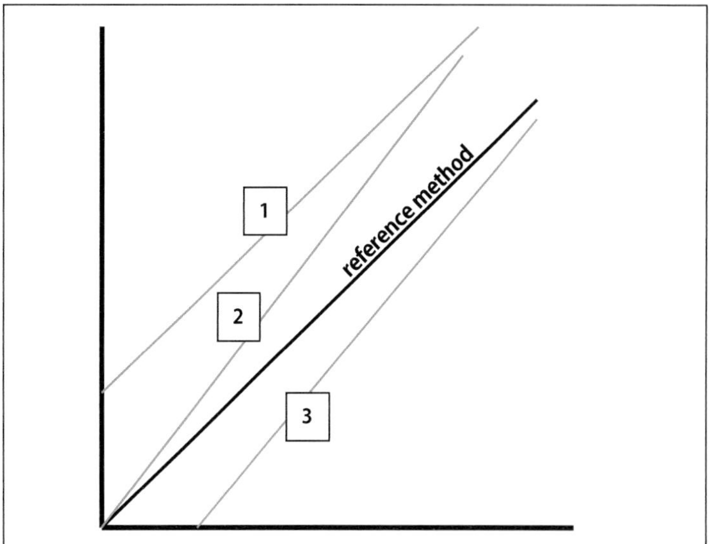

f7.5 Correlation study: 1 constant bias, 2 proportional bias, 3 mixed

rack	sample
1	low
2	low
3	low
4	high
5	high
6	low

f7.6 Example of carryover test: rack loading order

- Recovery experiment, in which certified reference materials of known quantity are analyzed
- Method comparison (method correlation) experiment, in which results obtained by the new method are compared with results from a previously validated method or a reference method
  - Recommended that at least 40 samples are used for comparison
  - Paired results plotted, with results from the new method on the y axis and those from the reference method on the x axis **f7.5**
  - The slope may indicate a proportional bias, one that is initially negligible but increases in magnitude in relation to the value of the result
  - The intercept may indicate a constant bias, one that is roughly the same throughout the range of values
  - A calculation of average bias, the difference between each result and the reference result, is compared to some preselected allowable limit
  - Linear regression analysis permits a line to be drawn that "best fits" the set of x and y datapoints
  - The correlation coefficient (*r*) is a number ranging from –1 to +1 that expresses the degree of linearity between the 2 data sets
  - Ideally, slope equals 1, intercept is 0, and *r* is 1. If the CV of variables is 0, there is no correlation between methods

- If more than 1 instrument is in service, then method comparison should be carried out between instruments (secondary method comparison); secondary method comparison must be performed initially and at least twice per year

7.4.2.4 Analytical specificity, interference & carryover

- Analytical specificity refers to the degree to which the analyte can be detected in the presence of interfering substances (bilirubinemia, lipemia, hemoglobinemia)
- Can be tested in "recovery" experiments, in which quantities of interferent are added to known samples, and the amount of analyte measured ("recovered") is compared to the known amount
- Types of interference
  - Heterophile antibody interference is a major problem in immunoassay-based testing
  - Serial dilutions of samples containing heterophile antibody do not lead to predictable changes in analyte measurement; in fact, the measurement may increase with dilution
- Solvent exclusion effect
  - Falsely low analyte concentration that results from a higher than normal "solid phase"
  - An "indirect ISE" instrument measures analyte concentration within the aqueous phase and calculates the concentration for the entire volume of blood; when the solid phase is increased as, for example, in lipemia or paraproteinemia, then the calculation underestimates the true value
- Carryover
  - A problem for analytes that can have a wide range of concentration, such as β-human chorionic gonadotropin (hCG)
  - Carryover from 1 sample into another could have major impact upon the second sample
  - Carryover studies are performed using a sample of known high analyte concentration and a sample of low concentration **f7.6**. Carryover of <1.5% is desirable

- High carryover suggests a problem in the dispensing/ pipetting system

7.4.2.5 Analytical sensitivity, limit of detection & functional sensitivity

- Analytical sensitivity refers to the lowest analyte concentration that is reliably detectable
- Limit of blank (LoB) and limit of detection (LoD) are similar, referring to the lowest concentration that can be distinguished from background (blank)
- Functional sensitivity, also called limit of quantitation (LoQ), is the lowest analyte concentration reliably quantified with an acceptable CV

7.4.2.6 Linearity, analytical measuring range & clinical reportable range

7.4.2.6.1 Analytical measuring range (AMR)

- Range over which reliable measurement can be obtained without manipulation (without dilution, concentration, or other manipulation)
- Usually determined by linearity experiment
  - Samples of known concentration serially diluted and assayed, and results plotted
  - At least 5 different points within the reportable range is ideal
  - The plot is examined for limits of linearity

7.4.2.6.2 Clinical reportable range (CRR)

- Also called maximum dilution/concentration (MD/C)
- Highest & lowest values that can be reported accurately
- The range of quantitative results that may be reported, considering the ability to dilute samples that fall outside the upper limit of the AMR, if applicable
- Low end of the CRR is typically identical to the low end of the AMR

7.4.2.7 Specimen stability

- *Specimen stability* refers to the length of time that a stored specimen will continue to produce reliable results
- May be assessed for specimens stored at room temperature, at refrigerator temperature, and/or for frozen specimens
- To determine, patient samples are tested immediately and at intervals under the defined storage conditions
- Maximum storage time is defined as the last time before significant, predefined, variation is noted. For example, one may choose to use 2 or 3 SD as defining significant variation

7.4.2.8 Laboratory information systems (LIS)

- Software system with features to support a laboratory's complex operations including specimen processing, storage, tracking and management of laboratory workflow data
  - LIS functionalities include audit management, data security, tracking of testing personnel, instrument integration (uni- and bidirectional interfaces, sample tracking, test order management, quality control data management, integration with electronic medical records via Health Level 7 (HL7), integration or interfaces to billing systems, and interfaces between laboratories
- The process of testing & documenting changes made to an LIS is called validation
- Utilization of barcode technology presents data in a machine-readable form and automates transactions & manual processes such as transcription
  - Barcode technology is rapidly expanding
- When verifying a new instrument or test, the reliability of interfaces should be verified
  - Key interfaces include those between the instrument and the LIS and those between any "middleware" (between instrument & LIS)
  - Autoverification transmits test results automatically via an instrument interface when the results are validated against established rules or parameters
  - Often, there is then an interface between the LIS and the hospital information system and possibly numerous additional proprietary information systems
  - A validation approach is to simply report several "test" patients across the various interfaces, originating with the instrument
  - A wide variety of possible results should be generated, for example, normal results, abnormal low, abnormal high, critical (if applicable)
  - Reports generated across each interface should be checked for fidelity and for integrity of interpretive comments, patient identification, units of measure & reference ranges
- Downtime processes must be established to receive test orders and return results in the event of a failure of the LIS, network, or interface

7.4.2.9 Written procedures

- Each test must have a written procedure, which must address all aspects of the testing process
- Should follow a standard format and include the information listed in t7.3

t7.3 Elements of a laboratory procedure

Element	Notes
Test principle	An overview of the analyte, the methodology the test is based on, and clinical utility of the test
Patient preparation	eg, fasting, nonfasting, preparation of venipuncture site
Specimen collection, labeling, handling & transport	What specimen is appropriate, how collected & into what container? Should the specimen be inverted several times immediately after collection? Can it be mailed, pneumatically tubed? Under what conditions & how quickly must it be transported to the laboratory?
Specimen storage, preservation & stability	Room temperature, refrigerator, or freezer storage, stability of analyte under various conditions, how quickly must it be centrifuged
Criteria for specimen acceptability	General "rejection criteria" are often discussed in a separate "labwide" procedure; herein list any criteria particular to this analyte or assay
Referral instructions	The laboratory must refer specimens for testing only to a CLIA certified or CMS approved laboratory If the laboratory accepts referral specimens, written instructions must be available to clients, and must include the items listed above
Reagents	List of reagents, including proper storage (as applicable, temperature, humidity), concentrations, expiration dates
Procedures for microscopic examinations	If applicable, including the detection of inadequately prepared slides
Test procedure	Step by step
Reportable range	Determined at time of method verification/validation
Test calibration	How performed, how often
Quality control (QC) procedures	How performed, how often
Steps to be taken when calibration or QC fails	eg, retest the unacceptable control (1 time only) If repeat acceptable, no further action; if the repeat unacceptable, what actions are to be taken? This should include evaluating all patient test results obtained since the last acceptable QC to determine if the patient test results were adversely affected (before reporting the results and if necessary issuing corrected reports); at what point to notify clinicians of an anticipated delay?
Limitations of procedure	eg, interfering substances
Reference range	Determined at time of method verification/validation
Critical values	A labwide procedure should address the steps to be taken in reporting critical values; herein list the values considered critical, if any
Results reporting & calculations, if any	How results are entered into laboratory information system and any calculations that must be carried out
References	Sources of information for the procedure, including product insert, standard texts, published studies

- Product or package inserts may be a source for some of the information in the procedure, but they should not be used instead of a procedure
- The medical director must review procedures initially, each time a major change is made, and biennially (every 2 years). After the initial review, the medical director may delegate subsequent reviews to qualified individuals
- Testing personnel must read and understand the procedures prior to testing and at regular intervals thereafter (annually, usually); every change to the procedure must, likewise, be read and understood
- Ideally, written procedures should be maintained on a computerized document control program
    - Such procedures are usually accessible through an "intranet"
    - A backup data source must be available for system downtimes
    - Printed copies should be avoided, but certain printed "work aids" may be necessary

7.4.2.10 Training, Competency assessment & continuing education

- Personnel requirements specific to laboratory role & responsibilities
    - Job descriptions defining minimum qualifications, duties & work tasks
    - Certification if required
    - Validation of educational qualifications (copies of diploma, transcriptions, primary source verification reports
    - Licenses if required
    - Training, competency assessment & continuing education records
- Training
    - Organized documented process to provide instructions to help a person attain or regain a required level of knowledge and skill required to perform a task or procedure
    - Training documentation alone does not satisfy the requirements for competency assessment
- Competency assessment
    - Confirms a person's ability to use his or her skill and knowledge to perform assigned duties correctly
    - Must be performed & documented for testing personnel for each test or test system that an individual is authorized to perform before reporting test results
        - Assessment must be performed before testing & reporting patient results

- Semiannually during the first year of testing then annually
- When methodology or instruments are changed
- When new test platforms are introduced
- Newly hired, transferred, or promoted personnel
- When an employee demonstrates repeated performance issues

- Required minimum qualifications of competency assessors
  - Waived—determined by medical director
  - Moderate complexity testing—a bachelor's degree with 2 years of medical laboratory experience
  - High complexity—a bachelor's degree with 4 years of medical laboratory experience
- Six elements of competency must be assessed at the minimum
  - Direct observation (handling, preparation, processing, testing)
  - Monitoring the recording & reporting of testing
  - Review of intermediate test results or worksheets, QC, PT results, and preventive maintenance records
  - Direct observation of performance of instrument maintenance & function checks
  - Assessment of problem-solving skills
  - Assessment of test performance using previously tested specimens, blind specimens, and external proficiency samples
- Documented retraining & reassessment of competency must occur when performance issues are identified

- Continuing education
  - Topics based on the needs of the employees

7.4.2.11 Recruitment, hiring practices & performance management

7.4.2.11.1 Regulation-defined policies

- Employers use policies & procedures to ensure compliance with local, state, and federal employment laws
  - Equal Employment Opportunity
    - Prohibits discrimination with respect to hiring or promotion of individuals, conditions of employment, disciplinary & discharge practices, or any other aspect of employment based on race, color, religion (creed), sex, gender identity or expression, sexual orientation, national origin (ancestry), disability, age, genetic information, marital status, citizenship, pregnancy or maternity, and protected veteran status
    - Unacceptable pre-employment questions
      - Marital status, age, national origin, race, sex, inquiries related to pregnancy, religion, number of children, citizenship or place of birth, arrest history, or medical history
    - Protection against unlawful harassment
    - Protection against retaliation for reporting noncompliance
    - Rights for safe work environment
    - Pay practices & job protection
      - Federal Fair Labor Standards Act (FLSA) establishes pay practices to lawfully compensate nonexempt (hourly) employees for overtime hours worked and practices premium pay eligibility and compensation. Workers are assigned to either a 40-hour or 8/80 overtime rule based on operational necessity
      - 40-hour: Overtime is paid at a rate of 1½ times regular pay for hours worked beyond 40 hours in a 7-day period
      - 8/80: Overtime is paid for hours beyond 8 hours/day or 80 hours within a 14-day period
    - Defined meal & rest periods
    - Exempt employees are not eligible for overtime
  - Collective bargaining
    - A process where terms of employment are negotiated between a labor union representing the collective interests of a group of workers and an employer
    - The terms may include base pay or wages, work hours, training requirements, health & safety, overtime, shift length, vacation & retirement benefits, health care coverage, working conditions, and grievance mechanisms
  - Family and Medical Leave Act (FMLA) requires that covered employers provide up to 12 weeks of unpaid, protected leave to eligible employees for:
    - Incapacitation because of pregnancy, prenatal medical care, or childbirth
    - Caring for an employee's child after birth or adoption
    - Caring for employee's spouse, child, or parent with a serious health condition
    - Serious health conditions in which employees are unable to perform the duties of their job
  - American with Disabilities Act (ADA)
    - Job accommodations: A reasonable adjustment to a job or work environment to help individuals with disabilities perform their job duties
  - Uniformed Services Employment and Reemployment Rights Act (USERRA)

ISBN 978-089189-6616

- Guarantees the rights of military service members to take a leave of absence for active military service and to return to their jobs with accrued seniority and other employment protections

7.4.2.11.2 Employer-defined policies

- Employer-defined personal policies can be very far-ranging
  - Attendance
  - Behavior expectations
  - Dispute resolution
  - Drug & alcohol-free workplace
  - Employment of relatives (nepotism)
  - Personal leaves of absences
  - Appearance and dress code including personal protective equipment (PPE)
  - Personal communication at work (eg, cell phone, email)
  - Solicitation
  - Verification of previous employment/reference checks
  - Smoking
  - Performance evaluations
  - Time away from work

7.4.2.11.3 Performance and change

- Performance management
  - Ongoing process toward the continuous alignment of expectations as it relates to key responsibilities and compliance with policies and procedures
  - Performance evaluation
    - Formal performance feedback that documents & summarizes an employee's overall performance against job expectations & performance standards
    - Progress toward previously established short-term or long-term goals are assessed and issues or corrective actions that may have been addressed throughout the year are documented
    - The process provides an opportunity for supervisor & employee to set future goals and individual development plans
    - The evaluation is one component of an ongoing competency assessment process
  - Performance management & performance issues
    - Immediate verbal counseling regarding unsafe work practices
    - Direct verbal feedback in the moment to reward excellent behavior or to address issues
    - Discussion with supervisor at regular intervals
    - Series of progressive steps if performance issues are not resolved with documented expectations
    - Examples of performance issues: Insubordination, falsifying or altering documentation, possession of unauthorized materials, failure to comply with employer's policies/procedures, incompetence, performing tasks outside scope of responsibilities, and lack of motivation
  - Formal corrective action
    - Counseling
    - Performance improvement plan
    - Written warning
    - Final written warning
    - Termination of employment
  - Employee intrinsic & extrinsic motivation and motivation techniques
    - Money & other rewards
    - Positive feedback or other nonmonetary rewards
    - Giving input to working conditions, personal and team goals, decision making
    - Job significance
    - Challenging vs boring & repetitive
    - Production of high-quality outputs
    - Job variety, expansion & enrichment
    - Learning opportunities
    - Contributing to quality & safety improvements
  - Change management
    - Prepare staff for organizational change
    - Describe what will be improved
    - Present pros/cons and business case for change
    - Encourage input from staff
    - Involve staff in decision making
    - Plan for change including required materials & resources
    - Communicate, communicate, communicate

7.5 Quality management

7.5.1 Definitions

7.5.1.1 Quality management, quality assurance & quality control

- The definition of quality is complicated with various definitions and inconsistent use in literature
- Many of the quality concepts used in the laboratory were derived from the quality movement in manufacturing
- Experts have defined quality from both a product specification & a customer perspective

- To achieve high quality, the focus has been on improving processes or systems to improve the product to meet desired specifications
- The elements of quality are interrelated but distinctly different

7.5.1.2 Quality management system (QMS)

- A process-oriented, coordinated & organized system of activities that encompass the totality of all functions involved in achieving quality and maximum customer satisfaction
- A quality management system or plan is designed to detect errors and prevent them from occurring and from recurring, however, it does not guarantee an error-free laboratory
- There are 12 essential elements or building blocks that should be addressed in a QMS to ensure quality
  - Organization: Roles/responsibilities
  - Personnel: Job qualifications, orientation, training, competency assessment, continuing education & job description that matches the content & requirements of specific tasks skills & abilities of the worker
    - Credential requirements: Employers may require specific credentials (formal recognition of professional or technical competence) and/or a license granted by an authority to engage in a specific occupation
    - Training: Documented training is required for newly hired, transferred, promoted employees. Employees who demonstrate performance issues require documented retraining
    - Competency: Must be assessed before testing, at 6 months, and annually thereafter
  - Equipment & instrument management: Acquisition, installation, validation, maintenance, calibration, trouble-shooting, repair, records
  - Purchasing & inventory: Vendor qualifications, supplies & reagents management (preparation, labeling, troubleshooting, lot-to-lot acceptability, expired products, inventory management
  - Process control: QC, sample management, test method validation, method verification, lot-to-lot acceptability
  - Information management: Confidentiality, requisitions, records, reports, laboratory information system (LIS)
  - Documents & records: Creation, revisions, approval, control & distribution, review, storage, retention
    - Information management: Data security, requisitions, data entry, records, patient reports & LIS
  - Occurrence management: Identification & correction of nonconformities, complaint resolution, investigations, implementation of corrective actions, development of preventive measures, complaints, mistakes, problems, root-cause analysis, immediate actions, corrective actions, preventive measures
  - Assessment: Internal & external audits or inspections
  - Process improvement: Customer feedback, ideas from staff, problem resolution, corrective action, monitoring of quality indicators or key performance indicators across the flow of work, identification of opportunities for operational improvement (ideas from staff), patient safety improvements
  - Customer service: Customer needs
  - Facilities & safety: Safe work environment, transportation management, containment, waste management, ergonomics

7.5.1.3 Quality improvement (QI)

- System or process interventions aimed at raising product quality
- Iterations of QI, known as continuous quality improvement (CQI), seek to cyclically identify opportunities, make changes, and measure improvement

7.5.1.4 Quality assurance (QA)

- *Proactive* systematic activities to provide confidence that the quality requirements will be met
- QA activities are designed to *prevent* defects and identify system variations or barriers to quality. Examples include:
  - Daily refrigerator & freezer temperature recording
  - Rigorous adherence to standard operating procedures (SOPs)
  - Internal & external audits (inspections)
  - Proficiency testing
  - Glasswash procedures to ensure removal of detergents
  - Quality monitors, eg, turnaround time, specimen acceptability, or critical value notification

7.5.1.5 Quality control (QC)

- Laboratory quality control refers to a process and procedures used to detect analytical errors before the release of patient test results
- QC measures accuracy, precision & reproducibility of a test system over time and under various operating conditions

 ISBN 978-089189-6616

Day	Interpretation	
2	Accept run	Control value is <2SD; run is in control
3	Accept run	Control value is <2SD; run is in control
4	Accept run	Control value is <2SD; run is in control
5	Accept run	Control value exceeds 2SD; No rules violated; run is in control
6	Reject run	Control value exceeds 2SD 2:2s rule violated
7	Accept run	Control value is <2SD; run is in control
8	Reject run	Control value exceeds 2SD 1:3s rule violated
9	Accept run	Control value is <2SD; run is in control
10	Accept run	Control value is <2SD; run is in control
11	Accept run	Control value is <2SD; run is in control
12	Accept run	Control value exceeds 2SD; no rules violated; run is in control
13	Reject run	Control value exceeds 2SD 2:2s (and 10:mean) rule violated
14	Accept run	Control value is <2SD; run is in control
15	Accept run	Control value is <2SD; run is in control
16	Accept run	Control value exceeds 2SD; no rules violated; run is in control
17	Accept run	Control value is <2SD; run is in control
18	Reject run	Control value exceeds 2SD; 4:1s rule violated

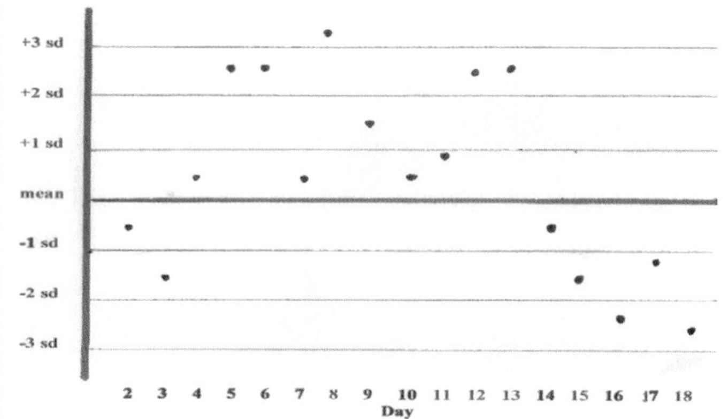

f7.7 Statistical quality control

7.5.2 Statistical quality control

- Walter Shewhart, an engineer introduced the concept of acceptable variation in manufacturing. Shewhart, sometimes referred to as the father of statistical quality control, introduced the quality control chart to keep variations controlled and detect system errors in manufacturing processes
- Variability is inherent in all processes; limits of acceptability should be defined by statistical means, and processes should not be adjusted when products fall consistently within them
- When outside defined limits, the process should be inspected for "assignable causes"
- To define limits, Shewhart plotted data on a control chart, a graph with lines demarcating the mean and several SD
- When Levey & Jennings proposed the use of Shewhart control charts in the clinical laboratory, the charts became known as "Levey-Jennings" charts
- The process became known as statistical quality control (SQC or simply QC)
- 6 Sigma is an extension of the SQC concept, the name referring to 6 SD from the mean
- The premise in 6 Sigma is that a process design in which limits of acceptability are 6 SD from the mean has a very low likelihood of failure; specifically, 3.4 defects per million (2 sigma produces 308,000 per million)
- Parallel testing of known samples in order ensures that the test system is working properly and that results obtained from patient samples are reliable
- Specimens used for QC are most often samples provided by an outside vendor
    - For each type of quantitative test, usually 2 or 3 controls are used: a "low" QC reagent and a "high" QC reagent, sometimes a "midrange" QC reagent, often referred to as level I, level II, and level III controls
    - When a new control lot is received, it is tested several times (usually 20). The results from these tests are used to calculate a mean and standard deviation (SD). Based on these, a Levey-Jennings (Shewhart) chart is created f7.7. Only 1 Levey-Jennings chart is illustrated, but usually there is 1 for each level of control
    - Frequency of control sample assay
        - Usually once per level per run but may be done only once per day, depending on the type of test and its frequency
        - At minimum, CLIA requires 2 levels of QC every 24 hours (if testing is performed during the 24-hour period) or as frequently as recommended by the manufacturer, whichever is more frequent, unless an alternative plan is implemented
    - Application of control sample test result
        - The result obtained is plotted on the Levey-Jennings chart
        - If the control sample result falls within 2 SD of the mean, the run is considered "in control," and the results of patient samples can be reported
        - If the result falls outside 2 SD of the mean, the Levey-Jennings chart is interpreted in terms of Westgard rules
        - Based on this, the run is determined to be "in control" or "out of control"
        - The results of "out of control" runs should not generally be reported

7.5.2.1 Westgard rules

- 2-SD rule
    - An indication for further review of the QC data
    - It is expected that about 5% of QC results will fall outside 2 SD

- Most commonly employed rules are described in **t7.4**
- The 2:2s, 4:1s, and 10 : mean rules are sensitive to systematic error, which could result in shifts or drifts (trends)

t7.4 Selected Westgard rules

Rule	Definition	Purpose
1:3s	1 value is found to be ±3 SD from the mean	Detects imprecision
2:2s	2 consecutive values found to be >2 SD on the same side of the mean	Detects imprecision & systematic bias
R:4s	2 values within the same run are found to be >4 SD from each other	Detects random error
4:1s	4 consecutive values are found to be >1 SD on the same side of the mean	Detects systematic bias
10:mean	10 consecutive values are found to be on the same side of the mean	Detects systematic bias

SD, standard deviation

  - Drift: Gradual movement away from the mean; causes of drift include slow deterioration in a light source, corrosion of electrodes, accumulation of debris within tubing, or reagent deterioration
  - Shift: Rapid & sustained move away from the mean; causes include altered temperature or humidity, lot changes, instrument maintenance, or failure in any number of system components
- The R:4s and 1:3s rules are most sensitive to random error
  - Random error may be caused by bubbles, underfilled tubes, technologist error & auto pipetting errors
- When an "out of control" run is detected
  - Evaluate the test system, including reagents & instrument
  - After doing this, it is acceptable to repeat QC testing on a new aliquot of the QC reagent
  - If this is substantially within acceptable limits, then it is possible that QC reagent handling or deterioration was the culprit, and patient results from the run may be reported
  - If repeat testing is not within acceptable limits:
    - A thorough check of the instrument and reagents must be undertaken
    - Suspected problems are corrected and QC reagents are retested to ensure resolution
    - If this corrects the problem, patient samples must be repeated before reporting
  - If QC results are still not acceptable, then the next step is to repeat calibration and repeat testing on the QC reagents, then repeat patient testing if appropriate
  - Persistence of an out of control assay may require formal instrument maintenance. Testing should be shifted to the backup instrument or sent to another laboratory in the meantime
- QC specimens
  - May demonstrate matrix effects
  - May require reconstitution or dilution, which can be a source of error
  - May undergo deterioration during storage
  - May be commutable or noncommutable; commutable QC reagents are those that are biologically like patient samples whose results are directly comparable to them, while noncommutable reagents have altered constituents such as the matrix

7.5.2.2 Alternatives to traditional QC

- Individualized quality control plans (IQCP) as an alternative to traditional QC
- IQCP: Three components: Risk assessment, quality control plan & periodic quality assessment
- A QC plan customized for a test based on risk assessment & management principles
- Risk analysis must be performed upon the test before implementation
- Risk analysis may justify & establish a QC plan that is less stringent than traditional QC
- Laboratories are required to perform 2 levels of liquid QC per day (or more if recommended by manufacturer) for all nonwaived tests unless an IQCP analysis has been conducted that permits an alternate plan (while still satisfying at a minimum the manufacturer's recommendation)
- The requirements for IQCP include ongoing risk assessment and effectiveness quality assessment monitoring

7.5.3 Proficiency testing (PT) & performance assessment

7.5.3.1 Regulatory-required external quality assessment

- CLIA requirement
  - Each laboratory must enroll in a proficiency testing (PT) program for each area in which it performs testing
  - PT must be administered by an agency approved by CMS

ISBN 978-089189-6616

- PT programs
  - Participants receive 3 surveys per year, each survey consisting of 5 samples
  - The laboratory performs the indicated testing and reports results to the surveying agency
  - The laboratory must treat the survey sample as it would a patient sample
  - The sample must not be sent out of the laboratory, even if under normal circumstances, confirmatory testing might be sought outside the laboratory
  - There must be no communication with other laboratories that do not share the same CLIA certificate
- PT grading
  - Samples
    - Commutable samples (preferred)
      - Commutable PT samples can be traced to a reference method, and a "true" value can be assigned to the sample
      - The mean & SD of the reference method is used to grade results
    - Noncommutable samples
      - The "peer group" includes all participating laboratories using the same methodology
      - The mean & SD of the peer group results is used to grade results
- Participant results are graded as acceptable (within 2 SD of the mean), needs improvement (2-3 SD) or unacceptable (>3 SD)
- Satisfactory performance on a PT survey is achieved if at least 4 of 5 (80%) sample results are graded as acceptable
- Unacceptable PT results must be investigated, even if satisfactory performance is achieved for a survey. Corrective action must be taken with appropriate documentation
- Ungraded or educational PT challenges must be assessed
- The causes of PT failure are like those that cause QC failure, eg, reagent problems, instrument malfunction, calibration problems & climate control problems
- Investigation should include evaluation of QC data, maintenance data & reagent logs around the time of PT performance
- In general, a laboratory's likelihood of failing PT on a purely analytical basis is statistically unlikely if the laboratory's SD for the surveyed analyte is <33% of the SD allowed
- Lastly, even successful PT performance can be a source of useful information. Is bias, drift, or shift implied by the reported SDs Cembrowski & colleagues recommend a Westgard-like method of evaluating the data **t7.5**
- For some assays, PT is not available (unregulated analytes). This may be the result of the nature of the sample tested or the novelty of the assay. In such instances, the laboratory must engage in an alternative means of ensuring proficiency

t7.5 Cembrowski rules for evaluation of proficiency testing data

Rule	Description	Implication
Screening rule	Do ≥2 of the 5 results exceed 1 SDI?	Proceed to evaluate data according to the following rules
Mean rule	Does the average of the 5 SDIs exceed ±1.5?	Systematic error is significant
3 SDI rule	Any result beyond 3 SDI?	Random error is significant
4 SDI rule	Any 2 results >4 SDI apart?	Random error is significant

SDI, standard deviation index

7.5.3.2 Alternative quality assessment

- For tests for which approved commercial external PT is not available or not required, the laboratory must conduct an alternative performance assessment system (APAS) at least semiannually to determine the reliability of analytical testing
  - The laboratory must maintain a list of tests requiring alternative assessments and records of those assessments and associated criteria and evaluation for acceptability. Examples of APAS include:
    - Split sample analysis with a reference laboratory or other laboratories
    - Split sample analysis with an established in-house method
    - Use of purchased assayed materials
    - Clinical validation by chart review
    - For some molecular-based testing, alternative assessment may be performed by method or specimen type rather than for each analyte or abnormality

7.6 Nonanalytical variables in laboratory medicine: Preanalytic & postanalytic

7.6.1 Preanalytic variables

7.6.1.1 Patient identification

- Both CAP & TJC established "patient safety goals" that require 2 unique patient identifiers when collecting specimens and on all sample labels
  - Specimens must be labeled in the presence of the patient
  - The most common patient identifiers are full name, date of birth & medical record number
  - The patient's room number is not an acceptable patient identifier

Nonanalytical variables in laboratory medicine: Preanalytic & postanalytic>Preanalytic variables

- "Wrong blood in tube" (WBIT) occurs when a sample tube is labeled with unique identifiers for one patient, but the blood in the tube was collected from a different patient
  - Wrong blood in tube is identified by the laboratory when the current ABO typing result disagrees with the historical blood type
  - δ checks may detect some specimen labeling errors
  - The estimated frequency of "wrong blood in tube" is 400 per million (1 in 2500) specimens

7.6.1.2 Other preanalytical variables

- Examples of preanalytical variables that can contribute to laboratory test error or influence test results
  - Patient's age & gender
  - Food intake (fasting) & medication interference
  - Exercise
  - Time of day, posture
  - Tightness of tourniquet
  - Collection site: Line draw vs venipuncture vs capillary puncture
  - Overly vigorous shaking of blood collection tubes or not adequately mixing collection tubes with anticoagulants
  - Specimen acceptability
  - Specimen container **t7.6**
  - Specimen labeling
  - Wrong order of collection tube draw **t7.7**
  - Specimen transportation delays
  - Temperature during transportation & storage

t7.6 Selected blood collection tubes

Tube	Additive	Used for
Red	Glass—none Plastic—silica clot activator	Serum chemistry & serology
Green	Heparin	Plasma chemistry
Blue	Citrate	Coagulation tests
Note: A 1:9 ratio of anticoagulant: Blood is ideal; higher ratios lead to increased coagulation times, affecting the aPTT>PT; for polycythemic patients with Hct>60%, the PT and PTT can be prolonged due to decreased effective plasma		
Black	Citrate (calcium chelation)	ESR
Lavender (purple)	EDTA (calcium chelation)	cell counts
Yellow	Citrate & dextrose (ACD)	blood bank tests, HLA typing
Gray	Sodium fluoride (inhibits glycolysis)	glucose, lactate

aPTT, activated partial thromboplastin time; ESR, erythrocyte sedimentation rate; HLA, human leukocyte antigen; PT, prothrombin time; PTT, partial thromboplastin time

t7.7 Order of draw

Priority	Glass	Plastic
First	Culture	Culture
	No additive tubes (red)	Coagulation test tubes
	Coagulation test tubes	No additive tubes (red)
	Serum separator tubes	Serum separator tubes
Last	Additive tubes (green then lavender then gray)	Additive tubes (green then lavender then gray)

- During storage, blood cells continue to metabolize and slowly undergo lysis, serum proteins progressively degrade, and adsorption to tubes may occur
  - Some tests are performed on anticoagulated whole blood (eg, hematology), others on serum (clotted whole blood), and others on plasma (clot inhibited centrifuged whole blood)
  - For most purposes, serum & plasma give essentially similar results; serum must be used for serum protein electrophoresis & serologic assays, whereas plasma is required for coagulation tests
- If not separated from blood cells, serum & plasma progressively change in several ways such that they no longer accurately reflect the in vivo state
  - For example, glucose progressively diminishes and lactate increases
  - Ideally, all tests should be run within 1-2 hours of blood collection, but this is not always practical
  - Blood specimens not tested immediately should be stabilized
  - In the case of plasma tests, for example, blood should be centrifuged within 1 hour and stored at 4°C-6°C
- Every test has defined storage requirements (room temperature, refrigerated, frozen at –20°C or frozen at –80°C)

7.6.1.3 Serum vs plasma

- For most measured analytes, serum & plasma are interchangeable
  - The clotting process in which plasma is converted to serum, results in the release of substances in which platelets are rich, including calcium, magnesium, LD & potassium
  - Thus, one should expect these analytes to be higher in serum than in plasma
  - Furthermore, the clotting process uses plasma proteins (notably fibrinogen), such that total protein is higher in plasma

ISBN 978-089189-6616

7.6.2 Postanalytic variables

7.6.2.1 The postanalytic phase

- This phase consists of reporting, results retrieval, and the interpretation of test results
- Postanalytical errors include errors in reports (transcription & proofreading errors), errors in reading reports (misreading or incorrectly hearing the result), errors in interpretation of the report, incorrect reactions to the information & failure to retrieve results

7.6.2.2 Result reporting

- CLIA requires the following elements in laboratory reports
  - Patient name & identification number or unique patient identifier
  - Date of specimen collection, and if appropriate, the time of collection
  - Specimen source
  - Test performed, test result(s) & units of measure when applicable
  - Reference intervals
  - Date & time of test result release
  - Name & address of the testing laboratory
  - Name of the physician or legally authorized person of record

7.6.2.3 Critical test result reporting

- A critical test result requires rapid communication of the result even if normal. Critical (alert or panic) laboratory values are those that deviate from defined medical criteria and indicate the presence of a condition that could be immediately life threatening
- The list of critical values is determined by the medical director of the laboratory in consultation with the medical staff. Critical value lists & notification expectations vary between institutions depending on patient populations
- TJC's patient safety goals requires that laboratories have a written procedure for critical values that addresses
  - The list of critical values for the laboratory
  - Who is responsible for reporting critical values, and who is authorized to accept them?
  - What is the acceptable length of time to report a critical value?
- Some laboratories require that critical values be written down and read back to ensure accurate communication of information

7.6.2.4 Notifiable Conditions

- Public health surveillance programs require reporting of certain conditions to identify and control sources of infection or disease, prevent disease, and describe health trends
  - Examples include various infectious diseases & lead contamination
- Reporting requirements vary by state. Notifications must be documented and disclosures of personal health information (PHI) must be tracked

7.7 Instrumentation/laboratory equipment

7.7.1 Balance

- A device or scale used to measure mass or weight
  - A traditional balance consists of 2 plates or bowls suspended from a fulcrum at equal distances. The weight of materials is compared to objects of known weights until the 2 plates are balanced, that is, in equilibrium
  - Springe balance uses springs of known stiffness to determine weight
  - Analytic balance is typically enclosed and used to precisely measure small masses

7.7.2 Centrifugation

- Use of centrifugal force (high speed rotation around a fixed axis) to separate lighter portions of a liquid from denser ones
  - Particles or denser components settle to the bottom while low density ones rise to the top
  - The acceleration (speed) can vary
  - Examples of how centrifuges are used in laboratories:
    - Separate cells from plasma or serum
    - Concentrate cells
    - Separate to remove precipitated protein or DNA
    - Separate fat from nonfat
    - Aqueous solutes into solvent
- Types: A large variety of laboratory centrifuges are used in specimen processing, chemistry, or hematology, ranging from large, small, room temperature, and refrigerated with various rotors, eg, horizontal head, swinging bucket, fixed angle
- Centrifugation protocols
  - specify the amount of acceleration applied to a sample achieved by varying rotational speed (revolutions per minute [RPM]), relative centrifugal force to create a relative centrifugal force [RCF] or G-force

Instrumentation/laboratory equipment>Centrifugation | Microscopy | Spectrophotometry

- G-Force (gravitational force equivalent) is a measurement of force exerted per unit mass
- The rotor radius is length from the center to the circumference of a circle
- A tachometer (revolution counter) is an instrument used to measure the rotation speed of a centrifuge rotor or RPM

- If the RPM is known, the equation to calculate G-Force in centimeters is:

$$0.00001118 \times \text{rotor radius} \times (\text{RPM})^2$$

- If the G-force is known, the equation to calculate RPM in centimeters is:

$$\sqrt{[\text{G-force}/(0.0000284 \times \text{rotor radius})]}$$

- Centrifuges vary in sizes and serve different purposes in the laboratory. Examples of specialized centrifuges include:
  - Benchtop & floor standing models are versatile and used for a variety of purposes
  - Refrigerated centrifuge: Used for temperature-sensitive applications
  - Microhematocrit: Used for rapid determination of volume or percentage of red blood cells (RBC) in blood by high speed centrifugation of blood contained in heparinized capillary tubes. After centrifugation, the volume of packed RBCs is divided by the total volume of blood
  - Cytocentrifuge: A low-speed, low-acceleration centrifuge used to separate cells without causing damage to the cellular components. Some cytocentrifuges use a closed system to prevent aerosolization of specimens. Some deposit the cellular material directly onto microscope slides
- Safe use of centrifuges
  - Centrifuges must be used on solid, level surfaces with the lid closed and secured
  - Appropriate containers must be covered or capped to prevent spills or areoles. Damaged or flawed containers should not be used
  - Hazardous & infectious materials require specific carriers
  - The items in the centrifuge must be balanced with the load/weight distributed evenly
  - The rotors should come to a complete stop before the centrifuge lid is opened
  - Centrifuges should be inspected periodically in addition to scheduled maintenance (cleaning, verification of speed, timer, commutator/brush replacement)

7.7.3 Microscopy

- A microscope is an optical instrument containing ≥1 lenses used for viewing very small objects that would not be visible to the naked eye
  - Microscopes require a light source or electrons to pass through a thin film of the subject of interest (eg, blood smears, bacteria, tissue structures, chromosomes)
  - Organic material is prepared and affixed to microscope slides before analysis
  - An ocular micrometer, glass disc with a ruled scale, is a device that can be inserted inside a microscope eyepiece to enable visualization of a specimen/sample and a micrometer scale at the same time to take direct measurements of a microscopic object
- Examples of different types of microscopes
  - Light or photon optical microscopes
    - Use condenser & objective lenses to capture light and form an image. Early microscopes used a mirror to reflect natural light before electric lamps were available
    - Use monocular or binocular eyepieces
    - Use a variety of stains to highlight specific structures
  - Electron microscope
    - Uses a beam of accelerated electrons for illumination and has a higher resolution power than a standard light microscope to see very small intracellular structures & viruses
  - Fluorescence microscope
    - Uses fluorescence to generate an image
  - Digital microscope
    - A type of optical scope that uses a digital camera to output an image to a computer monitor
    - Computer algorithms can perform analysis of blood cells or urine sediment and group similar objects to facilitate analysis by the user

7.7.4 Spectrophotometry

- Used for qualitative & quantitative measurement of the light properties of biological & chemical compounds as a function of wavelength
- The wavelength of light or radiant energy, expressed in nanometers (nm), is defined as the distance between 2 peaks as the light travels in a wavelike manner
- The wavelength of ultraviolet (UV) is <380 nm
- Visible light ranges from violet to red in the range between 380 nm & 750 nm, whereas infrared light (IR) is >750 nm

 ISBN 978-089189-6616

- The energy of light is inversely proportional to the wavelength; shorter wavelengths have greater energy
- Bandwidth specifications of a spectrophotometer indicates the spectral purity of the instrument
- A spectrophotometer uses a spectrometer to produce light at a specific color (wavelength) and a device (photometer) for measuring the intensity or absorption of light
  - A photodetector converts light into a measurable electrical signal
  - The concentration of a substance is directly proportional to the amount of light absorbed or inversely proportional to logarithm of the transmitted light (Beer law, the relationship between transmittance, absorbance & concentration)
- The components of a single beam spectrophotometer are arranged in this order:
  - Light source > entrance split > monochromator (a device to isolate light of a narrow bandwidth or specific wavelength) > exit slit > cuvette > photodetector > readout device or meter > data system
- Double beam spectrophotometers use a light beam chopper after the exit slit with a system of mirrors that measure light through a sample and a reference cuvette
  - The utilization of a reference cuvette can correct for variation in intensify of a specific light source
- Identifying the wavelength with maximum absorbance of a specific compound is typically the first step in developing an assay as the maximum absorbance decreases interferences
  - A specific wavelength can be selected (isolated or excluded) in several ways including the use of interference or dichroic filters, prisms & diffraction gratings
  - Reference filters such as didymium can be used to verify or calibrate wavelength settings on a broader bandpass instrument
  - Holmium oxide glass filters are used as a wavelength standard reference in narrow bandwidth spectrophotometers
- Bichromatic analysis is the spectrophotometric measurement of a reaction at 2 wavelengths
  - Bichromatic analysis is used to correct for background color or spectral interference of another compound
- Fluorescence spectroscopy (fluorimetry or spectrofluometry) uses a beam of light, typically UV light, to excite electrons in molecules causing them to emit light of a different wavelength

7.7.5 Atomic absorption spectrophotometry (AAS)

- This is a spectroanalytical method used for the quantitative determination of chemical elements (eg, aluminum, copper, lithium) by using the absorption of specific frequencies of light by free metallic ions or atoms
- The energy source for atomic absorption is a hollow cathode lamp
- The amount of energy absorbed by a substance correlates to its concentration

7.7.6 Osmometry

- Measures the concentration of solute particles (electrolytes, proteins, organic compounds) that contribute to the osmotic pressure of a solution
- Osmotic pressure is a factor in regulation of cellular & extracellular fluid equilibrium
- Total osmotic pressure is the total number of solute particles in a solution of a specific mass
- The movement of solute & permeable ions exerts osmotic pressure
- The most common method for measuring osmolality is freezing point depression
- Measurement of osmolality in plasma & urine can be used to assess the electrolyte & acid/base disorders

7.7.7 Nephelometry & turbidimetry

- Analytic techniques to measure light scattered by particles
- A nephelometer measures the concentration of suspended particles by employing a light beam and a detector set at 90 degrees from the source
- The intensity of scatted light is measured
- Turbidimetry measures the intensity of light transmitted through a sample

7.7.8 Electrophoresis

- The separation of compounds based on the movement of ions or charged solutes across various support mediums under the influence of a charged electrical field
  - Buffers are used as carriers of charged ions or ionized solutes
  - Support matrices used include gel, polyacrylamide & agarose
  - Depending on their charge, ionized solutes will migrate toward the negative electrode (cathode) or the positive electrode (anode)

- Electrophoretic mobility is inversely proportional to the size of a molecule and directly proportional to the net charge
- Net charge, shape, size, temperature, buffer ionic strength, properties of support medium & electrical field strength influence the motility of ions
- Ion-selective electrodes (ISE) selectively favor a single ion dissolved in a solution over other ions present. Ion-selective membrane support media increase the selectivity of the ISE
- Electrophoresis is commonly used to separate proteins from DNA
- Sample loading issues can lead to distorted zones of separation

7.7.9 Chromatography & extraction

- Chromatography describes various techniques used to separate a compound from a mixture
  - Chromatography can be used to determine if an analyte is present and to determine the concentration
  - A mobile phase carries an extracted analyte of interest through a stationary phase to separate it from a mixture, based on differential interactions or differential solubility
  - After separation, a detection system is used
- Various constituents can be separated using various methods such as:
  - Ion exchange chromatography: Separates ions & polar molecules based on their affinity to the ion exchanger
  - Steric exclusion chromatography: Separates compounds solely based on size
  - Partition chromatography: A process for the separation of mixtures in columns or on filter paper based on partition of a solute between 2 solvents, one of which is immobilized by the substance in the column or by the paper
  - Adsorption chromatography is a process of separation of components of a mixture based on the relative differences in adsorption of components to the stationary phase
- Types of stationary phases include:
  - Paper: Colored dissolved compounds are separated based on different migration rates across paper
  - Thin layer (TLC): Uses a thin stationary phase supported by a flat inert backing such as glass to separate compounds
  - Column: A mobile phase is applied to a stationary phase, which is packed into a vertical glass column to separate compounds. The retardation factor R_f is defined as the ratio of this traveled by a compound as compared to the front of the solvent. The R_f range is 0-1
  - Gas (GC): An inert gas is used to carry vaporized volatile compounds through a column to separate & analyze
  - Liquid: High-performance liquid chromatography (HPLC) relies on pumps to pass pressurized liquid solvents containing compounds of interest through a solid absorbent material that is packed into a column. Abnormally high pressures may be an indicator that the effluent line is obstructed
  - Gel: Substances are passed through a bed of porous, semisolid substance which separates compounds based on molecular weight & size
- A chromatography detector is used to detect and identify a compound that has been separated followed by a data acquisition system
  - Flame ionization
  - Nitrogen phosphorus
  - Electron capture
  - Flame photometric
  - Photoionization
  - Mass spectrometer: An analytical technique that involves the separation, ionization, and the mass to charge ratio analysis of compounds
  - Absorbance
  - UV
  - Fluorescence
  - Thermal conductivity
  - Electrochemical & conductivity

7.7.10 Electrochemistry & chemical sensors (blood gases)

- Measurement of blood gas tension (partial pressure of oxygen [PO_2] and partialpressure of carbon dioxide [PCO_2]) based on electrochemical phenomena plays an important role in the clinical management of respiratory, renal & metabolic disorders including acid-base imbalances
  - Electrochemistry involves the measurement of current or voltage in an electrochemical cell
  - The cell consists of ≥2 electrodes that interact with a chemical and that are connected to an electrical system

ISBN 978-089189-6616

Instrumentation/laboratory equipment>Electrochemistry & chemical sensors (blood gases) | Immunochemical techniques | Point-of-care testing (POCT)

- The Henderson-Hasselbalch equation is used to calculate the pH of blood using the bicarbonate & carbonic acid ratio as a measure of acidity using the acid dissociation constant, pKa

$$pH = pKa + \log \text{bicarbonate (salt)/carbonic (acid) or } pH = 6.1 + \log HCO_3/(0.03 \times PCO_2)$$

- In addition to blood gases, blood gas analyzers typically measure additional analytes t7.8

t7.8 Components of a blood gas analyzer

Sensor	Measurement technology
pH, Na^+, K^+, Ca^{++}, Cl^-	Potentiometric method using standard ion-selective electrode (ISE) technology
Reference	Silver/silver electrode in potassium chloride & silver chloride
pCO_2	Modified potentiometric method based on the principles of the Severinghaus electrode
PO_2	Amperometric measurement based on the principles of the Clark electrode
Glucose	Amperometric method using an enzyme electrode that contains glucose oxidase
Lactate	Amperometric method using an enzyme electrode that contains lactate oxidase
Hematocrit	Conductimetric method
Co-oximetry	Measures the absorbency of light at different wavelengths

7.7.11 Immunochemical techniques

- Immunoassays/immunochemical techniques use antibodies that specifically bind to an antigen of interest or vice versa
  - The extreme sensitivity & specificity of immunoassays enables the detection of and the concentration of analytes, even in low levels
  - Antibodies &antigens can be used as a reagent or the analyte of interest
  - Many assays include the linking of antibodies or antigens with a detectable label that allows for detection through various means such as a color change, fluorescence, light emission or absorption & radiation emission
- A large variety of qualitative & quantitative immunochemical methods are used in the laboratory to detect antigens and antibodies. For example:
  - Immunoprecipitation or agglutination: Clumping of antibody particles to which specific antigenic labels are attached
  - Immunoelectrophoresis: A type of immunoprecipitation in which antigens are separated by migration in an electrical field, followed by an antibody reaction by immunodiffusion
  - Immunodiffusion: Spreading movement of antibody and/or antigen in a support medium. Lowest sensitivity with high specificity
  - Immunofixation: Western blot
  - Heterogeneous immunoassay: Uses liquid & solid phases to separate reactive components from those that are unreactive
  - Homogeneous immunoassay: Labeled analyte does not require separation of bound & free antigen
  - Radioimmunoassay (RIA)
  - Enzyme-multiplied immunoassay technique (EMIT): Does not require a separation step
  - Enzyme-linked immunosorbent assay (ELISA)
  - Immunofluorescence or fluoroimmunoassay: Uses a fluorescent indicator label
  - Immunohistochemistry
  - Nephelometry: Measures the light scattering properties of antibody-antigen aggregation

7.7.12 Point-of-care testing (POCT)

- Laboratory testing performed by nonlaboratory personnel outside of the clinical laboratory, close to or near the patient is defined at point of care testing
  - Testing performed by laboratory staff in satellite laboratories near the patient are not considered to be POCT
  - There is a wide variety of POCT, ranging from simple manual dipsticks (waived) to several portable nonwaived tests or devices
  - Performing laboratory testing at the point of care eliminates the time required to transport specimens to the laboratory and thus reduces the total turnaround time for testing
  - POCT typically uses a smaller sample size than testing performed in the laboratory
- Point of care testing is typically performed by nonlaboratorians and nearly always subject to regulatory & accreditation standards that vary, depending on the location & test complexity; states vary in their requirements of POCT whether waived or nonwaived and whether performed in a physician office, treatment center, or hospital setting
- POCT compliance, while varying in degree, includes supply & device management, quality control, operator (testing personnel) training, competence assessment & management
- As more laboratory testing moves outside the laboratory, oversight of POCT by laboratory professionals is expanding to ensure quality & regulatory compliance

health hazard carcinogen mutagenicity reproductive toxicity respiratory sensitizer target organ toxicity 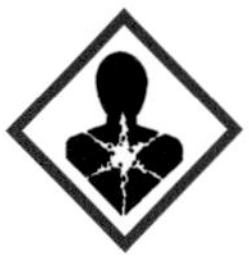	**flame** flammables pyrophorics self heating emits flammable gas self reactives organic peroxides 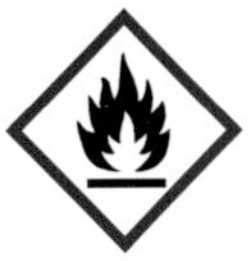	**exclamation mark** irritant (skin & eye) skin sensitizer acute toxicity narcotic effects respiratory tract irritant hazardous to ozone layer 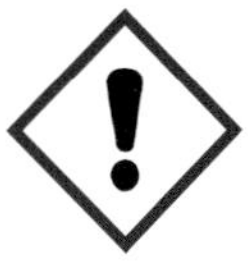
gas cylinder gases under pressure 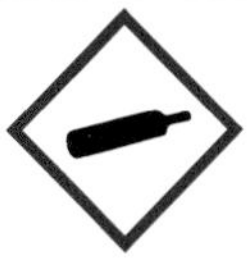	**corrosion** skin corrosion/burns eye damage corrosive to metals 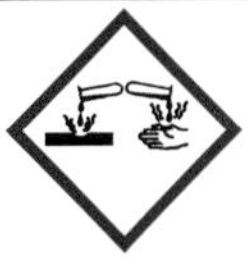	**exploding bomb** explosives self reactives organic peroxides 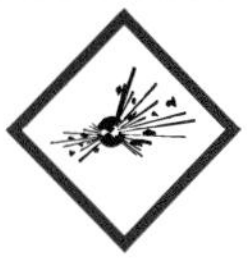
flame over circle oxidizers 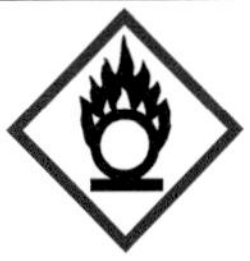	**environment** aquatic toxicity 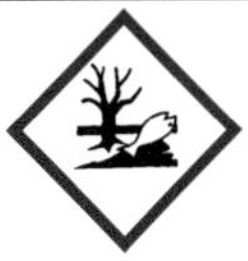	**skull & crossbones** acute toxicity (fatal or toxic) 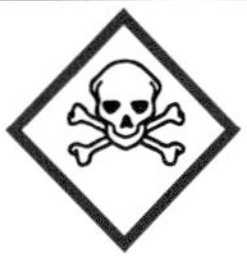

f7.8 GHS chemical hazard symbols & hazard categories

- Automation
  - Over the last half century, laboratories have evolved from using manual methods to highly automated & connected instruments. Laboratory information systems (LIS) now provide electronic workflow & data management

7.8 Laboratory safety

- The laboratory work environment is dangerous
- Multiple regulatory agencies, state, federal & international laws & guidelines establish a framework for workplace safety
- The strictest applicable regulation or standard must be followed
- Engineering & management controls, policy-driven safe work practices, and an array of personal protective equipment provide the foundation needed to minimize risk
- Maintaining a degree of cautious vigilance helps workers comply with safety requirements
- If workers normalize routine hazards, they may let down their guard and become careless

7.8.1 US regulatory agencies with legal jurisdiction over laboratories

7.8.1.1 OSHA

- Occupational Safety & Health Administration (OSHA) sets minimum standards for performing hazardous jobs, inspects compliance, and issues citations for failures to comply with standards
- OSHA requires employers to have a complete safety policy, provide appropriate safety equipment, and conduct safety training
  - Hazard Communication Standard: Requires employers to inform employees about potential chemical hazard exposure (right to know)
  - Hazardous Chemicals in Laboratories: Chemical Hygiene Plan (CHP)
    - Classification of hazardous chemicals: Pictograms
      - Physical hazards (flammable, corrosive, oxidizer, compressed gas, explosive)
      - Health hazards (acute toxic, corrosive, health hazard, irritant)
  - Environmental hazards chemical labeling (immediate warning to a container's contents with pertinent hazard information) f7.8
    - Chemicals in original containers shipped from manufacturer
      - Product identifier (chemical or common name)
      - Signal word (danger or warning)
      - Hazard statement(s)—describes the nature of the hazard including potential threat to target organ
      - Pictogram
      - Precautionary statement(s) (prevention, exposure, response, storage, disposal)
      - Name, address & phone number of manufacturer
    - Secondary container labels
      - Labeled with chemical name & appropriate hazard warning

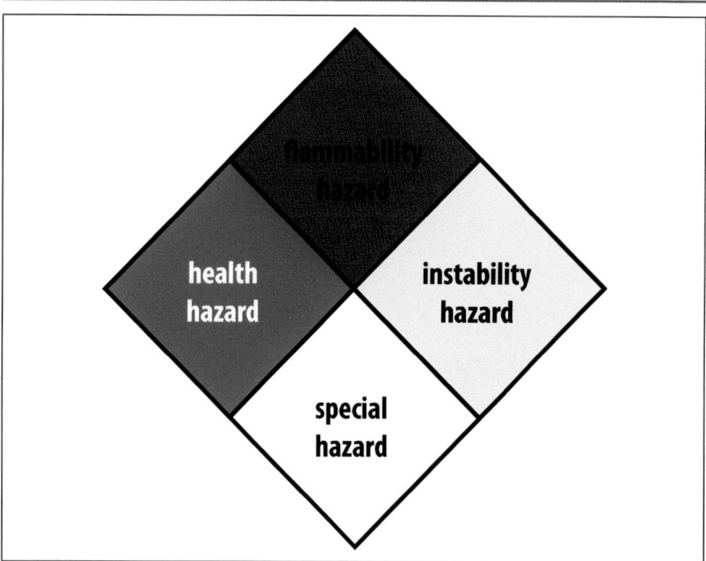

f7.9 Generic NFPA diamond

- May use National Fire Protection Association (NFPA) to convey chemical hazards f7.9
  - Flammability hazard 0-4, with 4 being the lowest temperature flash point
  - Instability hazard 0-4 with 4 = may detonate
  - Special hazard (OX, W, SA)
  - Health hazard 0-4 with 4=deadly
- Transfer of a hazardous chemical for immediate use from either primary or secondary container by the individual performing the transfer, does not require labeling

- Bloodborne pathogens
- Formaldehyde standard: Minimize formaldehyde exposure. Formaldehyde is a known carcinogen
- Baseline chemical exposure monitoring is required for substances such as xylene & formaldehyde. Repeat monitoring should be performed if procedures or equipment is changed
- Personal protective equipment (PPE) standard: Requires an annual hazard assessment of a workplace and addresses chemical & biological risks, physical & electrical hazards, sharps, and laser risks
- Ergonomics
  - Hearing loss
  - Repetitive motion disorders
  - Skeletomuscular disorders
- Slip, trips, falls

7.8.1.2 Other regulatory agencies

- Environmental Protection Agency (EPA): Hazardous waste disposal must be performed by licensed waste hauler (eg, xylene)
- Nuclear Regulatory Commission (NRC): Licensure and inspection of the use of radioactive materials and other sources of radiation in medical laboratories including blood irradiators
- US Department of Transportation (DOT), US Postal Service (USPS), and International Air Transport Association (IATA): Packaging & labeling requirements for the shipment of specimens, infectious agents, hazardous materials, and dangerous goods including dry ice
- Clinical Laboratory Improvement Amendments of 1988 (CLIA '88): Requires inspections of a broad set of standards including safety
- US Department of Homeland Security (DHS): Site-specific security requirements for chemical & biological agents to prevent acts of terrorism

7.8.2 Professional/research bodies for voluntary compliance

- Centers for Disease Control (CDC) & National Institute for Occupational Safety & Health (NIOSH): Organizations that do not regulate laboratories but define minimal accepted practice for handling biohazardous materials
- National Institutes for Health (NIH)
- National Fire Protection Association (NFPA): A professional organization that publishes fire prevention information
- Clinical Laboratory Standards Institute (CLSI): A private organization that produces peer-reviewed consensus guidelines
- Voluntary accrediting bodies
  - Centers for Medicare and Medicaid Services (CMS): Has granted deemed authority to ensure compliance with CLIA requirements
    - Accreditation is required for a health care organization to receive payment from the federal government for health care services provided
    - Accrediting bodies can establish additional requirements such as patient safety goals
  - College of American Pathologists (CAP)
  - Commission on Accreditation of Laboratories (COLA)
  - The Joint Commission (TJC) formerly known as JCAHO

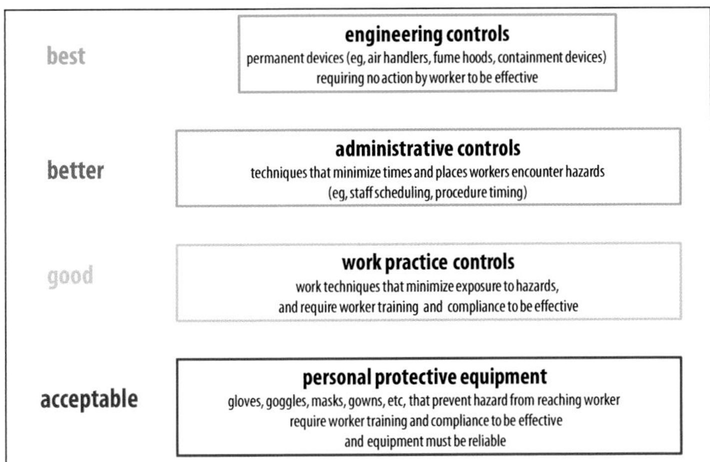

f7.10 Safety management tools

7.8.3 Staff training

- All staff must undergo through safety training at hire and when new policies and/or procedures are introduced or changed substantially
- Training must be documented and staff must demonstrate competence
- Staff must be knowledgeable of all safety-related policies & procedures
- Escalation of safety concerns or if an individual experiences symptoms of potential exposure should start with supervisors and have a clear chain of escalation if concerns are not addressed. A medical exposure evaluation should be paid by the employer on work time without loss of pay

7.8.4 Safety management (key elements)

7.8.4.1 Overview

- A formal safety program requires:
  - Policies & procedures
  - Staff training
  - Audit of safe work practices
  - Reporting systems for laboratory accidents & employee on-the-job injuries
  - Emergency preparedness
  - Evacuation
- Types of safety controls **f7.10**

7.8.4.2 Engineering controls

- Engineering controls are physical setups or devices that reduce exposure. They are the most effective measures for maintaining safety in many laboratory situations
  - Chemical fume hoods
  - Biological safety cabinets
  - Safe sharps
  - Sharps containers
  - Sound dampening materials
  - Adjustable height tables

7.8.4.3 Administrative controls

- Administrative controls are management strategies to reduce exposure (policies, procedures & audits)
  - Safety policies
  - Chemical hygiene plan (chemical safety)
  - Biological safety
  - Fire safety
  - Ergonomics program
  - Emergency preparedness
  - Evacuation plan
  - Dress code

7.8.4.4 Work practice controls

- Work practices are the least effective method (still indispensable, particularly for infectious agent protection)
  - Personal protective equipment (PPE) include face shields, goggles, disposable gloves, closed laboratory coats
  - Mouth pipetting is prohibited
  - Eating & drinking, applying cosmetics, and handling contact lenses are all prohibited

7.8.4.5 United nations recommended policies

- Documented policies & procedures for 9 classes of hazardous materials found in clinical laboratories are recommended by the United Nations (UN)
  - Explosives
    - Example: A chemical that is extremely volatile, flammable & capable of forming explosive peroxides on long-term contact with atmospheric oxygen such as diethyl ether
  - Gases
    - Compressed gases
      - Tanks should be stored away from flammable materials, have safety covers on when not in use, secured by chain to the wall, or chained to hard cart or dolly
      - Nature of compressed gas
      - Safe handling of compressed gas
    - Cryogens (liquid gases with boiling points of –100°F at 1 atmosphere of pressure)
      - Liquid nitrogen & helium
      - Extremely cold temperatures can cause physical injury; skin & eyes should be protected with appropriate shields or protective covering

ISBN 978-089189-6616

t7.9 Types of fire extinguishers

Class of fire	Traditional NFPA symbol	NFPA pictogram	Water extinguishers	Dry chemical & CO_2 extinguishers
Class A: ordinary combustibles (eg, wood, clothing, paper)	A		yes	yes, but CO_2 not considered optimal since gas dissipates
Class B: flammable liquids & gases	B		no (spreads liquid & fire)	yes
Class C: energized electrical equipment	C		no (risk of shock)	yes
Class D: combustible metals	D		no (intensifies fire)	no, sand or special extinguishing agents required
Class K: kitchen hot oil cookers	K		no (can cause oil explosion)	no (can cause oil explosion)

- Typically stored in metal tanks or Dewar flasks
- If cryogens convert from liquid to gas, the atmosphere can become anoxic. Room air oxygen monitoring with alarms trigger aggressive ventilation and/or evacuation of an enclosed space
- Materials to be frozen in a cryogen should be lowered into the liquid slowly to minimize splashing

- Flammable liquids: Storage requirements vary based on volume & volatility
  - Flammable liquids must always be stored in approved containers
  - Category 1, up to 1 gallon, and category 2-4, up to 5 gallons must be stored in metal flammable safety cans
  - Approved metal storage cabinets are required for larger volumes of flammable liquids
- Flammable solids
- Oxidizer materials
- Toxic materials
- Radioactive materials
  - Types of radioactive emissions
  - Radiation exposure
  - Safe handling & disposal of radioactive materials
- Corrosive materials can cause immediate visible damage to skin
- Miscellaneous materials not elsewhere classified

- Documented policies & procedures for chemical hygiene, bloodborne pathogen & tuberculosis exposure control and ergonomics are required
- Written policies & procedures for emergency preparedness and evacuation plans are required
- Written policies & procedures for reporting and documenting accidents and workplace injuries are required
- Compliance with regulatory requirements must be audited/assessed
  - To reduce workplace hazards, safe work practices must be audited & assessed at least annually
  - The assessment must include bloodborne hazard control & chemical hygiene
  - Any problem or risk identified must be investigated, with corrective actions taken to prevent reoccurrences or mitigate risks
- The incident data must be analyzed and preventive measures put in place to prevent recurrence

7.8.5 Fire safety

- Physical space management
  - Hallways, corridors & evacuation routes should be clear & free of obstruction
  - Fire exits, fire extinguishers, fire alarms & sprinkler heads should not be blocked
- Fire triangle or quadrahedron: Oxygen, heat, fuel, chemical chain reaction **f7.9**
- Fire equipment
  - Types of fire extinguishers (optimal type depends on the type/class of fire) **t7.9**
    - Class A: Fires involving ordinary organic combustibles like paper & wood

- Class B (CO_2): Fires involving flammable liquid, petrol, grease & gases
- Class C (dry chemical): Fires involving energized electrical equipment
- Class D: (Dry chemical & other agents for metal) fires involving combustible/reactive metals
- Class K (wet chemical): Fires involving hot cooking oil
- PASS describes steps for using a fire extinguisher:
  - ***P***ULL out the pin
  - ***A***IM the extinguisher
  - ***S***QUEEZE the double-handled trigger
  - ***S***WEEP the base of the fire

- Fire hose (water): Class A fires only
- Fire alarms: Scattered throughout a facility with audible & visual signals
- Fire blankets: Can be used to cover or wrap around a person's body to smother flames. The stop, drop & roll technique is used to prevent a chimney effect that occurs when a person is standing
- Sand buckets
- Respirators: Should be used if toxic fumes are generated by a fire

- Fire plan
  - RACE
    - ***R***ESCUE people in danger
    - ***A***LARM: Sound the alarm
    - ***C***ONTAIN: Close doors and windows
    - ***E***XTINGUISH or EVACUATE depending on fire size
  - Evacuation routes
    - Staff trained to plan (eg, relocation area, fire pull, fire extinguisher & exit locations)

7.8.6 Chemical safety

- Chemical Hygiene Plan (CHP)
  - Required by OSHA
  - Specifies the mandatory requirements to protect workers from harm due to hazardous chemicals
  - CHP includes policies, procedures & responsibilities that protect workers in a specific work environment
  - A chemical hygiene officer must be identified
  - Employers are required to establish a program that ensures that workers are provided with information regarding hazardous chemical dangers in the workplace
- Labels (see 7.8.1.1, f7.8)
- Storage & inventory
  - Incompatible chemicals should not be stored together as noted on the Safety Data Sheets (SDS)
    - Chlorine should not be stored with ammonia
    - Acetone should not be stored with bromine, chlorine, nitric acid, sulfuric acid or hydrogen peroxide
  - Desiccants are commonly used to protect chemicals and other goods against damage from moisture
    - Desiccants frequently contain a humidity indicator that shows a change in color
    - For example, cobalt chloride ($CoCl_2$) is blue when dry, and turns purple then pink as it absorbs water molecules
- Hazard Communication Safety Data Sheets or SDS (formerly called Material Safety Data Sheets or MSDS) is a standardized document that contains occupational safety and health data; SDS typically contain 16 sections, of which sections 1-8 are mandatory
  - Section 1: Identification includes product identifier; manufacturer or distributor name, address, phone number; emergency phone number; recommended use; restrictions on use
  - Section 2: Hazard(s) identification includes all hazards regarding the chemical; required label elements
  - Section 3: Composition/information on ingredients includes information on chemical ingredients; trade secret claims
  - Section 4: First-aid measures includes important symptoms/effects, acute, delayed; required treatment
  - Section 5: Fire-fighting measures lists suitable extinguishing techniques, equipment; chemical hazards from fire
  - Section 6: Accidental release measures list emergency procedures; protective equipment; proper methods of containment & cleanup
  - Section 7: Handling & storage lists precautions for safe handling & storage, including incompatibilities
  - Section 8: Exposure controls/personal protection lists OSHA's Permissible Exposure Limits (PELs); ACGIH Threshold Limit Values (TLVs); and any other exposure limit used or recommended by the chemical manufacturer, importer, or employer preparing the SDS (where available) & appropriate engineering controls; personal protective equipment (PPE)

ISBN 978-089189-6616

7.8.7 Electrical safety

- Electrical hazard management
  - Insulation, guarding, grounding, circuit protection devices & safe work practices including removing malfunctioning equipment from service
  - Laboratory instruments & appliances must be adequately grounded & checked for current leakage before installation, after repair or modification or when an issue raises suspicion. Exceptions are made for devices protected by marked double insulation
  - Electrical power should be turned off before repairs are attempted
- Emergency generators supply power during service interruptions
- Use of electrical equipment
  - Use only Underwriters Laboratories (UL) or other safety agency-rated electrical equipment
  - Ground fault circuit interrupter (GFCI) used near water sources to prevent electrocution
  - Surge protectors protect equipment from excess current
- Identification of electrical hazards

7.8.8 Equipment safety

- Glassware: Broken, cracked, chipped, and/or flawed glassware should be removed from service to prevent injury and disposed of in a puncture proof container. Mouth pipetting is prohibited
- Sharps pose both physical & biological hazards. Safety-engineered mechanical devices & safe work practices should be used to prevent accidental injury and/or exposure
- Centrifuge safety
- Sterilizer/autoclave safety

7.8.9 Biological hazards & bloodborne pathogens

7.8.9.1 Policies and procedures

- Written policies & procedures regarding occupational bloodborne pathogen & other biological hazards that are in compliance with national, state, and local guidelines and laws are required, ie, exposure control plan. Laboratory professionals exposed to blood & body fluids have highest infection rate of hepatitis B
  - Policies prohibiting smoking, eating, mouth pipetting & other hand-to-face manipulations are required
  - Procedures for responding to blood & body fluid spills are required. The choice of methods & products is based on the goals that need to be achieved. Disinfectants & antiseptics kill most organisms but do not eliminate them all (spores)
    - Before applying disinfectants, blood spills should be absorbed with a disposable material
    - Disinfectants—typically used on objects—a wide variety of products regulated by the EPA
      - Fresh 1:10 dilution of household bleach (5.25% sodium hypochlorite) effectively kills HIV & hepatitis B viruses
      - Blood or body fluid spills should be cleaned with a disinfectant such as sodium hypochlorite immediately
    - Antiseptics—typically used on skin—regulated by the FDA
      - Common examples include ethanol, isopropanol, and iodine
    - Sterilants kill all microorganisms and are regulated by the FDA
      - Boiling or incineration
      - UV light or ionizing radiation
  - Inactivation of suspected transmissible spongiform encephalopathy proteins or prions are an exception to standard decontamination procedures
    - All prion-contaminated waste including formaldehyde used to preserve tissue & heat-sensitive or disposable instruments should be incinerated
    - Reusable instruments should be decontaminated by using a combination of chemical & autoclaving methods before cleaning in a washer and routine sterilization
      - Autoclave heat-resistant instruments after submersion/soaking in a pan containing 1N sodium hydroxide (NaOH), or in some cases, sodium hypochlorite, followed by cleaning & sterilization
  - Biohazardous waste: Containers used to hold blood, tissue, or body fluids, items that are saturated with blood, possibly infectious, from a surgical procedure or contaminated room must be separated from regular waste. Infectious waste is also described as regulated medical waste
    - Red biohazardous bags
    - Specialized labeled cardboard boxes
    - Some states require specialized containers (plastic totes)

Laboratory safety>Biological hazards & bloodborne pathogens

- Appropriate personal protective equipment (PPE) must be provided by employers in work areas where blood & body substances are handled or in special circumstances where exposure might occur
  - PPE must be worn when performing vascular access. Gloves should be removed after each patient contact or after manipulating biological samples and hands cleaned using effective antimicrobial methods
  - Personnel must be trained in the proper use of PPE and training records retained
  - Gloves should be removed when touching clean surfaces or in designated clean areas (eg, telephone, keyboard, mouse)
- Biohazard symbol must feature an orange background **f7.11** and must be displayed whenever biohazards are present (eg, doors, equipment, waste, laundry and specimen receptacles). Red biohazard bags are an acceptable substitute

7.8.9.2 Assessment of exposure

- OSHA requires that any exposure, regardless of severity, be reported and documented as soon as possible. Employers are required to provide safety equipment, handwashing facilities, PPE, prevention training, and treatment and/or monitoring at no cost if an employee experiences an exposure
  - Specimens, tissues, animals, plants, insects, people—direct contact
  - Aerosols & droplets—inhalation
  - Mouth or other mucus membrane contact
  - Contaminated surfaces (fomites)
  - Inoculation (punctures, scratches): Contaminated sharps (eg, needles, scalpels, blades) are one of the most dangerous items in a laboratory and the most likely mode of bloodborne pathogen transmission; the highest risk of human immunodeficiency virus (HIV) exposure is from needle sticks
    - Employers must provide rigid, spill proof, puncture resistant containers for sharps disposal
    - Needles should be discarded in an impermeable container immediately after use without additional manipulation
    - In the case of an accidental needle stick, the wound should be washed immediately with soap & water
- CDC biosafety levels (BSL) for infectious agents
  - BSL1: Low-risk organisms, usually not pathogenic in healthy individuals
  - BSL2: Pathogenic organisms, usually only acquired by direct contract
  - BSL3: Pathogenic organisms, usually acquired via inhalation and/or can cause very serious illness
  - BSL4: Very dangerous organisms
- CDC risk assessment recommendations
  - Identify biological agents likely to be present. Assign a BSL category. If agent is unknown, assign BLS2
  - Review hazards of procedures performed. Implement steps to minimize risk
  - Determine final BSL category based on agents & procedures involved
  - Train staff on safety protocols. Inspect equipment
  - Review final risk assessment with knowledgeable professional
- Biosecurity is an extension of the biosafety concept
  - Physical & personnel security
  - Material control
  - Transportation security

7.8.9.3 Additional infectious disease considerations

- Laboratory-acquired infections can occur from a wide variety of bacteria, fungus, viruses & parasites. Biological safety cabinets are the most effective engineering control to prevent transmission. Infectious agents of greatest concern for laboratory acquired infection include:
  - *Mycobacterium tuberculosis*, *Neisseria meningitides*, *Brucella*, *Shigella*, *Salmonella* & SARS-CoV-2
  - Bloodborne pathogens in the order of infection frequency are hepatitis B (HBV), hepatitis C (HCV), and human immunodeficiency virus (HIV)
  - Emerging diseases: Severe acute respiratory syndrome (SARS), West Nile, Ebola

ISBN 978-089189-6616

Laboratory safety>Biological hazards & bloodborne pathogens | Waste & waste management | Work practices & safety equipment

- Universal, standard & transmission-based precautions
  - Universal: Applied to blood & fluids visibly or likely to be contaminated with blood
  - Standard: Every person & specimen should be considered infectious (except for sweat)
  - Transmission based: In addition to standard precautions, special protocols are used when a specific suspected or confirmed pathogen has a strong likelihood of person-to-person transmission
- Histology laboratories & autopsy suites
  - Tissues fixed in alcohol, formalin, or paraffin are considered low biohazard risk
  - Frozen tissue
  - Unfixed tissues, organs & bodies pose significant risk especially during dissection or procedures that cause aerosolization
  - Improper use of cryostat, bone saws, blenders, and tissue grinders increase risk of exposure
  - Decontamination with midlevel disinfection, special protocols for suspected prions; bleach/formaldehyde should not be used together
- Biological safety cabinets (BSCs) & air circulation
  - An enclosed ventilated workspace used to protect laboratory workers & surrounding environment from bacterial, viral & fungal pathogens
  - Class I, II & III depending on the degree of containment needed
  - Class II is the most common BSC that protects personnel and the environment from harmful/infectious agents inside of the cabinet
  - Exhaust air is filtered through a high-efficiency particulate air (HEPA) filter as it exits the cabinet before the air is exhausted to the outside or recirculated
  - Some BSCs are designed to protect a product from environmental contamination
- Accidental exposures
  - Common sources of aerosol exposure that require safety equipment/protocols, eg, decapping blood collection containers, pouring specimens from on container to another, centrifugation of uncapped or overfilled tubes, sterilization of inoculation loops in open flame, forcibly delivering liquids by blowing, vortexing of open containers
  - Pierced intact skin (eg, puncture, cuts)
  - Splash to mucous membranes or broken skin
  - Self-inoculation (eg, application of lip balm, touching eye)

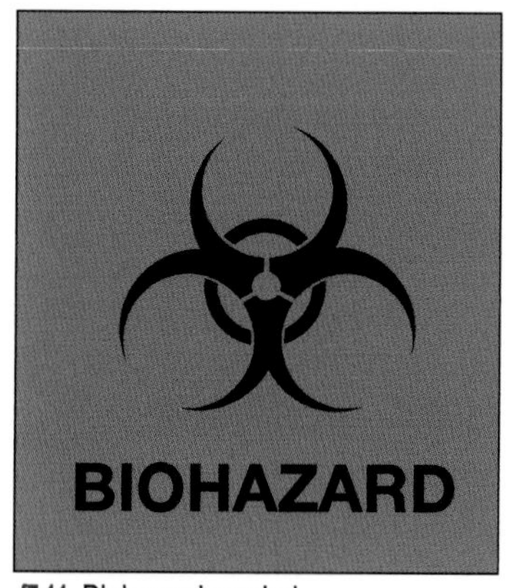

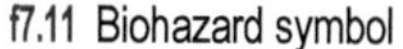
f7.11 Biohazard symbol

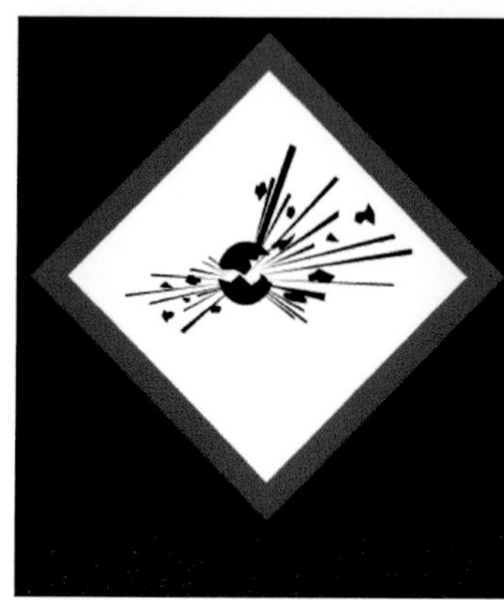
f7.12 Explosive symbol

7.8.10 Waste & waste management

- Hazardous waste categories: Ignitable, corrosive, reactive & toxic. In addition to the primary waste categories, special labeling, handling & disposal of radioactive, chemotherapy, and "e-waste" are required
- Handling of hazardous waste
- Infectious waste (separation of noninfectious & infectious waste)
- Accidental release of waste
- Basic waste management

7.8.11 Work practices & safety equipment

- Basic work practices
  - A formalized risk assessment should be conducted & documented
  - Controls should be put in place to minimize the risks identified
  - Periodic audits should be set up

7.8.11.1 Signage

- Required signage
  - Hazardous signage & safety instructions must be physically posted on entrance and storage cabinet doors, on walls, temperature storage devices, equipment, and laboratory walls **f7.11-f7.16**
    - Eyewash location & emergency showers (green & white) **f7.15**
    - Liquid nitrogen & dry ice
    - Biohazard symbol (orange) **f7.11**
    - Radiation hazard (yellow) **f7.13**
    - Prohibition of eating, drinking, or food storage
    - Clean vs dirty areas
    - Hand washing

Laboratory safety>Work practices & safety equipment

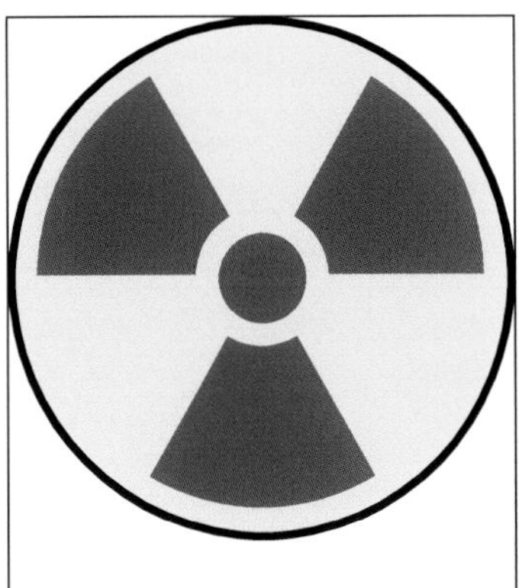
f7.13 Radiation hazard

f7.14 Electricity warning

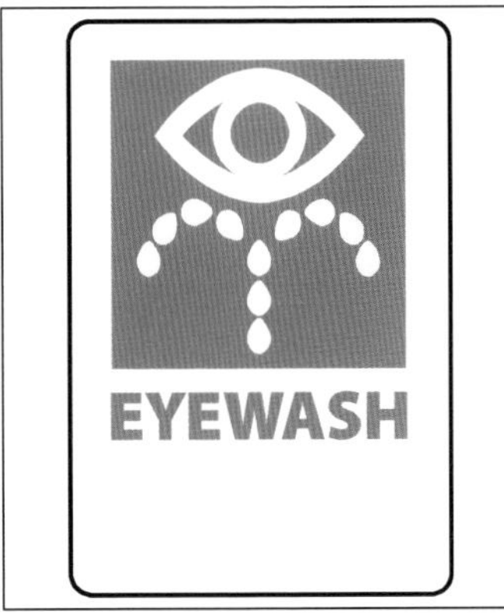

f7.15 Eyewash sign

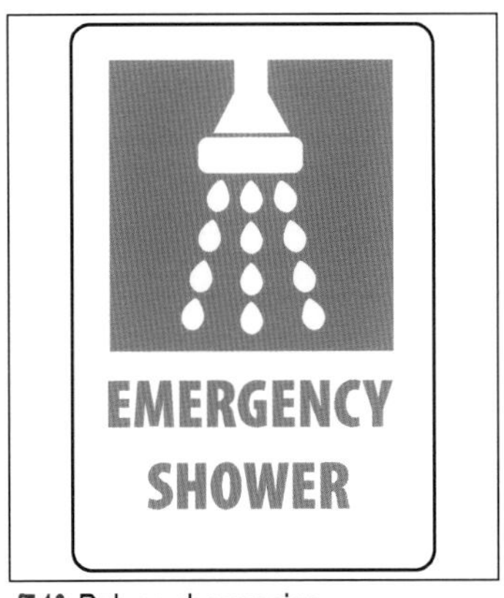

f7.16 Deluge shower sign

    - Standard danger signs (black, red & white for explosives **f7.12** or black/yellow for electric hazard) **f7.14**
    - Fire evacuation routes & exit signs
    - Temporary signs (spills, temporary route changes due to construction)
    - UV light exposure warning
    - Chemical hazards
    - Safety showers **f7.16**
- Telephones & computer terminals should be sufficient and conveniently located. Emergency phone numbers should be readily available to staff
- Safety shower: Required by OSHA & state regulations designed for quick drenching of the head and entire body that has come into contact with hazardous chemicals. The high pressure of water from a safety shower is not appropriate to use to flush eyes
  - There are 2 types of emergency showers
    - Plumbed to a continual source of potable tepid water capable of flowing 20 gallons/min
    - Self-contained with a limited supply of flushing liquid
  - Must be located at ≤10-second travel distance with no obstructions
  - Must be inspected annually
  - Signage required
- Eyewash
  - There are 2 types of eye wash stations:
    - Permanently plumbed to a continual source of potable tepid water
    - Self-contained with a limited supply of flushing liquid such as a gravity fed tank or squirt bottles specially designed for flushing eyes
    - Must be activated (plumbed) or inspected (self-contained) every week
  - Must be located at ≤10-second travel distance with no obstructions
  - Flow is provided to both eyes simultaneously
  - Must be inspected annually
  - Signage required
  - Eyes must be flushed with water for 15 minutes after chemical exposure
- Personal protective equipment (PPE) and personal protective practices: Dependent on degree of risk & type of procedure. Employee training specific to the job required
  - Face protection (eg, safety glasses, facial shields, masks should be worn when there is potential for splashing chemicals, blood specimens, body fluids)
  - Respiratory protection (respirators specific to the risk of breathing air contaminated with dusts, gases, fumes & vapors should be defined in policies)

ISBN 978-089189-6616

- Hand protection
  - Single-use disposable gloves should be worn during contact with blood or potentially infectious materials. Soiled gloves should be removed, and hands washed with soap
  - The appropriate chemical-resistant glove to be used is dependent on the type of potential chemical exposure as detailed on the safety data sheets
- Body protection
  - Shoes should be fluid impermeable and cover the entire foot
  - Fluid-resistant full-length laboratory coats
- Personal
- Hoods
- Sharps
- Hand hygiene is the most effective intervention to prevent the spread of infection including hospital acquired (nosocomial) infections
  - Hands must be washed after touching items in dirty or contaminated areas, after removing gloves, at the end of a work session, and before exiting the laboratory
  - Hand washing with soap and water: Hands should be wet with water when soap is applied and then scrubbed for 15-20 seconds on all surfaces of hands and fingers when:
    - Hands are visibly soiled
    - Caring for a person with potentially infectious diarrhea
    - After known or suspected exposure to spores
  - Alcohol-based hand sanitizers: After application of the hand sanitizer, hands should be rubbed together so that all surfaces are covered & dry
    - Before & after touching a patient
    - Before performing an invasive or sterile task
    - Touching environmental surfaces in patient care areas or in a laboratory
    - After contact with specimens
    - After glove removal
- Dress code and employee work habits
- Employers must establish policies that define acceptable attire such as closed toed shoes and where and when to don personal safety equipment (PPE)
- In addition to PPE compliance, employees must develop work practices to reduce risk of exposure or injury such as no eating/drinking in the laboratory, avoiding the application of lip balm or cosmetics, manipulation of contact lenses, and securing long hair

7.8.12 Accidents, emergencies & disasters

- Accident reports
- Emergency & disaster preparedness
- First aid & spill containment
- Evacuation if there is a significant spill of chemical with significant health hazard—clean up should be done by hazard professionals

7.8.13 Patient safety: A culture of safety

7.8.13.1 Inculcating a culture of safety

- Culture aligns with overarching tenets of an organization
- It is essential to define and conceptualize a culture of safety as culture is both context-specific and a local phenomenon
- In a broad context, a culture of safety in healthcare pertains to core values and behaviors aligned with elevating safety over other goals, while having vital commitment to the culture of safety by the entire team (leadership and frontline team members)
- Laboratory teams at a unit level should focus on contributions at all levels of safety culture—improving this across and within work teams contributes to the organization's overall culture of safety
- Transparency, accountability, honest and frequent communication, while following improvement models and continuously learning are keys to effective leadership at all levels to ensure a patient-centered culture of safety
- Improving the culture of safety within laboratories, is essential to elevating patient outcomes by reducing errors

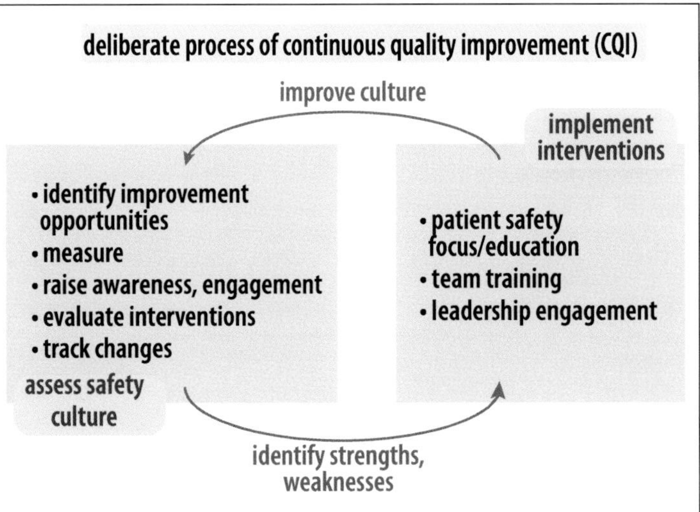
deliberate process of continuous quality improvement (CQI)
improve culture
implement interventions
• identify improvement opportunities
• measure
• raise awareness, engagement
• evaluate interventions
• track changes
• patient safety focus/education
• team training
• leadership engagement
assess safety culture
identify strengths, weaknesses

f7.17 Algorithm for continuous quality improvement implementation

- A culture of safety is committed to continuous quality improvement (CQI). As strengths, opportunities, and barriers are identified, an assessment of weaknesses should be vetted through proven quality improvement tools and with targeted interventions f7.17
- Research has shown that one of the most vital ways to promote a patient-focused culture of safety is to encourage open reporting and transparent communication of any mistakes, potential problems, and/or error laden workflows that are noticed. Resilient learning organizations utilize each mistake to improve patient care
- Contribute to the culture of safety by identifying and promoting quality standards that improve patient outcomes. Recognize meaningful contributions as a final safety net to intercept errors before they reach patients. Decrease process deviations that contribute to errors
- Advocate for a culture of safety by remaining open and transparent; honor fairness; cultivate trust and dissuade blaming. Promote willingness to identify and assure quality initiatives
- A step-wise, purposeful approach aligns a culture of safety with impactful change in our work processes, systems, behaviors and attitudes, making that culture of safety ever present

7.8.13.2 High-reliability laboratories

- Laboratories that generate and maintain high levels of safety, are high-reliability
- High-reliability starts with engaged, pro-active leadership, along with cultural awareness and advancement of patient-focused safety based on robust quality improvement
- Teamwork is essential to high-reliability. High-reliability laboratory teams exhibit a set of key characteristics:
    - They assure safety as a top priority
    - They are well-attuned to operations and intrinsic hazards, including workflows that may be hypercomplex
    - They recognize expertise vested in the many contributory decision makers in communication networks
    - They are engrossed or pre-occupied with potential failures
    - They continuously monitor and aim for a low failure rate
    - They willingly delve into quality challenges and are reluctant to accept simple explanations for problems (especially when risky or persistent)
    - They engage in timely, frequent feedback around decisions
    - They seek and align expertise across synchronized outcomes
    - They have a high level of accountability and resiliency

7.8.14 Ergonomics

- A scientific discipline focused on reducing or avoiding musculoskeletal disorders (MSDs) and other injury through workspace, equipment and process design
- Ergonomic injuries generally happen from doing common movements incorrectly
- Injuries can occur over a long time with gradual deterioration of a joint or tendons
- They may occur suddenly

 ISBN 978-089189-6616

- Ergonomic injury risk factors include:
  - Inflexible computer workstations (eg, chair, keyboard, mouse, monitor height)
  - Repetitive motion
  - A single event (lifting strain)
  - Repeated impact or vibration
  - Awkward lifting & lifting too much weight
  - Frequent reaching for materials
- Symptoms of MSDs should be recognized & reported to supervisors when they occur:
  - Pain/discomfort/stiffness, eg, in the back, neck, shoulders, hands, wrists
  - Numbness or tingling
  - Decreased strength or hand grip
  - Unusual muscle fatigue
  - Swelling, redness & other signs of inflammation
  - Limited range of motion
- Common MSDs injuries:
  - Carpal tunnel syndrome: Numbness, tingling & pain in the wrist, hand, and arm caused by a compressed nerve in the wrist
  - Swelling of tendons—tennis elbow

7.9 Selected readings

7.9.1 Books

Boyd JC. Laboratory statistics. In: Dufour DR, ed. *Professional Practice in Clinical Chemistry: A Companion Text.* Washington, DC: American Association for Clinical Chemistry; 1999 ISBN9781890883287a

Boyd JC. Reference limits in the clinical laboratory. In: Dufour DR, ed. *Professional Practice in Clinical Chemistry: A Companion Text.* Washington, DC: American Association for Clinical Chemistry; 1999 ISBN9781890883287b

Boyd JC. Statistical aids for test interpretation. In: Dufour DR, ed. *Professional Practice in Clinical Chemistry: A Companion Text.* Washington, DC: American Association for Clinical Chemistry; 1999 ISBN9781890883287c

Committee on the Quality of Health Care in America. *Crossing the Quality Chasm: A New Health System for the 21st Century.* Washington, DC: National Academies Press; 2001 ISBN9780309072809

Davis DL. *Laboratory Safety: A Self Assessment Workbook,* 2e. Chicago, IL: American Society for Clinical Pathologists; 2016 ISBN9780891896463

Dufour DR. Preanalytic variation, or what causes abnormal results (besides disease). In: *Professional Practice in Clinical Chemistry: A Companion Text.* Washington, DC: American Association for Clinical Chemistry; 1999 ISBN9781890883287d

Institute of Medicine, Committee to Design a Strategy for Quality Review and Assurance in Medicare; Lohr K, eds. *Medicare: A Strategy for Quality Assurance,* vol 1. Washington, DC: National Academies Press; 1990 ISBN9780309042307

Kaplan LA, Pesce AJ. *Clinical Chemistry: Theory, Analysis, Correlation, 5e.* Philadelphia, PA: Mosby Elsevier; 2010 ISBN9780323036580

Miller WG. Quality control. In: Dufour DR, ed. *Professional Practice in Clinical Chemistry: A Companion Text.* Washington, DC: American Association for Clinical Chemistry; 1999 ISBN9781890883287e

Pincus MR. Interpreting laboratory results: reference values and decision making. In: Henry JB, Todd, JC, ed. *Clinical Diagnosis and Management by Laboratory Methods,* 19e. Philadelphia, PA: WB Saunders; 1996 ISBN9780721660301

Rifai N. *Tietz Textbook of Clinical Chemistry and Molecular Diagnostics,* 6e. Philadelphia, PA: Elsevier; 2018 ISBN9780323359214

Valenstein P. *Quality Management in Clinical Laboratories: Promoting Patient Safety through Risk Reduction and Continuous Improvement.* Northfield, IL: College of American Pathologists Press; 2005 ISBN9780930304881

Westgard JO, Klee GG. Quality management. In: Burtis CA, Ashwood ER, Tietz NW, eds. *Tietz Textbook of Clinical Chemistry,* 3e. Philadelphia, PA: WB Saunders; 1999 ISBN9780721656106

Chapter 8

Immunology

ISBN 978-089189-6616

8.1 Principles of immunology

8.1.1 Immune system physiology

- Primary lymphoid organs: Bone marrow & thymus
- Secondary lymphoid organs: Lymph node, spleen, mucosal-associated tissue (MALT), and cutaneous-associated lymphoid tissue (CALT)

8.1.1.1 Innate immunity

- Nonadaptive and nonspecific, using physical (eg, skin, sweat, mucous, cilia) and chemical barriers to induce inflammation and phagocytosis, and activation of the adaptive immune system through antigen presentation
- Acute-phase reactants are components of normal serum that increase rapidly during infection, injury or trauma. **t8.1** lists the components & describes functions
- Cells of the innate immune system and their characteristics are listed in **t8.2**

t8.1 Acute-phase reactants with function

C-reactive protein (CRP)	Binds receptors on phagocytic cells, promoting phagocytosis Capable of opsonization, agglutination, precipitation and activation of complement via the classical pathway Binding is non-specific and calcium dependent; primary substrate is phosphocholine Increases rapidly with levels 100-1000× higher, peaking at 48 hours Median CRP increases with age
Serum amyloid A	Activates monocytes and macrophages to produce inflammatory molecules Increases up to 1000× in response to infection or injury Increases more in the setting of bacterial vs viral infection Produced in the liver, transported by HDL to the site of infection
Complement	Functions in opsonization, chemotaxis and lysis of cells
α_1-Antitrypsin	Predominantly produced in the liver Limits the harmful effects of the immune system by inhibiting proteases released from leukocytes and regulating expression of proinflammatory cytokines
Haptoglobin	Antioxidant, binds irreversibly to free hemoglobin
Fibrinogen	Promotes clot formation
Ceruloplasmin	Principle copper-transporting protein in plasma

8.1.1.2 Adaptive immunity

- Antigen specific with T-cell & humoral memory
- B cells
  - 10%-15% of circulating lymphocytes
  - Differentiation in the bone marrow
  - Antigen presenting cells
  - Precursor of plasma cells
  - Primary role is to produce immunoglobulin

t8.2 Cells of the innate immune system

Cell type	Characteristics
Neutrophils	Represent 50%-60% of circulating white cells
	Role is to phagocytize & destroy pathogens
	One of first cell types recruited to acute inflammation sites
	Short-lived (2-3 days)
Basophils	Represent 0.5% of circulating white cells
	Role in allergic reaction & parasitic infection
	Membrane receptors bind Fc portion of IgE, resulting in degranulation
	Granules contain histamine, heparin & peroxidase, resulting in vasodilatation, bronchoconstriction & chemotaxis
	Not phagocytic
Eosinophils	Represent 0.5%-6% of circulating white cells
	Role in allergic reaction & parasitic infection
	Express FcεRI receptors that bind Fc portion of IgE
	Granules containing, eg, MBP, ECP, EDN
Monocytes	Represent 5%-10% of circulating white cells
	Precursors to tissue macrophages & dendritic cells
	Phagocytic; primary role to remove particulates of foreign or self-origin
	Have surface receptors for C3b & Fc
Macrophages	Differentiation from monocytes occurs in tissues
	Phagocytic cells with surface receptors for C3b
	Initiate both innate & adaptive immune responses
Dendritic	Differentiation & cell division are localized to tissues
	Phagocytic cells with surface receptors for C3b
	Initiate adaptive immune responses by capturing, processing & presenting antigen to naive T cells
Mast cells	Released from bone marrow as mast cell progenitor cells; terminal differentiation occurs in tissues
	Long-lived tissue-resident cells
	Role in parasitic infection & allergic reactions
	Have Fcε receptors upon their surfaces, bind IgE
	The surface IgE may become crosslinked in presence of antigen, activating degranulation
NK cells*	Innate lymphocytes
	Kill virally infected cells & tumor cells
	May play an important role in pregnancy
	Distinguish healthy cells from infected or cancerous cells by recognizing the MHC class I complex
	Do not specifically bind to tumor antigens; can kill tumor cells without prior exposure to them
	Found in spleen & liver, and represent 5%-15% of circulating lymphocytes
$\gamma\delta$ T cells*	Innate lymphocytes; express heterodimeric T-cell receptor composed of and δ chains
	Represent small subset of T cells in circulation
	Mediate ADCC to combat viral infection and tumor cells

ECP, eosinophil cationic protein; EDN, eosinophil-derived neurotoxin; IgE, immunoglobulin E; MBP, major basic protein; NK, natural killer
**Sometimes classified as cells of the adaptive immune system*

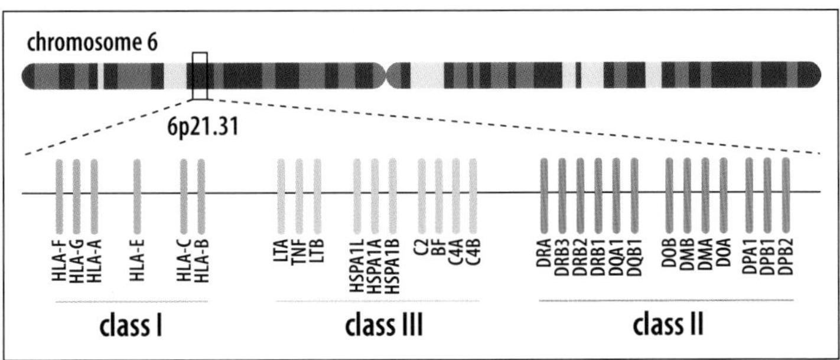

f8.1 HLA locus

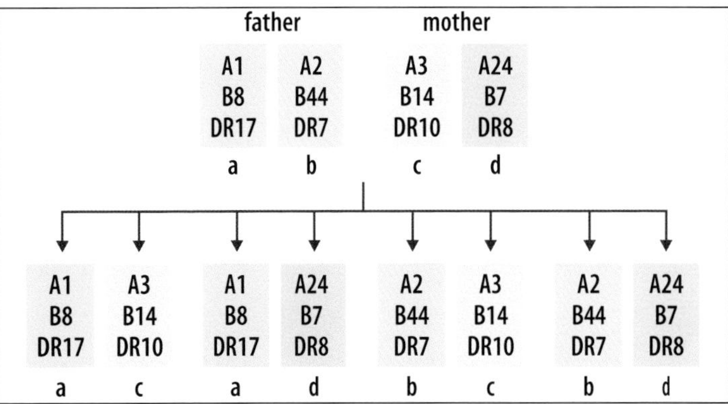

f8.2 Mendelian inheritance pattern of HLA locus

- T cells
  - 60%-80% of circulating lymphocytes
  - Differentiation in the thymus
  - Three subsets: helper, cytotoxic, and regulatory
  - Produce cytokines that stimulate the immune system
  - Assist in killing tumor cells or infected target cells

8.1.1.3 Genetics of the human leukocyte antigen (HLA) complex

- The HLA locus is composed of >200 genes located at 6p21, as shown in **f8.1**
- Class I major genes: HLA-A, HLA-B & HLA-C
  - Each locus (eg, HLA-A) has multiple alleles: eg, HLA-A*01, HLA-A*02
  - Highly polymorphic
- Class I minor genes: HLA-E, HLA-F, HLA-G
  - Display low polymorphism and include HLA-E, HLA-F, HLA-G
- Class II genes: HLA-DR, HLA-DQ, HLA-DP
  - Each locus (eg, HLA-DRB1) has multiple alleles: eg, DRB1*01, DRB1*02
  - Highly polymorphic
  - Gene products present exogenous antigens to the T-cell receptor
- Class II minor genes: HLA-DM & HLA-DO
  - Gene products function in internal processing & loading of peptides
- Class III gene products are involved in inflammation & other immune system activities
- Each HLA complex is closely linked and inherited
  - HLA antigens are inherited as a haplotype from each parent in a simple Mendelian inheritance pattern as shown in **f8.2**
  - One haplotype (A, B, C, DR, DQ, DP) is inherited from each parent; thus, the chance that 2 siblings will be HLA identical is 25%

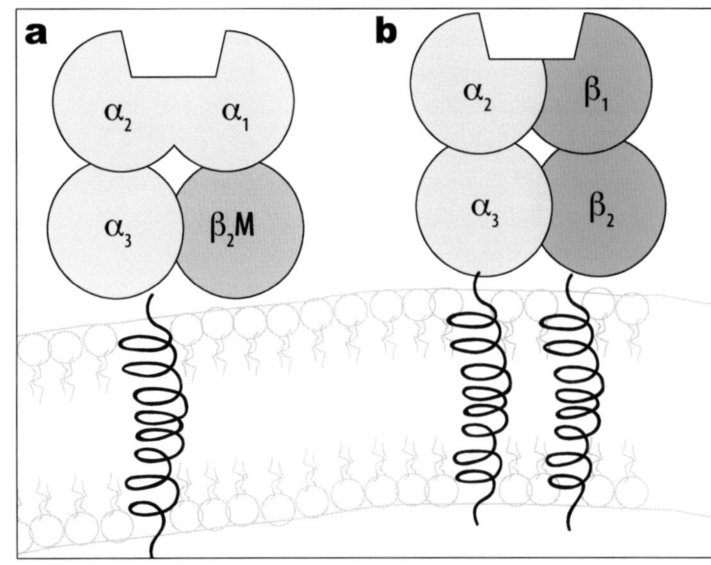

f8.3 Human leukocyte antigens: **a** class I, **b** class II

  - Certain alleles from different loci of HLA are found to occur more frequently and would be statistically expected by gene frequency studies; this linkage dysequilibrium is due to positive selection of haplotypes providing a survival advantage

8.1.1.4 Human leukocyte antigens

- The purpose of these proteins is to present antigens to the immune system to determine recognition of self vs non-self
- Class I (HLA-A, HLA-B & HLA-C)
  - Class I proteins are expressed on cell surface as heterodimer of HLA class I α chain and β2 microglobulin chain as shown in **f8.3a**
  - Found on the surfaces of most nucleated cells
  - Present **endogenous** antigens to CD8 (cytotoxic) T cells

ISBN 978-089189-6616

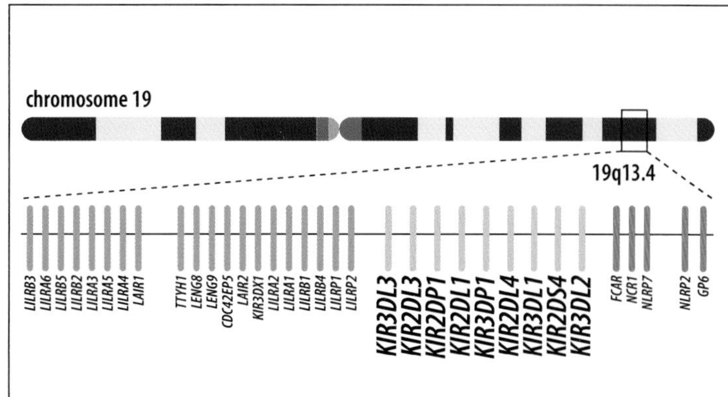

f8.4 Killer-cell immunoglobulinlike receptors

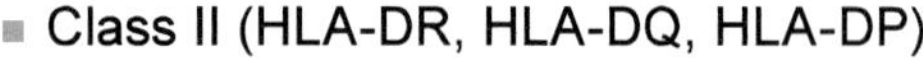

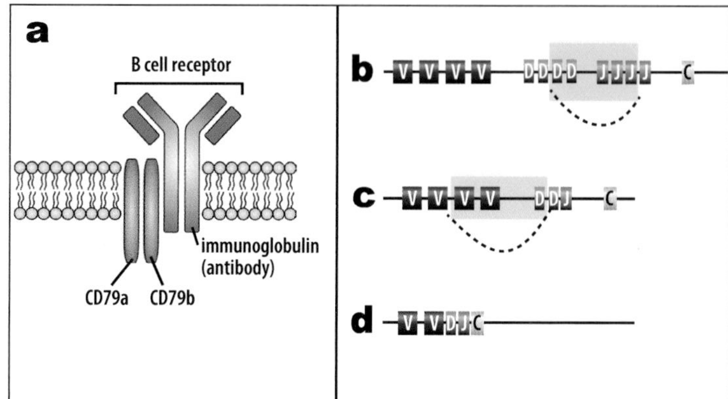

f8.5 B-cell receptor
C, constant region; V, variable region; D, D segment; J, J segment

- Class II (HLA-DR, HLA-DQ, HLA-DP)
  - Class II antigens are expressed on cell surface as heterodimer of one HLA class II alpha and one HLA class II beta chain as shown in **f8.3b**
  - Class II antigens are expressed on antigen-presenting cells, including B lymphocytes, monocytes, macrophages, dendritic cells. It can also be found on activated T lymphocytes
  - Present **exogenous** antigen to CD4 (helper) T cells
- Class III genes
  - Include several secreted molecules with immune function, such as components of complement, cytokines & heat shock proteins
  - Gene products are ligands NK cell receptors and are important for functions of both innate & adaptive immunity, as well as establishing fetal-maternal tolerance
- HLA antigens are known risk factors for autoimmune diseases & drug hypersensitivities; several well-established risk factors are presented in **t8.3**

t8.3 HLA disease & drug hypersensitivity associations

Disease or sensitivity	HLA association
Ankylosing spondylitis	B27
Behçet disease	B51
Celiac disease	DQ2, DQ8
Narcolepsy	DQB1*06:02
Rheumatoid arthritis	DRB1*04
Abacavir sensitivity	B*57:01
Carbamazepine sensitivity	B*15:02

8.1.1.5 Killer-cell immunoglobulinlike receptors (KIRs)

- KIR represents 9 exons located on 19q13.4 as shown in **f8.4**
- Encode for type I transmembrane glycoproteins
- Expressed on natural killer (NK) cells
- Regulate cell killing through inhibitory or activating KIRs
- Involved in protection against viral infection, autoimmune disease and cancer
- Individuals differ in number of KIR genes, inhibitory vs activating and allelic variation
- Naming convention is based on structure
  - First digit corresponds to the number of domains (D)
  - D is followed by L or S to indicate long or short cytoplasmic tail, or P, for pseudogenes
  - final digit indicates the number of the gene encoding a protein with this structure
  - 2 or more genes with very similar structure may be distinguished by final letter (eg, *KIR2DL5A* vs *KIR2DL5B*)

8.1.1.6 B-cell maturation & B-cell receptor (BCR)

- The BCR is composed of membrane bound immunoglobulin (Ig) and a signal transduction moiety as shown in **f8.5a**
- The immunoglobulin portion is composed of heavy and light chains, each containing both constant (C) and variable regions (V) as shown in **f8.7**
- Mature BCR is the result of VDJ gene rearrangements and somatic hypermutation occurring in the bone marrow
- Three genetic loci are involved Ig heavy (IGH), Ig κ (IGK) and Ig λ (IGL)
- Heavy chain genes on chromosome 14 rearrange first
  - Recombination occurs between a D and J segment and intervening sequences, highlighted in grey, are deleted as shown in **f8.5b**
  - V to JD recombination occurs and intervening sequences, highlighted in grey, are deleted as shown in **f8.5c**
  - Primary RNA transcript is generated containing VDJ and constant chain (V-D-J-C) as shown in **f8.5d**
  - Polyadenylated tail is added to the primary RNA after the constant chain

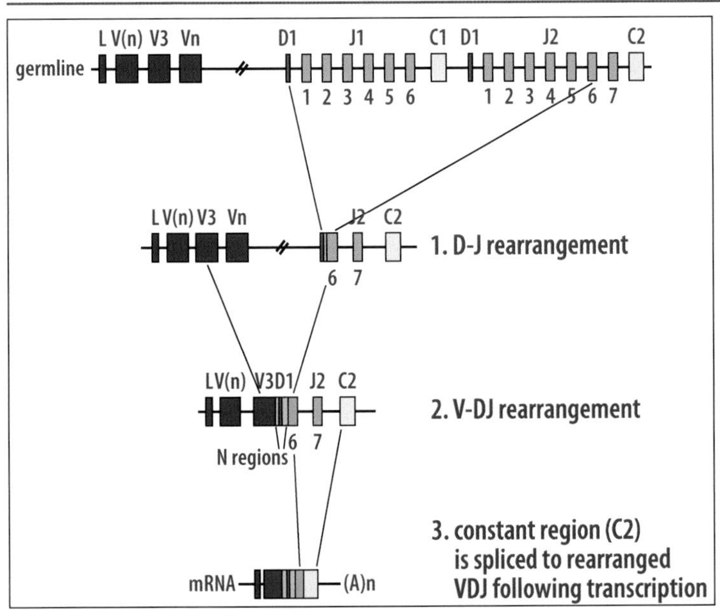

f8.6 T-cell receptor

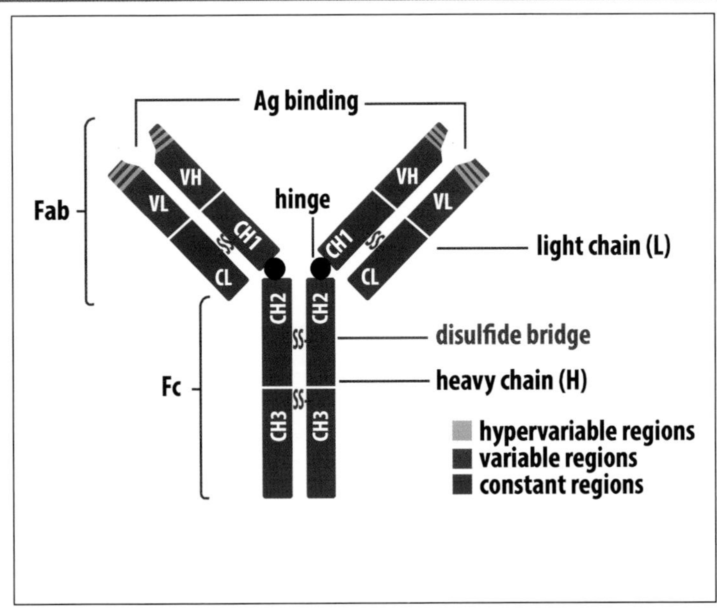

f8.7 Immunoglobulin structure

- Light chain genes on chromosomes 2 (IGK) and 22 (IGL) rearrange in a similar way except that light chains lack a D segment
- Ig heavy chains and light chains assemble to form the membrane-bound Ig that is expressed on the surface of the immature B cell
- Through interaction with stromal cells, B cells will undergo negative & positive selection processes to ensure that each cell has only 1 specificity and to delete self-reactive B cells

8.1.1.7 T-cell maturation & T-cell receptor (TCR)

- Stepwise maturation in the thymus involving somatic hypermutation of the T-cell receptor
  - α, β, γ, δ genes are located on chromosome 7
  - TCR β-chain D to J recombination occurs first, then V to DJ rearrangements as depicted in **f8.6**
  - Intervening sequences are deleted and a primary transcript is synthesized, including a constant domain
  - Full-length protein for the TCR β-chain is translated
  - TCR α chain follows in similar fashion
  - TCR α and β chains assemble to form the αβ-TCR
  - Majority of TCR (>95%) are αβ-TCR
  - TCR γδ cells are found primarily in mucosal surfaces & skin
- Differentiation into one of several types, identifiable by their surface antigen profile
  - T helper (Th) cells: CD3+, CD4+, recognize antigen presented by HLA class II
  - T cytotoxic (Tc) cells: CD3+, CD8+, recognize antigen presented by HLA class I
  - T regulatory (Tregs) cells: CD4+, CD25+
- T-cell receptor (TCR) is expressed in noncovalent association with CD3
- Usual CD4:CD8 ratio is approximately 2:1

8.1.2 Immunoglobulins (Ig)

8.1.2.1 Immunoglobulin function

- Fixation of complement
- Binding to receptors on cell surfaces

8.1.2.2 Immunoglobulin structure

- Immunoglobins are glycoproteins with a 4-chain structure (2 light; 2 heavy) as shown in **f8.7**
- Two domains per chain, 1 variable region and ≥1 constant regions
- Constant regions are unique to each Ig class
- Chains are bound together by interchain and intrachain disulfide bonds (disulfide bridge, **f8.7**)
- Light chains (L)
  - Consist of 2 domains: variable (VL) and constant (CL)
  - Classified as kappa (κ) or lambda (λ) based on differences in the amino acid sequence in the constant region
  - In normal individuals, ~65% of human immunoglobulin have κ chains and 35% have λ chains
  - Bence Jones proteins are light chains found in the urine of patients with multiple myeloma

ISBN 978-089189-6616

- Heavy chains (H)
  - 4-5 domains: 1 variable (VH) and 3-4 constant (eg, CH1, CH2)
  - Hinge region, located between CH1 & CH2 has high content of proline
- Papian cleavage can be performed in the laboratory
  - Cleaves IgG into Fab & Fc fragments, as indicated in **f8.7**
  - Fab fragment is the antigen-binding domain and is composed of variable regions of VL & VH
  - Fc fragment is composed of the constant regions & determines biological function

8.1.2.3 Immunoglobulin classes

- There are 5 primary classes of immunoglobulins: IgG, IgM, IgD & IgE as shown in **t8.5**
- Each class is distinguished by the type of heavy chain
- Function in different stages of the immune response & different types of responses
- Classes differ in valency as a result of different numbers of monomers forming the complete protein

8.1.2.4 Immunoglobulin classification as an antigen

- Antibodies can act as antigen if injected into different species or hosts
- Antibodies contain antigenic determinants
- Based on the location of the antigenic determinates, immunoglobulins can be divided into different types, as shown in **t8.4**

t8.4 Antibody classifiction based on location of antigenic determinates

Isotype	Different classes, eg, IgE vs IgG	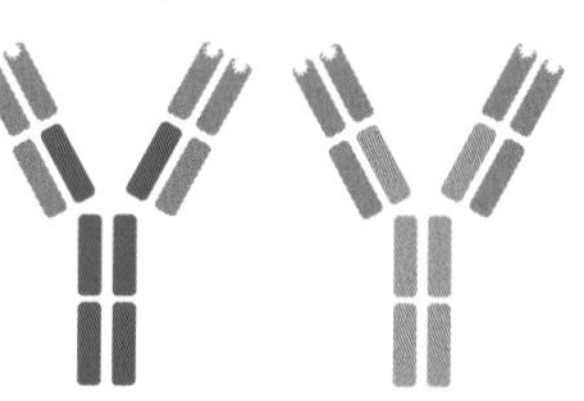
Allotype	Minor variations present in some individuals and not others; formed by constant regions of heavy & light changes	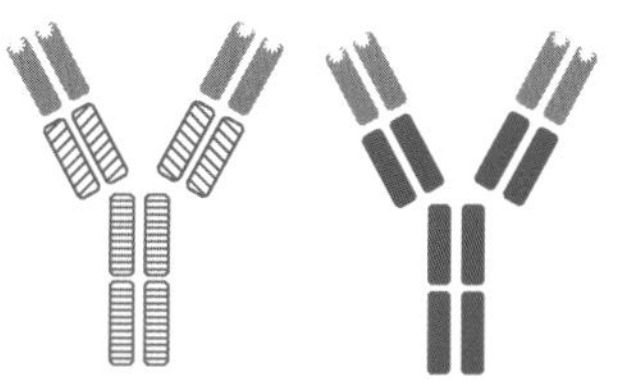
Idiotype	Epitope formed by the variable regions of the heavy & light chains of the antibody to create differences in antigen-binding site	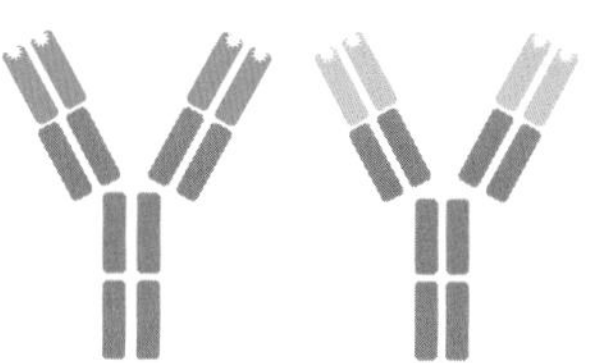
Anti-idiotype	Antibodies can be formed against the idiotype	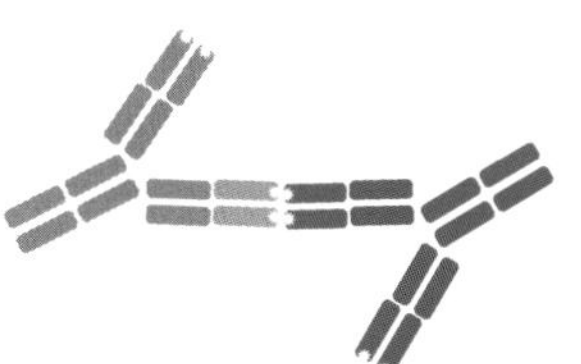

t8.5 Five classes of immunoglobulins (Igs)

	IgM	IgG	IgA	IgE	IgD
Immunoglobulin classes: purple indicates heavy chains, green indicates light chains & cyan indicates J (joining) chains	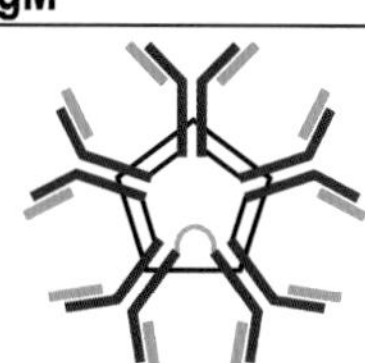	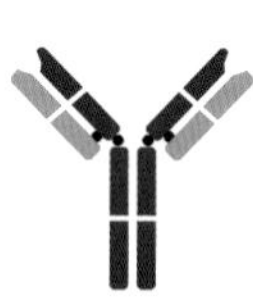	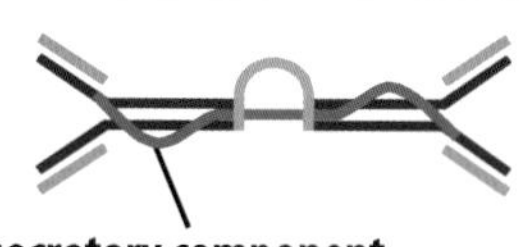 	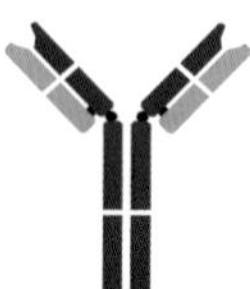	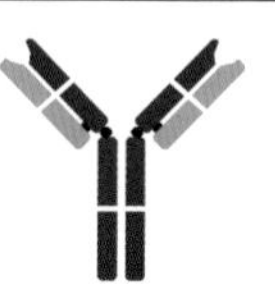
Form in blood	Pentamer 10 binding sites Held together by J chain	Monomer 2 binding sites	Monomer in blood (2 binding sites Dimer in secretions (4 binding sites) Held together by J chain	Bound to mast cells	Bound to immature B cells
Subclasses		IgG_1, IgG_2, IgG_3, IgG_4	IgA_1, IgA_2		
Average serum concentration	15 mg/dL	120 mg/dL	30 mg/dL	mg/dL	mg/dL
Activates complement (relative strength)	Yes (+++) Classic	Yes (++) Classic	Yes (+) Alternate	No	No
Heavy chains	μ	γ	α	ε	δ
Properties	First Ig made by fetus and naïve B cells; binds B cells; hemolytic; surface IgM anchored to cell membrane by 26 residue hydrophobic region	Placental transfer, especially IgG_1	Monomer in serum; dimer in secretions; most abundant Ig in saliva, tears and other secretions	Role in allergies and parasitic infection	Role in B cell development; anchored to cell membrane by 26 residue hydrophobic region

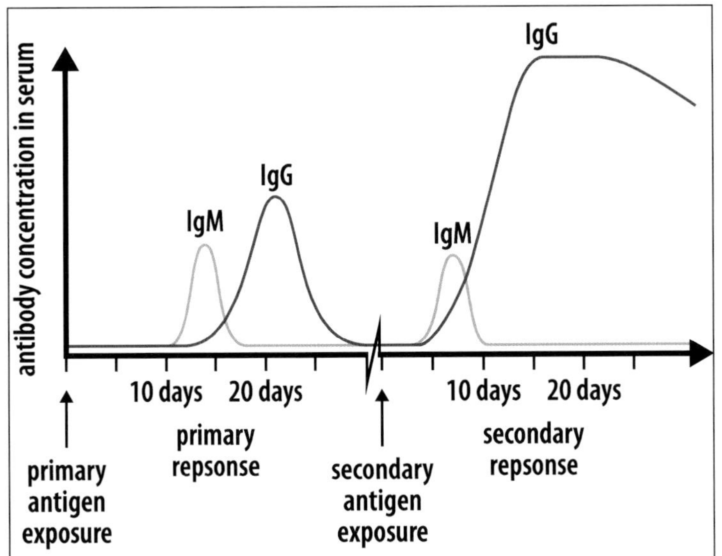

f8.8 Primary & secondary immune response

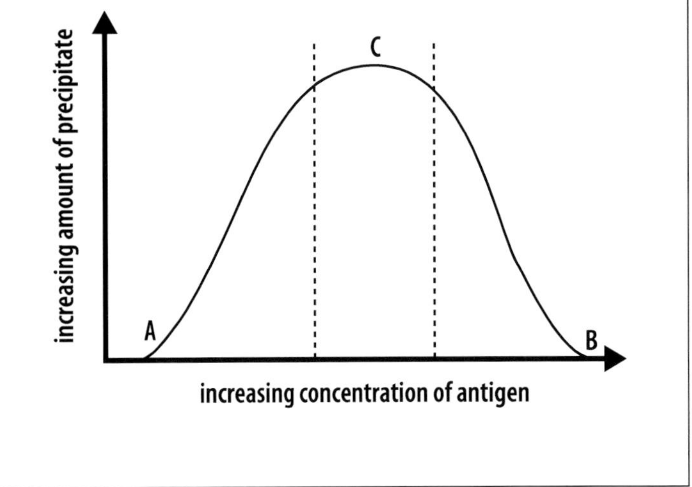

f8.9 Precipitin curve: A antibody excess, B antigen excess, C zone of equivalence

8.1.2.5 Primary & secondary antibody response

- The time course of antibody response that results from the culmination of primary & secondary immune response is presented in **f8.8**
- Primary immune response
  - Involves both B cells & T cells
  - Naïve B cells are stimulated by antigen and become activated
  - These cells differentiate into low-affinity antibody secreting cells specific to the antigen
  - A large amount of IgM and a small amount of IgG are produced
  - Different clones of plasma B cells will produce antibodies that interact with different epitopes on the same antigen. These are referred to as polyclonal antibodies, as observed with the numerous epitopes involved in the response to red cell antigens
  - Occurs primarily in lymph nodes and spleen
  - Antibody reaches peak in 7-10 days
- Secondary immune response
  - Not dependent on T cells
  - Usually a much stronger response compared to the primary response
  - The same antigen stimulates memory B cells for a second or subsequent time
  - Results in production of high-affinity antibodies
  - A large amount of IgG and a small amount of IgM, IgA & IgE are produced
  - Appears in bone marrow and later in lymph nodes and spleen
  - Antibody reaches peak in 3-5 days

8.1.3 Antigen-antibody interactions

8.1.3.1 Antibody testing purposes

- Detect antibody in response to infection, autoimmunity, transplantation, hypersensitivity, immunodeficiency, hematologic malignancy
- Differentiate between acute & past infection (IgM, IgG, IgE)
- Differentiate between passive antibodies & antibodies from vaccine or disease recovery

8.1.3.2 Definitions

- Affinity refers to the initial force of attraction between a single antigen epitope & a single Fab antibody site
- Avidity is the sum of the interactions between all interacting antigen epitopes & Fab sites
- A hapten is a substance that is only antigenic when coupled to a protein carrier
- Precipitation is the visible serologic reaction that occurs when soluble antigen is mixed with its specific antibody and precipitates out of solution
- A typical preciptin curve, in which antigen is added to antibody over time is represented in **f8.9**
  - Initially antibody is present in excess and little precipitation is visible. This is often referred to as the "prozone effect," when excess antibody prevents crosslinking between antigen & antibody
  - As more antigen is added, peak precipitation occurs. This is referred to as the "zone of equivalence." At this point, antibody and antigen multivalent sites are equal, leading to maximal precipitation of antigen-antibody complexes

 ISBN 978-089189-6616

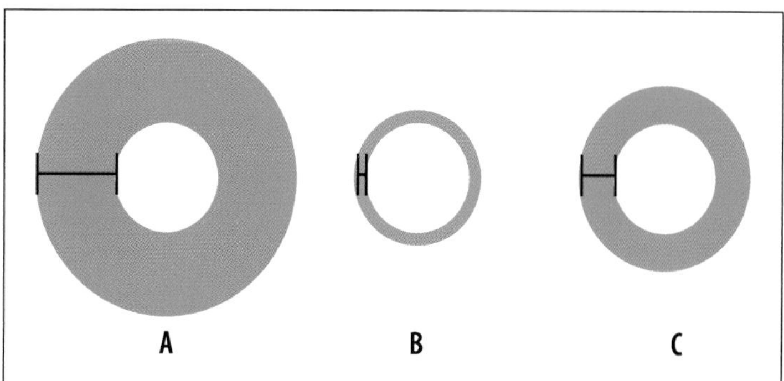

f8.10 Radial immunodiffusion: sample A contains the greatest amount of antigen & thus has the largest ring of antigen-antibody precipitation

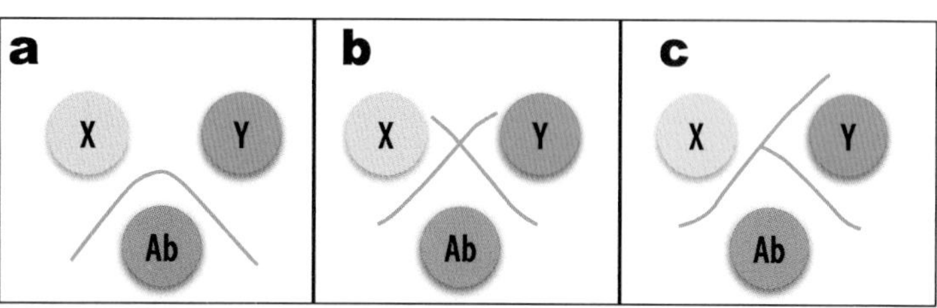

f8.11 Double immunodiffusion: **a** identity, **b** nonidentity, **c** partial identity

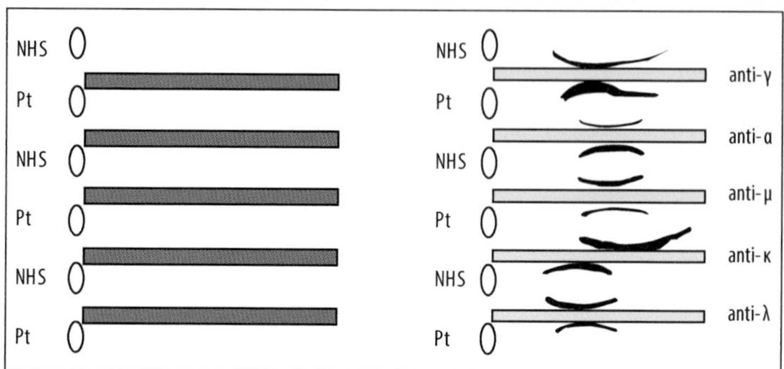

f8.12 Immunoelectrophoresis to detect gammaglobulinemia with uninoculated wells (left) & a gel following electrophoresis, diffusion, fixation & staining (right) demonstrating an IgG κ monoclonal protein

    - As antigen begins to exceed antibody, precipitation of antigen-antibody complexes is reversed

8.1.3.3 Light scattering

- Measure of antigen-antibody precipitin interactions through light scattering
- Turbidity: Measure the decrease in amount of light passing directly through the solution
- Nephelometry allows for quick detection and/or quantitation of immunoglobulins in a sample
    - Antibody is the reagent
    - Serum contains complement antigen
    - Measures the scattering of light as it passes through the solution
    - Results in milligrams per deciliter (mg/dL) or international units per milliliter (IU/mL)

8.1.3.4 Immunodiffusion

- Measurement of antigen-antibody precipitin interactions by diffusion
- Radial immunodiffusion (RID): Antibody in gel and antigen is added to the well, as shown in **f8.10**. The sample with the greatest radius has the greatest amount of antigen
- Ouchterlony double diffusion (passive double immunodiffusion): Antibody & antigen diffuse through gel in 2 dimensions; precipitin lines form where the moving front of antigen meets that of antibody at the point of equivalence, as shown in **f8.11**
    - Identity: Precipitin lines fuse, forming a single arc **f8.11a**
    - Nonidentity: Each antigen forms an independent precipitin line with the corresponding antibody at an equivalence point; precipitin lines cross, forming double spurs **f8.11b**
    - Partial identity **f8.11c**

8.1.3.5 Immunoelectrophoresis (IEP)

- No longer commonly used
- Measurement of antigen-antibody precipitin interactions using electrophoresis followed by immunodiffusion
- Serum is separated in agarose gel by electrophoresis
- A trough is cut parallel to the plane of electrophoresis
- Monospecific antiserum is placed in trough
- Antibody diffuses toward the serum proteins
- Arcs of antibody antigen precipitation occur as shown in **f8.12**

8.1.3.6 Immunofixation electrophoresis (IFE)

- Measurement of antigen-antibody precipitin interactions using electrophoresis
- Patient serum subjected to electrophoresis to separate out proteins
- Antibody is added to surface and incubated (eg, anti-IgG, IgA, IgM, κ and λ)
- Immunoprecipitants occur only where a specific antigen is located on the gel
- Normal serum should have a dark IgG, much lighter IgA and absent IgM, with denser κ compared to λ lane
- When a narrow band with sharp boards can be identified, it implies presence of a monoclonal protein
- Commonly used to detect gammopathy, such as the IgG κ monoclonal protein shown in **f8.13**

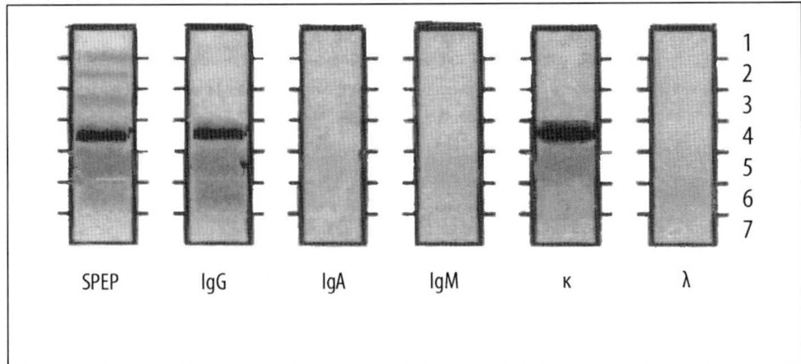

f8.13 Immunofixation electrophoresis demonstrating an IgG κ monoclonal protein

8.1.3.7 Agglutination

- Measurement of antigen-antibody precipitin interactions
- Particles suspended in liquid collect into clumps when antigen is mixed with antibody
- In a hemagglutination test red blood cells (RBCs) clump when antibody reacts with antigen on RBC surface, as shown in **f8.14a**
- In a latex agglutination test, antigen is mixed with antibody coated on surface of latex particles, or antibody is mixed with antigen-coated latex particles as shown in **f8.14b**
- Cold agglutinins are antibodies, usually IgM, to erythrocytes. A cold agglutinin titer is read as the last dilution showing agglutination at 39.2°F (4°C)

8.1.4 Complement

- Complement components constitute soluble & membrane-bound proteins that play a role to magnify the inflammatory response to destroy & clear foreign antigens
- This can be achieved through direct cell lysis via membrane attack complex (MAC), coating foreign entities with C3b to initiate phagocytosis, and directing the adaptive immunity to the site of infection as shown in **f8.15**
- There are 3 recognized pathways of complement activation, as discussed herein

8.1.4.1 Classic complement pathway

- Antibody dependent, activated by IgM, IgG1, IgG2, IgG3
- Components: C1q, C1r, C1s, C4, C2, C3, C5, C6, C7, C8, C9
- Three stages include recognition, activation & formation of the membrane attach complex (MAC)
  - Recognition: Fc portion of Ig interacts with C1 (3 subunits: C1q, C1r, C1s). C1q serves as the recognition piece

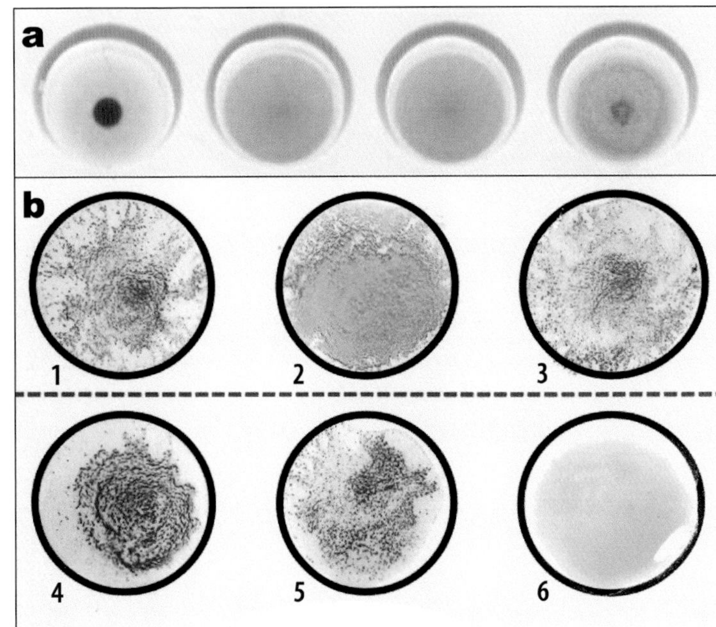

f8.14 Agglutination: **a** hemagglutination test; **b** latex agglutination test

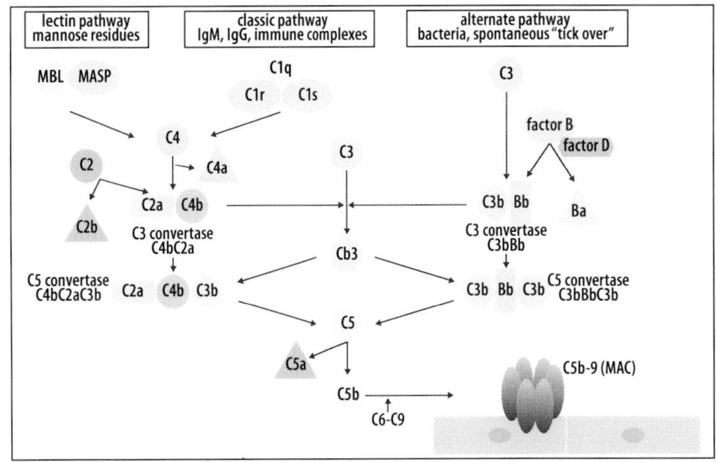

f8.15 Pathways of complement activation

  - Activation: Involves cleaving C4, C2, C3 into "a" and "b" fragments
    - C3a is small anaphylatoxin
    - C3b is larger, lands on target surface, and becomes part of C5 convertase, and is also a powerful opsonin; is inactivated by cleavage into C3c & C3d
  - Formation of MAC is initiated with C5, then C5a, C6, C7, C8, C9 form the complex
- C3a, C4a & C5a are anaphylatoxins and cause the release of histamine from basophils & mast cells
- C5a is both anaphylatoxin & chemotactic for neutrophils, basophils, mast cells & monocytes
- C3 & C4 are deposited on the target surface

ISBN 978-089189-6616

8.1.4.2 Alternate complement pathway (aka properdin pathway)

- Antibody independent, but can be initiated by IgA & IgE
- Unique components: factor B, factor D, properdin, shares C3
- Triggered by deposition of C3b on lipopolysaccharide in microbial cell walls, fungal cell walls, yeast, viruses, virally infected cells, and some parasites
- C3b factor B binds with C3b to make C3bBb
- C3bBb is cleaved by factor D to form the surface bound convertase, which is then stabilized by properdin
- Properdin increases the half-life of C3bBb
- Factor H limits the action of the alternative pathway by preventing C3 conversion

8.1.4.3 Lectin pathway

- Antibody independent
- Unique components: Mannose-binding lectin (MBL), MASP-1, MASP-2; shares C4 & C2
- Triggered by carbohydrates in microbial cell walls, such as MBL
- MBL-associated serine proteases (MASPs) activate the complement cascade by cleaving C4 & C2, leading to formation of MAC

8.1.5 Immune system function

8.1.5.1 Active humoral-mediated immunity

- Antibodies produced by an individual's own immune system
- Long-lasting immunity involving production of long-lasting memory cells
- Result of infection or vaccination

8.1.5.2 Passive humoral-mediated immunity

- The transfer of antibodies from 1 individual to another
- Naturally acquired, such as mother to child during fetal development or through breast milk
- Artificially acquired, such as intravenous immunoglobulin (IVIG), monoclonal antibodies, serum, or plasma; risk of hypersensitivity reactions
- Short-lived immunity because only antibodies are transferred

8.1.5.3 Cell-mediated immunity

- Immune response not involving antibodies
- Innate & acquired immunity cells are involved
- Primarily directed toward intracellular pathogens, also protect against fungi, protozoans & cancer
- Plays role in transplant rejection
- Macrophages phagocytose pathogens
- NK cells secrete cytotoxic granules
- Antigen-presenting cells (APC) present antigen to naïve T cells, converting to activated T cells
- Activated T cells include: Cytotoxic T cells, Th1 cells, Th2 cells

8.1.5.4 Immune privilege

- Certain areas of the body can tolerate the introduction of antigens without the usual inflammatory response
- Contributing factors include physical factors such as tight junctions, low expression of HLA class I, expression of other immunoregulatory molecules
- Immune privileged sites include eyes, placenta, fetus, testicles, central nervous system

8.2 Diseases of the immune system

8.2.1 Autoimmunity

- Breakdown of self-tolerance resulting in disease
- Generally most prevalent in women of reproductive age
- Onset often associated with recent infection
- Strong genetic component involving HLA and immune regulatory genes involved in tolerance & inflammation
- Either organ specific or systemic
- Organ specific: Thyroid, adrenal, stomach & pancreas
- Effectors of damage include antigen-driven self-reactive lymphocytes, autoantibodies & immune complexes

8.2.1.1 Mechanisms of autoimmunity

- Molecular mimicry, similarities between foreign and self-peptides results in cross-activation of autoreactive immune cells
- Direct stimulation of autoreactive cells by foreign antigen
  - The drug methyldopa can lead to autoimmune hemolytic anemia
  - Penicillamine is linked to systemic vasculitis
  - Procainamide, hydralazine & isoniazid are associated with drug-induced lupus
- Dysregulation of cytokines
- Increased MHC expression

8.2.1.2 Ankylosing spondylitis

- Organ-specific disease affecting the spine
- Begins in sacroiliac joints, causing vertebral fusion
- Inflammation can occur in other areas of body, commonly the eyes

- Affects males more than females
- HLA-B27 is a strong genetic risk factor

8.2.1.3 Autoimmune Addison disease

- Organ-specific disease affecting the adrenal gland
- Antibodies to adrenal antigens create adrenal insufficiency, leading to hormonal imbalances
- HLA-DRB1*04:04 is the most recognized genetic risk factor

8.2.1.4 Chronic active hepatitis

- Organ-specific disease affecting the liver
- Type 1 (classic)
  - Accounts for 96% of cases in the United States
  - HLA-DRB1*03 and HLA-DRB1*04 are genetic risk factors
  - Can occur at any age
  - Female-to-male ratio of 4:1
  - Characterized by presence of antinuclear antibody (ANA) and anti-smooth muscle antibody (ASMA)
- Type 2
  - Occurs most often in Europe
  - Common in children & young people
  - More severe disease compared to type 1
  - Characterized by anti-liver kidney microsomal antibody type 1 (anti-LKM1) and/or anti-liver cytosol type 1 (anti-LC1) autoantibodies

8.2.1.5 Graves disease

- Organ-specific disease affecting the thyroid
- Antireceptor antibodies to thyroid-stimulating hormone (TSH) receptor
- Mediated by thyroid-stimulating immunoglobulin (TSI)
- Autoantibody TSI binds to TSH receptor on thyroid follicular cells
- Stimulates thyroid hormone release, independent of TSH
- Serologic findings
  - Low TSH
  - Elevated thyroxine

8.2.1.6 Goodpasture syndrome

- Organ specific disease targeting the kidney & lungs
- Anti-glomerular basement membrane antibody targeting collagen
- Causes glomerulonephritis & bleeding in the lungs

8.2.1.7 Hashimoto thyroiditis

- Organ-specific disease targeting thyroid
  - CD4 T-helper cells react to specific thyroid antigens
  - CD4 cells recruit CD8 cytotoxic T cells that can destroy gland tissue
- Serologic findings
  - Elevated TSH
  - Low thyroxine in most cases
  - Antibodies against thyroid antigens
    - Antithyroglobulin
    - Antithyroid peroxidase

8.2.1.8 Myasthenia gravis

- Organ-specific neuromuscular disease
- Most commonly associated with antireceptor antibodies to acetylcholine receptor (AChR), may be binding, blocking, or modulating
- Leads to muscle weakness
- Circulating AChR antibodies are present in ~85% of patients
- Half of patients without anti-AChR antibodies will have muscle-specific tyrosine kinase (MuSK) antibodies
- MuSK is involved in forming the nerve-muscular junction

8.2.1.9 Pernicious anemia

- Organ-specific targeting gastric parietal cells
- Results in deficient adsorption of dietary vitamin B_{12}
- Type 1: Anti-intrinsic factor
- Type 2: Anti-parietal cell antibodies, found in 90% of cases

8.2.1.10 Primary biliary cirrhosis (PBC)

- Organ-specific disease targeting biliary epithelial cells of liver
- Antimitochondrial antibodies (AMA) are present in 90% of cases
- May also have highly PBC-specific antinuclear antibody

8.2.1.11 Primary sclerosing cholangitis (PSC)

- Organ specific disease targeting the bile ducts
- Affect males more than females
- Anti-neutrophil cytoplasmic antibodies (P-ANCA), antinuclear antibodies, and anti-smooth muscle antibodies are common in these patients but are not specific to PSC

ISBN 978-089189-6616

8.2.1.12 Progressive systemic sclerosis (aka scleroderma or CREST syndrome)

- Systemic disease affecting skin, subcutaneous tissues & smooth muscle
- Characterized by changes in texture & appearance of the skin because of increased collagen production
- Antinuclear antibodies, centromere antibody (ACA) & scleroderma antibody (Scl-70) are common in these patients

8.2.1.13 Rheumatoid arthritis (RA)

- Most common form of chronic inflammatory arthritis
- Systemic disease affecting the lining of the joints
- Other manifestations include interstitial lung disease, pleuritis, endocarditis & systemic vasculitis
- Women affected about twice as often as men
- Initial onset of symptoms between the ages of 30 & 50 years
- HLA-DR4 is a genetic risk factor
- Rheumatoid factor (RF)
  - Autoantibody that binds to the Fc portion of IgG
  - present in significant concentrations in about 80% of people with RA
  - Nonspecific not diagnostic for RA
- C-reactive protein (CRP) & erythrocyte sedimentation rate (ESR) are often elevated in RA, and can help differentiate from osteoarthritis
- Rheumatoid factor (RF) is positive in most patients, but up to 30% of patients are initially negative for RF
- Cyclic citrullinate peptide (CCP) antibody may be present before symptoms appear and are found in 60%-70% of RF-negative people with RA
- Antinuclear antibody (ANA) may also be present

8.2.1.14 Sjögren syndrome

- Systemic disease that attacks the glands that make tears & saliva, as well as other body systems including joints, thyroid, kidneys, liver, lungs, skin & nerves
- Most common in women >40 years of age
- Autoimmune antibody tests
  - Antibodies specific to Sjögren syndrome: Anti-SS-A (Ro) and anti-SS-B (La) are frequently positive
  - Antinuclear antibodies (ANA) are generally present
  - Rheumatoid factor (RF) may be positive
  - Anti-dsDNA can be seen in these patients

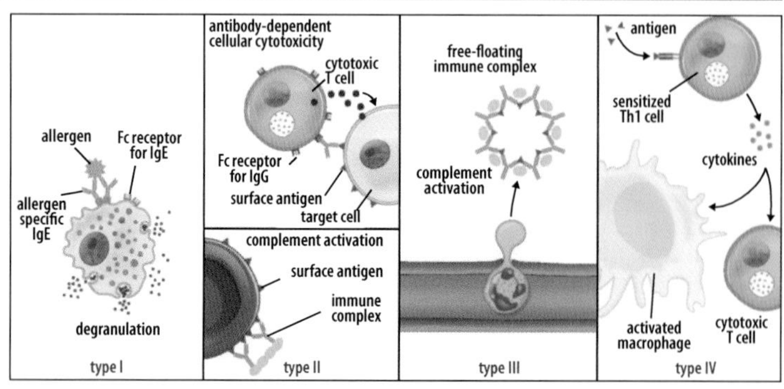

f8.16 Hypersensitivity reactions based on Coombs & Gell classification

8.2.1.15 Systemic lupus erythematosus

- Systemic rheumatic disorder
- Female-to-male ratio is approximately 8:1; greater prevalence in African Americans
- Most diagnosed between the ages of 15 and 45 years
- Hallmark is high anti-dsDNA antibodies; negative ANA essentially excludes lupus
- 20% of cases also have anti-Smith (Sm) antibodies which target a ribonucleoprotein found in the nucleus
- Complement C3 becomes depleted because of autoantibody C3-nephritic factor (C3NeF)
- Impaired ability to clear immune complexes
- Tissue injury is the result of large soluble complexes

8.2.1.16 Granulomatosis with polyangiitis (GPA) (aka Wegener granulomatosis)

- Systemic disease characterized by inflammation of blood vessels of respiratory tract & kidneys
- Affects men & women equally and can occur at any age
- Immune-related laboratory testing
  - C-reactive protein (CRP)
  - Erythrocyte sedimentation rate (ESR)
  - ANCA indirect immunofluorescence screen, antibodies are common, but not specific to GPA
  - Reflex positives to serine antiproteinase 3 (PRC) & myeloperoxidase (MPO)
  - Anti-PR3 predominate in GPA, whereas anti-MPO is less commonly associated

8.2.2 Hypersensitivity

- Hypersensitivity is overactivity of the immune system leading to tissue damage. Coombs and Gel devised a classification system for 4 types of hypersensitivity reactions, as show in **f8.16**

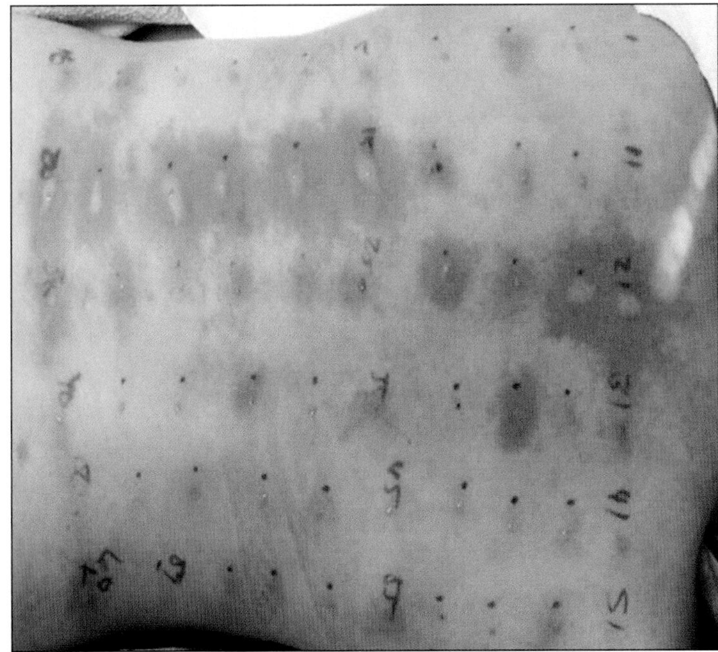

i8.1 Classic wheal & flare reactions generated during skin testing

8.2.2.1 Type I hypersensitivity: Immediate-type hypersensitivity

- IgE mediated
- Rapid reaction, 15-60 minutes after exposure
- Local or systemic reactions: Hay fever, allergic asthma, hives, anaphylaxis
- Antigens that trigger are referred to as allergens (eg, peanuts, eggs, pollen, penicillin, etc)
- Allergen binds IgE on surface of mast cells via the Fcε receptor causing mast cell degranulation and release of preformed mediators
- Preformed mediators include histamine, heparin, proteases & eosinophil and neutrophil chemotactic factors (ECF-A, NCF-A)
- Secondary mediators include leukotrienes, prostaglandins, cytokines & platelet-activating factor
- Characteristic wheal & flare as shown in i8.1
  - Wheal: Swelling caused by release of serum into tissue
  - Flare: Redness of skin caused by dilation of blood vessels
- Clinical manifestations include allergy, asthma, urticaria & anaphylaxis
- Testing involves skin tests (percutaneous or intradermal), total IgE measurement & allergen-specific IgE testing

8.2.2.2 Type II hypersensitivity: Antibody-mediated cellular cytotoxicity

- IgM & IgG mediated
- Anti-cell surface antigen reactions resulting in either:
  - Complement-mediated lysis via formation of membrane attack complex (MAC)
  - Cytotoxic T cell with an Fc receptor for the antibody; referred to as "antibody-dependent cell-mediated cytotoxicity" (ADCC)
  - Antireceptor antibodies
- Examples include blood transfusion reactions, erythroblastosis fetalis, various autoimmune diseases, and early transplant rejection
- Autoimmune reactions include rheumatic fever, myasthenia gravis, Goodpasture syndrome, Graves disease, multiple sclerosis

8.2.2.3 Type III hypersensitivity

- IgM & IgG mediated
- Immune complexes form & activate complement
- Complexes deposit on vasodilated vessels leading to platelet aggregation, chemotaxis of neutrophils
- Neutrophils release lysosomal enzymes, resulting in injury of surrounding cells
- Examples include systemic lupus erythematosus, arthus reaction, serum sickness

8.2.2.4 Type IV hypersensitivity: Delayed-type hypersensitivity (DTH)

- T cell-mediated response to antigen
- Initial sensitization phase of 1-2 weeks after first contact with antigen
- Antigen binds receptor T cells, causing T cell to release cytokines that activate macrophages, which in turn release inflammatory mediators
- Reaction begins after a latent period of several hours, peaks at about 48-72 hours after exposure to antigen
- Antigens are generally either contact or intracellular
  - Contact includes inorganic chemicals, poison ivy, nickel, etc
  - Intracellular can be bacteria, fungi, parasites, or viruses; aggregation & proliferation of macrophages results in granulomatous formation over 21-28 days and can persist for weeks
- Also includes transplant & tumor cell rejection
- Testing involves skin tests, such as the commonly administered test for tuberculosis exposures

ISBN 978-089189-6616

8.2.3 Immunoproliferative diseases

8.2.3.1 Monoclonal gammopathies (MG)

- Disorders characterized by abnormal proliferation of clonal plasma cells
- Produce protein; intact monoclonal immunoglobulin, free light chain or free heavy chain
- Protein is referred to as M protein, M band, M spike, monoclonal spike, paraprotein, Bence Jones protein
- Disorders range from low tumor burden, premalignancy & malignancy
- Quantification & identification of M proteins is important for diagnosis & monitoring
    - Protein electrophoresis, immunofixation, immunoglobulin quantitation, serum free light chain & heavy-light chain assays, matrix-assisted laser desorption/ionization time-of-flight mass spectrometer (MALDI-TOF)

8.2.3.2 Multiple myeloma (MM)

- MM develops in activated memory B cells or plasmablasts
- Chromosomal translocation between the immunoglobulin heavy chain and an oncogene are frequently involved
- A single plasma cell clone proliferates
    - Producing cytokines that cause localized damage
    - Producing antibodies that deposit in various organs

8.2.3.3 Light chain amyloidosis (AL amyloidosis)

- Clonal population of plasma cells producing monoclonal light chain of κ or λ type
- Amyloidogenic light chains misfold, forming β pleated sheets
- Deposit in the tissues in the form of amyloid fibrils
- Interferes with organ structure & function

8.2.3.4 Waldenström macroglobulinemia (WM)

- Lymphoplasmacytoid cancer
- Incurable, but treatable
- WM cells produce large amounts of IgM
- WM cells reside in the bone marrow, where they crowd out normal cells

8.2.3.5 X-linked lymphoproliferative disease (XLP)

- Duncan disease
- Affected individuals produce abnormally large numbers of T and B cells when infected with Epstein-Barr virus (EBV), causing a life-threatening reaction called "hemophagocytic lymphohistiocytosis"
- Inverted CD4:CD8 ratio & hypogammaglobulinemia common
- The underlying genetic abnormality is found in the *SH2D1A* gene, Xq25, which codes for an SH2 domain on a signal transducing protein called "SLAM-associated protein" (SAP)

8.2.4 Immunodeficiency

8.2.4.1 Primary immunodeficiency disorders

- Disorders characterized by poor or absent function in ≥1 components of the immune system
- Typically, congenital (present at birth) vs acquired
- May involve either adaptive (B-cell, T-cell) or innate immunity (phagocytic cells, complement)
- Often mutations in genes involved in the development of immune organs, cells & molecules
- Characterized by recurrent infections and a high risk of autoimmune disorders, allergy & malignancy

8.2.4.2 X-linked agammaglobulinemia (XLA) (aka Bruton agammaglobulinemia

- X-linked disorder of acquired immunity affecting B cells
- Characterized by the absence of mature B cells, antibody deficiency & recurrent bacterial infections
- Serum immunoglobulin levels (IgG, IgA & IgM) are markedly reduced
- Caused by mutation in Bruton tyrosine kinase (*BTK*) gene
- *BTK* gene encodes a protein tyrosine kinase important for pro- to pre-B transition

8.2.4.3 Selective IgA deficiency

- The most common primary immunodeficiency; disorder of acquired immunity
- Characterized by lack of IgA with normal IgG & IgM levels
- Most individuals with deficiency are asymptomatic whereas others have recurrent sinopulmonary infections, giardiasis, allergies, or autoimmune disorders
- Anti-IgA antibodies may develop after transfusion, IVIG or other blood products, leading to transfusion reactions
- Associated with an increased incidence of autoimmune disease

8.2.4.4 DiGeorge syndrome

- Disorder of acquired immunity caused by abnormal migration and development of cells & tissues during fetal development, causing the thymus gland to be affected
  - In the most complete form, children with this syndrome have no detectable thymus
- Characterized by T-cell deficiency, characteristic facies, congenital heart disease & hypocalcemia
- No cellular immune response
- 22q11.2 deletion

8.2.4.5 Severe combined immunodeficiency (SCID)

- Disorder of acquired immunity caused by mutations in genes of the immune system
- Decreased or absent T-cell function, low to undetectable immunoglobulin & thymic dysplasia
- Characterized by severe infections that are fatal within the first 2 years of life without treatment
- Increased risk for transfusion-associated graft vs host disease

8.2.4.6 Wiskott-Aldrich syndrome (WAS)

- X-linked recessive disorder of acquired immunity affecting white cells & platelets
- Characterized by thrombocytopenia, eczema, recurrent infections & abnormal or nonfunctional white cells
- *WAS* gene mutations on X chromosome disrupt the function of cytoskeleton in developing cells

8.2.4.7 Ataxia telangiectasia (Louis-Bar syndrome)

- Autosomal recessive disorder of acquired immunity involving both B & T cells
- Characterized by chronic sinopulmonary disease, cerebellar ataxia, small, dilated blood vessels of the eyes & skin, malignancy, progressive neurodegeneration
- Degree of immunodeficiency varies greatly from one individual to the next
- Laboratory abnormalities include deficient IgA, along with very high serum α-fetoprotein (AFP) & carcinoembryonic antigen (CEA)
- Caused by mutations in the *ATM* serine/threonine kinase gene, reducing or eliminating the enzymes DNA repair activity
- The *ATM* gene is located on 11q22.3

8.2.4.8 Chronic granulomatous disease

- X-linked recessive or autosomal recessive disorder of the innate immunity
- Characterized by recurrent bacterial & fungal infections, granuloma formation
- X-linked disease is associated with mutations in *CYBB* gene
- Autosomal recessive disease is associated with mutations in CYBA, NCF1, NCF2, or NCF4

8.2.4.9 Hereditary angioedema

- X-linked recessive disorder of innate immunity
- Characterized by recurrent episodes of severe swelling of limbs, face, intestinal tract & airway
- Types I, II & III distinguished by underlying causes and levels of C1 esterase inhibitor
- Mutations in *SERPING1* gene lead to type I and II abnormal C1 inhibitor function
- Affected individuals are susceptible to fulminant meningococcal disease

8.2.5 Complement deficiencies

- Deficiencies in complement can affect all 3 complement pathways as shown in **t8.6**

t8.6 Diagnosis of complement abnormalities

Impaired function or deficiency	Classic pathway	Lectin pathway	Alternative pathway
C1q, C1r, C1s	Low	Normal	Normal
C4, C2	Low	Low	Normal
MBL, MASP2	Normal	Low	Normal
B, D, P	Normal	Normal	Low
C3, C5, C6, C7, C8, C9	Low	Low	Low
C1-INH	Low	Low	Low
Factor H & I	Low	Low	Low
Improperly handled sera	Low	Low	Low

8.2.5.1 Deficiency of classic pathway

- C1q, C2, or C4
- Primarily manifested by autoimmune phenomena such as lupus

8.2.5.2 Deficiency of C2, C3

- Leads to recurrent infections with gram-positive encapsulated organisms
- C2 is the most common deficiency
- C3 is associated with life-threatening infections

ISBN 978-089189-6616

8.2.5.3 Deficiency of membrane attach complex

- Complement C5-9
- Symptoms include recurrent serious systemic infections, especially *Neisseria meningitidis* and *Neisseria gonorrhea*

8.2.5.4 Deficiency of C1 esterase inhibitor (C1 INH)

- Autosomal dominant disease
- Hereditary angioedema (HAE)
- Urinary histamine levels & serum C1 levels are elevated during attacks, whereas serum CH50, C4 & C2 are decreased. Between attacks, C4 is always low, whereas C2 levels are normal
- First-line therapy is recombinant C1 inhibitor concentrate

8.3 Transplantation

8.3.1 Types of transplants

8.3.1.1 Solid organ

- Liver
- Kidney
- Pancreas
- Heart
- Lung
- intestine

8.3.1.2 Hematopoietic stem cells

- Peripheral stem cell
- Bone marrow stem cell
- Cord blood

8.3.1.3 Categories of transplant donors

- Autologous: Patient receives own cells or tissue back
- Allogeneic: Patient receives graft from a family member or unrelated individual
- Syngeneic: Patient & donor are identical twins
- Xenograft: Patient receives a graft from another species

8.3.2 Sensitization to HLA

- Antibodies to non-self HLA arise in conditions such as pregnancy, transfusion, allografts
- Anti-HLA antibodies are responsible for humoral rejection in solid organ transplantation
- Anti-HLA antibodies can cause failure to engraft in hematopoietic stem cell transplantation

8.3.3 HLA testing

8.3.3.1 HLA typing by serologic methods

- Cell-based cytotoxicity assay requiring live cells
- Assesses presence of HLA antigen on cell surface
- Lymphocytes are tested with a panel of serum specimens containing well-characterized HLA-specific antibodies
  - Serum specimen is placed in microtiter plate
  - Cells to be typed are added
  - After incubation, complement is added, and cells bound to antibody lyse
  - Dye is added to discriminate live vs dead cells; plates are read under microscope
- Less commonly used method
- Misassignment of type is not uncommon because of low-expression antigens and lack of well-defined serologic reagents

8.3.3.2 HLA typing using molecular methods

- Molecular typing
  - DNA is extracted from samples
  - Polymerase chain reaction is performed using HLA specific primers
  - Various detection platforms, including DNA sequencing, are available for determination of sequence variation at low (eg, A*02) to high resolution (eg, A*02:01:01:01)

8.3.3.3 HLA antibody screen & identification

- Cytotoxic antibody detection
  - A panel of characterized cell lines is placed in microtiter plate
  - The serum to be tested is added to all wells
  - After incubation, complement is added; cells bound with antibody lyse
  - Dye is added to discriminate live vs dead cells; plates are read under microscope
- Bead array detection
  - More sensitive than cytotoxic method
  - Purified HLA antigens are loaded onto individual polystyrene beads with unique dye signatures
  - Beads for multiple antigens are then pooled
  - The serum specimen to be tested is added to the pooled beads
  - After incubation, beads are washed and labeled with fluorescent anti-human IgG
  - Antibody is detected based on fluorescent signal

- Panel reactive antibody (PRA)
  - Assessment of the proportion of the donor population to which the recipient's antibodies will react
  - A recipient with no HLA antibodies is assigned a PRA of 0%
  - A highly sensitized patient, for example with a PRA of 80%, would be expected to be HLA incompatible with 80% of the donor population

8.3.3.4 HLA crossmatch

- Purpose is to detect pre-existing HLA donor-specific antibodies in the serum of the recipient
- Cell-dependent cytotoxicity crossmatch
  - Donor cells are isolated and separated into T & B cells
  - Donor cells & patient serum are mixed together
  - After incubation, complement is added; cells bound with anti-HLA antibody will lyse
  - Cell death indicates that the donor is incompatible with the recipient; transplantation could result in hyperacute rejection
  - Several variations of this technique exist to enhance sensitivity
- Flow cytometric crossmatch
  - Donor cells & patient serum are mixed together
  - After incubation the cells are washed to remove unbound sera
  - Fluorescently labeled antihuman IgG as well as antibodies to discriminate T & B cells are added
  - The amount of bound donor-specific HLA antibody is assessed with flow cytometry
  - This represents the most sensitive HLA crossmatch technique

8.3.4 HLA matching for transplantation

8.3.4.1 Solid organ

- Match ABO
- Avoid donor-specific HLA antibodies

8.3.4.2 Hematopoietic stem cell transplantation

- Determine high-resolution HLA match status at a minimum of 4 loci (HLA-A, B, C, DRB1)
- Minimum HLA matching criteria for unrelated stem cell transplantation is 7 of 8 alleles
- Haploidentical (4 of 8 alleles) transplant may be used for related donor transplantation
- HLA mismatches between donor and recipient can lead to graft-vs-host disease
- Donor & recipient do not necessarily need to be ABO compatible

8.3.5 Solid organ transplant rejection

- Also referred to as host-vs-graft disease (HVGD)
- The host immune system attacks the transplanted organ

8.3.5.1 Hyperacute rejection

- Occurs within minutes to hours of transplantation
- Mediated by preformed high titer antibodies to ABO or HLA antigens expressed by donor graft endothelium
- Immunoglobulin is deposited along vessel walls, inducing complement-mediated vascular injury
- The result is the formation of fibrin & platelet thrombi, causing ischemic necrosis

8.3.5.2 Acute cellular rejection (ACR)

- Evolves over days to weeks after transplantation
- Mediated primarily by cytotoxic T cells
- Recipient T cells recognize foreign HLA antigens and stimulate a powerful cellular cytotoxic response

8.3.5.3 Acute humoral rejection (AHR)

- Presents within days to weeks after transplantation
- Mediated by donor-specific HLA antibodies
- Like hyperacute rejection, the endothelium is the primary target
- Depending on the organ involved, immunohistochemistry may reveal deposition of C4d in vessel walls

8.3.5.4 Chronic rejection

- Presents months to years after transplantation
- Often includes both antibody & cell-mediated components
- Eventually leads to graft failure
- Histologic findings include interstitial fibrosis, narrowing and arteriolosclerosis of vessels, and complement deposits in peritubular vessels

8.3.6 Transplant-associated graft-vs-host disease (GVHD)

- This occurs when donor lymphocytes react with the host tissue, proliferating and damaging the host tissue
- GVHD occurs most commonly in hematopoietic stem cell transplants and can be life threatening
- Can occur in solid organ transplants when graft contains large numbers of carrier lymphocytes

8.3.6.1 Requisites for the development of GVHD

- Immunocompetent donor T cells
- Immunosuppressed recipient
- Antigenic differences between donor & recipient

ISBN 978-089189-6616

8.3.6.2 Classification of GVHD based on severity

- Acute GVHD
  - Occurs within the first 100 days after transplantation
  - Primary targets include skin, intestinal tract, hepatobiliary tract
- Chronic GVHD
  - Occurs after the first 100 days
  - Affects skin, hepatobiliary tract, intestinal tract, and the mucosa of the mouth, vagina, eye, and respiratory tract
  - Leads to cutaneous sclerosis, esophageal strictures, bronchiolitis obliterans, scarring ocular lesions, and chronic liver damage

8.3.7 Tumor immunology

8.3.7.1 Cellular transformation

- Involves loss of normal controls over cell division & longevity resulting from DNA damage
- Point mutations, insertions, deletions, translocations
- Benign: When the cancer does not spread to other tissues
- Malignant: When it spreads to other tissues and potentially other sites in the body
- Oncogenes drive abnormal cell proliferation

8.3.7.2 Immune surveillance

- Process of the immune system to detect and destroy neoplastically transformed cells
- Success depends on cancer cells expressing antigens not found on normal cells
  - Oncogenic viral proteins (eg, Epstein-Barr virus [EBV], human papilloma virus [HPV], hepatitis B virus [HBV])
  - Inappropriately expressed host cells (eg, melanoma-associated antigen [MAGE], human epidermal growth factor receptor 2 [HER2])
  - Altered proteins caused by somatic mutation in host genes

8.3.7.3 Immunoediting

- Elimination
  - Innate & adaptive immune system detect and destroy tumors before they are clinically visible
- Equilibrium
  - Tumor cells begin to evade the immune system
  - Tumor cells are unstable and rapidly mutating
  - Longest phase of tumor progression
  - Tumor cells undergo selective pressure, creating more resistant variants
- Escape
  - Immune system fails to restrict tumor growth
  - Evade immune recognition through, eg, loss of tumor antigens, major histocompatibility complex (MHC), or costimulatory molecules
  - Increased expression of survival & immunosuppression markers
  - Cytokine production to enhance angiogenesis

8.3.7.4 Tumor suppressor genes

- Two-hit hypothesis: Both alleles of the gene must be affected before gene product function is lost
  - DNA surveillance & repair
  - Inhibition of cell cycle progression
  - Induction of apoptosis
  - Regulation of the cellular environment to prevent unregulated proliferation
- Retinoblastoma protein (pRb): Prevents cell cycle progression from G1 into S phase to prevent replication of damaged DNA
- p53: DNA repair, inducing apoptosis, transcription, cell cycle regulation
- BCL2: Family of proteins involved in induction or inhibition of apoptosis through maintenance of mitochondrial membrane

8.3.7.5 Tumor antigens

- Protein or other molecule found only in cancer and not on normal cells
- Useful in both diagnosis & therapy
- Can help immune system in mounting immune response against cancer
- Tumor-associated antigens: Relatively restricted to tumor cells

- Tumor-specific antigens: Unique to tumor cells
- Carcinoembryonic antigen (CEA)
  - Normally produced only in early fetal development
  - Bowel cancers, occasionally lung or breast cancer
- α-fetoprotein (AFP)
  - Glycoprotein produced in early fetal life by liver
  - Testicular, ovarian & hepatocellular carcinoma
  - Elevated levels can occur with benign liver disease & gastrointestinal tumors
  - Failure of AFP to return to normal within 1 month of surgery suggests residual tumor
- *MUC-1* gene encoded antigens
  - Frequently produced by carcinoma of the breast
  - Large molecular weight glycoproteins with O-linked oligosaccharide chains
  - Include NAM6, milk mucin antigen, cancer antigen (CA) 27.29 and CA 15-3
- Cancer antigen 125 (CA-125)
  - Ovarian cancer
  - Not predictive enough to use for cancer screening
  - Used to monitor therapy response
- Prostate-specific antigen (PSA)
  - Produced by both normal & malignant cells of the prostate gland
  - Levels are usually elevated in men with prostate cancer
  - Basis of test for screening & therapy monitoring of prostate cancer
- Programmed death ligand (PD-L1)
  - Immune checkpoint proteins important for T-cell self-tolerance
  - Overexpressed by some cancer cells to evade immune T-cell attack, eg, non-small cell lung cancer (NSCLC), melanoma, urothelial carcinoma
  - Demonstrated therapeutic target
- Human epidermal growth factor receptor 2 (HER-2)
  - Expression is frequently increased in breast cancer
  - Promotes the growth of cancer cells
  - Associated with high risk for relapse & shortened survival
- Melanoma-associated antigen (MAGE)
  - Protein family, mostly restricted to expression in reproductive tissue
  - Expressed in a wide variety of cancer types
  - Oncogenic activity

8.3.7.6 Immunotherapy

- Stimulation of immune system to treat cancer
- Exploits the presence of either normal or tumor antigens
- Antibody therapy
  - Alemtuzumab: Anti-CD52 monoclonal binds to peripheral blood lymphocytes, for treatment of CD52 positive lymphomas and leukemias such as chronic lymphocytic leukemia (CLL)
  - Ipilimumab: Anti-CTLA4 to prevent negative regulation of T cells by melanoma cells
  - Nuvolumab: Anti-programmed cell death ligand 1 (PDL-1) binds to cancer cells, preventing T-cell inactivation in advanced melanoma, metastatic renal cell carcinoma, advanced lung cancer, etc
  - Rituximab: Anti-CD20, targets mature B cells, for the treatment of certain B-cell malignancies
- Dendritic cell therapy
  - Aids in cancer targeting
  - Sipuleucel-T: Dendritic cells are collected from prostate cancer patient through leukapheresis, incubated with fusion protein of antigen prostatic acid phosphatase and granulocyte-macrophage colony-stimulating factor (GM-CSF), then reinfused into the patient
- Chimeric antigen receptor (CAR) T-cell therapy
  - Modifies T cells to recognize cancer cells
  - Tisagenlecleucel: Chimeric T-cell receptor that targets CD19-positive B cells for treatment of acute lymphocytic leukemia (ALL)
- Cytokine therapy
  - Stimulates the immune system
  - Interleukins (ILs) such as IL-2 are used to treat malignant melanoma and renal cell carcinoma
  - Interferons (IFNs) such as IFN-α for melanoma, hairy cell leukemia, chronic myeloid leukemia (CML)
- Success limited by plasticity of the cells, which will decrease expression of targeted antigens
- Combination therapies
  - Goal is synergistic response
  - Combines multiple therapeutic modalities, eg, ablation therapy, checkpoint immunotherapies, immunostimulatory drugs

ISBN 978-089189-6616

8.4 Infectious disease

8.4.1 *Treponema pallidum* stages of infection

- Causative agent of syphilis (see Microbiology 6.1.6.6.1)

8.4.1.1 Primary syphilis

- One week to 3 months after initial exposure
- Chancre formation usually at the site of entry
  - Painless ulceration most often on genitalia
  - After 4-6 weeks, it heals by itself without any other symptoms

8.4.1.2 Secondary syphilis

- If left untreated, 25% of primary cases develop second stage within 1-6 months
- This is the most contagious stage
- Symptoms include enlarged lymph nodes, fever, loss of weight, sore throat, headaches, stiffness in head & neck, light sensitivity, overall discomfort or illness

8.4.1.3 Latent stage

- Follows secondary syphilis
- No symptoms
- Early & late stages
  - In utero infection can occur
  - Spontaneous abortion, stillbirth, premature birth, death of newborn
- Following untreated latent-stage syphilis ~50% develop tertiary syphilis
  - Occurs as early as 1 year after initial exposure, more typically decades later
  - Gummas, a type of granuloma, form throughout the body as a result of unsuccessful immune reaction to clear organism

8.4.1.4 Tertiary syphilis

- Cardiac abnormalities, including ruptured aneurysms & heart failure are common causes of death
- Gradual degeneration of neurons: "general paralysis of the insane"

8.4.2 *Treponema pallidum* identification

8.4.2.1 Direct visualization

- Dark field microscopy (rarely performed)
  - Requires live, motile organisms from active lesions
  - Requires expeditious & careful processing
  - Other treponemes may be detected

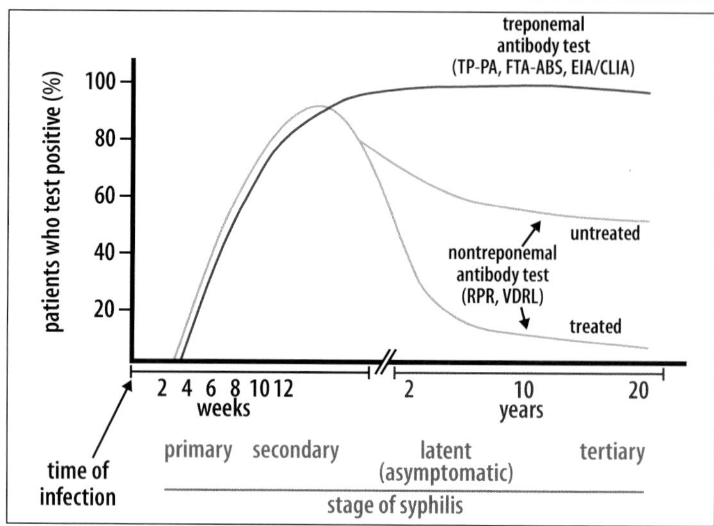

f8.17 Typical course of antibody patterns in syphilis

- Fluorescent antibody detection
  - Detection using antibody to *T pallidum*
  - Can be either direct or indirect labeling technique
  - Does not require live specimens
  - Monoclonal antibodies may cross-react

8.4.2.2 Nontreponemal serologic tests

- Include the VDRL and rapid plasma reagin (RPR) tests
- Nonspecific screening tests that detect IgM and IgG anti-cardiolipin antibodies (aka reagin) arising from cardiolipin release from damaged cells
- Antigen complex used in testing includes cardiolipin, lecithin & cholesterol
- Based on flocculation reactions, antigen clumps together in positive reaction
- High sensitivity, low specificity
- Antibodies detectable 1-4 weeks after appearance of primary chancre
- Titers decline in response to therapy & late latent syphilis
- False-negative tests can occur during secondary syphilis, when extremely high titers may cause a prozone (hook affect)
- False positives occur with hepatitis, herpesvirus infections, measles, malaria, leprosy, Lyme disease, autoimmune diseases, pregnancy, connective tissue diseases
- Typical course of both nontreponemal & treponemal antibody patterns are shown in **f8.17**

8.4.2.3 Nontreponemal VDRL test

- Qualitative & quantitative microscopic flocculation assay
- Acceptable for both serum & spinal fluid

- It is the only test used to analyze cerebrospinal fluid (CSF) for neurosyphilis
- Antigen for test prepared daily
- Serum heated at 132.8°F (56°C) for 30 minutes to inactivate complement prior to test
- Test must be performed at a room temperature with the range of 23°C to 29°C
- Slide is read microscopically

8.4.2.4 Nontreponemal RPR test

- Modification of VDRL test involving macroscopic agglutination
- Cardiolipin-coated charcoal particles
- Reagents stable for up to 3 months after opening
- Serum treatment to inactivate complement is not necessary
- Test performed and read on plastic-coated cards

8.4.2.5 Treponemal serologic tests

- Detect anti-*T pallidum* organism or specific treponemal antigens
- Usually positive before nontreponemal tests
- 100% reactive in secondary & latent syphilis, remains positive for life
- Highly specific for syphilis, used for confirmatory testing
- Not appropriate for congenital syphilis or neurosyphilis due to lack of sensitivity
- Fluorescent treponemal antibody adsorption (FTA-ABS)
  - Heat-inactivated serum samples are adsorbed with nonpathogenic strains of *Treponema* (Reiter strain) to remove cross-reactive antibodies
  - Incubate test serum with Nichols strain of *T pallidum* on test slides
  - Add fluorescent labeled antihuman immunoglobulin
  - Fluorescence intensity reported on scale of 0 to 4+, with 0 being negative and 2+ or higher reported as reactive
  - A beaded pattern is indicative of a false positive result in patients with systemic lupus erythematosus (SLE)
- *T pallidum* hemagglutination assay (TPHA)
  - Classic agglutination test, manual
  - RBCs coated with *T pallidum* antigens
  - Gel particles can be used instead of RBCs
- Microhemagglutination assay for *T pallidum* antibody (MHA-TP)
  - Sheep RBCs coated with *T pallidum* antigen
- *T pallidum* particle agglutination (TP-PA) test
  - Patient serum or plasma is incubated with colored gelatin particles coated with treponemal antigens in microtiter plates
  - Presence of antitreponemal antibodies results in formation of mat covering the surface of the well

8.4.2.6 Enzyme immunoassays (EIAs) for *T pallidum*

- Competitive
  - *T pallidum* antigen is bound to well
  - Patient treponemal antibody competes with enzyme-labeled antitreponemal antibody
- Immune capture
  - Wells coated with anti-IgM or IgG
  - Patient serum added
  - Enzyme labeled *T pallidum* antigen added
  - Useful for diagnosis of congenital syphilis (IgM)
- Sandwich
  - Patient antibodies bind to *T pallidum*-coated wells
  - Enzyme-labeled antibody or antigen is added to detect binding

8.4.3 *Borrelia burgdorferi* stages of infection

- Causative agent of Lyme disease (see Microbiology 6.1.6.6.2)
- Common tickborne disease transmitted to humans by deer tick

8.4.3.1 First stage

- Most cases involve localized rash, erythema migrans (EM)
- Appears between 2 days and 2 weeks after bite
- Patient may be otherwise asymptomatic
- Rash fades within 3-4 weeks
- Most patients are negative on serologic testing; antibody response takes up to 6 weeks

8.4.3.2 Second stage

- Spread to multiple organ systems via the bloodstream
- Without treatment neurologic or cardiac involvement may develop

8.4.3.3 Late stage

- Occurs in a subset of untreated patients, months to years after infection
- Symptoms are numerous & diverse; include arthritis, peripheral neuropathy & encephalomyelitis
- Normally responses well to antibiotics

ISBN 978-089189-6616

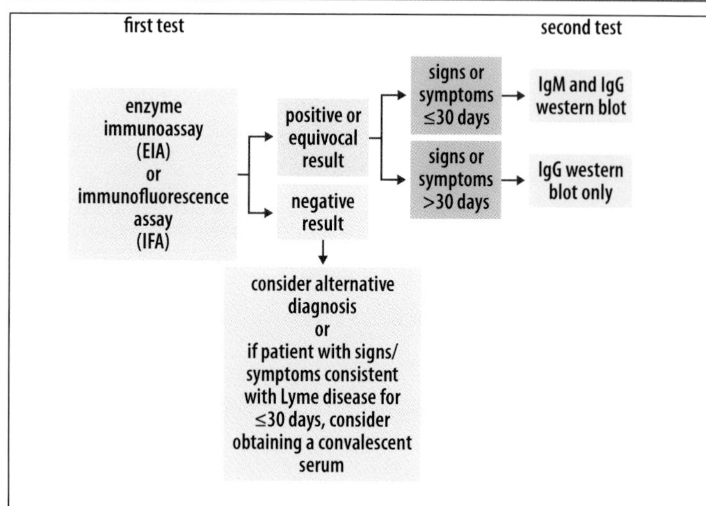

f8.18 Centers for Disease Control and Prevention recommendations for testing for Lyme disease

8.4.4 *Borrelia burgdorferi* identification

8.4.4.1 Early stages of infection

- Antibody response may take up to 6 weeks to develop
- Diagnosis is based on clinical symptoms
- Early treatment includes a course of antibiotics when the EM rash is seen
- In early stage, false-negative results on serologic testing are >30%

8.4.4.2 Later stages of infection

- Screen with immunofluorescence assay (IFA) or EIA test
- IFA
  - Commercially prepared slides coated with antigen
  - Incubated with doubling dilutions of patient serum
  - Antibody is detected with antihuman globulin conjugated with fluorescent tag
  - Cross-reactivity with similar microorganisms
- EIA
  - Mixture of *Borrelia* antigens is coated to wells or strips
  - Incubated with patient serum
  - Antibody is detected with antihuman globulin conjugated with enzyme tag
- The Centers for Disease Control and Prevention (CDC) recommend initial EIA or IFA followed by specific Western blot testing for confirmation of disease as shown in **f8.18**

8.4.4.3 Confirm positives with western blot (immunoblot)

- Nitrocellulose *Borrelia* antigen strips are reacted with patient serum
- Anti-*Borrelia* antibody is detected with antihuman globulin (IgM or IgG)
- Assesses antibody to specific *Borrelia* antigens
- Reactivity is scored to 10 proteins using a complex algorithm
- The CDC defines positive as:
  - At least 2 of 3 critical IgM bands reactive on strip
  - At least 5 of 10 critical IgG bands reactive on strip

8.4.4.4 Confirm positives with polymerase chain reaction (PCR)

- Detects genetic material from *Borrelia burgdorferi*
- Very specific, no cross-reactivity issues
- PCR is used only when diagnosis is very difficult
- Not approved for routine testing

8.4.5 Babesiosis

- Babesiosis is caused by apicomplexan parasites of the genus *Babesia*
  - Although more than 100 *Babesia* species have been reported, relatively few have caused documented cases of human infection, eg, *B microti*, *B divergens*, and *B duncani*

8.4.5.1 The *Babesia microti* life cycle **f8.19**

- Involves 2 hosts
  - Rodent, primarily the white-footed mouse, *Peromyscus leucopus*
  - Tick in the genus *Ixodes*
- *Babesia*-infected tick introduces sporozoites into the mouse host during a blood meal
- Sporozoites enter erythrocytes
  - Asexual reproduction (budding) occurs within erythrocytes
- In the blood, some parasites differentiate into male & female gametes, although they are indistinguishable by light microscopy
- The definitive host is the tick
  - Once ingested by an appropriate tick, gametes unite and generate sporozoites via a sporogonic cycle
  - Vertical, or hereditary, transmission has only been documented for large *Babesia* species not for *B microti*

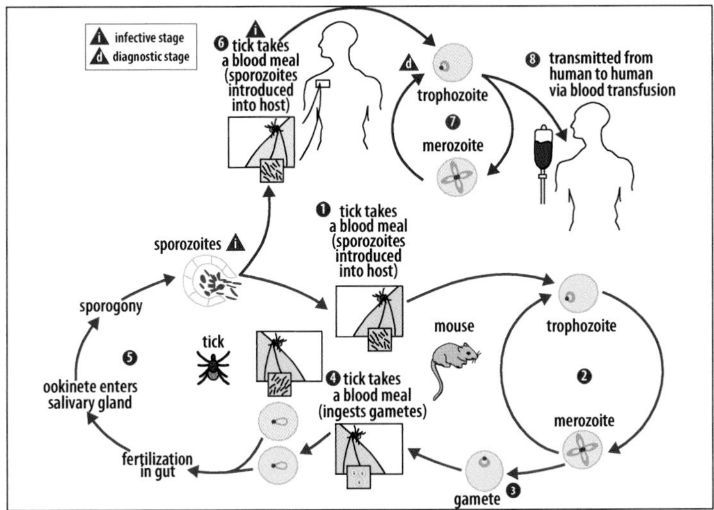

f8.19 Life cycle of in babesiosis

- Humans enter the cycle when bitten by infected ticks
  - During a blood meal, a *Babesia*-infected tick introduces sporozoites into the human host
  - Sporozoites enter erythrocytes
    - Asexual replication (budding) occurs
    - Multiplication of the blood-stage parasites is responsible for the clinical manifestations of the disease
  - Humans are naturally dead-end hosts
    - Blood transfusions with contaminated blood result in human-to-human transmission

8.4.5.2 Diagnosis

- Examine blood specimens under microscope to observe parasites inside red blood cells
- Antibody tests may be useful in indivuduals with very low levels of parasitemia
- IFA detects antibodies in 88%-96% of patients with *B microti* infection; cross reactivity may occur in patients with malaria infections

8.4.6 *Herpesviridae* & other serologically diagnosed viruses (see Microbiology 6.6.4)

8.4.6.1 Human herpesviruses (HHV)

- DNA viruses
- Capable of establishing latent infection
- Lifelong persistence in the host; capable of opportunistic reactivation

8.4.6.2 Herpes simplex virus 1 (HSV-1) (see Microbiology 6.6.4.1)

- Primarily oral herpes, can also cause genital herpes
- Rarely encephalitis or keratitis
- Viral culture has low sensitivity, not appropriate for CSF or late lesions
- Serologic testing is approved by the US Food and Drug Administration (FDA) but may show false-negative results in immunocompromised individuals
- Molecular testing is sensitive & specific and can differentiate between HSV-1 and HSV-2

8.4.6.3 Herpes simplex virus 2 (HSV-2) (see Microbiology 6.6.4.1)

- Primarily genital herpes, can also cause oral herpes
- Neonatal herpes
- Viral culture has low sensitivity, not appropriate for CSF or late lesions
- Serologic testing is FDA approved but may have false-negative results in immunocompromised individuals
- Molecular testing is sensitive & specific and can differentiate between HSV-1 and HSV-2

8.4.6.4 Varicella zoster virus (VZV, HHV-3) (see Microbiology 6.6.4.2)

- Causative agent for varicella (chickenpox) & herpes zoster (shingles)
- Primary infection results in varicella and is characterized by blisterlike itchy rash & fever
- Infection is usually self-limiting in healthy children, though complications such as bacterial infection and central nervous system (CNS) infection can occur
- Infection in adults, neonates & pregnant women are more severe
- Infection during the first trimester of pregnancy can result in congenital malformations
- Immunocompromised individuals may develop disseminated disease, including neurologic conditions, pneumonia, hepatitis, and nephritis
- Virus remains latent in sensory neurons where it can reactivate & cause herpes zoster

ISBN 978-089189-6616

- Primary route of transmission is inhalation of respiratory secretions or aerosols from skin lesions
- Vaccine for varicella was introduced in 1995 and since then US infection rates have continued to decline
- Vaccine for persons aged ≥60 years was introduced in 2006 for prevention of herpes zoster
- Infection diagnosed by direct immunofluorescence, viral culture, serology, molecular
  - Viral culture to detect cytopathic effect takes >1 week to yield results and has low sensitivity
  - Antibody testing
    - High-titer IgM indicates acute infection
    - IgG titer is used to determine immunity to VZV
    - Compare IgG titers to standard reference serum
  - PCR is sensitive & specific and does not require live organism

8.4.6.5 Epstein-Barr virus (EBV, HHV-4) (see Microbiology 6.6.4.4)

- Implicated in infectious mononucleosis, Burkitt lymphoma, nasopharyngeal carcinoma, and post-transplantation lymphoproliferative disease (PTLD)
- Most common route of transmission is salivary secretions
- Infection usually occurs during childhood, with seroprevalence of 95% in adults
- Mononucleosis spot test
  - Serologic test in which patient's serum specimen is mixed with sheep or horse RBC; agglutination represents presumptive positivity for mononucleosis
  - Detects heterophile antibodies
  - Largely replaced by more sensitive methods; not recommended by the CDC for general use
  - May indicate infectious mononucleosis, but does not confirm EBV infection
- Mononucleosis differentiation test
  - Differentially diagnose patients with infectious mononucleosis vs serum sickness or Forssman antibodies
  - Two types of heterophile antibodies, Forssman & non-Forssman
  - Infectious mononucleosis is caused by production of non-Forssman heterophile antibodies
  - Serum is mixed with 2 different antigen suspensions, guinea pig kidney antigen & beef red blood cell stroma; then tested with horse RBC
  - Agglutination occurs in serum mixed with guinea pig kidney antigen in infectious mononucleosis
  - Recent modifications of test use antigen-coated beads or immune-chromatographic strips in place of RBC
- EBV antigen-specific serologic tests
  - Antiviral capsid antigen (VCA), IgM, and IgG
  - Anti-early antigen (EA)
  - Anti-EBV nuclear antigen (EBNA)
  - A summary of serologic responses at different stages of infection is provided in **t8.7**

t8.7 Serologic responses of patients with EBV-associated disease

Condition	Anti-VCA			Anti-EA			
	IgM	IgG	IgA	EA-D	EA-R	Anti-EBNA	IgM*
Uninfected	–	–	–	–	–	–	–
Acute IM	+	++	±	+	–	–	±
Convalescent IM	–	+	–	–	±	+	±
Past infection IM	–	+	–	–	–	+	–
Chronic active infection IM	–	+++	±	+	++	±	–
Post-transplant lymphoproliferative disease	–	++	±	+	+	±	–
Burkitt lymphoma	–	+++	–	±	++	+	–
Nasopharyngeal carcinoma	–	+++	+	++	±	+	–

**Heterophile antibody*

8.4.6.6 Cytomegalovirus (CMV, HHV-5) (see Microbiology 6.6.4.3)

- Self-limiting disease in healthy individuals
- After initial infection, remains latent in the body, re-emerging later with compromised immune system
- Disease involving gastrointestinal tract, CNS, and hematologic abnormalities in immunocompromised individuals
- Ubiquitous, with seroprevalence from 40%-100% depending on the population
- Broad transmission routes
- The presence of virus may be found by viral culture, identification of CMV antigens, or PCR
  - Viral culture cytopathic effect may take a few days to several weeks; shell vial method uses rapid centrifugation to reduce detection time to <24 hours
  - Antigenemia tests use immunocytochemical or immunofluorescent staining to detect CMV lower matrix protein pp65
  - Viral culture & antigenemia have been replaced by real-time PCR in many laboratories, which can also be used to monitor response to therapy
- Serologic testing for IgM or IgG distinguishes acute infection, reactivation, or immunity
  - Typically performed with EIA
  - Frequently used to screen blood, stem cell & solid organ donors

8.4.6.7 Rubella (see Microbiology 6.6.15)

- Single-stranded RNA virus, member of the *Togoviridae* family
- Also known as German measles
- Generally benign infection except in the case of pregnant women
- Infection in pregnant woman can lead to miscarriage, stillbirth or congenital rubella syndrome, with risk highest in the first trimester
- Congenital rubella syndrome may include deafness, eye defects, cardiac abnormalities, and others
- Vaccine is included in routine childhood immunization schedules, thus incidence is low
- Detected on viral culture, viral protein by IFA or EIA, or reverse transcriptase PCR
- Antibodies to rubella are detected on hemagglutination inhibition, latex agglutination, or EIA
    - IgM or 4-fold rise in IgG titers in samples collected 10-14 days apart indicates acute infection
    - IgM antibodies appear ~5 days after onset of rash
- Antibody testing commonly used for women of childbearing age to determine immune status and need to vaccinate

8.4.6.8 Rubeola (see Microbiology 6.6.11.2; Molecular 9.3.3)

- Single-stranded RNA virus, member of *Paramyxoviridae* family
- Causative agent for measles
- Several genetically distinct strains, but only 1 is pathogenetic
- Systemic infection with symptoms during prodromal period mimicking the common cold with the presence of Koplik spots on the mucous membranes, with rash appearing around day 14 after exposure
- Can rarely cause fatal subacute sclerosing panencephalitis (SSPE), resulting from persistent virus replication in the brain
- Can cause complications of pregnancy, including spontaneous abortion, premature labor & low birth weight
- Transmitted by respiratory droplets
- Vaccine is included in routine childhood immunization schedules, thus incidence is low
- Presence of virus may be detected by culture or PCR using nasal or throat swab
- EIA is used to test for measles antibodies to determine immune status
    - IgM antibodies present with acute infection
    - 4-fold increase in IgG between acute & convalescent sera

8.4.6.9 Mumps (see Microbiology 6.6.11.3; Molecular 9.3.4)

- Single-stranded RNA virus, member of Paramyxoviridae family
- Systemic infection, with inflammation of the parotid glands occurring in 30%-40% of cases
- Infection in pregnant women increases fetal death risk in the first trimester of pregnancy
- Transmitted by respiratory droplets, saliva & fomites
- Vaccine is included in routine childhood immunization schedules, thus incidence is low
- Preferred sample source for virus detection is buccal swab or saliva samples collected within 3 days of onset of symptoms
- Viral culture is the gold standard for detecting mumps virus, and molecular testing is becoming the primary method in most laboratories
- Viral genotyping may be performed for outbreak tracking
- Antibody testing to confirm current infection are usually EIA based
    - IgM antibodies can be detected within 3-4 days of onset of symptoms; negative result does not rule out mumps infection
    - IgG antibodies can be detected within 7-10 days; 4-fold increase in IgG between specimens collected in acute & convalescence phases

8.4.6.10 West Nile virus (WNV) (see Microbiology 6.6.16; Molecular 9.3.4)

- RNA virus, member of the *Flaviviridae* family
- Transmitted from infected birds via mosquitos; leading cause of mosquito-borne disease in the United States
- One in 5 infected individuals will become symptomatic with fever, joint pain, etc
- One in 150 infected individuals develop severe illness such as encephalitis or meningitis; ~1 in 10 of these individuals will die
- No vaccination available for humans
- Diagnostic testing is most commonly performed on serum or CSF specimens for WNV-specific IgM antibodies, which develop 3-8 days after onset of illness and persist for 30-90 days; may cross-react with other flaviviruses
- The presence of IgG antibodies alone indicates previous infection
- IgG test is performed on CSF when encephalitis or meningitis occurs
- Viral culture, reverse transcriptase (RT) PCR, and IHC tests are also available
- Nucleic acid testing (NAT) is performed on all blood products before release

8.4.6.11 Human influenza virus (see Microbiology 6.6.10.1)

- Enveloped RNA respiratory virus belongs to the Orthomyxoviridae family
- Three types, based on hemagglutinin & neuraminidase surface proteins, known to infect humans (types A, B, C)
- Type A and type B cause seasonal epidemics; type A is associated with global pandemics of flu
- Most cases are mild, but flu complications, including pneumonia, bronchitis, sinus & ear infections, and sometimes death, may occur
- Seasonal influenza vaccines include both type A and type B viruses
- Antibody testing is not recommended because of the seasonal nature of influenza
- Acceptable specimens include nasopharyngeal (NP) swab, aspirate, wash, sputum
- Various tests available, including direct & indirect immunofluorescence, viral culture, shell vial, rapid antigen detection, RT-PCR
- Rapid influenza tests detect influenza antigens in respiratory specimens; low sensitivity & specificity

8.4.6.12 Human coronavirus (see Microbiology 6.6.11.14; Molecular 9.3.4)

- Common human coronaviruses
  - Subdivided into α, β, γ, and δ based on crownlike spikes on the virus surface
  - Humans are known to be infected by coronavirus 229E, NL63, OC43, HKU1
  - Worldwide infection is common & generally mild
- Middle East respiratory syndrome (MERS)
  - Caused by the coronavirus MERS-CoV
  - Respiratory virus emerged in Fall 2012 in or near the Arabian Peninsula
  - The risk of contracting MERS in the United States is low
  - Spreads through close contact
  - Causes severe respiratory illness as well as diarrhea and nausea/vomiting in a subset of individuals
  - Approximately 3-4 of every 10 individuals with MERS have died, most commonly, individuals with pre-existing medical conditions
  - RT-PCR tests are available for diagnosis
  - Serologic tests are primarily used for disease surveillance
- Severe acute respiratory syndrome (SARS)
  - Caused by the coronavirus SARS-CoV
  - Respiratory virus emerged in Asia in the Spring of 2003 and became a global outbreak
  - No known cases since 2004 laboratory-acquired infections
  - Spreads through close contact
  - Available laboratory tests include RT-PCR and EIA for respiratory, blood & stool specimens
  - Positive predictive value of testing is low in current environment
- COVID-19 (see Molocular 9.3.4)
  - Caused by the coronavirus SARS-CoV-2
  - Respiratory virus emerged as global pandemic in the Fall of 2019
  - Special precautions, as outlined by the CDC, should be taken during specimen collection
  - Viral tests of respiratory specimens are recommended to diagnose acute infection
  - RT-PCR tests are the predominant viral test
  - Because of the newness of the virus, antibody results should not be used to determine an individual's immune status

8.4.6.13 TORCH panel

- *TO*xoplasma, *R*ubella, *C*MV, *H*SV
- Detects the presence of antibodies to infectious diseases that can cause illness in pregnant women and may cause birth defects
- Infants tested at birth for IgG antibodies will exhibit the mother's antibodies
- Infants tested at >6 months of age for IgG antibodies demonstrate postbirth infection
- Other infectious diseases may be included in the panel

8.4.7 *Mycobacterium tuberculosis* (see Microbiology 6.2.1.5)

8.4.7.1 Infection

- *M tuberculosis* is inhaled, enters macrophages, and is disseminated throughout the body
- Macrophages present mycobacterial antigens to CD4-positive T cells
- Th1 cells are generated and IFN-γ is released, activating macrophages
- Recruited monocytes & macrophages are converted to epithelioid histocytes, forming granuloma

8.4.7.2 Primary pulmonary tuberculosis

- Ghon focus develops as bacilli settle in lower part of upper lobe or upper part of lower lobe
- Ghon complex refers to the Ghon focus plus the regional draining lymph nodes where bacilli also drain

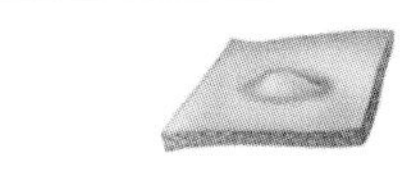

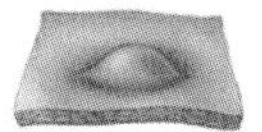

• recent contact with an active TB patient
• nodular or fibrotic changes on X-ray

• recent arrivals (<5 yrs) from high-prevalence countries

• resident/employee of high-risk congregate settings
• mycobacteriology lab personnel

• children <4 yrs old
• infants, children, and adolescents exposed to high-risk categories

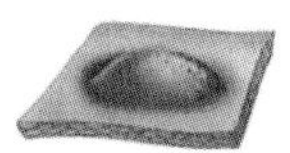
≥15 mm
• persons with no known risk factors for TB

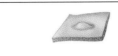

f8.20 Interpreting tuberculin thresholds

- Bacilli are effectively walled off and remain dormant
- Progressive primary tuberculosis will occur in immunocompromised patients, resulting in pneumonia as well as disseminated disease, including meningitis & miliary tuberculosis

8.4.7.3 Secondary TB

- Occurs in <5% of individuals with primary tuberculosis
- Occurs if an infected individual becomes immunocompromised
- Cavitation formation in the lung is a key feature

8.4.7.4 Tuberculin skin test (aka Mantoux test)

- Screening test to determine if an individual has been exposed to *M tuberculosis* or related organism
- Purified protein derivative (PPD): Soluble antigen from *M tuberculosis* cell wall
- PPD injected intradermally
    - The site is examined between 48 and 72 hours for induration resulting from cell-mediated delayed hypersensitivity reaction (type IV hypersensitivity) **f8.20**
- Positive results do not necessarily indicate active tuberculosis infection
- Persons who have received the bacillus Calmette-Guérin (BCG) vaccine for tuberculosis will have a positive reaction

8.4.7.5 Interferon-γ release assays (IGRAs)

- Test measures the release of interferon (IFN) γ by T cells stimulated with antigen to *M tuberculosis*
- Number of IFN-γ producing cells or amount of IFN-γ may be quantified

QuantiFERON-TB Gold In-Tube (QFT-GIT) assay: ELISA whole blood test measuring IFN-γ

T-SPOT.TB assay: Enzyme-linked immunospot assay measuring IFN-γ producing T cells

- Detects both latent & active tuberculosis infection
- Diagnosis of latent tuberculosis infection that may benefit from treatment
- Prior BCG vaccination does not interfere; sensitivity decreased in human immunodeficiency virus (HIV) infection

8.4.8 Acquired immunodeficiency

8.4.8.1 Human immunodeficiency virus

- Genus *Lentivirus*
- Single-stranded retrovirus
- Infects CD4-positive cells, CD4-positive T cells, monocytes, macrophages, dendritic cells, microglial brain cells
- Reverse transcriptase converts viral RNA to DNA

8.4.8.2 HIV antibodies

- Used for diagnosis
- Seroconversion occurs within 1-3 months after exposure
- Early antibody responses target Gag proteins (eg, p24)
- Limit viral replication
- Keep virus in check during early asymptomatic stage
- Late antibody responses are to viral envelope and some regulatory proteins

8.4.8.3 ELISA

- Screening test for HIV antibodies
- High sensitivity & high specificity
- Early testing detects antibodies against viral lysates from HIV-1 viruses
- Detects anti-HIV antibodies of different isotypes
- CDC requirements
    - A positive ELISA test result should be confirmed by a 2nd and 3rd identical ELISA test on the same individual
    - If 2 of 3 are positive, then a confirmatory Western blot must be carried out

8.4.8.4 Rapid tests

- Screening test for HIV antibodies
- Easy-to-perform qualitative immunoassays using lateral flow technology

ISBN 978-089189-6616

- Do not require laboratory equipment, technical staff, or complicated procedures
- Used for blood, plasma, oral exudates
- Performed where resources are scarce
- As sensitive as ELISA
- Always followed by confirmatory test

8.4.8.5 Confirmatory testing

- Western blot evaluates presence of antibodies to >1 viral component
- The CDC suggests reactivity against 2 viral components (p24, p31, gp41, gp120/160) be considered a positive confirmatory test
- If test shows some bands but less than suggested, it is an intermediate result
- Should be repeated at a later date
- Most intermediates test positive when retested later

8.4.8.6 Nucleic acid testing

- Reverse transcriptase polymerase chain reaction (RT-PCR) (see Molecular 9.3.4)
- Real-time qPCR (see Molecular 9.3.5)
- Very sensitive, can detect all subtypes of HIV
- Allows measurement of viral load
- Assesses success or failure of treatment

8.4.9 Hepatitis

8.4.9.1 Hepatitis A virus (HAV) (see Microbiology 6.6.9.1)

- Not chronic
- Antibody is protective so reinfection does not occur
- Recovery is nearly 100%
- Physical signs/symptoms of hepatitis are quite similar regardless of the virus
- Laboratory diagnosis is very important for treatment & prognosis
- Reportable infection
- National surveillance
- Screen for IgM antibody to HAV using IgM capture technique
- Test for total anti-HAV antibody using indirect enzyme immunoassays

8.4.9.2 Hepatitis B virus (HBV) (see Microbiology 6.6.9.2)

- Acute & chronic infections
- Antibody is protective against reinfection
- Reportable infection

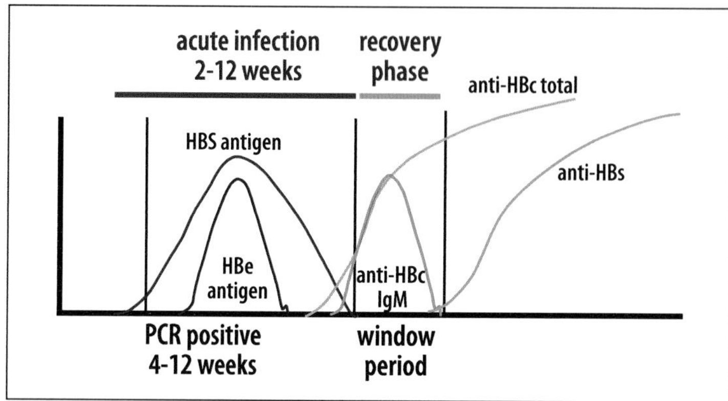

f8.21 Typical infection course for hepatitis B virus (HBV)

- Virus structure
  - Partially double-stranded circular DNA associated with polymerase
  - Surrounded by a nucleocapsid composed of the core protein (HBc)
  - Lipoprotein envelope containing the hepatitis B surface antigen (HBsAg)
  - Excess HBsAg exists in particles, known as the Australian antigen
  - Between nucleocapsid & lipoprotein envelope is the hepatitis B e antigen (HBeAg)
  - Hepatitis B surface Ag (HBsAg)
- Infection
  - Incubation period from 60-150 days
  - May take 6 months to clear the virus. Individuals with spontaneous recovery will test negative for HBsAg and HBV DNA at ~15 weeks after the appearance of symptoms
  - Typical course of infection & expected serologic results are presented in t8.8 & f8.21

t8.8 Interpretation of serologic results

HBsAg	anti-HBc	IgM anti-HbC	anti-HBs	Interpretation
–	–		–	Susceptible
–	+		+	Immune due to natural infection
–	–		+	Immune due to hepatitis B vaccination
+	+	+	–	Acutely infected
+	+	–	–	Chronically infected
–		+	–	Interpretation unclear; 4 possibilities: 1. Resolved infection (most common) 2. False-positive anti-HBc, thus susceptible 3."Low level" chronic infection 4. Resolving acute infection

- HBV IgM detection with EIA capture
  - IgM antibody captured by antihuman IgM
  - Hepatitis antigen is added
  - Enzyme-labeled antibody to the antigen is added
- Detected with direct competitive assays
  - Antigen is coated on plate
  - Patient serum (antibody) is added
  - Enzyme labeled (reagent) antibody is added
  - Patient antibody competes with kit antibody for binding antigen
- Hepatitis B surface antigen (HBsAg)
  - Produced in high levels during acute & chronic infection; presence indicates active infection
  - First serologic marker to appear in acute infection, detected weeks 1-9 of infection
  - This antigen is used to make HBV vaccine
- Hepatitis B surface antibody (anti-HBs)
  - Detectable after the disappearance
  - Disappearance of this marker is generally interpreted as recovered & immune; positive in vaccinated individuals
- Total hepatitis B core antibody (anti-HBc)
  - Appears during onset of symptoms and can occur during an acute flare in chronic HBV infection
  - Persists for life; may represent previous or ongoing infection
  - IgM anti-HBcAg and HBsAg are used for blood product screening
  - IgG anti-HBc remains positive and serves as a marker of past infection

8.4.9.3 Hepatitis D virus (HDV)

- Small circular single-stranded RNA
- Spread by percutaneous and, to a lesser extent, mucosal contact with blood or other body fluids
- Satellite virus: Requires coinfection or prior infection with HBV virus to replicate
- The term "superinfection" is applied to HDV infection occurring in an individual already having chronic HBV infection
- Uses envelope proteins of HBV to assemble into new particles and attach and enter new cells
- Causes acute or long-term infection; can lead to lifelong liver damage & death
- It is uncommon in the United States
- There is no vaccine for HDV; however, vaccination for HBV protects against future HDV infection

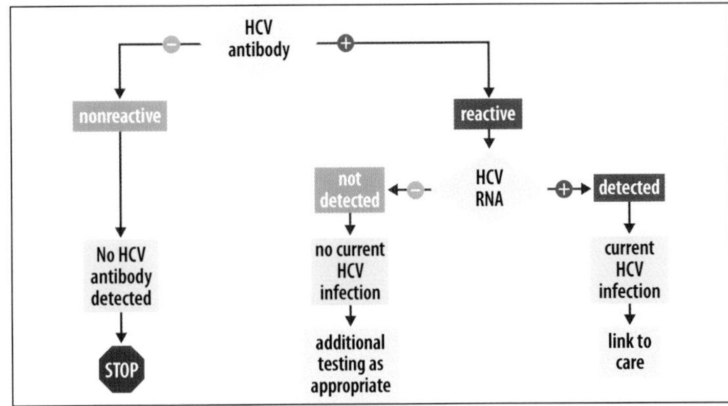

f8.22 Hepatitis C virus (HCV) testing algorithm recommended by the Centers for Disease Control (CDC)

8.4.9.4 Hepatitis C virus (HCV) (see Microbiology 6.6.9.3)

- RNA virus, 7 genotypes and at least 67 subtypes
- Spread by contact with blood from an infected person, previously as the result of blood or organ transplantation; currently most commonly by sharing needles
- Estimated 2.4 million people in the United States are HCV positive, with genotypes 1a, 1b, 2, and 3 being the most common
- In ~50% of infected individuals, the infection will spontaneously resolve
- For every 100 people infected with HCV, 5%-25% will develop cirrhosis within 10-20 years without treatment; cirrhosis patients have a 1%-4% annual risk for developing hepatocellular carcinoma
- There is no vaccine for HCV; effective treatments have recently become available
- The CDC recommends universal HCV screening for all US adults and all pregnant women during every pregnancy wherever HCV prevalence is >0.1% according to the algorithm presented in **f8.22**
- Screening tests for anti-HCV antibody
  - Available platforms include various EIA approaches, such as chemiluminescence and immunochro-matographic assay
  - False-negative results may occur after acute HCV infection before seroconversion or may occur in immunocompromised individuals
  - False-positive results occur because of cross-reactivity with other vial antigens or the presence of immunological disorders

ISBN 978-089189-6616

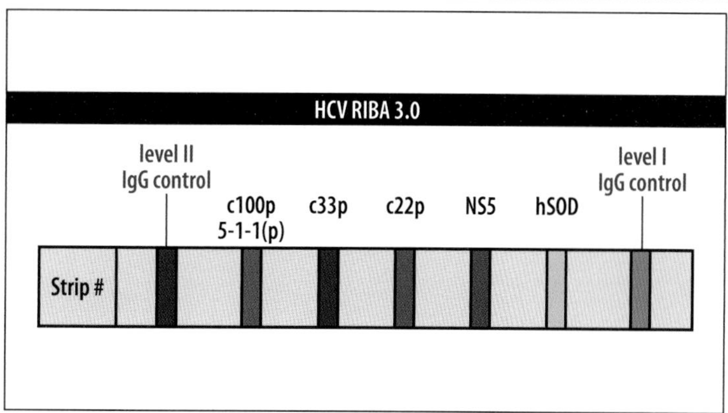

f8.23 Recombinant immunoblot assay (RIBA) to detect hepatitis C virus (HCV)–specific antibodies

- HCV confirmatory testing
  - HCV RNA nucleic acid tests (NAT); currently required
  - Recombinant immunoblot assay (RIBA); no longer available in the United States
    - Similarities with Western Blot
    - Recombinant antigens or synthetic peptides are applied to a nitrocellulose strip f8.23
    - Indirect enzyme immunoassay
    - Patient antibody binds to antigens
- HCV RNA nucleic acid tests (NAT)
  - Qualitative confirmatory tests include RT-PCR and transcription-mediated amplification (TMA)
  - Quantitative viral load
- HCV genotyping
  - Helpful to predict spontaneous clearance & therapy selection
  - Most tests target the 5' untranslated region of the viral genome
  - Molecular methods include reverse hybridization, RT-PCR, and sequencing
- HCV drug resistance testing
  - Detect mutations in HCV that provide resistance to direct-acting antivirals (DAAs)
  - Molecular methods include PCR sequencing

8.5 Serologic & molecular procedures (see chapter 9 Molecular Biology)

8.5.1 T-cell function

- T-cell subsets can be determined with flow cytometry
- Response to mitogenic proteins can be assessed using T-cell proliferation assays
  - Expose T cells to mitogens such as phytohemagglutinin or concanavalin A
  - Proliferation is measured by uptake of tritiated thymidine
- Tuberculin-type skin testing can assess delayed-type hypersensitivity

8.5.2 B-cell function

- Antibodies raised to protein antigens require orchestration of T- and B-cell function, whereas B cells are capable of autonomous production of antibody to carbohydrate antigen
- Poor response to a protein antigen such as tetanus or diphtheroid toxoid could indicate either a B cell or a T cell defect
- Poor reaction to carbohydrate antigens (pneumococcal or meningococcal vaccine) is indicative of a B-cell defect
- Abnormal immunoglobulin levels may indicate:
  - IgA is the most observed deficiency
  - IgG subclass deficiency is less frequent
  - Total IgE may be elevated in a subset of conditions, such as Job syndrome

8.5.3 NK-cell function

8.5.3.1 Chromium release assay

- Incubate target cells with ^{51}Cr
- Incubate target cells with effector T cells
- If effector cells kill target cells, ^{51}Cr will be released
- ^{51}Cr in lysate is measured in a gamma counter

8.5.3.2 Granzyme B (GrB) detection

- Serine protease present in granules of NK cells & cytotoxic T cells
- Test contains fluorescent substrate that is hydrolysable by granzyme B
- Results in release of quench of fluorescent group
- Detected fluorometrically

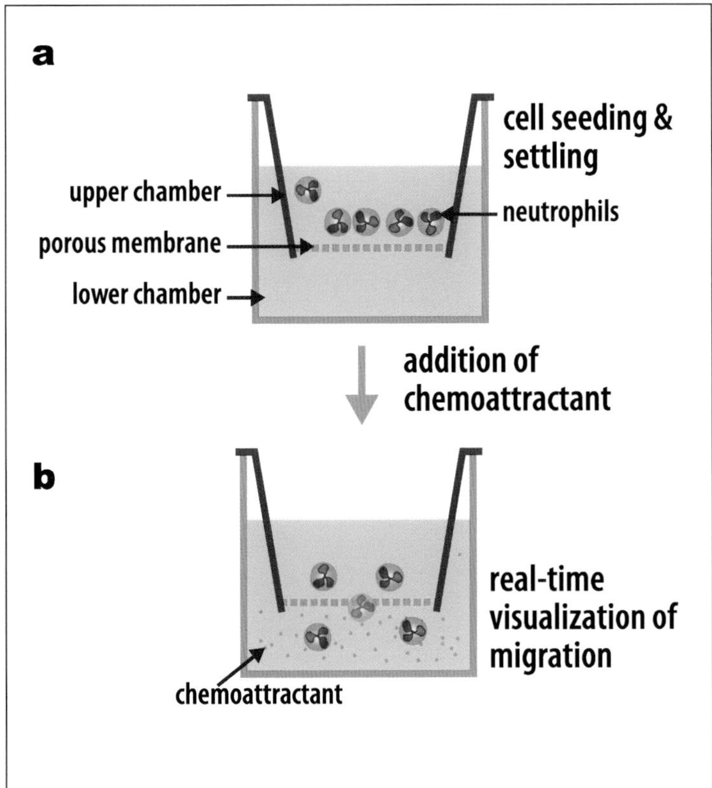

f8.24 Neutrophil chemotaxis; **a** cells are seeded onto insert of upper chamber of well on porous membrane; **b** chemoattractant is added to lower chamber; real-time visualization of migration is captured by live cell imaging

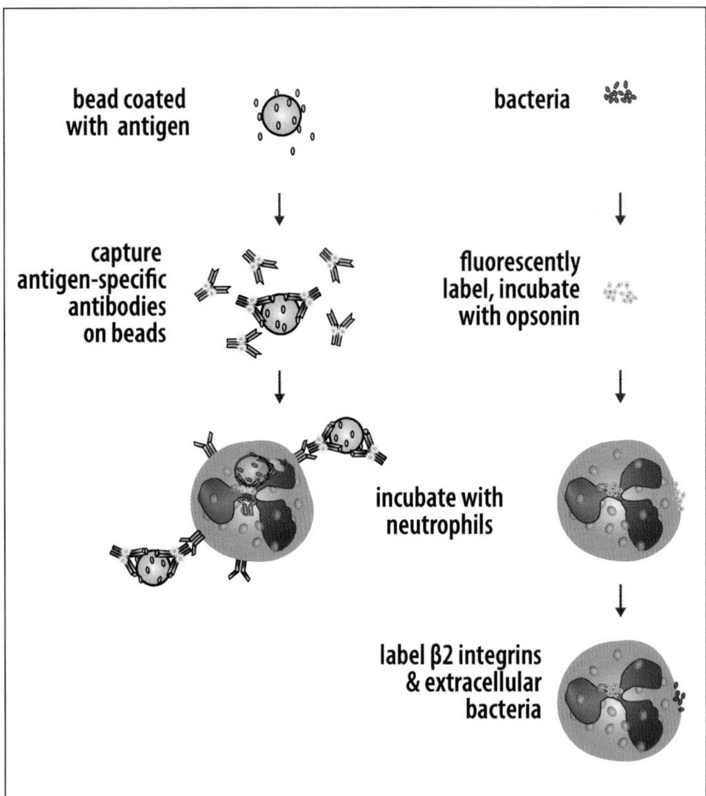

f8.25 High-throughput methods to measure antibody-dependent phagocytosis. Results may be read with either flow cytometry or fluorescent microscope

8.5.4 Neutrophil function

8.5.4.1 Neutrophil adhesion & chemotaxis

- Adhesion deficiency may be assessed by measuring cell surface adhesion molecules on neutrophils using flow cytometry (eg, CD11b, CD15, CD18)
- Chemotaxis can be evaluated by assessing the migration of neutrophils through permeable membranes **f8.24**

8.5.4.2 Neutrophil phagocytosis assay

- Neutrophil suspensions are incubated with bacteria or coated beads as shown in **f8.25**
- Aliquots are collected and fixed at various time points
- Flow cytometry is performed, collecting forward & side scatter data to separate neutrophils from bacteria or beads
- Fluorescent markers within bacteria or beads is used to quantitate phagocytosis

8.5.4.3 Respiratory burst

- Neutrophil oxidative burst assay aids in screening for chronic granulomatous disease
- White blood cells are incubated with dihydrorhodamine 123 (DHR) & catalase
- Cells are then stimulated with phorbol 12-myristate 13 acetate (PMA)
- DHR oxidation by respiratory cell burst to rhodamine is measured using flow cytometry

8.5.5 Cytoplasmic antibodies

8.5.5.1 Antineutrophil cytoplasmic antibody (cANCA)

- Screening test for ANCA-associated vasculitis
- Commonly performed by indirect immunofluorescence (IIF)
- Positive cases may be reflexed to titer and to detection of MPO/PR3 antibodies

ISBN 978-089189-6616

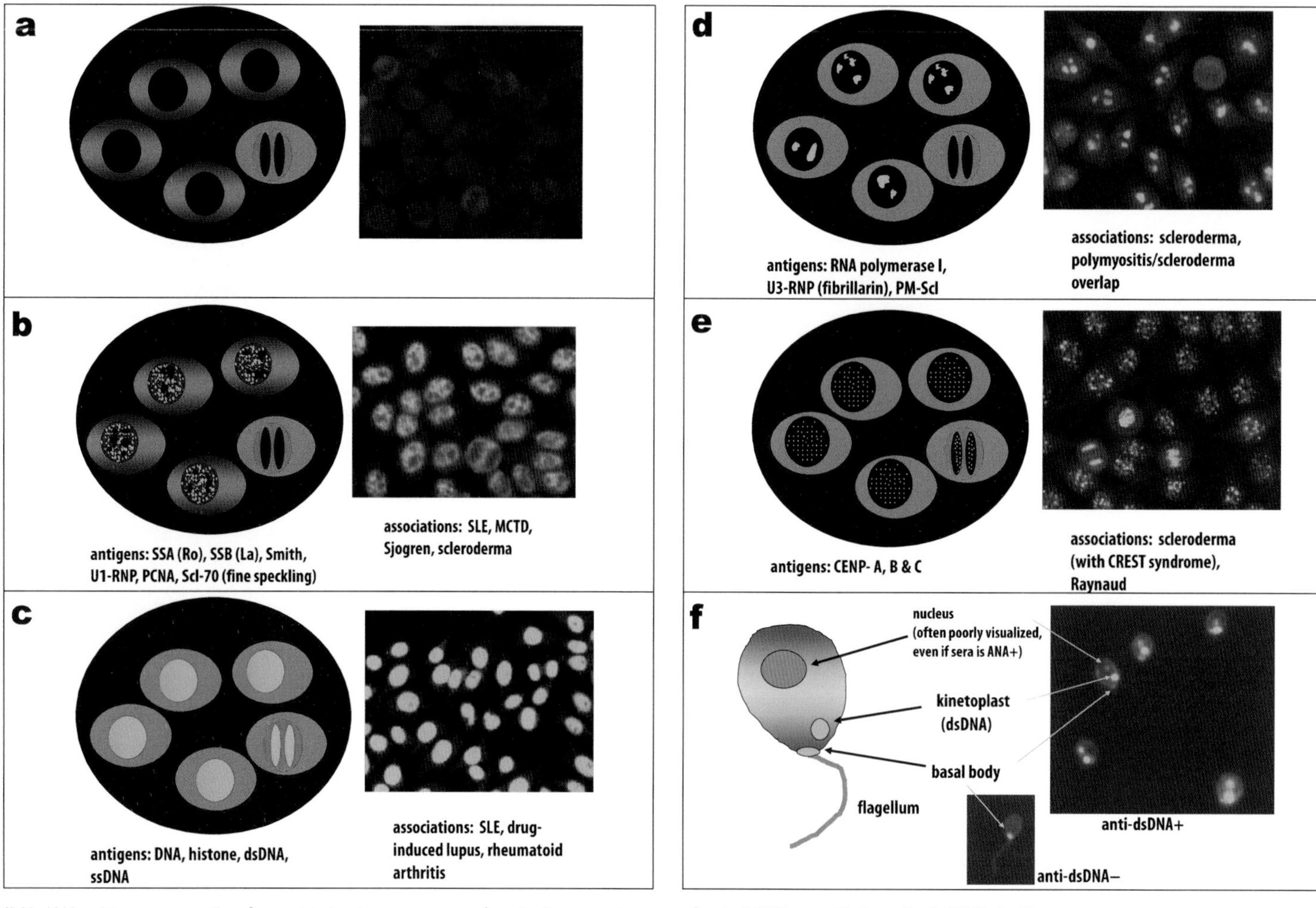

f8.26 ANA patterns: a negative, b speckled, c homogeneous, d nucleolar, e centromere , f anti-dsDNA quantitation with *Crithidia luciliae*

8.5.5.2 Islet cell cytoplasmic antibody

- Used to evaluate autoimmune diabetes mellitus
- Usually performed in combination with another antibody test
- Commonly performed by indirect immunofluorescence (IIF)

8.5.5.3 Liver cytosolic antigen type 1 (LC-1) antibody

- Detected in patients with autoimmune hepatitis type 2
- Commonly performed on serum by qualitative immunoblot or EIA
- Performed in combination with liver-kidney microsome-1 antibody, IgG

8.5.6 Antinuclear antibodies (ANAs)

- ANA are a group of antibodies that react to different nuclear, nucleolar, or perinuclear antigens
- ANA damage tissue by reacting with nuclear substances released from injured or dying cells
- ANAs are associated with several autoimmune disorders

8.5.6.1 Indirect immunofluorescence (IIF) for ANA using Hep-2 cells

- Indirect immunoassays use an unlabeled antigen, unlabeled antibody & labeled antiglobulin
- The unlabeled antigen is found on fixed Hep-2 cells
- The unlabeled antibody is anti-ANA found in the patient serum
- The labeled antiglobulin is fluorescently labeled antihuman immunoglobulin
- Pattern of staining provides antigen specificity & disease association **f8.26** and **t8.9**
- Negative ANA virtually excludes systemic lupus erythematosus (SLE)

8.5.6.2 Enzyme immunoassay (EIA) for ANA

- Antigen mixture is adsorbed to a solid surface
- ANAs are detected through an enzyme-labeled anti-human immunoglobulin **f8.27**
- Can determine the presence of specific autoantibodies

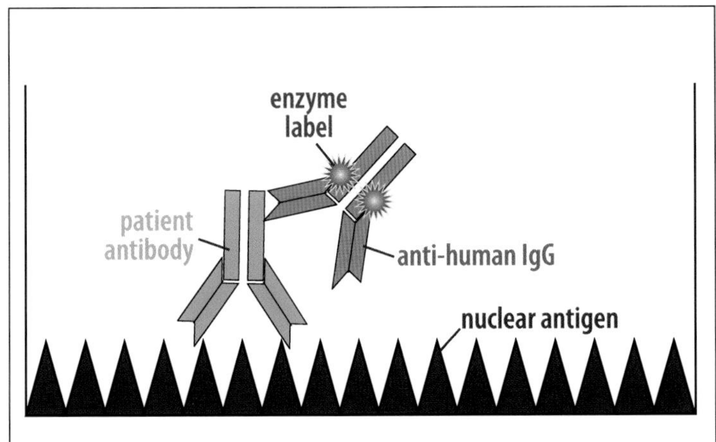

f8.27 Indirect ELISA to detect anti-nuclear antigens. Addition of enzyme substrate creates color that can be measured by spectrophotometer

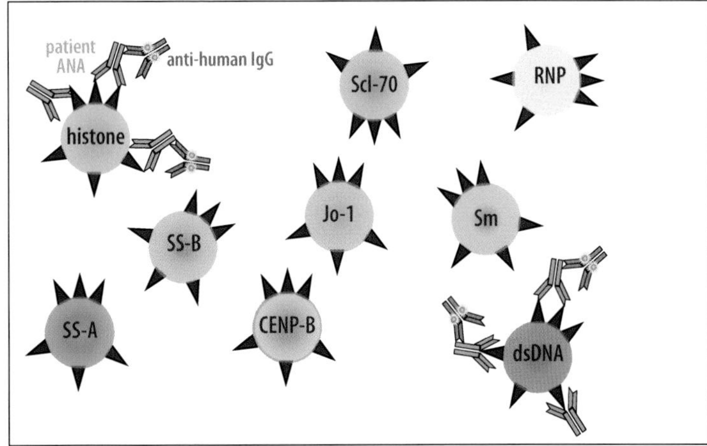

f8.28 Multiplex immunoassay for ANA. Each bead is coated with different antigen, indicated by navy triangles. Patient ANA (cyan) binds specific antigens. Fluorescently labeled anti-human IgG is added. Fluorescence is detected by flow cytometry

t8.9 ANA patterns

Fluorescent staining pattern	Antigen specificity & disease associations
homogeneous or peripheral (rim pattern), mitoses +	fluorescent mitotic figures distinguish this from a finely speckled pattern homogeneous pattern: indicate antibodies to ssDNA & histone rim pattern: indicate anti-dsDNA, which are antibodies to nuclear envelope antigens or lamins disease associations: suggestive of SLE, especially if titer is high. Low titer homogeneous pattern: Sjögren syndrome, mixed connective tissues disease (MCTD) & rheumatoid arthritis rim pattern: Primary biliary cirrhosis, chronic liver disease, drug induced SLD
speckled (mitoses–)	anti-Sm, RNP, Ro/SS-A, La/SS-B, PCNA (extractable nuclear antigens) disease associations: this pattern occurs in CREST, SLE, mixed connective tissue disease (MCTD), Sjögren syndrome, rheumatoid arthritis & scleroderma
nucleolar (mitoses–)	antibodies to RNA polymerase I & proteins of small nucleolar RNP complex (fibrillin, hU3-55K, Mpp10) Th/To, B23, PM-Scl & NOR-90 disease associations: scleroderma
centromere (mitoses+ in centromeric pattern)	antibodies to Scl-70, the centromeres of chromosomes, specifically on active centromere proteins: CENP-A, CENP-B, CENP-C **f8.28** disease associations: CREST (50%-80% patients are positive), idiopathic Raynaud phenomenon (25% patients are positive)

CREST = syndrome of calcinosis, Raynaud, esophageal sclerosis, sclerodactyly & telangiectasia

8.5.6.3 Multiplex immunoassay (MIA) for ANA

- Polystyrene beads are conjugated to a known ANA antigen
- Bead sets are distinguished from one another based on their fluorescent signature
- Beads with different antigens are mixed together
- Patient's serum sample is incubated with the beads
- Patient antibody binding is detected using fluorescently labeled antihuman immunoglobulin as shown in **f8.28**

8.5.7 Thyroid antibodies

8.5.7.1 Normal thyroid function

- Follicle cells release thyroglobulin, from which thyroid hormones triiodothyronine (T3) and thyroxine (T4) are synthesized upon stimulation by thyroid-stimulating hormone (TSH) produced by the pituitary gland
- Thyroperoxidase enzyme oxidizes iodine before linking to thyroglobulin
- T4 provides feedback to downregulate TSH
- Thyroiditis has multiple causes

8.5.7.2 Thyroid autoimmunity

- Development of autoantibodies against proteins involved in thyroid hormone production
  - Anti-thyroglobulin (Tg)
  - Anti-thyroperoxidase (TPO)
  - Anti-thyroid-stimulating hormone (TSH) receptor (TRAb)
  - Initial screening involves measurement of TSH levels using chemiluminescent immunoassays

8.5.7.3 Hashimoto thyroiditis (aka chronic lymphocytic thyroiditis)

- Most common autoimmune disease, affecting 8 of every 1,000 individuals
- Women are 5-10 times more likely to get the disease
- Patients develop a rubbery goiter
- Immune destruction leads to hypothyroidism

- TPO antibodies are present in 90%
- TRAb is not present
- Tg antibodies are present in 60%-80%
- Most patients with Hashimoto thyroiditis have high levels of both TPO and Tg antibodies

8.5.7.4 Graves disease

- Among the most common autoimmune diseases
- Women are 5 times more likely to get the disease
- Most often presents in the fifth and sixth decades of life
- Patients develop a firm goiter
- Exophthalmos, bulging eyeballs, occurs in about 35% of patients
- Hyperthyroidism, TRAb antibodies bind to TSH receptor, resulting in uncontrolled receptor stimulation
- TPO antibodies are present in 80%
- TRAb antibodies are present but are not diagnostic by themselves
- Tg antibodies are present in 40%-70%
- TRAb antibody-binding assays involve competitive binding between a labeled TRAb reagent and patient antibody for TSH receptor
- TRAb bioassays require tissue culture; can distinguish between TRAbs with stimulatory activity and those with inhibitory activity

8.5.8 Rheumatoid arthritis (RA)

- Chronic, symmetric erosive arthritis of peripheral joints
- Affects about 0.5%-1% of the population
- Presents most often between the ages of 25 and 55 years
- Smoking doubles risk
- Women are 3 times more likely to be affected
- Strongest genetic association is with certain HLA-DRB1 alleles
- Lesions show formation of a pannus, a sheet of granulation tissue growing in the joint space, invading cartilage

8.5.8.1 Rheumatoid factor (RF)

- IgM antibodies reacting to the Fc portion of IgG is common
- Previously detected with latex agglutination assays, largely replaced by other methods with greater sensitivity and can detect additional isotypes
- Contributes to the formation of immune complexes
- Found in >70% of all RA subjects
- Nonspecific, also found in low titers in healthy people and in ~20% of people >65 years
- Not a conclusive diagnosis

8.5.8.2 Antibodies to cyclic citrullinated proteins (ACPA)

- ACPA are a collection of autoantibodies with different isotypes that recognize citrulline in proteins
- Second major antibody associated with RA
- Presence is associated with disease severity

8.5.9 Immunoglobulin quantitation

8.5.9.1 Nephelometry measure of serum immunoglobulins

- Antibody to IgA, IgM, or IgG serves as the reagent
- Serum contains M proteins
- Reagent antibody & M-protein antigen are mixed in concentrations such that small aggregates form
- Measure the scattering of light as it passes through the solution and compared to the scatter of known mixtures to determine the amount of M-protein present
- Endpoint nephelometry allows antibody-antigen reaction to run to completion. If large complexes form, they will fall out of solution causing a false scatter reading
- Kinetic nephelometry involves addition of reagent at a constant rate while scatter is being measured. The rate of change is directly related to the amount of antigen present

8.5.9.2 Turbidimetry measure of serum immunoglobulins

- Similar to nephelometry, but measures decrease in the amount of light passing directly through the solution

8.5.9.3 Serum free light chains (sFLC)

- Latex-enhanced assays performed on either nephelometric or turbidimetric instruments
- Assess individual sFLC concentration & the κ:λ ratio
- Appropriate diagnostic screening, when used in combination with serum protein electrophoresis (SPE), to diagnose high tumor burden monoclonal gammopathies
- This method has highest analytical sensitivity for identifying moloclonal sFLCs

8.5.9.4 Immunoglobulin heavy-light chain (HLC) assays

- Separately quantify different light chains using either nephelometric or turbidimetric instruments
- IgGκ, IgGλ, IgAκ, IgAλ, IgMκ, and IgMλ
- Assessed in pairs to produce HLC ratios
- Useful to overcome issues of comigration and dye saturation observed with protein electrophoresis

8.5.9.5 Protein electrophoresis (SPE, UPE)

- Serum protein electrophoresis (SPE) and urine protein electrophoresis (UPE)
- Serum is separated in agarose gel according to size and charge into albumin and globulin fractions
  - Albumin forms a dense band close to the anode
  - Globulin is subdivided into 5 regions closer to the cathode
- After electrophoresis proteins are fixed in gel and stained
- Gels are examined or may be scanned with a densitometer to product an electropherogram
- Scanning densitometry can determine concentration of each band
- Detection of the M protein as narrow peaks
- Monoclonal fractions & normal protein fractions may both be reported
- Initial identification of abnormal protein by SPE or UPE should be examined using immunofixation electrophoresis (IFE)

8.5.10 Immunotyping

8.5.10.1 Immunofixation electrophoresis (IFE)

- Serum, urine, CSF
- Electrophoresis followed by immunodiffusion against monospecific antisera to immunoglobulin and individual heavy & light chains
- Separates albumin & globulin subgroups based on size & electrical charge
- Detection of the M protein as discrete bands
- α1-globulin, α2-globulin, β-globulin, γ-globulin
- Used to help diagnose or monitor monoclonal gammopathies, lymphoma, leukemia, kidney & liver disease, autoimmune & neurologic disorders, and malnutrition & malabsorption
- For suspected monoclonal gammopathy
  - Patient sample undergoes electrophoresis in 5 lanes
  - Immunodiffusion of each lane is performed with different monoclonal antibodies
  - Gel paper is washed & stained
  - Normal result does not exclude multiple myeloma, may require 24-hour urine IFE or immunoassay
- Urine immunofixation may produce step ladder pattern, indicative of polyclonal hypergammaglobulinemia with spillage into the urine

8.5.10.2 Immunosubtraction

- Antibodies against IgG, IgA, IgM, κ, or λ are bound to solid-phase beads
- Beads are incubated with patient serum
- Capillary zone electrophoresis (CZE) is performed to determine which beads remove an electrophoretic abnormality
  - Protein separation is performed in liquid buffer system
  - Proteins in capillaries pass ultraviolet source and absorbance as 200-215 nm is measured
- Can be used in place of IFE, but is less sensitive and may require a complementary method

8.5.10.3 Matrix-assisted laser desorption ionization time of flight (MALDI-TOF) mass spectrometry

- Detects, isotypes, and quantitates M proteins in a single assay
- Possible because of unique light chain masses that result from immunoglobulin light chain rearrangements in B cells
- Immunoaffinity purification is performed to separate immunoglobulin G, A, M, κ, and λ
- Isolated immunoglobulins are reduced to separate heavy & light chain subunits
- Analyzed using MALDI-TOF mass spectrometry analysis
- Individual spectra are overlaid & analyzed for anomalies
- Useful for monitoring patients receiving therapy because it is more sensitive and specific than electrophoresis-based methods
- Helps avoid interference of biologics

8.5.11 Complement testing

8.5.11.1 Radial hemolysis

- Classical pathway
- Radial immunodiffusion (RID)
- Agarose gel with specific anticomplement factor antibodies
- Add serum to wells
- Antigen & antibody diffuse toward one another, precipitation occurs at the zone of equivalence
- Diameter of precipitin ring relates to concentration

8.5.11.2 Nephelometry

- Antibody is the reagent
- Serum contains complement antigen
- Measures the scattering of light as it passes through the solution
- Results obtained in milligrams per deciliter (mg/dL) or international units per milliliter (IU/mL)

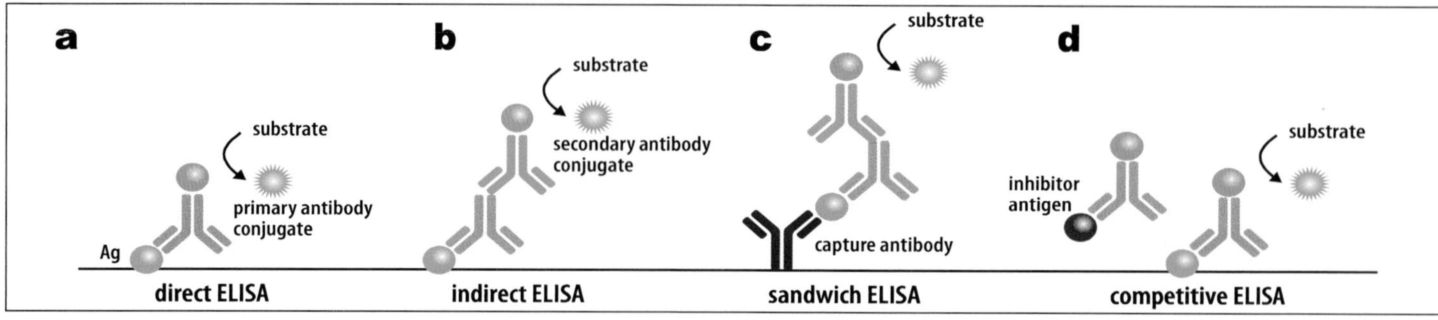

f8.29 Labeled immunoassay variations: **a** direct, **b** indirect, **c** sandwich, **d** competitive

8.5.11.3 Turbidimetry

- Measures decrease in amount of light passing directly through the solution

8.5.11.4 ELISA

- For classical pathway, microtiter wells are coated with IgM
- For alternative pathway, microtiter wells are coated with bacterial polysaccharide

8.5.11.5 Strip tests

- For classical pathway, IgM
- For alternative pathway, bacterial polysaccharide
- For mannose-binding lectin (MBL), coat with mannose

8.5.11.6 CH50

- Functional assay for classical pathway
- Ig-coated sheep RBC; CH50 units: the reciprocal of the dilution that lyses 50% of RBCs
- Enzyme-filled liposomes; measures amount of serum to lyse 50% of liposomes

8.5.11.7 AH50

- Alternative pathway
- Similar to CH50, using rabbit RBC
- Buffer added to chelate calcium, blocking classical pathway

8.5.11.8 Interpretation of complement results

- Decreased levels of C3 reflect either primary C3 deficiency or activation of the alternative pathway
- Levels of C4 or C1q are typically used to look at the classical pathway

8.5.12 Direct detection methods for pathogens

8.5.12.1 Direct immunofluorescence assay (DIFA)

- Can be used to detect various pathogens, commonly used for viral antigens on swabs from lesions
- Infected cells are placed on a glass slide
- Cells are fixed & permeabilized
- Cells are incubated with fluorescence-linked antibody to specific pathogen proteins
- Staining reflects the localization of the pathogen within the cells
- Visualized under a fluorescence microscope

8.5.12.2 Indirect immunofluorescence assay (IIFA)

- Similar in methodology to direct immunofluorescence
- Unlabeled antipathogen antibody followed by a fluorescently labeled secondary antibody

8.5.13 Labeled immunoassay (EIA/ELISA/RIA)

- Enzyme immunoassays (EIAs) use labeled antibodies to increase sensitivity as shown in **f8.29**
- The constant region of the antibody is covalently bound with an enzyme or fluorophore that allows the antigen or antibody in the test to be visualized and/or quantified

8.5.13.1 Immunoblots

- Antigens are immobilized on membrane
- Labeled antibodies are used to detect the presence of specific antigens (eg, detection of HIV peptides)

8.5.13.2 Immunostaining

- Antigens are on or in cells
- Labeled antibodies are used to detect & localize antigen
- Direct immunofluorescence (DIF) involves incubation of tissues with fluorescently labeled antibodies. In the case of autoantibody detection, this could be labeled antihuman globulin (AHG)
- Indirect immunofluorescent (IIF) for autoantibodies involves incubation of tissues first with unlabeled antigen and then with labeled AHG

8.5.13.3 Direct ELISA

- Antigen is immobilized on surface
- Antigen is detected with labeled antibody

8.5.13.4 Indirect ELISA

- Antigen is immobilized on surface
- Primary antibody within patient serum binds to antigen
- Secondary antihuman-labeled antibody detects patient antibody to antigen

8.5.13.5 Sandwich ELISA

- Uses 2 antibodies that bind to different places on the target antigen
- Capture antibody is immobilized on surface
- Antigen is added
- Labeled detection antibody is applied in the last step

8.5.13.6 Competitive ELISA

- Measures the concentration of an antigen by detection of signal interference
- Antigen is immobilized on surface
- Sample antigen competes with a reference antigen for binding to a specific amount of labeled antibody
- Either antibody or antigen may be labeled
- Often used in lateral flow assays

8.5.14 Chemiluminescent immunoassay

- Variation of standard EIA
- Uses chemiluminescent endpoints generating photons of light
- More sensitive than colorimetric & fluorometric alternatives
- Reagents are stable, relatively nontoxic & inexpensive
- Labeling can be attached to either antigen or antibody
- Detection systems consist of photomultiplier tubes
- Therapeutic drug & hormone levels
- Electrochemiluminescence immunoassay (ECLIA) **f8.30**
  - Uses electrochemical compounds that generate light because of an oxidation-reduction reaction
  - Ruthenium (Ru) is a commonly used indicator
  - Tripropylamine (TPA) regenerates Ru after photon release
  - Magnetic beads are commonly used as solid phase to capture labeled antibody

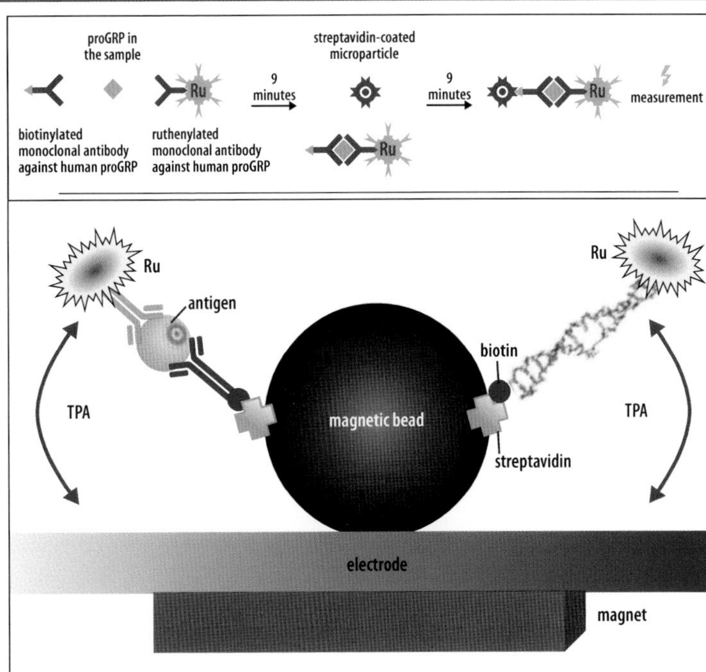

f8.30 The development of electrochemiluminescence immunoassays is based on the use of a ruthenium-complex and tripropylamine (TPA); TPA regenerates the ruthenium complex after it releases a photon

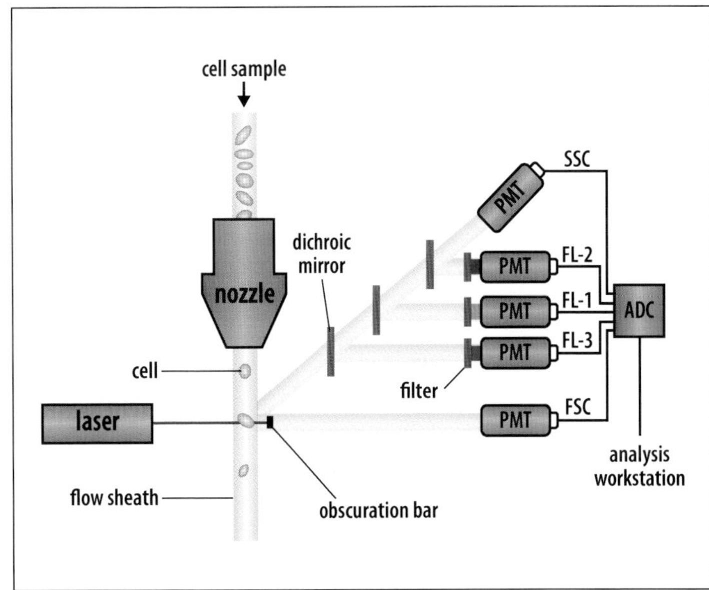

f8.31 Flow cytometer components

8.5.15 Flow cytometry

- Cell-associated proteins are fluorescently labeled with monoclonal antibodies to identify cells of interest
- Cells suspended in solution are individually analyzed for light scattering properties and the presence of fluorescently labeled intracellular or cell surface molecules **f8.31**
- Can be used for cell counting, cell sorting, biomarker detection, microorganism detection

ISBN 978-089189-6616

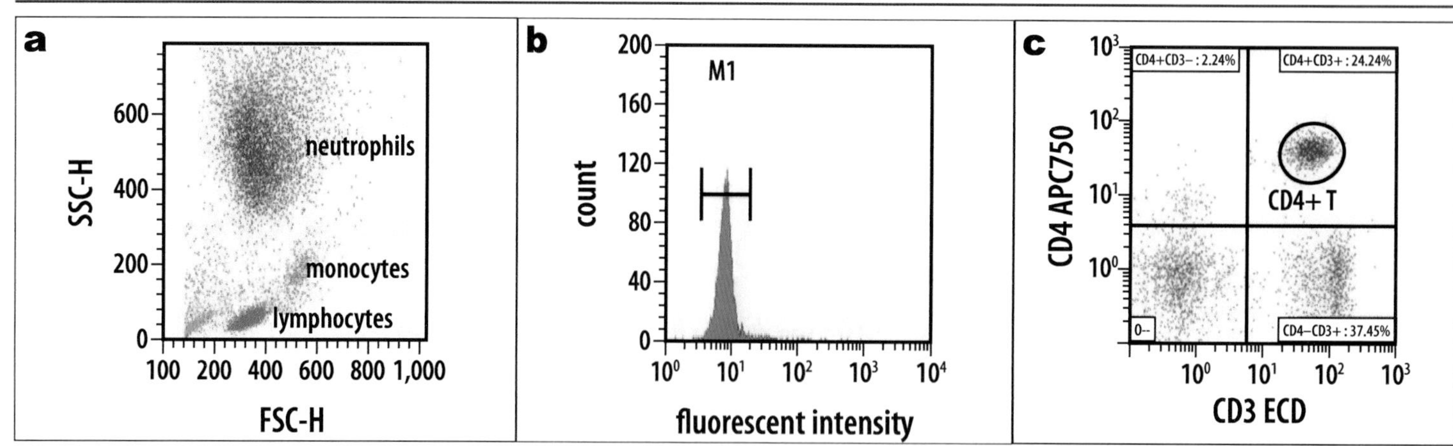

f8.32 **a** Forward & side scatter profile of pheripheral blood leukocytes; **b** single parameter histogram; **c** quadrant analysis

8.5.15.1 Instrumentation

- Instrument fluidics draws cell suspension into sheath fluid, allowing cells to pass through laser 1 at a time
- The light source is typically solid-state diode laser(s); the use of multiple lasers expands the number of fluorochromes that can be used in the assay
- Light scatter is detected by photodiodes
- Fluorescence is detected by photomultiplier tubes, creating an electrical current that is converted into a voltage pulse and then to a digital signal
- Intensity of signal is measured on a relative scale, typically 1-256 channels

8.5.15.2 Data acquisition

- Cells pass by laser & detection system 1 cell at a time. Fluorescence, forward scatter (FSC), and side scatter (SSC) data are collected
  - Forward light scatter allows discrimination of cell size
  - Side scatter provides information about internal complexity, such as granularity
- Data are typically collected for ≥10,000 events
- Data are gated based on fluorescence intensity and forward & side scatter to produce histograms
- Gated data may be represented as a single parameter histogram, dual-parameter dot plot, or quadrant analysis, as shown in f8.32

8.5.15.3 Applications

- Immunophenotyping for cancer characterization & immunodeficiency
- DNA ploidy status
- CD34 cell enumeration
- Functional assays such as oxidative burst analysis
- Characterization of leukemias & lymphomas
- Transplantation crossmatch
- Antibody detection by bead array, in which labeled beads are used in place of cells and incubated with patient serum

8.6 Selected readings

8.6.1 Books

Delves PJ, Martin SM, Burton DR, Roitt RM. *Roitt's Essential Immunology (Essentials)*. 13th ed. Wiley. 2017. ISBN 978-1118415771

Detrick B, et al, eds. *Manual of Molecular & Clinical Laboratory Immunology*. 7th ed. ASM Press. 2006. ISBN 978-1555813642

Stevens CD, Miller LE. *Clinical Immunology and Serology: A Laboratory Perspective*. 4th ed. FA Davis. 2016. ISBN 978-0803644663

Tan S-L. *Translational Immunology*. Elsevier. 2016. ISBN 978-0128015773

Wanger A, Chavez V, Huang R, Wahed A, Dasgupta A, Actor JK. *Microbiology and Molecular Diagnosis in Pathology: A Comprehensive Review for Board Preparation, Certification and Clinical Practice*. Elsevier. 2017. ISBN 978-0128053515

8.6.2 Journals & online

Quinn MT, DeLeo FR, Bokoch GM. Neutrophil methods & protocols. *Methods Mol Biol*. 2007; 412:vii-viii. doi 10.1007/978-1-59745-467-4

Centers for Disease Control and Prevention (CDC) [2020] CDC recommendations for testing for Lyme disease. https://www.cdc.gov/lyme/healthcare/clinician_twotier.html

Centers for Disease Control and Prevention (CDC) [2020] Hepatitis C virus (HCV) testing algorithm recommended by the CDC. https://www.cdc.gov/hepatitis/HCV/PDFs/hcv_flow.pdf

Centers for Disease Control and Prevention (CDC) [2020] Interpretation of serologic results. https://www.cdc.gov/hepatitis/HBV/PDFs/SerologicChartv8.pdf

Chapter 9

Molecular Biology

ISBN 978-089189-6616

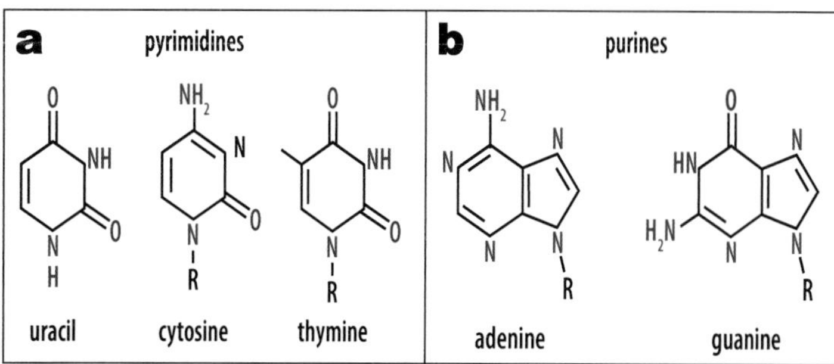

f9.1 Nitrogenous bases: **a** pyrimidines, **b** purines

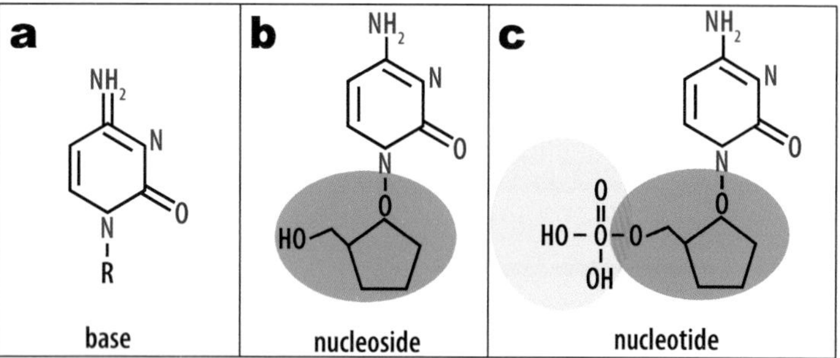

f9.2 Difference between **a** base, **b** nucleoside, and **c** nucleotide structure

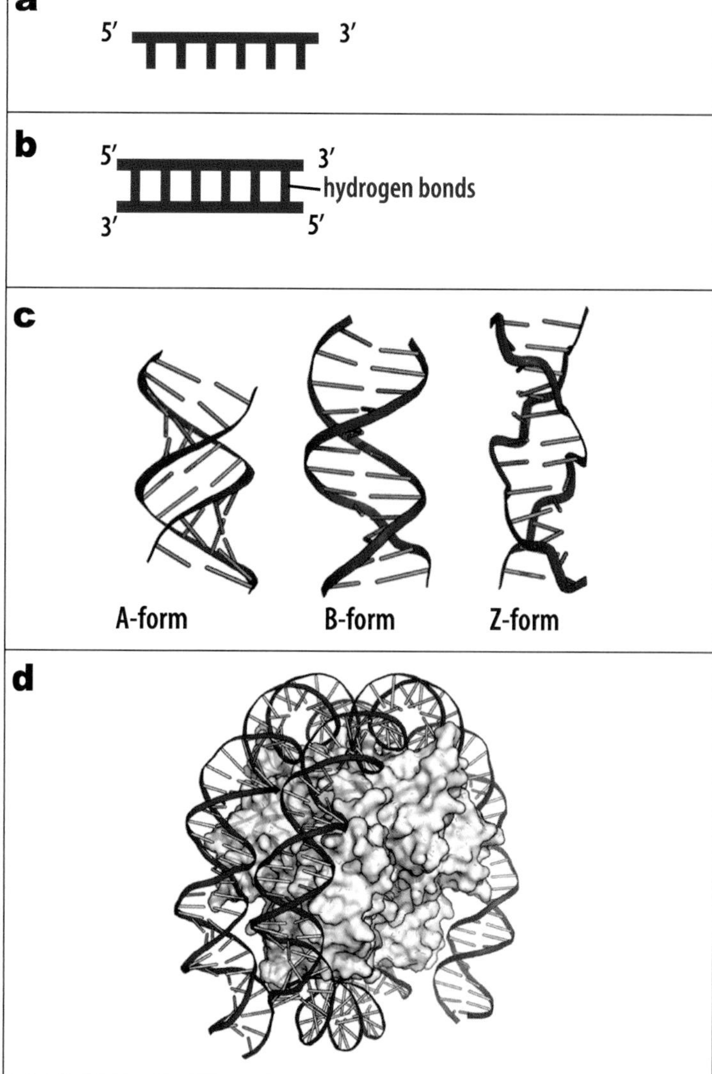

f9.3 DNA structure, including **a** primary, **b** secondary, **c** tertiary & **d** quaternary

9.1 Molecular biology

9.1.1 Structure of nucleic acids

9.1.1.1 Bases, nucleosides & nucleotides

- Bases
  - The primary building blocks of nucleic acids and can be subdivided, based on ring structure; the pyrimidines uracil (U), cytosine (C) and thymine (T), shown in **f9.1a**, have a single ring structure. The purines adenine (A) and guanine (G), shown in **f9.1b** have a double ring structure
  - Nitrogenous bases are adenine (A), thymine (T), uracil (U), cytosine (C), and guanine (G)
  - A, T, C and G are present in deoxyribonucleic acid (DNA)
  - A, U, C, and G are present in ribonucleic acid (RNA)
- Nucleosides
  - Composed of a base **f9.2a** plus sugar as shown in **f9.2b**, with the sugar structure highlighted in blue
  - The pentose sugar is ribose in RNA and deoxyribose in DNA
- Nucleotides
  - Composed of a base, sugar, and phospate as shown in **f9.2c**, with the sugar structure highlighted in blue and the phosphate group highlighted in yellow

9.1.1.2 DNA structure

- Primary structure
  - Consists of phosphodiester bond links nucleotides between the 5' triphosphate of 1 nucleotide and the 3' hydroxyl group of another on 1 strand of DNA, as shown in **f9.3a**
- Secondary structure
  - Refers to the formation of hydrogen bonding between complementary bases of 2 strands of DNA as shown in **f9.3b**
  - Two hydrogen bonds form between A:T
  - Three hydrogen bonds form between C:G
- Tertiary structure
  - Refers to the stacking interactions between 2 polynucleotide strands resulting a in double helix **f9.3c**

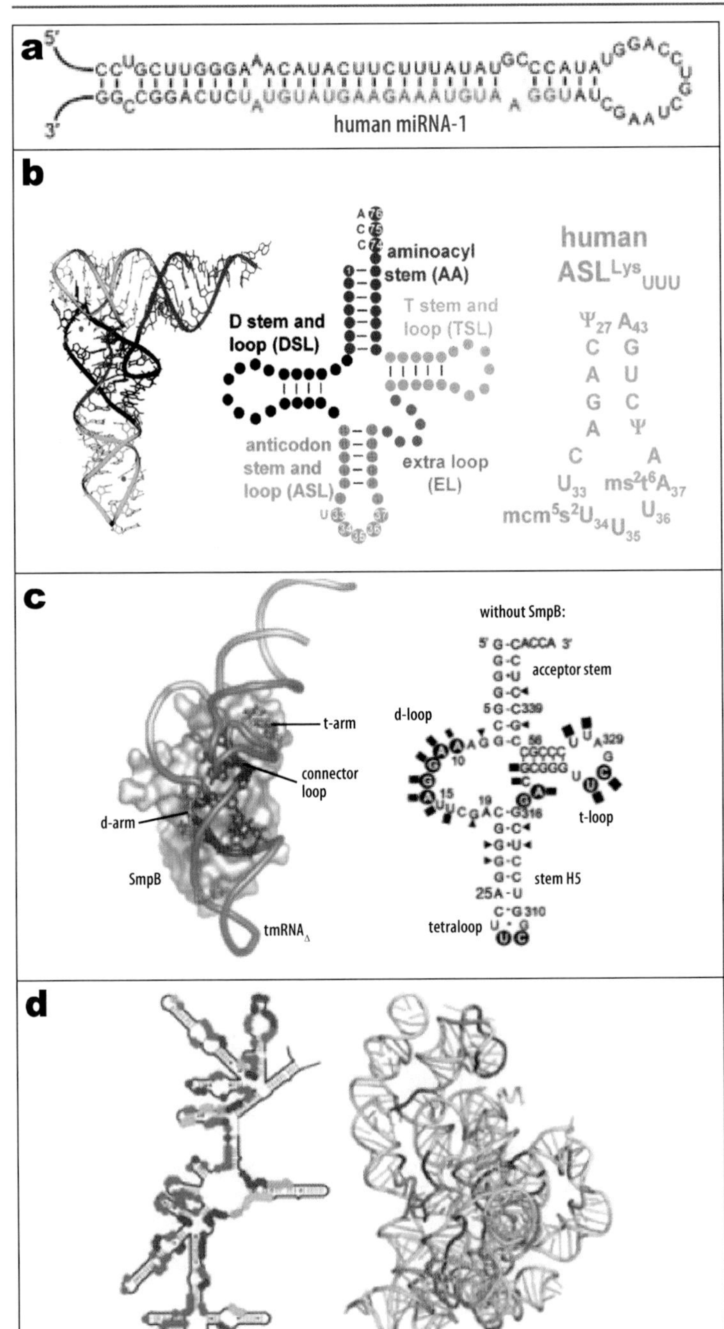

f9.4 RNA secondary & tertiary structure as relates to function: **a** miRNA forming a stem loop, **b** tRNA, **c** mRNA & **d** rRNA

- There are 3 conformations of the double helix that occur
  - B-DNA is the common form possessing wide major grooves accessible to proteins
  - A-DNA forms under dehydrating conditions
  - Z-DNA occurs at high salt concentrations and does not have a functional major groove
- Quaternary structure
  - Refers to the interactions of the strands with other molecules, such as proteins & nucleosomes **f9.3d**

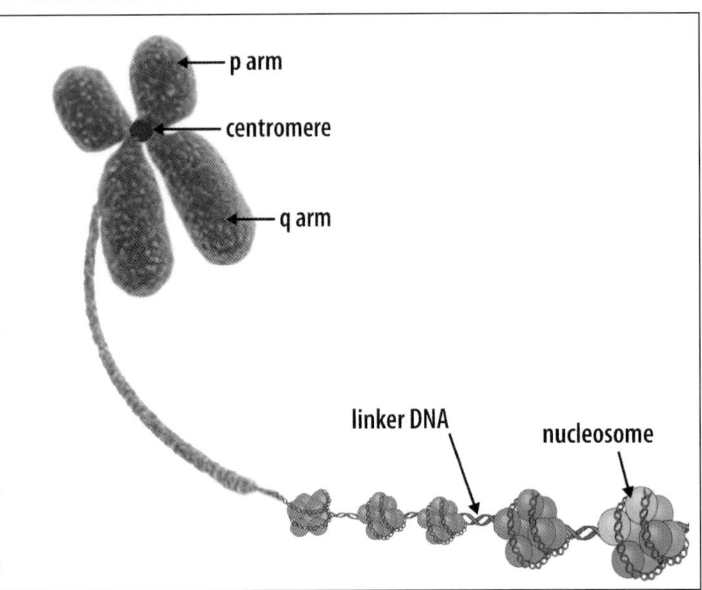

f9.5 Chromosome structure is composed of DNA wound onto nucleosome beads, tightly compacted

9.1.1.3 RNA structure

- RNA is inherently less stable than DNA because of structural differences
- RNA primary structure is similar to that of DNA
  - RNA contains uracil instead of thymine
  - The sugar is ribose instead of deoxyribose
- Secondary structure
  - Result of localized base pairing as the strand folds on itself
  - Stem-loop, or hairpins, are composed to a run of paired bases with a short unpaired loop
  - Pseudoknots consist of at least 2 stem loop structures. Pseudoknots can form structures with catalytic activity
- Secondary and tertiary structure varies by function **f9.4**
  - microRNA (miRNA) regulates mRNA levels to control protein expression
  - transfer RNA (tRNA) delivers specific amino acids to the growing peptide chaine
  - ribosomal RNA (rRNA) is involved in both the structure and the catalytic activity of the ribosome

9.1.2 Chromosome

- A chromosome is an exceptionally long strand of DNA that contains hundreds to thousands of genes wrapped with proteins to form a compact structure as shown in **f9.5**

Molecular biology>Chromosome | Gene structure

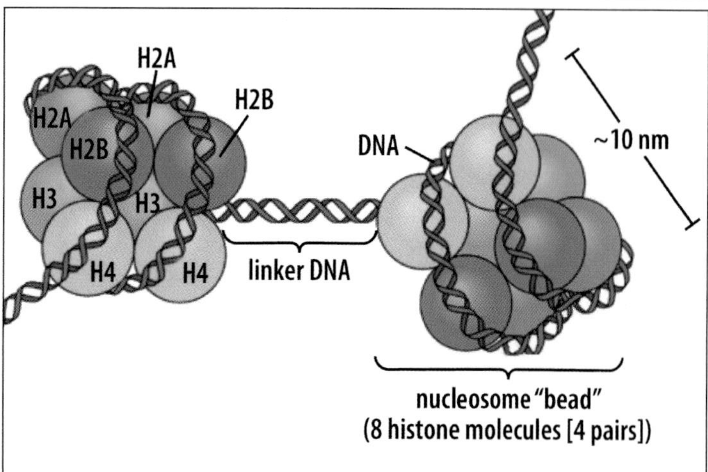

f9.6 Nucleosome structure: 146 base pairs of DNA wrap each nucleosome and they are connected one to another by 20-150 base pairs of linker DNA

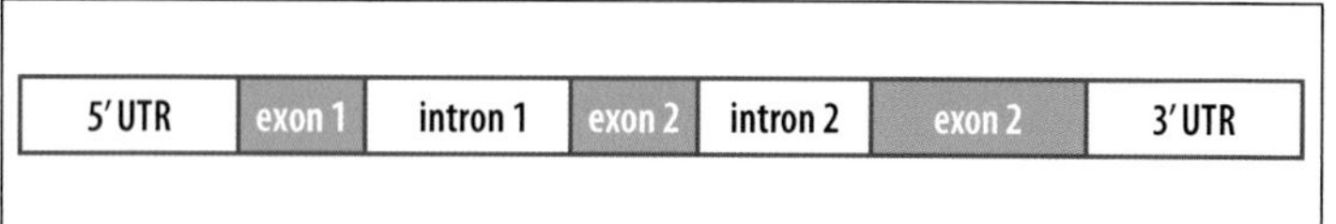

f9.7 Gene structure

9.1.2.1 Nucleosome structure

- The nucleosome is an octamer of positively charged histone proteins; 2 each of histones 2A, 2B, 3, and 4, as shown in **f9.6**
- There are 146 bases of negatively charged DNA wraps around each octamer
- There is a 20-150 bp DNA linker between adjacent nucleosomes
- Nucleosomes are stack with 6 nucleosomes per turn, further compacted by looping, to form a chromosome, as shown in **f9.5**
- Modification of histone charge, primarily through acetylation, affect the binding properties and is involved in the regulation of gene expression

9.1.2.2 Chromosome nomenclature

- Chromosomes are generally numbered according to length, from longest (1) to shortest (22). However, chromosome 21 is the shortest
- Chromosomes classified by the location of the centromere
  - Subcentric chromosomes have 1 short arm (p) and a long arm (q)
  - Metacentric chromosomes have arms of approximately the same length
  - Acrocentric chromosomes have a very long (q) and 1 very short (p) arm
- Chromosomal staining methods are used to establish banding patterns as shown in **t9.1**

t9.1 Chromosomal staining & banding patterns

Type of banding	Staining summary
G	Geimsa stain AT-rich regions stain darker than GC-rich regions
Q	Quinacrine fluorescent dye stains AT-rich regions
R	Banding pattern is opposite G-banding
C	Stains heterochromatic regions close to the centromeres Usually stains the entire long arm of the Y chromosome

- Identifying specific chromosomal location based on banding patterns
  - Regions of arms are numbered relative to the centromere; nearest region labeled 1
  - Each region of the arms is further divided into bands and, possibly, sub-bands
  - The nomenclature used is [chromosome][arm][region][band][sub-band], for example 22.q.11.2 as shown in **t9.2**
- Heterochromatin regions retain constitutively higher levels of compaction and associated with gene inactivation
- Euchromatin regions are less compacted and associated with increased gene expression

t9.2 Chromosomal nomenclature based on banding patterns

22q11.2	
22	Chromosome 22
q	Long arm of chromosome (q)
1	Region 1
1	Band 1
2	Sub-band 2

9.1.3 Gene structure

- The transcribed region of a gene includes 5' and 3' untranslated regions, exons, and intervening introns as shown in **f9.7**

9.1.3.1 Untranslated regions

- Two per gene: 5'UTR and 3'UTR
- Untranslated regions are sequences that occur before the first and after the last exon
- They contain regulatory elements that influence regulation of transcription, translation, polyadenylation, translation efficiency, localization, and stability of the mRNA

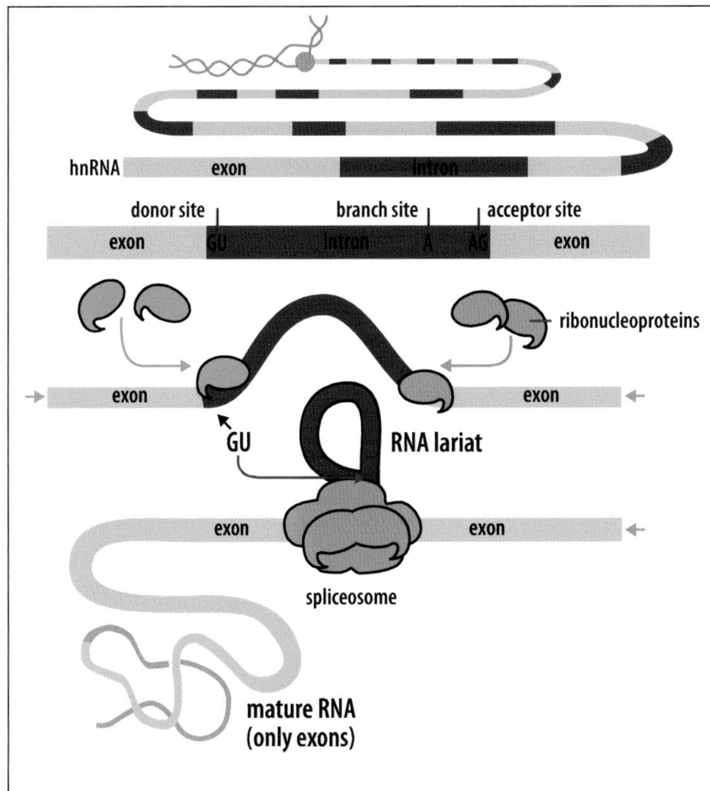

f9.8 Introns & RNA splicing
hnRNA, heterogeneous nuclear RNA

9.1.3.2 Exons

- Exons are sequences that occur in the mature mRNA and code for the amino acids that form the protein
- Referred to as exon when referring to either the DNA or RNA

9.1.3.3 Introns

- Sequences within a gene that are integral to regulation of expression
- Introns are not translated into protein
- Introns are removed by RNA splicing as shown in **f9.8**
- Alternative splicing of introns increases the repertoire of proteins that can be produced from a single gene

9.1.3.4 Start & stop codons

- The start codon is the first codon of the messenger RNA translated on the ribosome
  - RNA sequence AUG, codes for methionine in eukaryotes
  - Rare non-AUG codons occur in both prokaryote and eukaryotes, still code for methionine but use unique t-RNA for initiation
- The stop codon (aka termination codon) signals termination of translation of the protein
- Stop codons bind to factors that cause the ribosomal subunits to dissociate
  - The 3 standard recognized RNA stop codons are UAG, UAA, UGA
  - Alternative stop codons have been described in mitochondrial genomes

9.1.4 Mitochondrial DNA

9.1.4.1 Mitochondrial genome

- Composed of double stranded circular DNA existing outside the nucleus
- Endosymbiotic theory states that mitochondrial DNA evolved separately from nuclear DNA, originally derived from circular genomes of bacteria
- The mitochondrial genome consists of 37 genes including proteins coding for oxidative phosphorylation complex as well as transfer RNA and ribosomal RNA necessary for translation of mitochondrial genes
- Additional mitochondrial proteins are encoded in the nuclear genome
- Replication is independent of cell cycle

9.1.4.2 Mitochondrial heteroplasmy & homoplasmy

- Eukaryotic cells contain hundreds of copies of mitochondrial DNA
- Homoplasmy
  - All mitochondria in a cell are genetically identical
  - This is expected in normal cells, though homoplasmy mutations can lead to disease
- Heteroplasmy
  - Refers to the state when not all mitochondrial DNA within a given cell are genetically identical
  - Arises because of mitochondrial DNA replication errors
  - Mutation in mitochondrial DNA contributes to variable penetrance of mitochondrial genetic disorders

9.1.4.3 Maternal inheritance

- In gametogenesis, mitochondria come exclusively from the egg
- Disorders are inherited from the mother's side

9.1.5 DNA replication & cell cycle

9.1.5.1 DNA replication

- Occurs during the S phase of cell cycle

ISBN 978-089189-6616

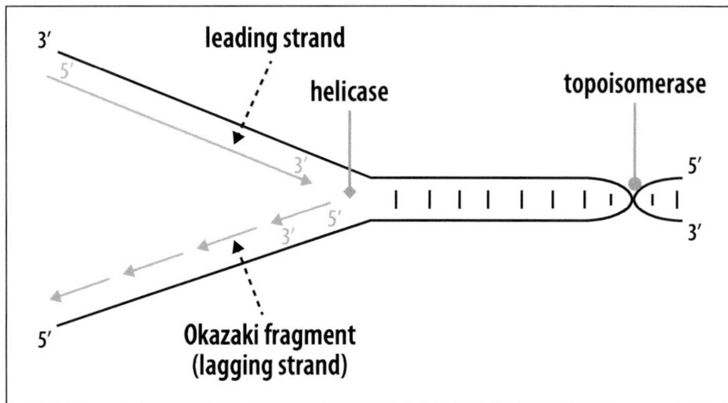

f9.9 DNA replication fork

- Semiconservative replication
- DNA helicase & DNA topoisomerase unwind the double helix
- DNA polymerase catalyzes strand synthesis in the 5' to 3' direction as shown in **f9.9**
  - The 'leading' strand is synthesized in uninterrupted fashion
  - The 'lagging' strand is synthesized in a discontinuous fashion, creating Okazaki fragments

9.1.5.2 Cell cycle

- Interphase is shown in **f9.10**
  - Occurs between mitotic/meiotic phases
  - In the first gap phase (G1), cellular contents, excluding chromosomes, are copied
  - Synthesis (S) phase, all chromosomes are duplicated (2N-4N chromosomes)
  - In the second gap phase (G2), the cell checks for and repairs DNA replication errors. Not present in meiosis

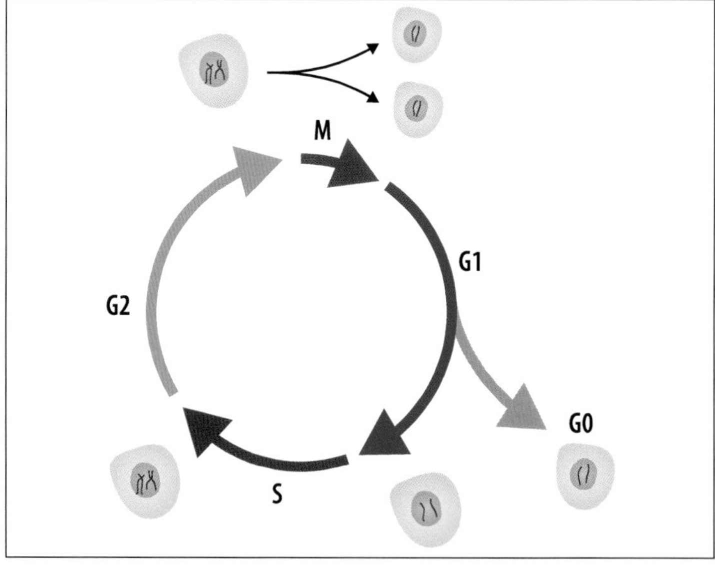

f9.10 Interphase

- Mitosis (M)
  - Cell divides its copied DNA, organelles, and cytoplasm to make 2 cells
  - Prophase, the centrioles move to opposite poles in the nucleus, and the microtubule apparatus begins to form
  - Metaphase, the nuclear envelope disappears, and chromosomes begin to condense and align with the central metaphase plate. This is the period of maximal chromosome condensation, explaining why karyotype analysis relies on the "metaphase spread" of chromosomes
  - Anaphase: Separation of sister chromatids (duplicated chromosomes)
  - Telophase: Chromosomes are located at the opposite poles, nuclear envelope reforms, and cytokinesis physically divides the cell in 2
- Resting stage (G_0)
  - The cell is not actively preparing to divide and may be terminally differentiated

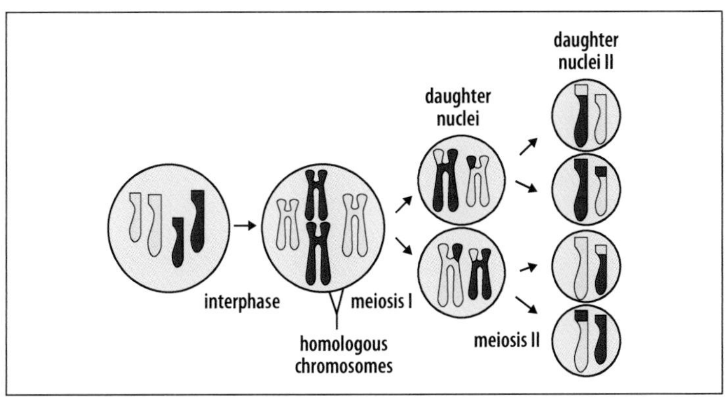

f9.11 Meiosis overview

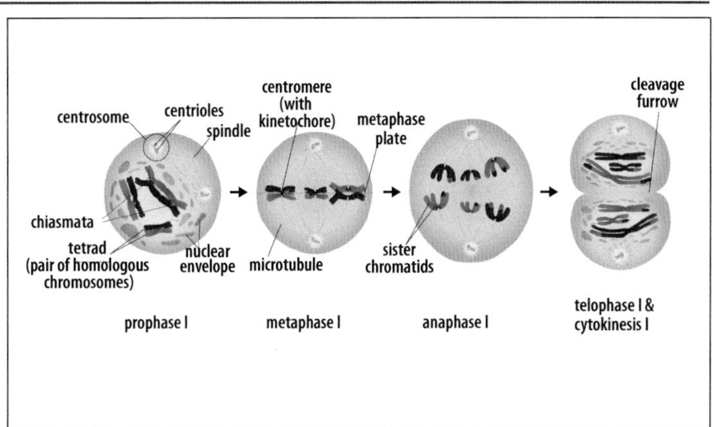

f9.12 Phases of meiosis I

9.1.5.3 Meiosis

- Cell division of reproductive cells to produce gametes. Diploid germ cells (2N) produce 4 haploid gametes at the end of meiosis as shown in **f9.11**
- Subdivided into 2 processes: meiosis I and meiosis II
- Before meiosis starts, DNA of each chromosomes replicate in S phase
- Meiosis I is shown in **f9.12**
  - Prophase I: The longest phase, subdivided into 5 steps—leptotene, zygotene, pachytene, diplotene, and diakinesis. During prophase, homologous chromosomes forms pairs (synapse) and exchanges genetic information (genetic recombination)
  - Metaphase I: Paired homologous chromosomes aligned along an equatorial plane and microtubule spindle attached to the chromosomes of each pair
  - Anaphase I: Chromosomes segregation occurs because of shortening of microtubule spindles
  - Telophase I: Each pole receives half of the chromosomes consist of sister chromatids (haploid). Nuclear membrane surrounds each haploid set of chromosomes
- Meiosis II is shown in **f9.13**
  - Four phases: prophase II, metaphase II, anaphase II, and telophase II
  - Each haploid (N) nuclei divide and produce 2 similar haploid (N) nuclei
  - At the end of meiosis II, original parent (2N) cells produce 4 haploid cells (N)

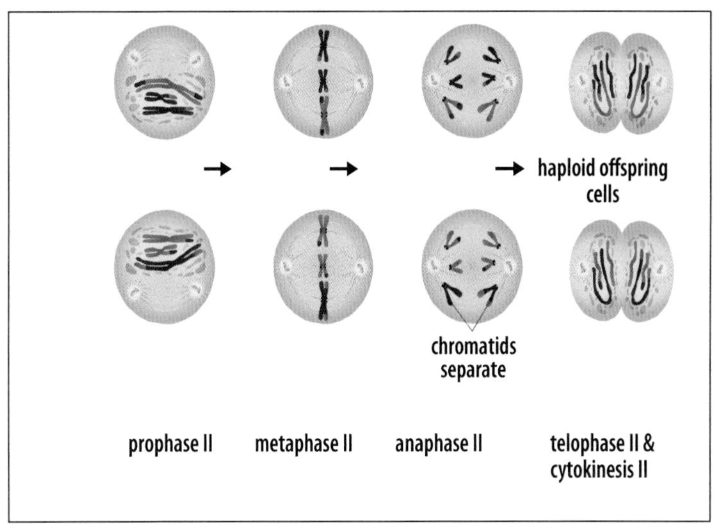

f9.13 Phases of meiosis II

9.1.6 Gene expression

- The process of making functional gene products, including proteins, rRNA, and tRNA

9.1.6.1 Epigenetic regulation

- Involves changes in gene expression without any changes in the nucleotide sequence of the genome
- Examples are DNA methylation of gene promoters & histone modifications

9.1.6.2 Alternative mRNA splicing

- The process of making multiple different proteins product from a single gene
- Involves alternate joining of different exons of a gene to form different isoforms of a protein

ISBN 978-089189-6616

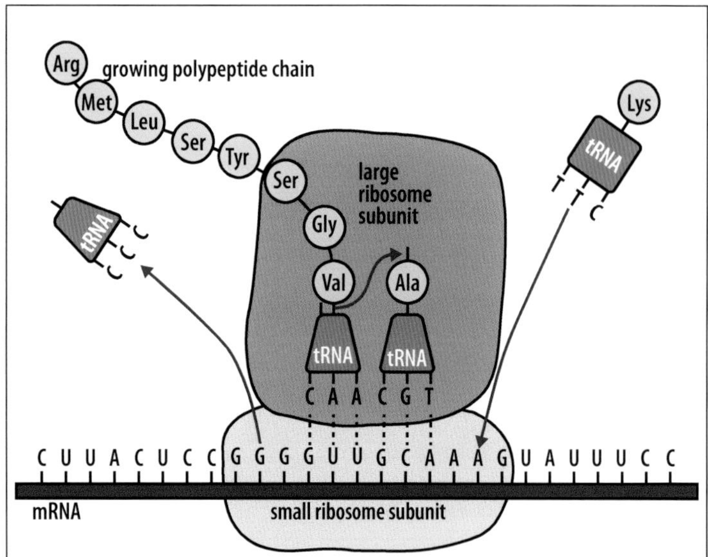

f9.14 Docking of tRNA (TTA) onto the mRNA within the ribosome, as AGG tRNA is released

first letter	U (second letter)	C	A	G	third letter
U	UUU Phe	UCU Ser	UAU Tyr	UGU Cys	U
U	UUC Phe	UCC Ser	UAC Tyr	UGC Cys	C
U	UUA Leu	UCA Ser	UAA Stop	UGA Stop	A
U	UUG Leu	UCG Ser	UAG Stop	UGG Trp	G
C	CUU Leu	CCU Pro	CAU His	CGU Arg	U
C	CUC Leu	CCC Pro	CAC His	CGC Arg	C
C	CUA Leu	CCA Pro	CAA Gln	CGA Arg	A
C	CUG Leu	CCG Pro	CAG Gln	CGG Arg	G
A	AUU Ile	ACU Thr	AAU Asn	AGU Ser	U
A	AUC Ile	ACC Thr	AAC Asn	AGC Ser	C
A	AUA Ile	ACA Thr	AAA Lys	AGA Arg	A
A	AUG Met	ACG Thr	AAG Lys	AGG Arg	G
G	GUU Val	GCU Ala	GAU Asp	GGU Gly	U
G	GUC Val	GCC Ala	GAC Asp	GGC Gly	C
G	GUA Val	GCA Ala	GAA Glu	GGA Gly	A
G	GUG Val	GCG Ala	GAG Glu	GGG Gly	G

f9.15 Genetic code table: each 3-letter sequence of RNA nucleotides corresponds to a specific amino acid, or to a stop codon

9.1.6.3 Protein translation

- Processed RNA transcripts are transported from the nucleus to the cytoplasm for translation by ribosomes
- The mRNA enters ribosome until a start site (AUG) is encountered
- A tRNA charged with methionine recognizes the AUG sequence and binds mRNA
- A tRNA recognizing the next 3 nucleotide sequence, coding for the next amino acid docks and its amino acid becomes covalently linked to the methionine and so on, as shown in **f9.14** and **f9.15**

9.1.6.4 Translational control

- Control of the amount of protein synthesized from mRNA in the cell
- Includes ribosomes recruitment on the initiation codon, modulation of elongation, termination of protein synthesis, ribosomes, tRNA biogenesis, availability of translation factors
- Translational control can change the rate of synthesis faster than pretranslational regulations

9.1.6.5 Protein degradation rate

- Different proteins degrade at different rates
- The N-end rule, intrinsic disorders, flexibility, presence of carbohydrate/phosphate group, and physiological state determine the half-life of proteins in the cell
- Proteins are degraded by proteasome complex in the cell

9.1.7 Genetic anomalies

9.1.7.1 Polymorphism

- A genetic change that is not deleterious and is present in at least 1% of the population
- Examples include blood groups & histocompatibility antigens
- May consist of a single or multiple alternative nucleotide at a locus
- Variable length of microsatellites
  - Single nucleotide polymorphism (SNP)
  - Occur at a frequency of approximately 1 in 600 base pairs
- May alter restriction endonuclease digestion sites

9.1.7.2 Mutation

- A genetic change with a deleterious outcome, may result in loss or gain of function
- There are multiple classifications of mutations as shown in **f9.16** and described below
- Point mutation
  - A single nucleotide change, insertion or deletion, leading to nonsense, missense, silent, frameshift or splice site mutations
  - Nonsense mutations result in premature truncation of translation
  - Missense mutations lead to changes in protein sequence
  - Silent mutations change the nucleic acid sequence, but do not result in the production of either a stop codon or different amino acid

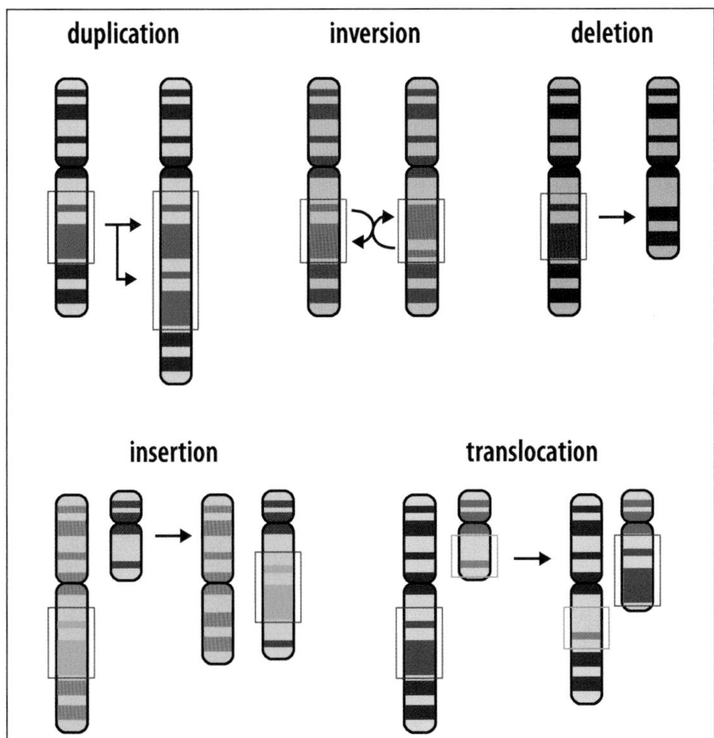

f9.16 Various types of mutations

- Splice site mutations are caused by point mutations of splicing donor or acceptor sequences
- Frameshift mutations lead to changes in the reading frame of the ribosome in translation and are most commonly the result of insertions & deletions

- Insertion mutations
  - Addition of ≥1 nucleotide base pair in the DNA sequence
  - It is deleterious if it happens in the exon region of a gene, which results in alternation in reading frame (frameshift mutation) of the codon
- Deletion mutations
  - Deletion of ≥1 nucleotide base pair in the DNA sequence
  - It is deleterious if it happens in the exon region of a gene which may result in alternation in reading frame (frameshift mutation) of the codon
- Duplication mutations
  - Duplication of a portion of DNA resulting in multiple copies of that region in the genome
- Inversions
  - Reversal of the segment of a gene or chromosome
- Translocations
  - Interchange of the segment of chromosomes between nonhomologous chromosomes

9.1.7.3 Inherited vs acquired genetic disorders

- Disorders that result from a gene defect are generally considered genetic disorders, but not all genetic disorders are inherited
- Some genetic defects are sporadic; that is, the defect is absent in both the paternal and maternal genome, and is somehow acquired during oogenesis, spermatogenesis, or early embryogenesis
- For most genetic disorders, there are both inherited and sporadic forms, the latter termed "simplex cases." Such sporadic defects are usually "germline" nevertheless; that is, the defect is present in all cells of the organism
- Other genetic defects arise within a differentiated cell; such "somatic" defects are not found in germline DNA and are unlikely to be passed on to offspring
- Constitutional mutation
  - Mutation acquired in germ cells and present in every cell of an offspring
- Somatic mutation
  - Mutation acquired in somatic cells during cell division
  - Somatic mutations are not transferred in next generation of an organism

9.1.7.4 Common inheritance patterns

- Autosomal dominant disorders
  - Often involve genes that encode structural proteins, receptor proteins, or transmembrane channels
  - At least 1 parent is usually affected
  - Boys & girls are affected with equal frequency
  - Both men & women have a 50% chance of transmitting the condition to offspring
  - Conditions are modified by penetrance & expressivity
    - Penetrance: The proportion of patients with the mutation who manifest a phenotypic abnormality. Genetic defects that always result in abnormal phenotype are said to have 100% penetrance
    - Expressivity: The severity & range of manifestations
- Autosomal recessive disorders
  - Skips generations (parents are usually unaffected, but both parents are implied carriers)
  - Boys & girls are equally affected
  - For a couple with an affected child, the likelihood of a second affected child is 25%
  - Rare autosomal recessive genetic defects rely heavily on consanguinity for survival in the population

ISBN 978-089189-6616

- In general, autosomal recessive conditions do not vary in terms of penetrance or expressivity. Autosomal recessive genetic defects usually involve genes that encode enzymes
- X-linked recessive disorders
  - Expressed almost exclusively in males
  - Females may be affected in regions of very high mutant gene frequency, such that a homozygous female patient becomes a statistical likelihood. Girls may also be affected on the basis of asymmetric lyonization or Turner syndrome (monosomy X)
  - Men cannot pass the trait to their male offspring, but their daughters are obligate carriers. Women have a 50% chance of passing the trait to their male offspring (who will be affected) and to their female offspring (who will be carriers)

9.2 Molecular science principles

9.2.1 Enzymes & nucleic acid chemistry in molecular techniques

9.2.1.1 Polymerases

- DNA polymerase
  - Catalyze DNA replication in the 5' to 3' direction
  - Some polymerases have exonuclease activity in 5' to 3' and/or 3' to 5'
  - DNA Pol I includes a large fragment carrying polymerase activity (Klenow fragment) and a small fragment with exonuclease activity that bestows proofreading capacity
  - Must be stable at high temperature
  - Commonly used Taq polymerase originates from *Archaebacterium Thermus aquaticus*
- DNA-dependent RNA polymerase
  - Copy a template strand of DNA into RNA
  - Prokaryotes share a single multi-subunit RNA polymerase
  - Eukaryotes have 3 types of RNA polymerase (Pol I, Pol II & Pol III)
  - Pol I & Pol III synthesize noncoding RNA
  - Pol II synthesizes messenger RNA (mRNA)
- RNA dependent RNA polymerase
  - Copy a template strand of RNA into RNA

9.2.1.2 DNA ligase

- Catalyzes formation of phosphodiester bonds between nucleotides
- Can act on both DNA & RNA

EcoRI (sticky ends)	SmaI (blunt ends)
5′ - G|AATTC - 3′	5′ - CCC|GGG - 3′
3′ - CTTAA|G - 5′	3′ - GGG|CCC - 5′

f9.17 Sticky & blunt ends generated by endonucleases

9.2.1.3 Endonuclease

- Cleave the sugar-phosphate bonds within a strand of DNA, generating either blunt ends or a 5' and 3' overhang as shown in **f9.17**
- Restriction endonucleases occur naturally in bacteria as a defense against invading DNA
- Cleaves DNA at specific recognition sequences, which are usually a palindrome, same sequence in both 5' to 3' and 3'-5' direction
- Methylation sensitive enzymes recognize CpG motifs and cannot cleave if the cytosine residue is methylated

9.2.1.4 Exonuclease

- Removes nucleotides from ends of single stranded DNA
- Enzyme is often used to create blunt ends during molecular cloning procedures

9.2.1.5 Reverse transcriptase

- RNA-dependent DNA polymerase
- Isolated from RNA viruses
- Requires a sequence-specific primer
- Copies RNA single strand to an RNA-DNA hybrid
- Uses a hairpin formation on the end of the newly synthesized DNA strand to prime synthesis of the complimentary DNA strand, resulting in cDNA

9.2.1.6 Primers

- Short sequences of DNA (15-30 bases) that will hybridize to a target and direct polymerases to the target sequence to be copied by the polymerase
- Synthesized chemically
- Used in *pairs* for most polymerase chain reaction (PCR) applications
- May be either unlabeled or labeled with a reporter dye, depending on application
- Primer design is essential to test performance
  - Primer pairs should have similar melting temperatures (T_m)

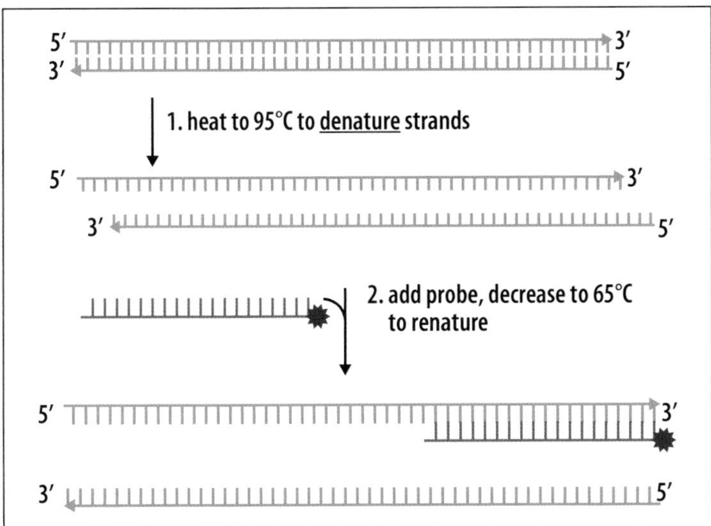

f9.18 Nucleic acid hybridization

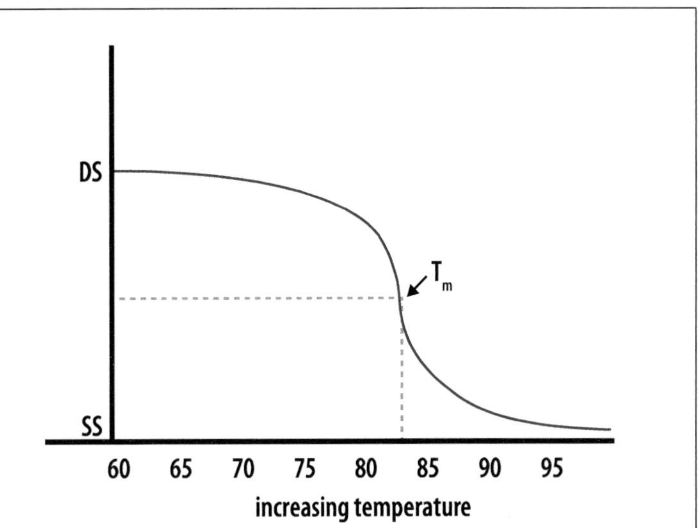

f9.19 Typical DNA melt profile

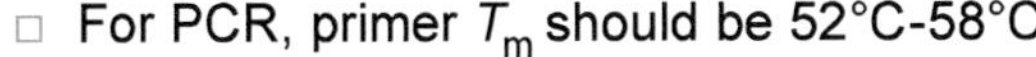

- For PCR, primer T_m should be 52°C-58°C
- If the primer T_m is too high compared to annealing temperature, false-positive reactions may occur because of mis-hybridization
- If the primer T_m is too low compared to annealing temperature, false-negative reactions may occur because of lack of hybridization

9.2.1.7 Probes

- A segment of nucleic acid, most commonly DNA, complimentary to the target sequence, with a covalently attached reporter molecule
- Hybridizes to its target sequence to allow for detection of the target sequence
- Probe length varies depending on the application
  - Chemically synthesized oligonucleotides (15-200 bases)
  - Fragments of genomic DNA (100s to 1,000s bases)

9.2.2 Molecular processes

9.2.2.1 Hybridization of nucleic acids

- The process of hybridization is depicted in **f9.18**
- Any nucleic acid can be detected by hybridizing a *probe*
- Probe is a complementary DNA fragment
  - Must be labeled with radioactive isotope or fluorescent dye
- Hybridization temperature is ~5°C below the T_m
- Complex sequences may take longer to reanneal
- Hybridization is commonly used in PCR, solid array, and blotting techniques
  - Southern blotting detects DNA
  - Northern blotting detects mRNA
- Formamide may be included in some hybridization techniques to help denature secondary structure
- Dextran sulfate, polyethylene glycol, or polyacrylic acid may be included to accelerate hybridization of long probes

9.2.2.2 Melting temperature (T_m)

- The temperature at which half of a particular DNA duplex will dissociate
- A simple T_m calculation can be used for short sequences (14-20 bases)
  - T_m= (4°C × number of GC pairs) + (2°C × number of AT pairs)
- For longer sequences, calculation of T_m considers salt concentration, G-C content and base-pair length
- A typical DNA melt profile is shown in **f9.19**

9.2.2.3 Stringency

- Conditions that dictate how accurately and tightly a probe binds to its target sequence
- Low stringency conditions allow for probe binding in the presence of target sequence mismatch
- If stringency is too high, a probe will not bind to its target sequence
- Controlled by several factors
  - Temperature of hybridization: Low temperature is low stringency
  - Salt concentration: High salt is low stringency
  - Concentration of denaturant
  - Probe length and G-C content

ISBN 978-089189-6616

9.3 Molecular techniques

9.3.1 Isolation of nucleic acid

- Extraction methods isolate nucleic acid from other cell components including proteins & lipids, while rendering the sample noninfectious

9.3.1.1 Silica/solid-phase isolation method

- Nucleic acid will adsorb to silica certain pH & salt concentrations
- Appropriate for somewhat fragmented DNA, large DNA fragments are subject to shearing
- Sample is applied to the column, washed with buffer, and DNA is eluted with water
- Also used in downstream molecular techniques to remove proteins, RNA, primers, unincorporated nucleotides, enzymes & salts, phenol, chloroform

9.3.1.2 Salting out method

- Appropriate for isolating large amounts of high-molecular-weight DNA for Southern blot, etc
- Cells are lysed with detergent
- Low pH & high salt conditions to precipitate proteins
- DNA is precipitated with alcohol, washed & dissolved in the appropriate solution

9.3.1.3 Organic: Phenol/chloroform

- Can be used to isolate the DNA, RNA, or protein fraction
- Use high salt, low pH & organic reagents
- Recovers large quantities of nucleic acid
- Suitable for recovery of fragmented nucleic acid
- DNA will be in the aqueous phase, proteins in the interphase & RNA in the organic phase

9.3.1.4 Organic: Phenol/chloroform/guanidinium thiocyanate

- Recovers large quantities of RNA
- Guanidinium thiocyanate denatures proteins, including RNases, and separates ribosomal RNA from the ribosomes
- RNA will be in the aqueous phase, DNA in the interphase, and proteins & lipids in the organic phase **f9.20**

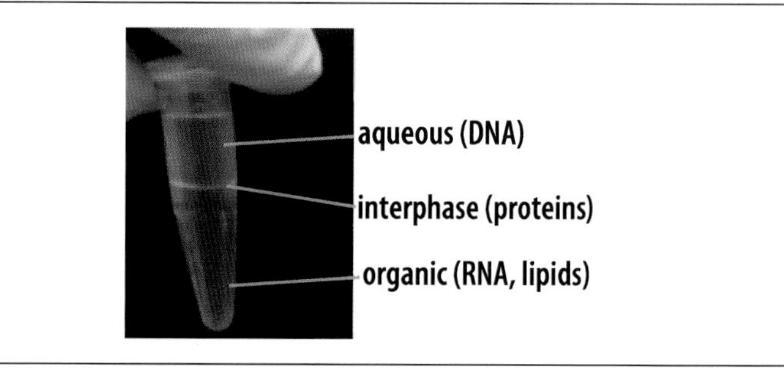

f9.20 Aqueous, interphase & organic phases formed during organic extraction

9.3.2 Assessing nucleic acid quantity & quality

9.3.2.1 Spectrophotometry

- Quantitation is based on the principle that, because of adenine residues, nucleic acids adsorb light at 260 nm

concentration (ug/mL) = (OD_{260} × [dilution factor] × [absorptivity constant])

- Absorptivity constants: DNA = 50 µg/mL; RNA = 40 µg/mL; single stranded oligo = 33 µg/mL
- Traditional spectrophotometer gives reliable absorbance readings 0.1-1.5 OD
- Protein adsorbs light at 280 nm. Assessment of purity is achieved by examining the 260/280 ratio. The ratio for good quality DNA should be 1.6-2.0. The ratio for RNA should be 2.0-2.3
- Microvolume instruments use fiber-optic technology and rely on surface tension between 2 optical pedestals
- Requires minimal sample (0.5-2 µL)
- Quantitative range approximately 2,000-3,000 ng/µL
- Nucleic acid contamination can be assessed by measuring adsorption at additional wavelengths. Common contaminants are listed in **t9.3**

t9.3 Common contaminants detectable with spectrophotometry

Contaminant	Wavelength of peak absorbance
Phenol	270 nm
Thiocyanates	230 nm
Protein	280 nm

9.3.2.2 Fluorometry

- Measures nucleic concentration in association with specific dyes
- Dyes are specific to intact double stranded DNA or single stranded DNA or RNA
- Readings may vary from those obtained by adsorption and may be considered more accurate for some downstream applications such as next-generation sequencing
- Hoechst 33258 is the most common fluorescent dye used for DNA concentration measurement

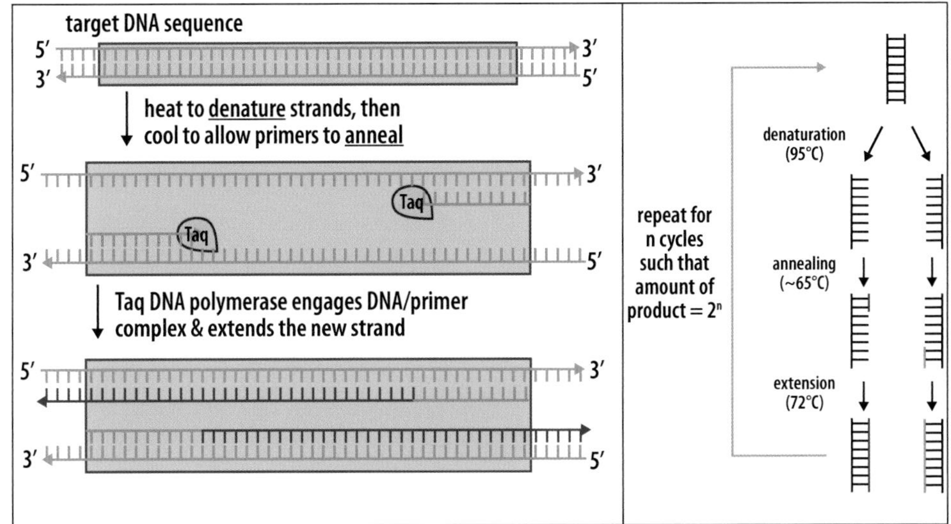

f9.21 Polymerase chain reaction showing strand separation, primer annealing, engagement of Taq and elongation of the complementary strands

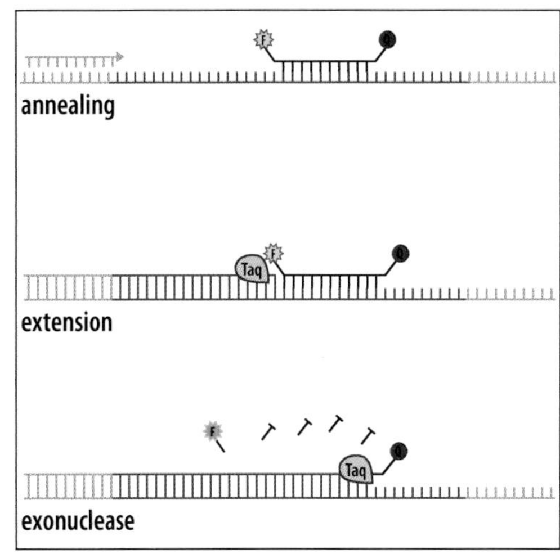

f9.22 Dual-labeled hydrolysis probes in real-time PCR. The probe anneals to the target. Taq continues to add nucleotides to the growing strand until it reaches the probe. Taq has exonuclease activity and digests the probe, allowing the fluorescence to be detected

9.3.2.3 Electrophoresis

- Quality of nucleic acid can be assessed with agarose gel electrophoresis
- High-molecular-weight DNA or RNA will produce strong bands with low mobility
- Smearing of bands is generally indicative of nucleic acid degradation and may indicate that the quality is unacceptable for downstream molecular applications

9.3.3 DNA amplification by PCR

- Uses thermostable polymerase with repeating cycles of DNA synthesis to amplify a target sequence as shown in **f9.21**
- Can make up to 10^{12} copies per reaction
- Components include DNA polymerase, primers, deoxynucleotides, divalent cation, and pH buffer
- Amplify a target sequence through repeated cycles of synthesis in thermocycler
    - Denature at 95°C to separate DNA strands containing target
    - Anneal complementary primer at lower temperature specified by primer & target sequences
    - Extension of the DNA strand by DNA polymerase occurs at 72°C
    - Repeat for 30-40 cycles
- The amount of DNA produced under optimal conditions: [DNA] = 2^n, where n = number of cycles. A 10-fold amplification takes place every 3.3 cycles ($2^{3.3}$=10). If there are 100 copies in cycle 7, then there will be 1,000 copies in cycle 10

9.3.4 Reverse transcriptase PCR (rt-PCR or RT-PCR)

- Used to detect specific RNA sequences
- Template RNA is converted to cDNA in the first step by reverse transcriptase
    - Primer hybridizes to complementary RNA sequence
    - Reverse transcriptase enzyme engages RNA/DNA hybrid as the start site for reverse transcription
    - Reverse transcriptase enzyme creates a DNA copy (cDNA) of RNA
    - Occurs at 50°C
- PCR proceeds using the cDNA as the template

9.3.5 Real-time PCR (QPCR, qPCR)

- Uses fluorescent dyes or probes to detect the formation of PCR amplicons during PCR
- Requires target specific primers & probe(s)
- Frequently uses hydrolysis probes (eg, TaqMan dual labeled probes) and fluorescence resonance energy transfer (FRET) as shown in **f9.22**
- With FRET, the inhibition of 1 dye is caused by second dye in close proximity; hydrolysis of the probe allows the labeled nucleotides to move away from one another and the previously inhibited signal becomes detectable
- Commonly used to detect infectious disease targets
- Allows for quantitation of targets, often used to assess efficacy of antiviral therapy and to monitor for the development of drug resistance

ISBN 978-089189-6616

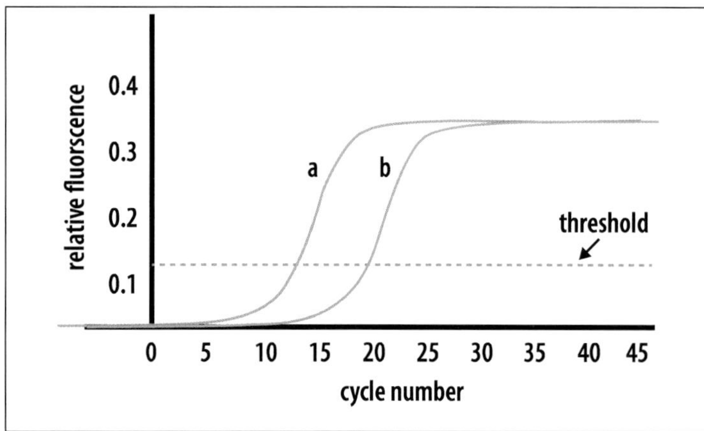

f9.23 Real time PCR amplification plot

- Data are represented on amplification plots comparing the cycle number to the fluorescence signal as shown in **f9.23**
  - The *threshold* is a horizontal line, set by the user, at the point at which the fluorescence enters the logarithmic phase of amplification
  - The *Ct* is the cycle number that the amplification curve for a sample crosses the threshold
  - Samples with more template cross at an earlier Ct value
  - Samples that differ in template concentration by a factor of 10 will be about 3.3 Ct apart, as demonstrated by curve A and curve B in **f9.23**
- Post PCR melt curve analysis may be performed to further subtype the pathogen

9.3.6 Melting point analysis

- Following PCR, using nonhydrolyzable probes or intercalating dye, florescence is measured while incrementally increasing the temperature
- The melting point is the point at which 50% of the DNA is single stranded
- Data are plotted as fluorescence vs temperature, with the melting point as the point of the maximal change in rate of melting; **f9.24** shows the melt profiles for a 200-base pair PCR product for 10 different enterovirus serotypes
- Melting point is dependent on length, G:C content, and the amount of mismatch
  - AT-rich regions denature first (2 H bonds)
  - GC-rich regions denature last (3 H bonds)

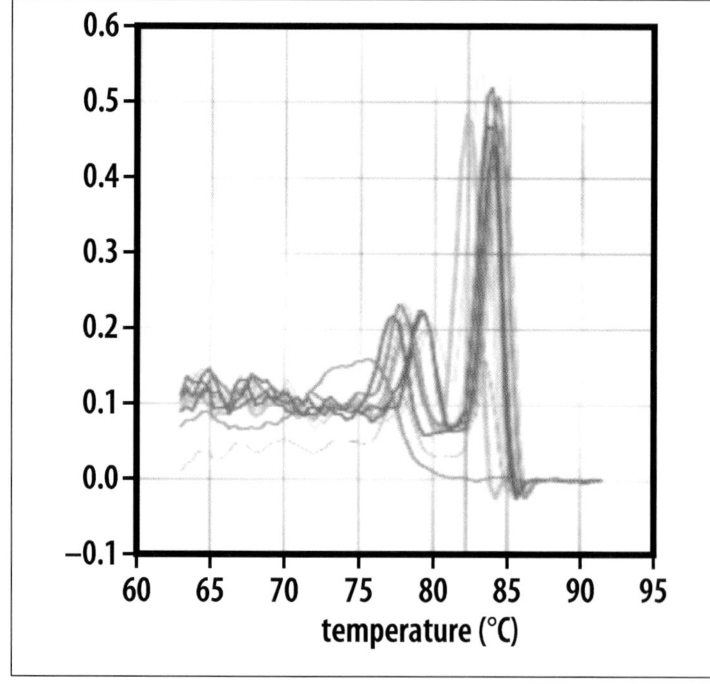

f9.24 SYBR green PCR melt curves for 10 different enterovirus serotypes

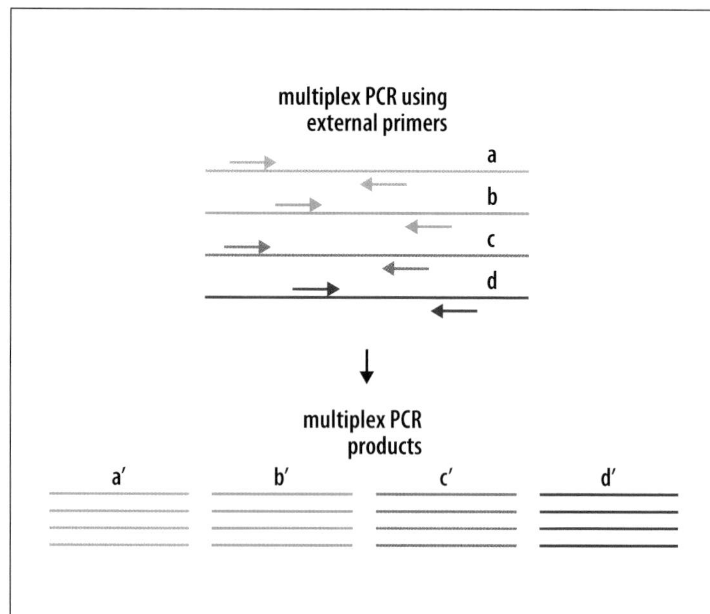

f9.25 Multiplex PCR

9.3.7 Multiplex PCR

- Multiple primers for different targets are added to the reaction mix and run in a single tube, as shown in **f9.25**
- Allows for the identification of multiple targets within the same sample

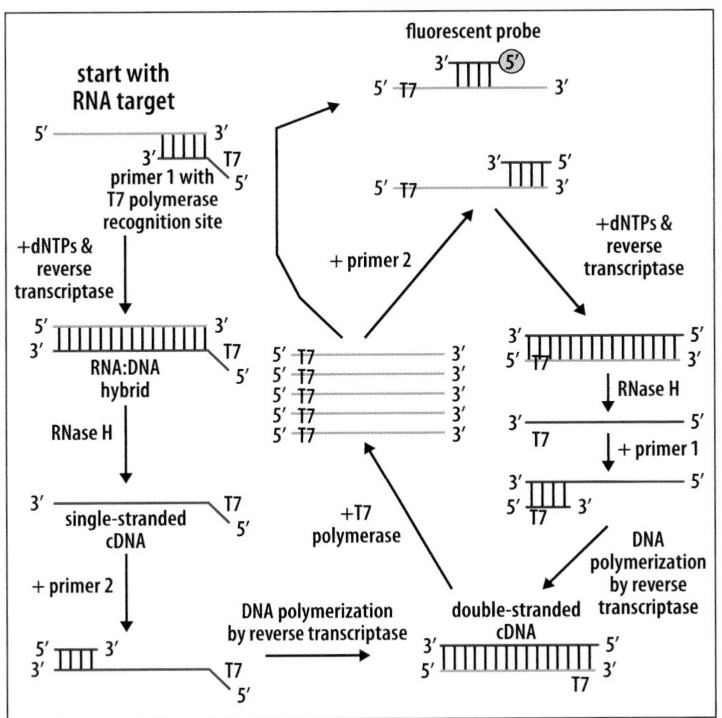

f9.26 TMA & NASBA isothermal amplification

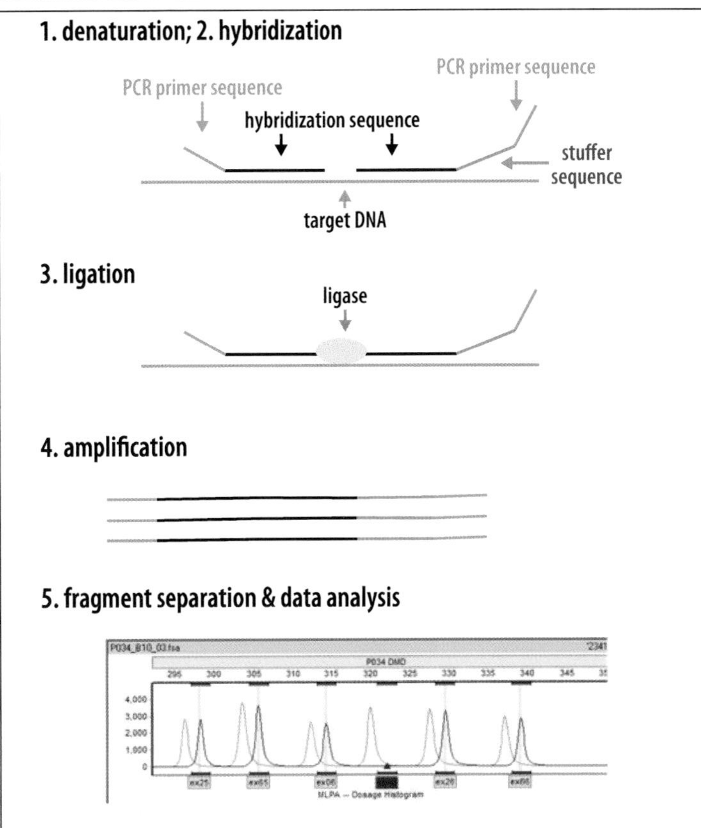

f9.27 Multiplex ligation-dependent probe amplification

9.3.8 Transcription-mediated amplification (TMA) & nucleic acid sequence-based amplification (NASBA)

- For isothermal amplification of RNA targets, primarily used for infectious disease applications
- Use specific sequences that are recognized by bacteriophage RNA polymerase to make more RNA copies
- Technique is presented for each method in **f9.26**
- RNA copies produced can then be probed

9.3.9 Multiplex ligation-dependent probe amplification (MLPA)

- Used to interrogate multiple mutations at the same time
- Quantitative method useful to quantify, detect copy number changes, identify methylation status, detect SNP, and quantify mRNA
- Uses hybrid nucleic acid sequence that contains probe hybridization sequence, stuffer sequence, and PCR primer sequence, as shown in **f9.27**
- For each possible mutation, there is a specific probe & adjacent anchor probe separated by a single base
- Only when the 2 probes anneal adjacent to each other are they able to be subsequently ligated and then amplified with probe-specific primers

9.3.10 Signal amplification

- Techniques that amplify signal rather than the target sequence

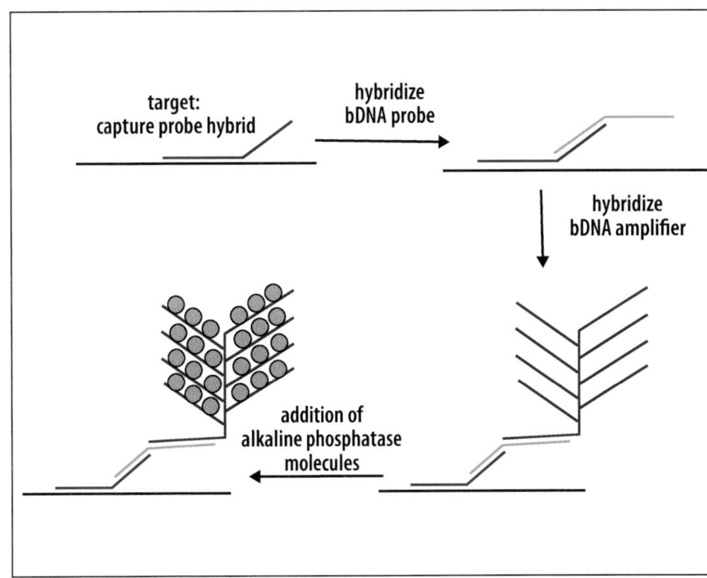

f9.28 Branched DNA detection is an example of signal amplification technique

- Less susceptible to contamination, but not as sensitive as target amplification
- Cleavage-based amplification or ligation amplification reaction amplifies the probe
- Branched DNA or hybrid capture techniques amplify the signal as shown in **f9.28**

ISBN 978-089189-6616

Molecular techniques>Restriction fragment length polymorphism (RFLP) analysis | Blotting | Methylation-specific PCR

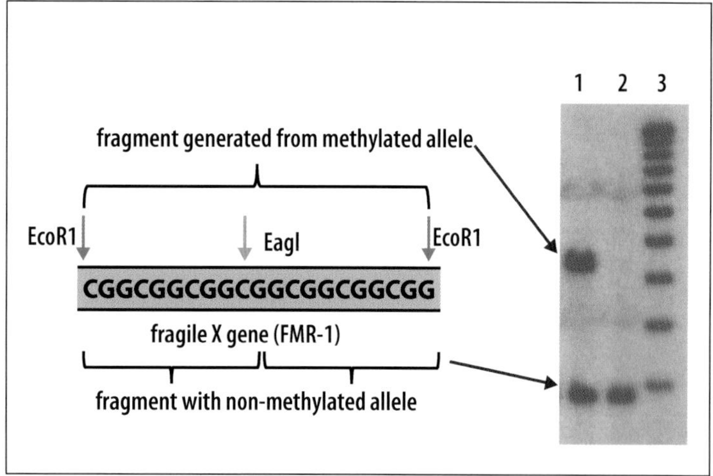

f9.29 Restriction fragment length polymorphism (RFLP) analysis of Fragile X gene. Endonuclease cut sites for EcoRI & EagI are indicated in **a**. EagI is methylation sensitive & will not cut if the site is methylated. **b** shows resulting from double digestion (EcoRI & EagI) digestion of the *FMR-1* gene from a female in lane 1 & a male in lane 2. Females have 2 copies of the X chromosome, 1 is active & the second is methylated. Digestion of the female DNA results in a large fragment generated by only EcoRI cuts & 2 more fragments, migrating in the same position in the gel. The male sample does not have the large methylated fragment

1 electrophoresis gel
nitrocellulose filter
2 blotting paper
3 DNA transferred to filter
4 hybridize with unique nucleic acid probe
5 probe hybridized to complimentary DNA sequence
6 expose x-ray to filter
autoradiogram

f9.30 Southern blot technique

9.3.11 Restriction fragment length polymorphism (RFLP) analysis

- Use of restriction endonucleases to produce sequence-specific maps of DNA
- Restriction enzymes must be used at defined conditions to ensure high specificity of recognition and cutting
- Pattern of fragments produced can be used to determine identity between 2 individuals or to identify differences, eg, mutation, translocation, or trinucleotide expansion
- Fragments can be assessed by agarose gel or capillary electrophoresis as shown in **f9.29** for agarose gel analysis

9.3.12 Blotting

9.3.12.1 Southern blot

- The Southern blot technique is used to detect DNA
- Before blotting, genomic DNA is digested with restriction enzymes and separated by size by electrophoresis
- The resulting DNA fragments are transferred to nitrocellulose membrane has shown in **f9.30**
- DNA fragments are cross-linked to the membrane before incubation with hybridization probes

9.3.12.2 Northern blot

- The northern blot technique is used to detect cellular RNA or RNA transcripts
- The blotting process is similar to that of Southern blot
- Can be used to observe gene expression patterns of normal or oncogenes

9.3.12.3 Western blot

- The western blot technique is used to detect protein
- Also known as *protein immunoblot*
- Proteins are denatured & electrophoresed
- Protein is transferred to a membrane
- Membrane is washed in a solution containing antibodies to protein targets of interest

9.3.13 Methylation-specific PCR

- Also known as *bisulfate sequencing*
- Used to detect methylation of genes
- Sodium metabisulfite will reduce methylated cytosine residues to uracil
- After pretreatment with metabisulfite, PCR primers that are specific to a sequence containing uracil are used to selectively amplify the methylated sequence
- DNA is then sequenced by one of the various methods described herein

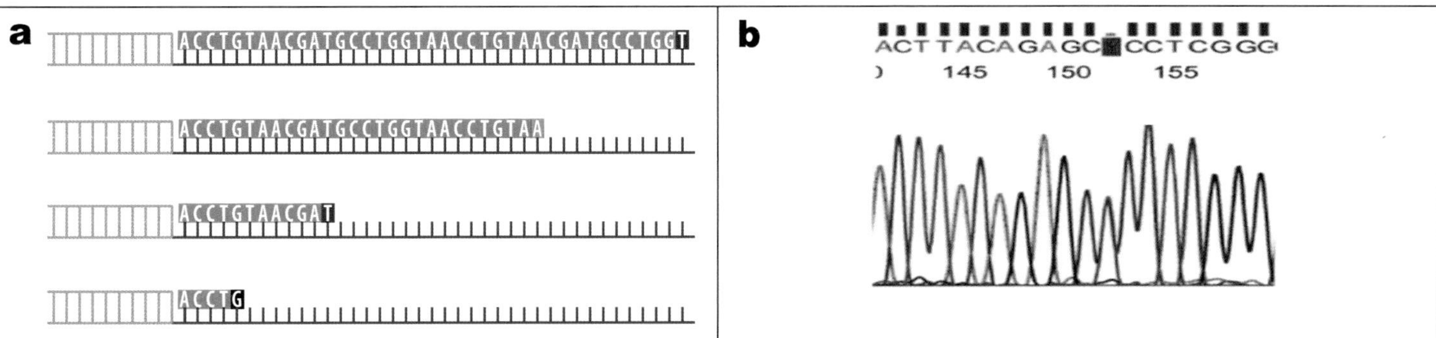

f9.31 Sanger dideoxy sequencing example: **a** PCR products generated during the sequencing reaction. The dideoxy terminators are indicated as the colored nucleotide at the end of the growing strands. **b** electropherogram output, including a heterozygous position (Y)

t9.4 Common nucleotide ambiguity codes used in sequence analysis

Symbol	Description	Symbol	Description
A	adenine	R	purines (A,G)
C	cytocine	Y	pyrimidines (C, T)
T	thymine	K	keto (T, G)
G	guanine	M	amino (A, C)
W	A or T	B	C, G or T
S	C or G	D	A, G or T
H	A, C or T	V	A, C or G
N,X	A, G, C or T	–	gap symbol

9.3.14 DNA sequencing

9.3.14.1 Sanger dideoxy sequencing

- Based on termination of strand elongation when a dideoxy base (ddNTP) is incorporated, resulting in a mixture of strands of varying length as shown in **f9.31a**
- ddNTPs lack a 3' hydroxyl group so further bases cannot be added by polymerase
- Sequencing reaction is performed in a single tube with differentially colored fluorochrome labeled ddNTPs (fluorescent chain terminators) and subjected to capillary electrophoresis
- Sequencing software displays data in the form of an electropherogram **f9.31b**. This can differentiate homozygous vs heterozygous sequence as indicated at position 152 where both C and T are present as overlapping red (T) and blue (C) peaks. This is also indicated in the text translation as Y, which is the C/T ambiguity code
- Additional common ambiguity codes are listed in **t9.4**

9.3.14.2 Pyrosequencing

- The molecular basis is shown in **f9.32**
  - PCR primer is designed to anneal near the mutation site
  - DNA polymerase elongates the single stranded template from the sequencing primer

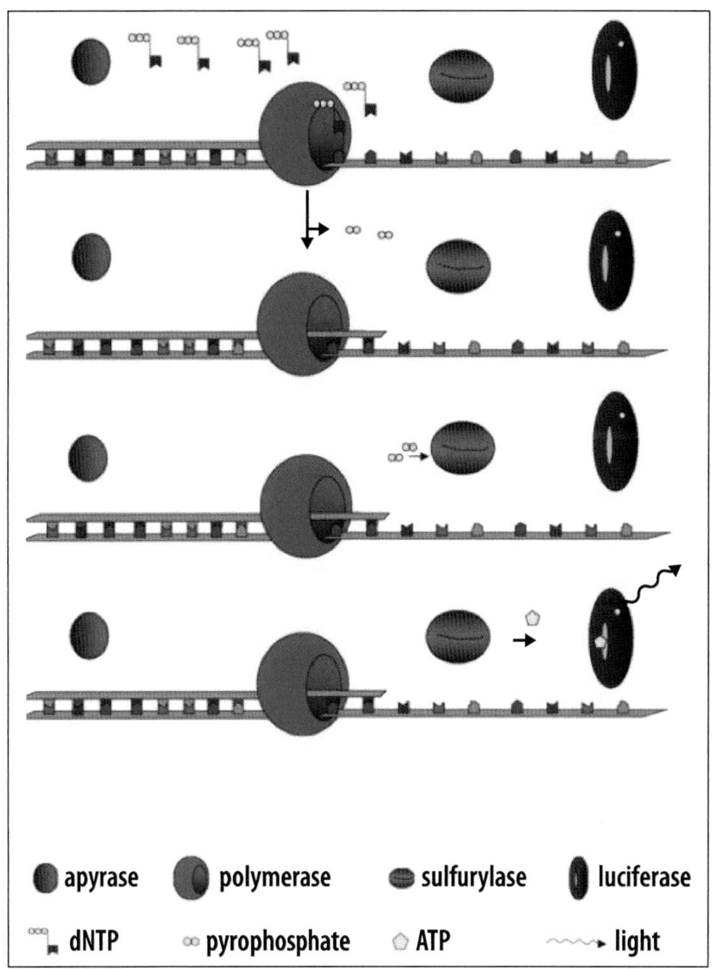

f9.32 Molecular basis of pyrosequencing

  - Incorporation of dNTPS results in the release of pyrophosphate molecules
  - Pyrophosphate molecules are converted to adenosine triphosphate (ATP) and then to detectable light
  - After each cycle, enzyme is added to degrade unincorporated dNTPs
  - Then the next dNTP is added and the cycle repeats
- Quantitative measurement of the pyrophosphate released whenever a phosphodiester bond forms

 ISBN 978-089189-6616

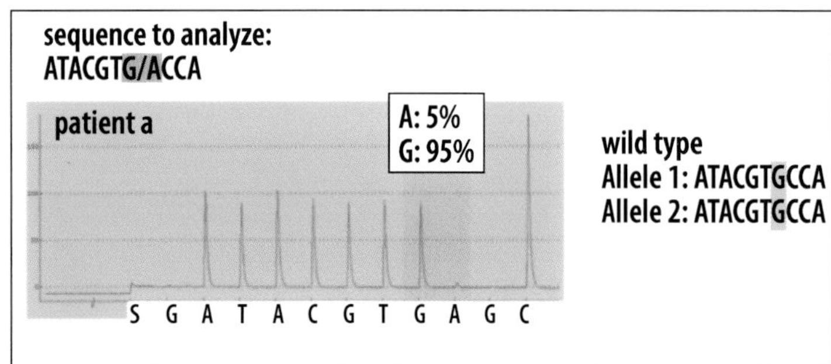

f9.33 Pyrosequencing data output

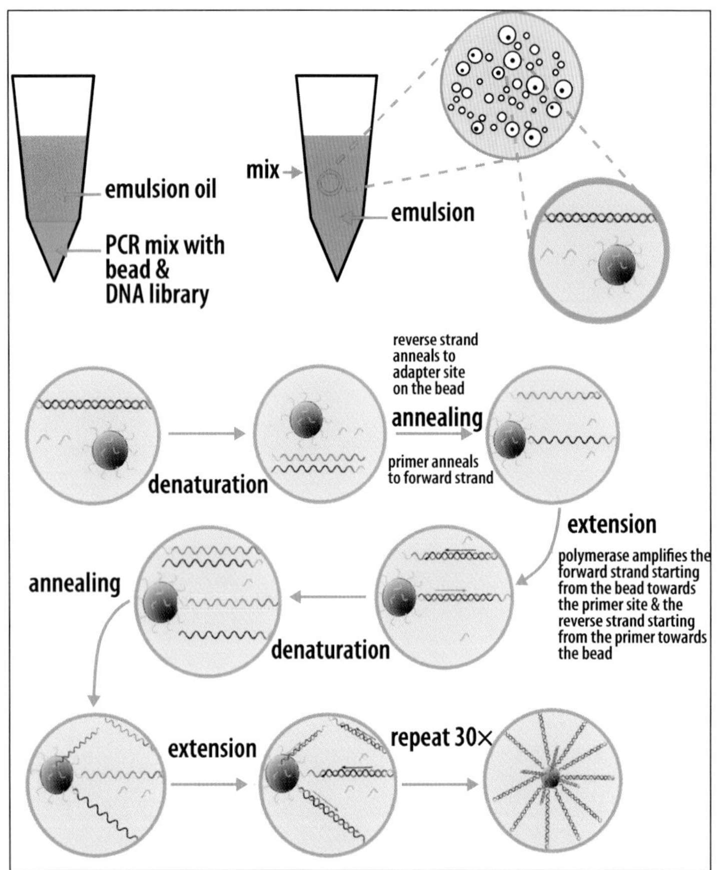

f9.34 Emulsion polymerase chain reaction (PCR)

- Because the pyrophosphate is released in a stoichiometric amount in relation to the number of bases incorporated, the sequence of a target DNA can be inferred
- **f9.33** is representative pyrosequencing data: 6 conserved nucleotides were sequenced before interrogation of the mutation site; in this case the patient expresses the wild type allele, as indicated by detection of 95% G nucleotides at that position

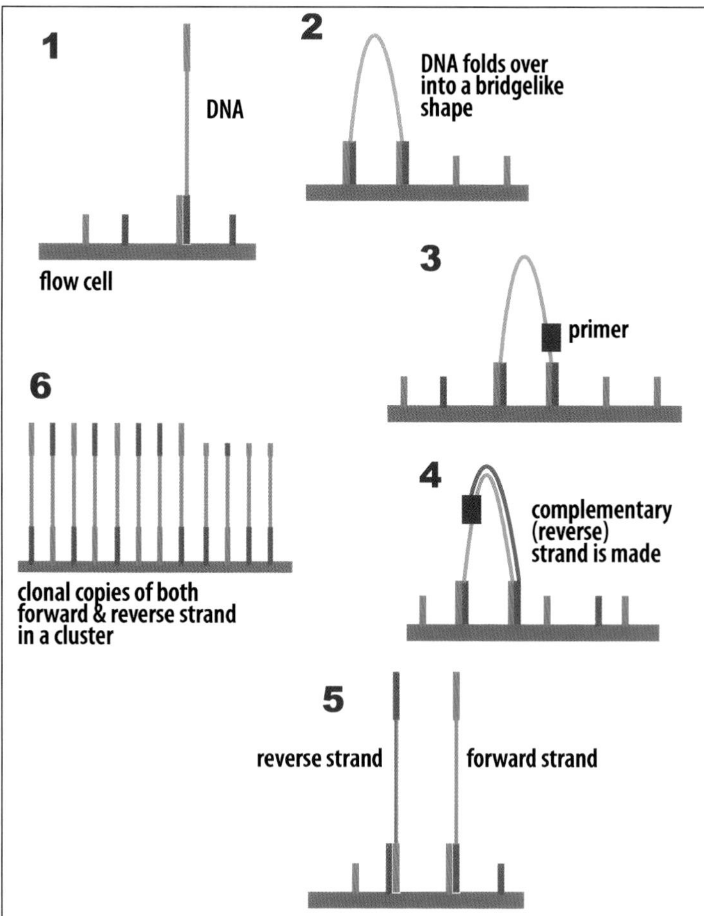

f9.35 Next-generation sequencing (NGS) polymerase chain reaction (PCR) on solid substrate (aka bridge PCR): The DNA attaches to the the flow cell via complementary sequences. The strand bends over and attaches to a second oligo forming a bridge. A primer synthesizes the reverse strand. The 2 strands release and straighten. Each forms a new bridge (bridge amplification). The result is a cluster of DNA forward & reverse strands clones

9.3.14.3 Next-generation sequencing (NGS)

- Massively parallel sequencing followed by computer-mediated contiguous sequence alignment
- DNA is typically fragmented, ligated to an adapter sequence, barcode, and primer
- Individual DNA strands are clonally amplified through emulsion PCR, shown in **f9.34**, or PCR on solid substrate as shown in **f9.35**
- May be applied to whole exome sequencing, or selective sequencing of exons
- Multiple platforms exist employing a broad range of chemistries, including pyrosequencing, reversible dye terminator, oligonucleotide chained ligation, proton detection and phospholinked fluorescent nucleotides
- NGS technologies represent a major leap in sequencing technology; the field continues to evolve rapidly

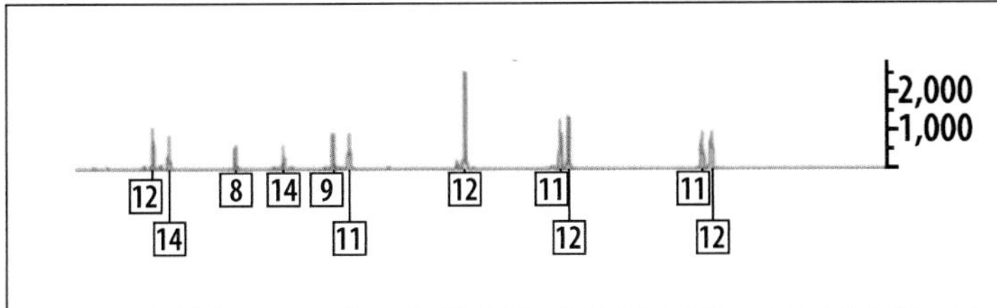

f9.36 STR electropherogram

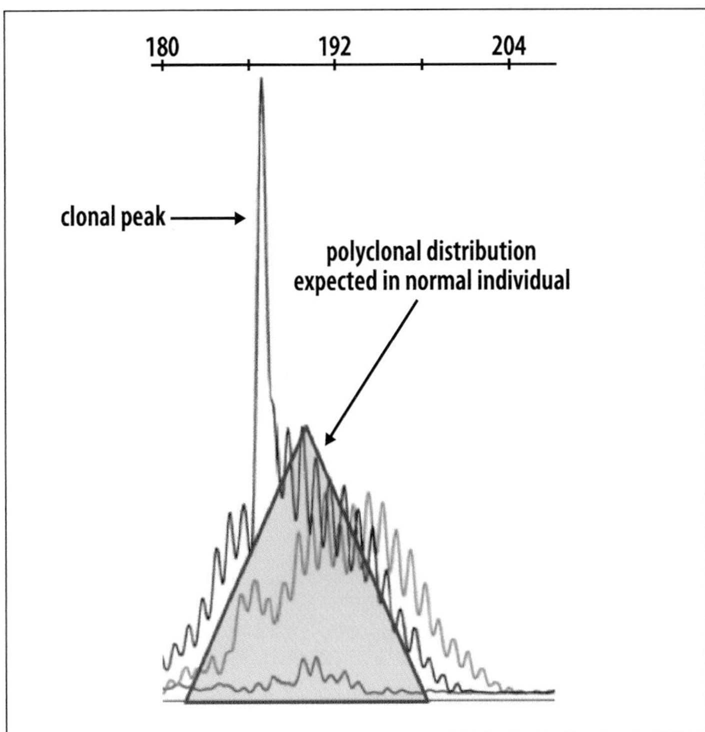

f9.37 T-cell clonality

9.3.15 Fragment analysis

9.3.15.1 Short-tandem repeat (STR) analysis

- Short tandem repeats (STR), runs of repeated oligonucleotides (2-8 bp) that are normally present in the genome
- The copy number of STRs is stably inherited and is normally stable from cell to cell, but differs from person to person
- Identity testing (forensics, paternity, bone marrow engraftment, tissue providence)
- Does not require large segments of intact genomic DNA, allowing testing of partially degraded samples
- Uses PCR primers that flank the STRs with capillary electrophoresis detection, as shown in **f9.36**
- The profile of the specimen is the collection of all alleles tested
- The individual allelic frequencies for all loci tested can be multiplied together to determine the overall frequency of the profile in the general population

9.3.15.2 Clonality analysis

- Rearrangement of BCR and TCR create diversity
- These PCR-based tests use PCR primers which flank VDJ regions, amplifying the repertoire of rearranged TCRs of various length in a given patient
- PCR product is analyzed using capillary electrophoresis and is visualized as a normal distribution in healthy patients as shown by the green histogram in **f9.37**
  - During infection or during malignancy, a single clone may become more predominant, creating a single peak of greater amplitude compared to the polyclonal distribution as shown in the black electropherogram in **f9.37**
  - Height of peak over background defines results

9.3.16 Cytogenetics & karyotyping

- Dividing cells are arrested in metaphase
- Stained with DNA-binding dyes to visualize banding patterns
- G banding is the result of Giemsa staining, AT-rich areas are stained more intensely compared to GC-rich regions
- Q banding is the result of quinacrine staining
- R banding produces a reverse staining pattern to G banding, can be achieved by several different techniques

9.3.16.1 Probes

- Using fluorescence in situ hybridization (FISH), chromosome enumeration probes (CEP) are targeted to conserved regions near centromeres
  - Locus-specific probes are targeted to a specific nucleotide sequence
  - Fusin probes are useful for well-defined translocations with conserved break/fusion points

ISBN 978-089189-6616

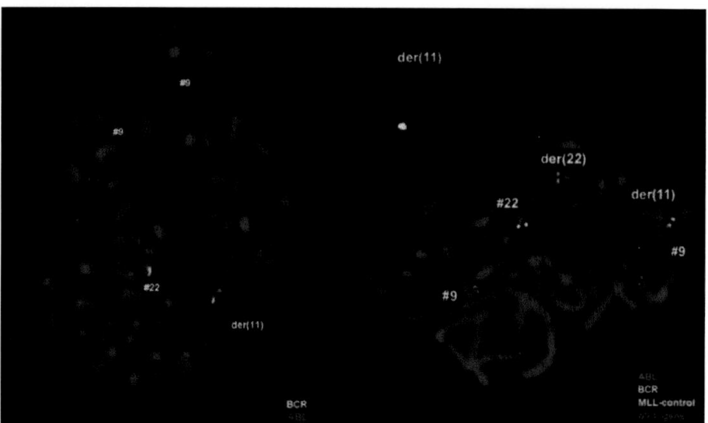

f9.38 Chromosome enumeration probes

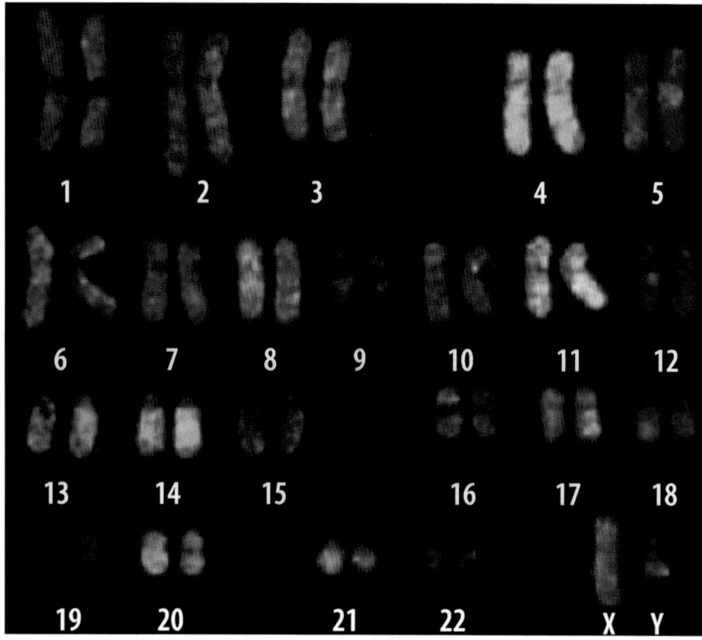

f9.39 Whole chromosome paint probes

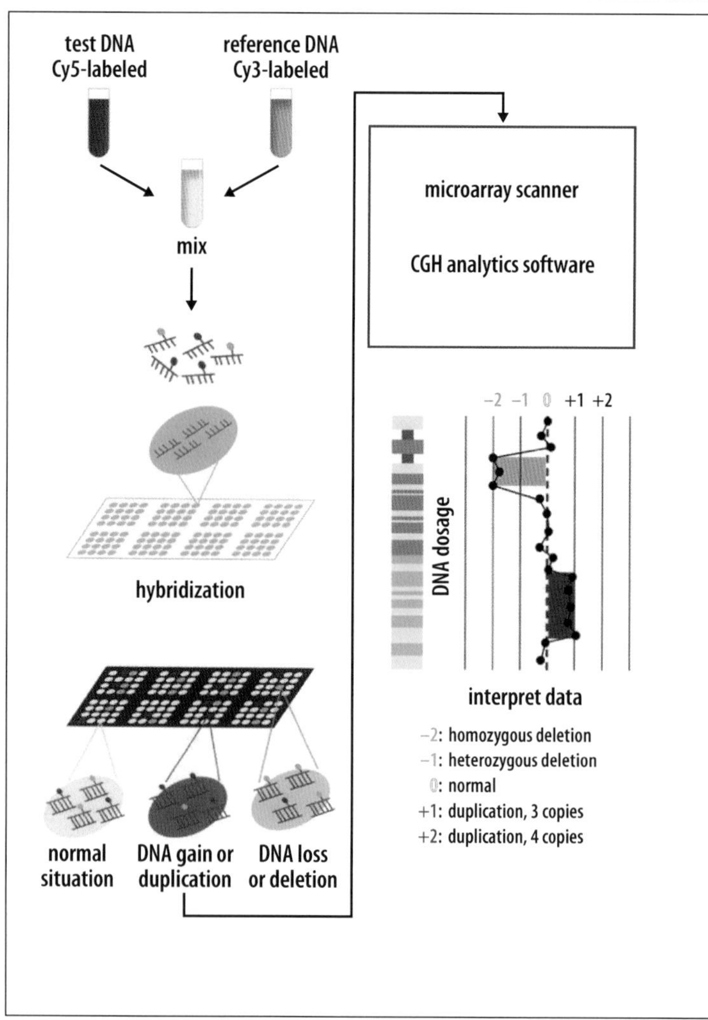

f9.40 Comparative genomic hybridization array. Array profile mapping copy number loss or gain across a chromosome, with loss of chromosome represented in green & duplication indicated in red

- Break-apart probes are useful when gene may be translocated with a variety of partners as shown in the acute myelogenous leukemia case presented in **f9.38**
- Whole chromosome paint probes are designed to provide full coverage of a chromosome, as shown in **f9.39**

9.3.16.2 Comparative genomic hybridization (CGH)

- Conventional CHG
  - Probes are applied to metaphase chromosomes for determining chromosomal/subchromosome copy number
  - Commonly used for genetic characterization of chromosomal anomalies in children and in tumor cells
  - Not able to detect balanced translocations; only unbalanced abnormalities
- Array CGH
  - Used for detection of chromosomal copy number changes on a genome wide scale, as shown in **f9.40**
  - Often used in the workup of a developmentally delayed patient with a normal-appearing karyotype
  - Provides higher resolution than conventional CGH

9.4 Appropriate samples for molecular testing

9.4.1 Preservatives, fixatives & processing reagents

- Preservatives & fixatives are used to maintain biological samples during collection, transport & storage
  - Common fixatives include aldehydes, oxidizing agents, protein denaturants & cross-linking agents

- Common preservatives include acid citrate dextrose (ACD), ethylenediaminetetraacetic acid (EDTA), and heparin
- Certain reagents are incompatible with some or all molecular procedures
  - Fixation with formalin will result in fragmented DNA which is not suitable for some molecular procedures
  - Heavy metals & heparin may produce false negative or under quantified PCR results
  - Decalcified samples are not suitable for molecular procedures
- Reagents highly compatible with molecular procedures include ACD, ETDA & reagents marketed specifically for the preservation of RNA and/or DNA
- Solid tissues are best analyzed from fresh or frozen samples, if precise morphology is not required to identify suitable sampling

9.4.2 Sample barriers to molecular testing

9.4.2.1 Hemolysis

- Free hemoglobin present in hemolyzed samples is a recognized inhibitor of PCR

9.4.2.2 Cellularity

- Extraction methods are sensitive to the amount of cellular content; overloading of the extraction may result in decreased nucleic acid yield as well as increased impurity
- Addition of excess nucleic acid to amplification reactions may inhibit PCR

9.4.3 Molecular inhibitors

- Naturally occurring substances or chemicals introduced during specimen preservation or processing can interfere with downstream testing processes

9.4.3.1 Sources of inhibition

- Common inhibitors for molecular techniques are either present in the sample or are acquired during sample processing **t9.5**

t9.5 Common PCR inhibitors

Native to sample	Processing related
Hemoglobin	Heparin
Urea	Heavy metals
Melanin	SDS
Complex polysaccharides	Alcohol

- Inhibitors exert action through 1 of 3 mechanisms:
  - Direct interaction with nucleic acid, which prevents primer, probes, or enzymes from access to the nucleic acid strand. For example, heparin is a charged polymer that will associate tightly with DNA
  - Direct interaction with polymerase. For example, the presence of denaturing agents or proteolytic enzymes can reduce or destroy the function of polymerase
  - Reduction in availability of enzyme cofactors (eg, Mg^{2+})

9.4.3.2 Detection of the inhibitor

- The presence of inhibitors is assessed by either amplifying genomic DNA targets within the sample or amplification of nongenomic target DNA that is spiked into the sample before extraction or into the amplification reaction
  - Inhibitor checks may be performed before performing downstream testing or may be included as a component of the testing
  - The use of genomic DNA targets is dependent on the presence of adequate intact cellular material and is not the appropriate approach for acellular samples such as cerebrospinal fluid (CSF)
  - Spiked controls allow for sensitive, semiquantitative detection of inhibition and a more subjective determination of specimen suitability for qualitative or quantitative downstream testing. Spiked controls are commonly included in infectious disease testing

9.5 Molecular applications (see also chapter 6 Microbiology; chapter 8 Immunology)

9.5.1 Pathogen detection

9.5.1.1 Rapid detection

- A rapid detection method is a diagnostic test that is quick and easy to perform. It can provide results on same day and sometimes in <20 minutes
- Rapid tests are suitable for preliminary or emergency medical screening and for use in medical facilities with limited resources

9.5.1.2 Scalability

- Scalability refers to flexibility in scale as per the need, eg, thermocyclers for PCR are commonly available in 96/384/1596-well formats; multiple samples can be tested simultaneously or as per the need

ISBN 978-089189-6616

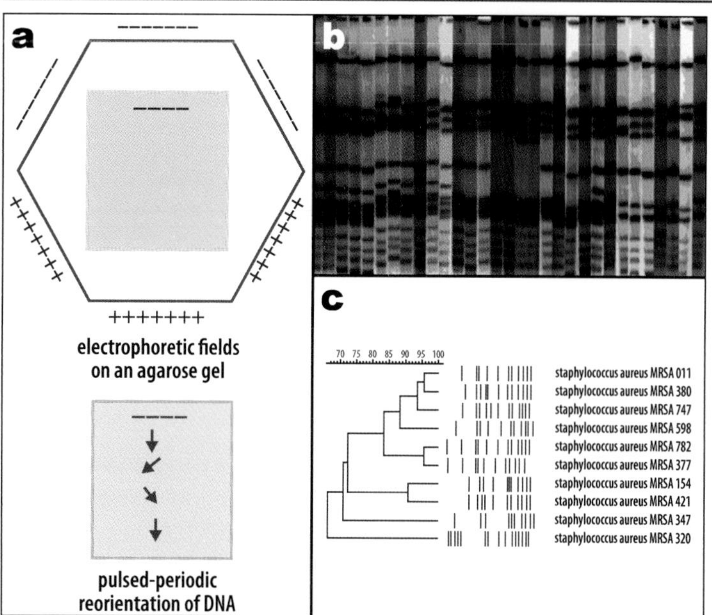

f9.41 Pulsed-field gel electrophoresis generates a highly discriminatory genetic fingerprint

- Automated extractors may allow for the extraction of only a few samples, to provide nucleic acid as quickly as possible. Other platforms are designed for high throughput with very few manual steps. Samples may be on board the platform for an extended time before becoming available for subsequent testing

9.5.1.3 Multiplex

- Multiplexing refers to analyzing multiple targets in a sample in 1 assay
- Multiplexing saves cost and sample volume, and provides increased output with data on several markers

9.5.1.4 Direct detection

- Identification of specific genetic sequences (genotype) in a sample that correspond to a disease (phenotype) Most common methods used for direct detection are PCR based and sequencing

9.5.1.5 Quantitation

- Quantitation refers to quantitative analysis of the target of interest. For example, HIV viral load is used to monitor response to therapy over time

9.5.2 Microbial identification & antimicrobial resistance (AMR) detection

9.5.2.1 Pulsed-field gel electrophoresis (PFGE)

- Genotyping method that separates DNA by applying electrical current that periodically changes direction in 3 dimensions **f9.41a**
- The fingerprint of an isolate can be used for phylogenetic analysis based on percentage of genetic similarity of an isolate to previously characterized strains as shown in **f9.41b, c**

9.5.2.2 Multilocus sequence typing (MLST)

- Genotyping method that involves sequencing fragments of DNA (400-500 base pairs) of 7 different conserved genes
- Sequence data are compared to a database
- Can detect small variations within a species

9.5.2.3 Ribotyping

- Examines the 16S and/or 23S rRNA genes
- Genes are cut with enzymes and subjected to electrophoresis
- Results are compared to known databases
- Alternatively, ribosomal genes can be amplified by PCR and then subjected to Sanger sequencing

9.5.2.4 DNA microarray

- Genotyping method that uses numerous DNA probes attached to a solid substrate
- Pathogen DNA is hybridized to the probes and pathogen is identified by probe binding pattern
- Useful for both genotyping & anti-microbial resistance (AMR)

9.5.2.5 Whole genome sequencing (WGS)

- A relatively new approach that uses next-generation sequencing technology
- This allows for the entire genome of a microbial isolate to be sequenced
- Useful for both genotyping & AMR detection

9.5.2.6 Matrix-assisted laser desorption ionization-time-of-flight mass spectrometry (MALDI-TOF MS)

- Either intact cells or cell extracts are ionized to gas phase
- Pathogen protein ions are separated on basis of mass to charge ratio as shown in **f9.42**
- Rapidly & sensitively identifies pathogens

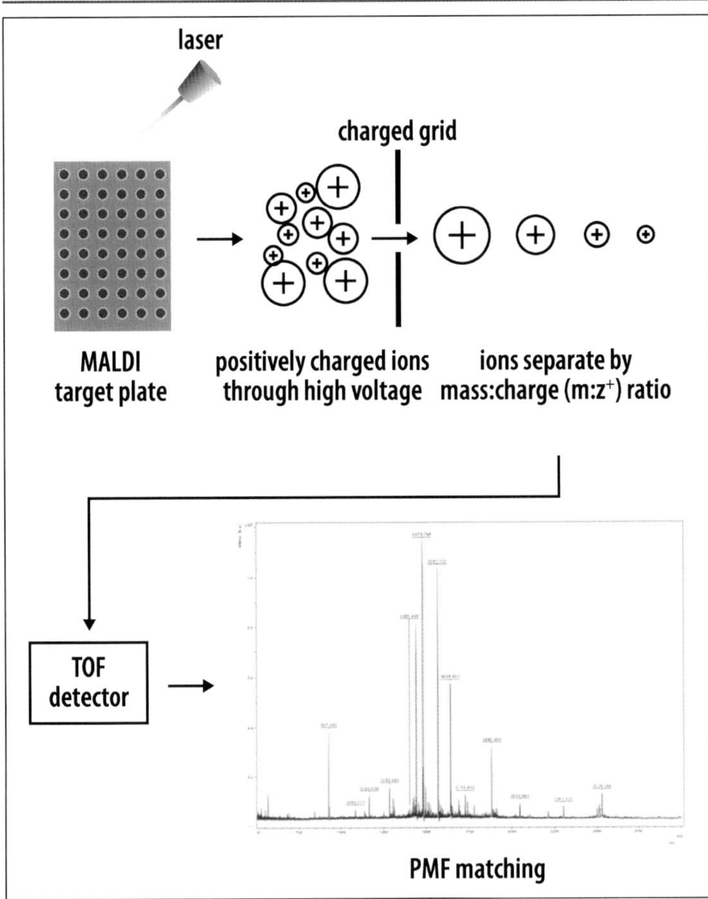

f9.42 Matrix-assisted laser desorption ionization-time-of-flight (MALDI-TOF) data acquisition & resulting in peptide mass fingerprinting (PMF) matching output

- The technology is limited to the currently available databases of peptide mass fingerprints

9.5.2.7 Targeted ARM detection

- Standard or real-time PCR can be used to target well-described resistance markers, such as those listed in t9.6
- For example, bacterial resistance to vancomycin is commonly tested with real-time PCR using primer and probe combinations to detect *van*A & *van*B genes

t9.6 Antimicrobial-resistant genes

Organism	Antimicrobial agent	Gene conferring resistance
Staphylococcus aureus	Oxacillin	*mecA*
Streptococcus pneumoniae	Penicillin	*pbp1 a and pbp1 b*
Gram-negatives	β-lactams	*tem, shv, oxa, ctx-m*
Enterococcus	Vancomycin	*vanA, vanB, vanC, vanD, vanE, vanG*
Salmonella	Quinolones	*gyrA, gyrB, parC, parE*
Mycobacterium tuberculosis	Isoniazid, rifampin	*katG, inhA, rpoB*

9.5.3 Mutation

- A polymorphism is DNA variation that occurs in at least 1 in 100 individuals. Can be either single nucleotide polymorphism (SNP) or copy number variation such as is seen with short tandem repeat polymorphism (STRP)
- A mutation is a change in a DNA sequence. Germline mutations can be passed to offspring. Somatic mutations occur later in development within an individual tissue compartment and are not passed on
- Mutations are detected using various methods as shown in t9.7. Method of choice depends on sample source, target size, clinical specificity & sensitivity requirements, and available platforms in a given laboratory

t9.7 Molecular methods applicable to mutation testing

Sequencing
Single-strand confirmation polymorphism
Denaturing gradient gel electrophoresis
Allele specific oligomer hybridization
High-resolution melt curve analysis
Multiplex inversion probe
Heteroduplex analysis
Denaturing high-performance liquid chromatography
Array technology
Sequence-specific PCR
Dideoxy DNA fingerprinting
Dye terminator
Protein truncation test
PCR-RFLP (restriction fragment length polymorphism)
Base excision sequence scanning
Nonisotopic RNase cleavage assay
Invader assay
Chemical cleavage of mismatches

9.5.4 Pharmacogenomics

- Pharmacogenomics is the study of the role of the genome in an individual's response to drugs
- The goal is to ensure optimum drug efficacy with minimum side effects
- The following is a subset of pharmacogenomic-relevant drugs

9.5.4.1 Warfarin

- Some individuals are slow metabolizers of the anticoagulant warfarin

ISBN 978-089189-6616

- Polymorphisms in 2 genes, *CYP2C9* and *VKORC1*, account for most variation in metabolism, either increasing or decreasing sensitivity, as shown in **t9.8**
- Genotyping may help guide dosage in treatment-naive individuals and predict time to clear the drug before surgery
- VKORC1*2 is associated with reduced expression of the warfarin target and a reduced dose requirement
- CYP2C8/9 variants are associated with a reduced rate of warfarin catabolism, thus a reduced dose is required
- Dose calculators, such as the one available at *www.WarfarinDosing.org* are necessary to account for the contribution of both genetic & nongenetic factors

t9.8 Warfarin sensitivity associated with genes

Warfarin sensitivity	*CYP2C9* genotype	*VKORC1* genotype
Normal	*1/*1	C/A
Less than normal	*1/*1, *1/*2	G/G
Mild	*1/*3, *2/*2, *2/*3 *1/*2	G/G G/A
Moderate	*1/*1 *1/*3, *2/*2 *3/*3	A/A G/A G/G
High	*1/*2, *2/*2 *2/*2, *3/*3	A/A G/A
Very high	*1/*2, *2/*3, *3/*3	A/A

9.5.4.2 Clopidogrel

- Some individuals are intermediate or slow metabolizers of the antiplatelet drug clopidogrel
- Effectiveness depends on conversion to an active metabolite by the cytochrome P450 system
- Polymorphisms in CYP2C19 account for most variation in response to clopidogrel

9.5.4.3 Abacavir

- Some individuals have a severe reaction when taking the antiretroviral drug abacavir
- Individuals positive for HLA-B*57:01 have a higher risk of developing skin reactions such as toxic epidermal necrolysis (TEM) and Stevens-Johnson syndrome
- Abacavir sits in major histocompatibility complex (MHC)–binding groove of HLA-B*57:01, altering self-peptide presentation, leading to activation of the immune system
- Reactions affect 5%-8% of patients during the first 6 weeks of therapy

9.5.4.4 Thiopurine S-methyltransferase (TPMT)

- Some individuals have a reduced ability to metabolize the thiopurines azathioprine, mercaptopurine & thioguanine, which are used to treat leukemias & autoimmune disorders
- *TPMT* & *NUDT15* polymorphisms account for variable activity
- Poor metabolizers have 2 loss-of-function alleles of *TMPT*, representing 0.3% of population
- Intermediate metabolizers have 1 loss-of-function allele of *TMPT*, representing 10% of the population

9.5.5 Extended molecular RBC genotyping (see also chapter 1 Blood Banking)

- Red blood cell (RBC) genotyping is used to predict the expression of human erythrocyte antigens (HEA)
- Extended panels are used to genotype multiple blood groups: Rh, Kell, Duffy, Kidd, MNS, Lutheran, Dombrock, Landsteiner-Wiener, Diego, Colton, Scianna & hemoglobin S
- Clinical sensitivity & specificity vary between blood groups, and rare variants may not be accurately genotyped because of limitations of primer/probes
- Helpful in patients with a recent history of transfusion or with conflicting serologic antibody results
- RBC genotyping is a common practice in transfusion medicine to prevent hemolytic transfusion reactions or hemolytic disease of the fetus and newborn (HDFN)
- Single nucleotide polymorphism (SNP)–based assays, Sanger sequencing & next-generation sequencing are common methods used

9.5.6 Histocompatibility (see also chapter 8 Immunology)

- The major histocompatibility complex (MHC) comprises a group of genes present on the short arm of chromosome 6
- In humans, MHC gene products are called human leukocyte antigens (HLAs)
- HLAs are divided into 3 classes (I, II, and III). HLA class I products are HLA-A, HLA-B, and HLA-C. HLA class II products are HLA-DP, HLA-DQ, and HLA-DR. HLA class I proteins are expressed in all nucleated cells whereas class II proteins are expressed only in professional antigen-presenting cells such as B lymphocytes, dendritic cells & macrophages
- HLA matching is performed to check the compatibility of organ donor & recipient. If organ donor and recipient are not HLA matched, then the recipient immune system (B and T lymphocyte) recognizes the donor organ as nonself and mounts an immune response that results in graft failure

- HLA matching is also required to prevent graft-vs-host disease (GVHD). GVHD is the reciprocal of graft rejection in which donor immune cells attack recipient body organs, which results in significant morbidity & mortality to the recipient
- HLA loci are very complex and have several thousand alleles
- HLA alleles follow standard World Health Organization nomenclature for specifying allele names
- Serologic assays or DNA-based typing (sequence-specific oligos or sequencing) methods are used for identification and resolution of HLA alleles
- Proteins that are out of the MHC and influence graft failure are minor histocompatibility antigens

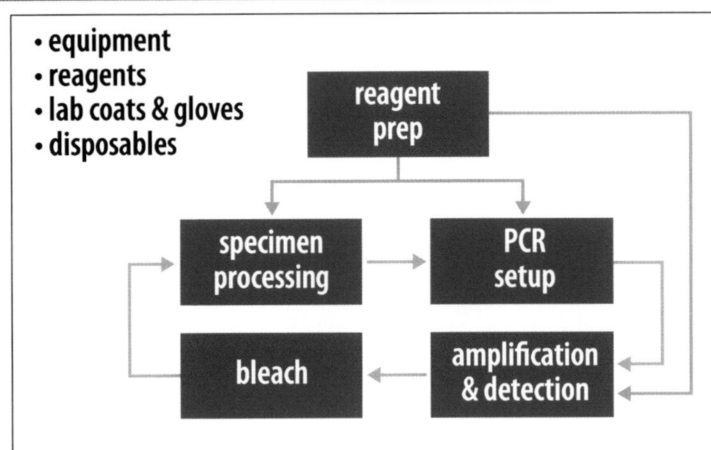

f9.43 Physical containment to prevent PCR amplicon contamination

9.5.7 Tumor detection & minimal residual disease (MRD) detection

- Cancer is a complex genetic disease. Mutations in oncogenes & tumor suppressor genes are frequently observed in different cancers
- Several translocations are found in certain types of tumor, for eg, t(14;18)(q32;q21) in B-cell leukemia & lymphoma or B-cell chronic lymphocytic leukemia (CLL)/lymphoma
- Molecular technologies have been developed to differentiate normal cells from the tumor cells using genetic variation markers
- Minimal residue disease (MRD) detection is used to survey for small number of cancerous cells that remain in the body after treatment; they are the major cause of relapse in cancer
- Sensitive methods like PCR, sequencing, or flow cytometry are used in MRD detection
- Treatments to eradicate MRD is different from those used during primary treatment

9.6 Contamination considerations

9.6.1 Avoiding nucleic acid contamination

9.6.1.1 Comingling specimens

- Leaky containers can cross-contaminate surfaces, gloves, etc
- Segregate samples known to contain high vs low titer of pathogens, for example:
  - High titer vesicle or respiratory swabs should not be stored alongside CSF
  - Stool samples should not be stored alongside blood
- Slides may be contaminated with other tissues "floaters" during the preparation process

9.6.1.2 Aerosols

- Aerosols or splashes from positive specimens or positive control are a source of contamination
- Centrifugate tubes briefly to pull contaminants from lids
- Use extreme caution & rubber-backed wipes when opening containers
- Use proper pipettes & pipetting technique to prevent aerosolization as well as direct contamination
- Ensure proper seal for centrifuge tubes; treat all centrifuge surfaces as contaminated
- Change gloves frequently, especially between potentially high-titer samples

9.6.1.3 Reagent contamination

- Aliquot reagents into daily or weekly aliquots when feasible
- Perform extraction & amplification blanks to detect the presence of contamination

9.6.1.4 Good laboratory practices

- The work environment should be routinely decontaminated with reagents capable of degrading DNA & PCR products
- Practice unidirectional workflow in combination with physical containment, as shown in **f9.43**
- Follow strict separation measures in work areas (reagent vs specimen)

ISBN 978-089189-6616

9.6.1.5 Topical inactivation of nucleic acid contamination

- Sodium hypochlorite solution
  - Stability affected by storage conditions
  - Protect from light
  - Prepare fresh
  - Wet surface & allow to air dry
  - Prevent skin & eye exposure
- Ultraviolet lights
  - Effective for small amounts of nucleic acid (<100 pg)
  - The light must be within 2 feet of work surface
  - Time of exposure important, longer times are more effective
  - Lamps should be checked periodically to ensure that proper intensity of UV light is emitted
  - Protect eyes & skin

9.6.1.6 Dedicated equipment & specialized consumables

- Use separate pipets for reagents, samples & PCR products
- Use aerosol-resistant pipet tips

9.6.2 Specimen sources containing high quantities of target

- Use lowest concentration of positive control possible that will amplify consistently, to prevent cross-contamination during test set-up
- Sequester high contamination risk specimens during initial processing & extraction, as skin & respiratory swabs, stool, and urine specimens

9.6.3 Enzymatic degradation of PCR product

- Amplification techniques produce large numbers of copies of a sequence (up to 10^{12} copies per reaction)
- Accumulation of amplified product that can result in contamination of reagents, buffers, equipment, ventilation systems
- Uracil-N-glycosylase (UNG) chemistry
  - A system to degrade low-level PCR contamination from a PCR reaction before initiation of the PCR cycling
  - Enzymatic amplicon inactivation
    - dUTP is substituted for dTTP in the PCR reaction mix
    - UNG is also added to the reaction mix and will recognize & degrade PCR product generated with dUTP, but not genomic template DNA
    - UNG is inactivated by heating the PCR reaction to 94°C before the initiation of PCR cycling
  - UNG chemistry optimization
    - Products should be large enough to be efficiently inactivated (100-500 bp)
    - GC-rich products are more difficult to inactivate (less uracil residues)
    - UNG will regain activity if temperatures drop below 55°C; PCR reactions should be held at 72°C until analysis
    - dUTP substitution may reduce affinity of probes

9.6.4 Identifying contamination

- Detecting target contamination
  - Run parallel extraction reagent blanks, containing everything except template nucleic acid
  - Run parallel negative controls, containing nontarget nucleic acid
  - Dispense negative controls last during setup
  - Critically review results when high-titer samples are on the run
  - Perform routine wipe tests to detect target DNA
- Detecting PCR amplicon contamination
  - Run parallel reagent blanks
  - Run parallel negative controls
  - Dispense negative controls last
  - Perform routine wipe tests to detect amplified DNA from each amplification assay

9.7 Selected readings

9.7.1 Books

Buckingham L. Molecular Diagnostics: *Fundamentals, Methods & Clinical Applications*. 3rd ed. FA Davis. 2019. ISBN 978-0803668294

Coleman WB, Tsongalis GJ (eds). *The Molecular Basis of Human Disease*. 2nd ed. Humana Press. 2016. ISBN 978-0128027615

9.7.2 Journals & online

Association for Molecular Pathology [2020] Molecular in My Pocket Guides. https://www.amp.org/education/education-resources/ molecular-in-my-pocket-guides/, last accessed 21 September 2020

Index

Page numbers with f indicate figures; with i indicate images, and t indicate tables.

ISBN 978-089189-6616

ISBN 978-089189-6616

B

ISBN 978-089189-6616

 ISBN 978-089189-6616

C

 ISBN 978-089189-6616

ISBN 978-089189-6616

D

 ISBN 978-089189-6616

F

 ISBN 978-089189-6616

False—FY

G

ISBN 978-089189-6616

H

 ISBN 978-089189-6616

ISBN 978-089189-6616

I

J

K

ISBN 978-089189-6616

L

 ISBN 978-089189-6616

M

ISBN 978-089189-6616

N

 ISBN 978-089189-6616

O

P

ISBN 978-089189-6616

S

ISBN 978-089189-6616

 ISBN 978-089189-6616

V

ISBN 978-089189-6616

W

X

Y

Z